Principles of
Dental Imaging

Principles of Dental Imaging

OLAF E. LANGLAND, DDS, MS, FACD

Professor, Department of Dental Diagnostic Science
The University of Texas Health Science Center at San Antonio Dental School
San Antonio, Texas

ROBERT P. LANGLAIS, DDS, MS, FACD

Professor, Department of Dental Diagnostic Science
The University of Texas Health Science Center at San Antonio Dental School
San Antonio, Texas

Consultants:

Joan Gibson-Howell, RDH, MSEd
Assistant Professor, Department of Dental Hygiene
Robert C. Byrd Health Sciences Center of West Virginia University
Morgantown, West Virginia

Dorothea M. Cavallucci, CDA, RDH, EFDA
Director, Dental Assisting
Harcum College
Bryn Mawr, Pennsylvania

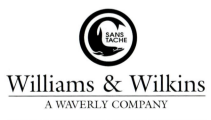

Williams & Wilkins
A WAVERLY COMPANY

BALTIMORE • PHILADELPHIA • LONDON • PARIS • BANGKOK
HONG KONG • MUNICH • SYDNEY • TOKYO • WROCLAW

Editor: Sharon R. Zinner
Managing Editor: Tanya Lazar
Marketing Manager: Rebecca Himmelheber
Production Coordinator: Danielle Hagan
Book Project Editor: Thomas Lehr
Designer: Artech
Cover Designer: Nick Lang
Typesetter: BI-COMP, Inc.
Printer and Binder: Edwards Brothers, Inc.

Copyright © 1997 Williams & Wilkins

351 West Camden Street
Baltimore, Maryland 21201-2436 USA

Rose Tree Corporate Center
1400 North Providence Road
Building II, Suite 5025
Media, Pennsylvania 19063-2043 USA

Accurate indications, adverse reactions and dosage schedules for drugs are provided in this book, but it is possible that they may change. The reader is urged to review the package information data of the manufacturers of the medications mentioned.

Printed in the United States of America

Library of Congress Cataloging-in-Publication Data

Langland, Olaf E.
    Principles of dental imaging / Olaf E. Langland, Robert P.
Langlais.—1st ed.
      p.   cm.
    Includes bibliographical references and index.
    ISBN 0-683-18241-2
    1. Teeth—Radiography. I. Langlais, Robert P. II. Title.
    [DNLM: 1. Radiography, Dental—methods. 2. Diagnostic Imaging—
methods. WN 230 L282pa 1997]
    RK309.L358   1997
    617.6'07572—dc21
    DNLM/DLC
    for Library of Congress   97-2361
                                            CIP

The publishers have made every effort to trace the copyright holders for borrowed material. If they have inadvertently overlooked any, they will be pleased to make the necessary arrangements at the first opportunity.

To purchase additional copies of this book, call our customer service department at (800) **638-0672** or fax orders to (800) **447-8438**. For other book services, including chapter reprints and large quantity sales, ask for the Special Sales department.

Canadian customers should call (800) **665-1148**, or fax (800) **665-0103**. For all other calls originating outside of the United States, please call (410) **528-4223** or fax us at (410) **528-8550**.

Visit Williams & Wilkins on the Internet: http://www.wwilkins.com or contact our customer service department at **custserv@wwilkins.com**. Williams & Wilkins customer service representatives are available from 8:30 am to 6:00 pm, EST, Monday through Friday, for telephone access.

98 99 00
2 3 4 5 6 7 8 9 10

To my wife, Gwendolyn Stokes Langland, whose encouragement, help, and sacrifices made this book possible.

—Ole Langland

To Denyse Paré Langlais. Once again, merçi beaucoup!

—Bob Langlais

Preface

Make no mistake: the principles described herein must be understood by all dental health care workers whose goal is to learn and perfect the techniques of dental imaging. The skills required to expose and process radiographs are exactly the same for all types of dental professionals. Additionally, the risks of radiation exposure are the same for all. Therefore, this text is meant to be used by all students who are required to learn dental imaging techniques.

ORGANIZATION: This text is organized into five sections, and each section is subdivided into several chapters. With the material subdivided into these smaller packages, students will find that their learning goals are more easily achieved. Course directors may wish to alter the order of the various sections to conform with different subject sequencing by various instructors. Section 1 is concerned with the concepts of radiologic imaging; Section 2 deals with radiographic techniques and procedures; Section 3 discusses special imaging techniques; Section 4 involves radiation health; and Section 5 describes assessment and interpretation.

LEARNING/TEACHING DEVICES: The authors of this textbook have used numerous pedagogic methods to enhance the learning process and to stimulate student interest in this sometimes difficult and confusing subject. The resulting content helps students correlate classroom and laboratory learning with assigned clinical experiences. For example, the first nine chapters and Chapter 11 include laboratory/workshop sessions to enhance the learning of concepts and clinical techniques; Chapters 10 and 12 through 18 contain case-based questions to further the cognitive skills necessary to assess and interpret the images. The full complement of these teaching devices is as follows:

Chapter Learning Objectives: At the beginning of each chapter, a list of objectives defines what the student should learn upon completion of the chapter. These objectives also emphasize the goals of the instructor.

Key Terms and Phrases: Key terms and phrases used within the text are listed at the beginning of each chapter. This list can be used as a quick reference to the material learned.

Illustrations and Tables: In many instances, concepts are illustrated with a combination of line drawings, clinical photographs, and radiographs, as well as tables where applicable. The authors have made extensive use of these aids to help the student visualize principles more clearly and to clarify complex ideas or to summarize important areas of the narrative, such as a series of steps in a technique. This book contains many unique illustrations copyrighted by the authors and publisher.

Boxed Information: Lists of key points, steps in a technique, or short paragraphs, set off in boxes, appear within the text throughout the book. These boxes will help apply information and ideas to clinical situations and also serve to highlight important information for future reference or review and study.

Practical Laboratory Workshops (Application of Knowledge): Workshops are found at the end of the first nine chapters and Chapter 11 to allow the student to practice a technique in a clinical setting, visualize a concept, or solve a problem. These practical applications are used to reinforce the previously presented information, which may have been only partially assimilated by the student in reviewing class notes and textbook information.

Sample Examination Questions: Sample examination questions are presented at the end of each chapter. Some questions are constructed so that answers will require only recall of simple concepts or facts. Other questions require more complex understanding and may have more than one correct answer. Other testing formats are added from time to time, including matching columns or basing questions on a diagram, a radiograph, or a case-based question. Many of the questions will help the student gain experience in applying information to clinical situations and will test their preparedness in answering examination questions.

Sample Examination: We have provided a sample National Board/State Board Certifying Examination, which is based on the content of the whole book. All of these questions may serve as topics for discussion with other students or with the instructor. Answering these questions correctly, however, does not necessarily test for problem-solving skills.

PROBLEM SOLVING: Problem solving is the mental process that we use to arrive at a "best answer" to an unknown, subject to a set of constraints. The problem situation is usually one that has not been encountered before, and the student must mentally process learned information to obtain the "best" answer. Our *first* objective in teaching problem-solving is that the student acquire an essential body of knowledge in dental imaging. This has two dimensions: **what** the students should learn and **how** the body of knowledge should be learned. It is later retrieved as useful information to perform clinical tasks. Our *second* objective concerns the students' ability to apply that knowledge effectively to assess, understand, and evaluate dental imaging problems. Students with only encyclopedic information are less effective, if not unsafe, because they do not have problem-solving skills necessary to approach dental imaging problems. Problem-solving skills encompass the skills needed to (*a*) evaluate the problem, (*b*) decide what is wrong, and (*c*) make decisions to manage the problem with appropriate actions. Our *third* objective in problem solving is to ensure that students are able to extend their knowledge base to remain contemporary in the field and be able to provide appropriate solutions for new or unique problems they may face in the future.

READABILITY: Readability is one of the highest priorities of the authors. We have therefore engaged the services of some of our colleagues, whose names appear in the **contributors list**. It has been our intent to make this book more readable so that a student may begin to learn without the added confusion created by a complex narrative format. This is one of the most important duties of our valued contributors.

APPROPRIATENESS OF CONTENT: To ensure appropriate content, we consulted the Oral and Maxillofacial Radiology guidelines published by the American Association of Dental Schools (AADS). We also studied the survey responses of 95 instructors of dental imaging to help us achieve the best design for the book. This book has **not** been diluted to create an artificial separation between the various types of dental professionals aspiring to learn oral and maxillofacial radiologic imaging.

FORMAT: Apart from the use of bold headings and fonts of various sizes to clearly delineate subheadings from major headings, the authors have used individual boxed subject highlights to further enhance divisions in the subject material and readability. All of these format variations are designed to stimulate the student in the learning process, to give the student a feeling of comfort and ease in reading the book, and to impart a feeling of satisfaction as the material is being learned in an organized fashion.

GLOSSARY: A glossary of pertinent terms and definitions is included at the end of the book. Review of the glossary is a helpful tool to identify weak areas requiring further study in preparing for examinations.

INDEX: The text contains a complete and "user-friendly" index for students and teachers to use in searching for specific information.

Olaf E. Langland
Robert P. Langlais

ACKNOWLEDGMENTS

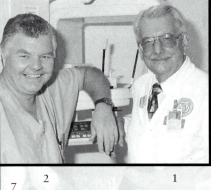

2   4   6   8

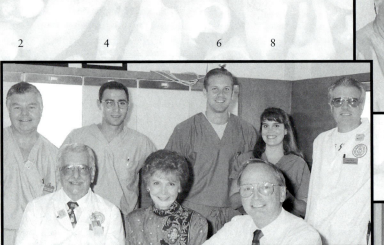

7   2   1

1   3   5

8   9   10

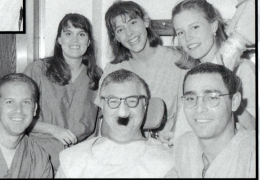

1

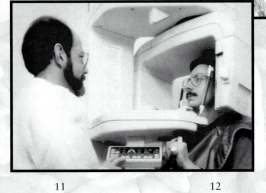

6   2   4

11   12

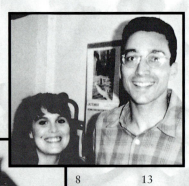

5

8   13

3

14

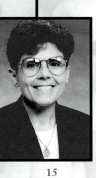

15

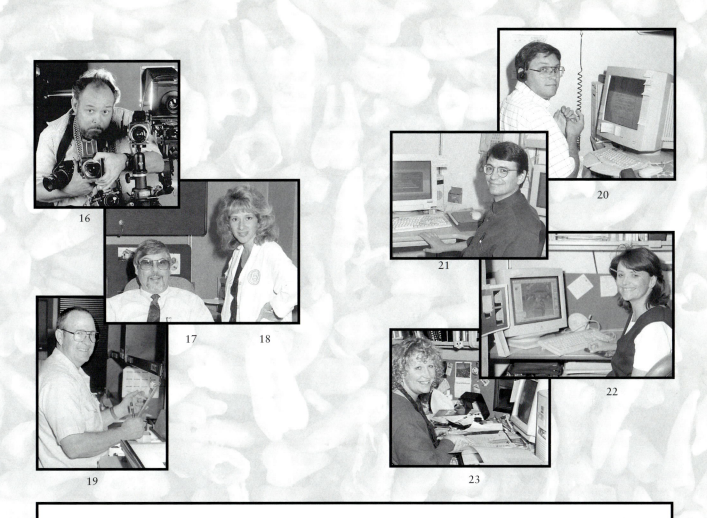

16

17 18

19

20

21

22

23

We, Ole Langland (1) and Bob Langlais (2) would especially like to recognize Gwen Langland (3) for the endless amount of word processing and editing she did during the preparation of the manuscript, and the dozens of little things needed to get the job done. We are also grateful to some of our favorite students who acted as models for the photographs of the various techniques. These include Mike Suhler (4), Brad Revering (6), Heidi Ritsco (8), Isabel Britain (9), Stacy Morgan (10), and David Tasch (13). Other persons who were photographed include Dr. Scott Makins (11) Univ. of Texas at Houston, TX; Dr. Michael McNally (12), Univ. of Nebraska; Dr. Craig Miller, Univ. of Kentucky at Lexington; Dr. Raghunath Puttaish, Baylor Univ., Dallas, TX; Dr. Cliff Thornell, private practice in Austin, TX; David Greer, (7) computer technologist at UTHSCSA; and Michelle Kirby, radiology technician at UTHSCSA. The book would not have been complete without our own Dr. John Precce's (5) exceptionally clear chapter on Radiation Biology. We also had the invaluable input of our two collaborators, Dorothea Cavallucci (14) Harcum College, Bryn Mawr, PA, and Joan Gibson-Howell (15) West Virginia Univ., at Morgantown, WV, who judiciously read and reread the manuscript several times, offered suggestions relating to terminology, assessed the comprehensibility of the text, critiqued the stated objectives, suggested the case based questions, and multiple other inputs which made the book better. Also, we are deeply indebted to those 95 wonderful dental radiology educators from every corner of the United States who answered our Dental Radiology Survey and offered us so many marvelous suggestions and advice. We are totally indebted to Lee Bennack (16), photographer extraordinaire who created the skull photos and the other special effect photos, and just about all of the other photos in the text. We also had the support of Al Julian (17) director of photography, April Cox (18) the photo lab technician who personally critiqued just about every photo and x-ray print in the text, and Thurman Hood (19), the photographic technician who was responsible for the lab work resulting in the exquisite illustrations, many of which were drawn by Nick Lang (20) who also designed and drew the cover illustration and the unfolding panoramic image drawings of technique errors. Other medical illustrators who helped include David Baker (21), Brian Neuenschwander and Chuck Whitehead, who drew the first illustrations depicting the unfolding of the panoramic image. We are also grateful to Nancy Place (22), Medical Illustrator and Kris Doyle (23), Publishing Coordinator. There are many others who helped with the book and we thank them also, including the editors and production team at Williams & Wilkins, most notably, Sharon Zinner, who believed in us from the start; Danielle Hagan, Production Coordinator; and Tanya Lazar, who formed the direct, but tactful liaison between the authors and the production team. Finally, Denyse Langlais, who has had numerous textbooks dedicated to her for her unfaltering support of Bob Langlais' book projects.

OEL and RPL

Contributors

Joan Gibson-Howell, RDH, MSEd
Assistant Professor, Department of Dental Hygiene
Robert C. Byrd Health Sciences Center of West Virginia University
Morgantown, West Virginia

Dorothea M. "Dossie" Cavallucci, CDA, RDH, EFDA
Director, Dental Assisting
Harcum College
Bryn Mawr, Pennsylvania

John W. Preece, DDS, MS
Associate Dean, School of Allied Health Sciences
The University of Texas Health Science Center at San Antonio
San Antonio, Texas

And all other persons who answered the dental radiology educational survey sent out by Drs. Langland and Langlais. You are the educators who make this textbook possible.

Contents

SECTION 5: RADIOGRAPHIC IMAGE INTERPRETATION

SECTION 1:

Concepts of Radiologic Imaging

Production of X-Rays

1

OBJECTIVES

Upon successful completion of this unit, the student will be able to:

1. *Identify the components of the x-ray tube on a diagram.*

2. *Discuss the steps that take place to produce radiation.*

3. *List and identify the 10 properties of x-rays.*

4. *Identify by written description and discuss bremsstralung and characteristic radiation.*

5. *Discuss the wave concept of electromagnetic radiation.*

6. *Identify the two types of ionizing radiation.*

7. *Discuss briefly the history of radiology.*

8. *State examples of electromagnetic radiation.*

9. *Discuss the components of an atom.*

10. *Complete a workshop demonstrating the properties of x-rays.*

11. *Learn the basic parts of the x-ray machine and how it works in a workshop format.*

12. *Complete a workshop/laboratory exercise regarding basic radiation safety.*

13. *Test his or her knowledge by solving a problem dealing with the properties of x-rays, including radiation protection.*

14. *Test his or her knowledge by answering the review questions.*

KEY WORDS/PHRASES

alpha particle	filament	orbital electrons
angstrom unit	focusing cup	particulate radiation
anode	frequency	photon
atom	gamma rays	propagate
beta particle	general radiation	proton
binding energy	hertz	quantum
bremsstrahlung radiation	heterogeneous radiation	radiograph
cathode	homogeneous radiation	radiography
cathode rays	ion	radiology
characteristic radiation	ionization	Roentgen, Wilhelm Konrad
corpuscular radiation	ion pair	roentgenology
dental radiography	kiloelectron volts	target
electromagnetic radiation	kilovoltage peak	useful beam
electron orbits	kinetic energy	valence electrons
electrons	nanometer	wavelength
electron-volt	negatron	wave propagation
excited state	neutron	x-rays
element	nucleus	Z number

HISTORICAL BACKGROUND

DISCOVERY OF X-RAYS

X-rays were discovered on November 8, 1895, by **Wilhelm Konrad Roentgen** (pronounced Rentken), Professor of Physics and Director of the Physical Institute of the University of Wurzburg in Bavaria, Germany. After Roentgen discovered x-rays, he determined that x-rays could darken a photographic plate. By placing objects between the source of the rays and the plate, he took permanent x-ray photographs, exploiting the differing abilities of materials to transmit the rays. In taking these photographs, he pioneered three key areas of x-ray imaging. First, an x-ray photograph of his closed wooden box of weights clearly revealed its contents, thus presaging the security application found at **every airport check-in**. Second, an x-ray image of his hunting rifle revealed a flaw inside the metal of the gun. This was the first time a **hidden structural flaw** had been exposed without destroying the object. Third and most startling, he took a permanent x-ray photograph of his wife Bertha's left hand, revealing the bones and the rings that she was wearing. To produce this image, Bertha held her hand still against the plate for about 15 minutes, which gave her a dose of x-rays that dangerously exceeded the limits set in modern health and safety standards. In recognition of his outstanding contribution to science, Roentgen was awarded the first Nobel Prize for Physics in 1901.

EARLY DENTAL RADIOGRAPHY

Supposedly, the first dental radiograph ever made was completed by Otto Walkhoff, DDS, MD, of Braunschweig (Brunswick), Germany, on January 14, 1896, 14 days after the publication of the experimental results of the discovery of x-rays by Roentgen. Walkhoff made the first dental radiograph by placing in his own mouth an unexposed photographic glass plate that was wrapped in black paper and covered with a rubber dam. He lay on the floor, submitting himself to 25 minutes of x-ray exposure. This dangerous experiment indicated the reckless ignorance of some of the early pioneers in the use of radiation. When Roentgen announced to the world the discovery of a new kind of ray in 1895, he called it the "X-ray" after the algebraic symbol for unknown quantity. The scientific world, for the most part, called it the "roentgen ray" in honor of the discoverer.

NATURE OF THE ATOM

To understand the nature of x-rays, it is important to be familiar with matter and the structure of the atom. Matter is a physical manifestation possessing mass (occupies space and has weight) and having form or shape. Matter is composed of substances, which are any materials that have a definite constant composition, such as pure salt. Simple substances are called **elements** and cannot be decomposed by ordinary means. At present, there are 105 known elements. The **atom** is the smallest particle of an element that has characteristic properties of that element.

The structure of the atom can be described as a miniature solar system. Each atom consists of a small **nucleus**, which has a positive charge, and a number of lighter particles with negative charges called **electrons**, which move around the nucleus in definite orbits. The atom is said to be neutral when the net number of positive charges of the nucleus (protons) equals the negative charges of the orbital electrons. The electrons are kept in their orbits by the balance between (1) the electrostatic attraction of unlike charges and (2) the centrifugal forces of the fast-moving electrons.

COMPOSITION OF THE NUCLEUS

The nucleus is composed of protons and neutrons. These particles are called **nucleons**. Protons carry a positive charge (+), which is equal in size to the neutrons but opposite in sign to the charge carried by the electrons (−). The neutrons carry no electrical charge (±) (Fig. 1.1).

ATOMIC NUMBER

Atoms differ from one another in the constitution of their nuclei and in the number and arrangement of their electrons. The atomic number, or Z number, is the number of protons in the nucleus or the number of electrons out-side the nucleus. Z numbers range from 1 for the simplest atom (hydrogen) to 105 for the most complex atom yet discovered (hahnium). The chemical properties of an atom are determined by the atomic number.

ORBITAL ELECTRONS

Electrons are very small particles carrying 1 unit of negative charge. They revolve around the nucleus in well-defined shells that exist at varying distances from the nucleus. The arrangement of the electrons around the nucleus determines the way atoms interact with each other. A maximum number of seven potential electron-containing orbits or shells exist. No known atom contains more than seven shells. These seven shells are designated as K, L, M, N, O, P, and Q in order of increasing distance from the nucleus (Fig. 1.2). Electrons in the outermost shell are termed **valence electrons** and determine the chemical properties of the atom (Fig. 1.3).

ELECTRON ORBITS OR SHELLS

The electrons in an atom do not spontaneously fly off from the nucleus by **centripetal force** or, on the other hand, drop into the nucleus by **electrostatic attraction** (unlike charges attract), because in the normal atom there is a balance between **centripetal** force and **electrostatic** force. This balance results in a definite electron path or orbit for each electron around the nucleus. Each shell has a different energy level, which is dependent on the atomic number of the atom and the distance the electron is from the nucleus. For each element, these orbital energy levels are different and characteristic. Because the nucleus carries

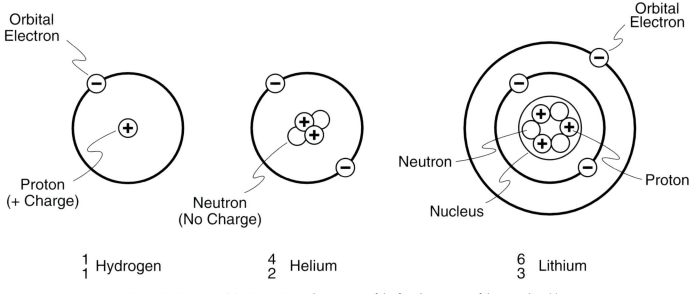

Figure 1.1. Structure of the Atom. Note the structure of the first three atoms of the periodic table.

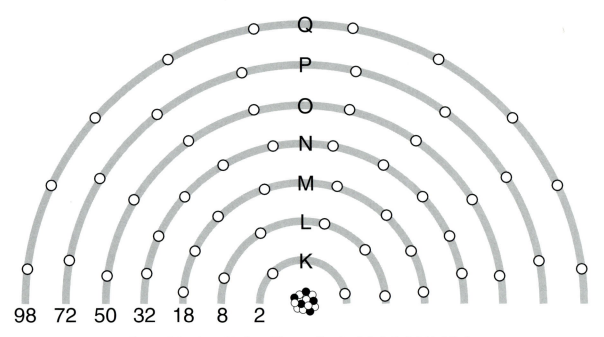

Figure 1.2. Maximum Number of Electrons That Can Exist in Each Orbital Shell.

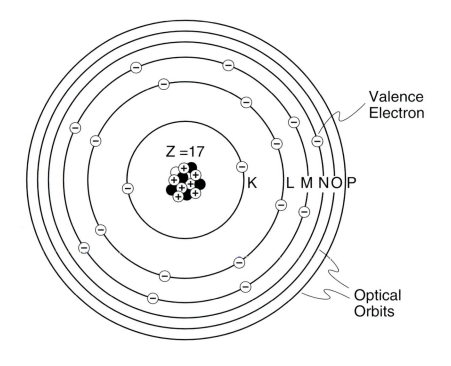

Potassium (K)

Figure 1.3. Electron Orbits of Potassium (Z = 17). For x-ray purposes, one is interested in the motion of the tightly bound K, L, and M shells, whereas the motion of the outer electrons is important in determining the chemical properties and optical spectrum of the atom.

a positive charge, it exerts an electric force of attraction on orbital electrons. The attraction force is greater when the electron shell is nearer the nucleus. Thus, it would require *more work* (energy) to remove an electron from the K shell and out of range of the nuclear electric field than to remove an electron from one of the outer shells.

BINDING ENERGIES

The energy required to remove an electron from a particular shell is designated as *binding energy* of that shell. The *binding energy* is largest for the K-shell because of its proximity to the positively charged nucleus, decreasing progressively for successive shells. The binding energy is characteristic of a given element and shell. Because of the relatively large amount of energy needed to remove an electron from the inner shell, the electron is said to be bound more tightly than the electrons of the outermost shells.

ELECTRON-VOLT

Energy is measured by the amount of work done or the amount of work capable of being done. The most useful unit of energy for our purposes is the *electron-volt*. This is the kinetic energy of an electron accelerated through a potential difference of 1 volt. Larger multiple units of the electron-volt are frequently used: **keV** for 1000 or kiloelectron volts, and **MeV** for 1 million or megaelectron volts.

BINDING ENERGIES IN ELECTRON-VOLTS

The binding energies of the K, L, and M shells of tungsten are 70 keV, 12 keV, and 3 keV, respectively. To remove a K-shell electron from tungsten would require an energy of 70 keV (Fig. 1.4). Because the electrons in the inner shells have greater binding energies, it takes x-rays, gamma rays, or high-energy particles to remove

Carbon $^{12}_{6}$C

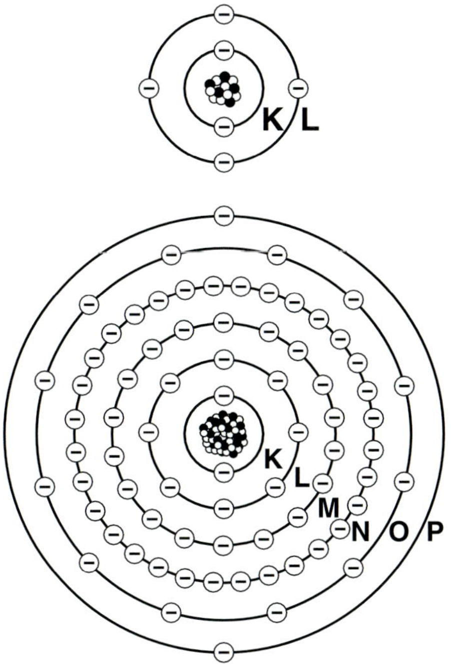

Tungsten $^{184}_{74}$W

Shell	Number of Electrons	Approximate Binding Energy (keV)
K	2	0.284
L	4	0.006
K	2	69.525
L	8	12.100
M	18	2.820
N	32	0.595
O	12	0.077
P	2	—

Figure 1.4. Binding Energies of Tungsten and Carbon (Two Important Elements in Radiology). Note that binding energies are greater for each element for the inner shell electrons. Also, tungsten is a more complex element than carbon and has higher binding energies in each shell.

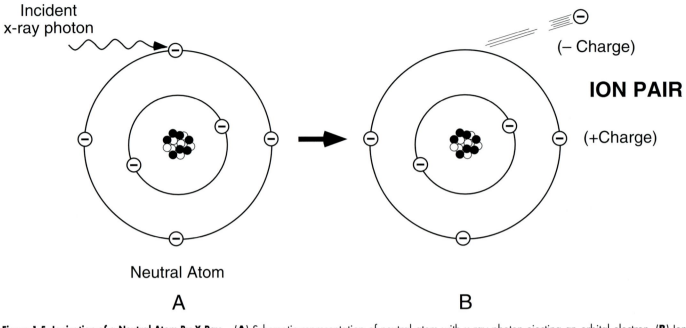

Figure 1.5. Ionization of a Neutral Atom By X-Ray. (**A**) Schematic representation of neutral atom with x-ray photon ejecting an orbital electron. (**B**) Ion pair formed by ejected electron (− charge) and the ionized atom with more protons than electrons (+ charge).

electrons from these shells. Electrons in the outer shells are not held so tightly to the nucleus and therefore can be affected by lesser energies, such as visible light rays and ultraviolet rays.

IONIZATION

Ionization is the process by which a neutral atom or molecule acquires either a positive or a negative charge. When an atom loses or gains an electron, it is said to be ionized. An ionized atom (called an ion) is not electrically neutral but carries a charge equal to the difference between the number of protons and electrons. Many elements have incompletely filled outer shells, which tend to capture electrons quite readily from adjacent atoms. Of course, when this occurs, the atom has more electrons than it should and it becomes a negative atom. When atoms lose electrons, they become deficient in negative charges and therefore will behave as positively charged atoms. An atom that is not electrically balanced is called an **ion**. In any ionization process, **ion pairs** are formed; it is this process that elicits chemical changes in matter.

X-rays are a form of energy that can form ion pairs in atoms. When an x-ray transfers its energy to an orbital electron, it ejects it from the atom, and an ion pair is formed. The atom becomes a positive ion (+1 charge) because it has lost an electron, and the ejected electron

has a negative charge (-1). Thus, an ion pair has been formed (Fig. 1.5).

IONIZING RADIATION

TYPES OF IONIZING RADIATION

There are two forms of ionizing radiation: (1) **corpuscular or particulate radiation** and (2) **electromagnetic radiation**.

Particulate Radiation

Particulate radiations are actually minute particles of matter that travel in straight lines at high speeds from their sources. Although incredibly small, they possess mass. All are charged electrically, except the neutrons, and they all move extremely fast—sometimes almost as fast as light. Examples of particulate radiation follow.

Alpha Particles Alpha particles are composed of a combination of two protons and two neutrons. It is the helium nucleus without orbital electrons. Alpha particles are emitted only from the nuclei of heavy metals. Compared with the other particles, the *alpha particle* is enormous and exerts a large electrostatic attraction. They have little ability to penetrate tissues and give up their large energies within a very short distance in air (5 cm) and in soft tissue (100 μm).

Electrons Electrons have a very small mass compared with protons. Electrons abound in nature. We are interested in the following two: beta particles (negatrons) and cathode rays (electrons).

Beta Particles (Negatrons) Beta particles are emitted from the nucleus of radioactive atoms and possess 1 unit of negative charge. They have very small atomic masses. Beta particles (negatrons) are more penetrating than alpha particles and may penetrate 10–100 cm of air and approximately 1–2 cm of soft tissue.

Cathode Rays (Electrons) Cathode rays are streams of electrons passing from the hot filament of the cathode to the target of the anode in an x-ray tube. They differ from beta particles in their place of origin. *Beta particles* come from the nucleus of radioactive atoms, whereas the cathode rays originate from *orbital electrons* of the atoms of the filament material for an x-ray tube.

Protons Protons are accelerated hydrogen nuclei. They are approximately 2000 times the mass of the electron. Because protons are heavy, charged particles, they lose kinetic energy rapidly as they penetrate matter.

Neutrons The neutrons carry no electron charge and have nearly the same mass as a proton. The characteristic of being electrically neutral has proved of great importance in nuclear physics, because such a particle can penetrate into the nucleus of an atom without being subjected to the enormous forces of repulsion that resist the entrance of a positively charged particle.

Electromagnetic Radiation

X-rays and **gamma rays** belong to a group of radiations called *electromagnetic radiations*. Electromagnetic radiation is the propagation of energy through space accompanied by electric and magnetic force fields (hence the name electromagnetic radiation). X-rays and gamma rays are identical except for their origin. X-rays are produced outside the nucleus in the electron orbital system. Gamma rays are emitted from the nucleus of a radionuclide, which is a species of atom that disintegrates with the emission of corpuscular and electromagnetic radiations (Fig. 1.6). In nuclear medicine, alpha particles, beta particles, and gamma rays are of prime importance. In diagnostic radiol-

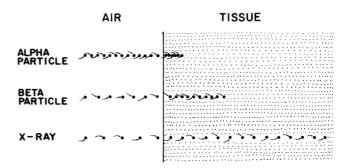

Figure 1.7. Particulate and Electromagnetic Radiation. Particulate radiation ionizes matter differently than electromagnetic radiation. An alpha particle has an enormous electrical charge and mass that ionize matter rapidly and penetrate tissue for very short distances. A beta particle does not ionize matter as readily as an alpha particle and penetrates tissue farther than an alpha particle. X-rays have no electrical charge or mass and do not ionize matter rapidly. This allows x-rays to penetrate matter for long distances.

ogy, x-rays are of prime importance because they do not seriously irradiate local tissue as particulate radiation does, and x-rays penetrate tissue for long distances (Fig. 1.7).

NATURE OF X-RAYS

As mentioned previously, x-rays are a form of electromagnetic radiation. To understand the production of a radiograph, we must first understand the nature of x-rays.

The interactions of electromagnetic radiations are difficult to understand. Some interactions are best explained by the theories of wave propagation, whereas other interactions are only explained if they are assumed to be particles or bundles of energy called "quanta" or "photons." It is necessary to discuss electromagnetic radiations as if the radiations were both waves and particles. The method used to detect x-rays or the way x-rays are being used determine which aspect (waves or photons) is the more useful concept. The wave concept of electromagnetic radiation explains why it may be reflected, refracted, diffracted, and polarized. The particle concept is used to describe the interactions between radiation and matter.

WAVE CONCEPT OF ELECTROMAGNETIC RADIATION

Electromagnetic radiation is the propagation of wave-like energy through space or mass at the speed of light (186,000 miles/sec or 3×10^8 m/sec). A wave can be defined as a variation or disturbance that transfers radiant energy progressively from point to point in a medium. (Energy is the capacity to perform work.) It is called electromagnetic radiation because the energy that is radi-

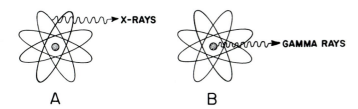

Figure 1.6. X-Rays and Gamma Rays. **(A)** X-rays are produced outside the nucleus of stable atoms. **(B)** Gamma rays are emitted from the nucleus of radioactive atoms.

ated is accompanied by oscillating electric and magnetic fields.

Each field is in phase with and perpendicular to each other and perpendicular to the direction of wave propagations (Fig. 1.8).

EXAMPLES OF ELECTROMAGNETIC RADIATION ARE:

1. The radio waves that we hear.
2. The light waves we see.
3. The infrared waves that can take pictures in the dark.
4. The ultraviolet rays that cause sunburn.
5. The x-rays studied in this text.
6. The gamma rays of the atomic bomb.
7. The cosmic rays that hinder travel in space.

The waves we are familiar with are like waves traveling down a stretched rope while one end of the rope is moved up and down in rhythmic motion. Sound waves traveling in water or air must be propagated in a medium. Electromagnetic waves need no such medium, as they can be propagated within and transmitted through a vacuum. All waves have an associated **wavelength** and **frequency**. The wavelength of a wave is the distance between two successive crests, or valleys, and is given the symbol λ (the Greek letter *lambda*, the symbol for length) (Fig. 1.9).

The number of waves passing a particular point during a specific period is called the **frequency** and is given the symbol ν (the Greek letter *nu*, the symbol for number).

It is usually identified as oscillations per second or cycles per second. The unit of frequency measurement is the **hertz** (Hz). One hertz equals 1 cycle/sec, and 60 Hz is the standard 60 cycle/sec alternating electrical current used in North America. Other parts of the world use 50-cycle current. Because the velocity is always known, the wavelength of the radiation can be determined if the frequency is known; conversely, the frequency can be determined if the wavelength is known. It also holds true that if the frequency of the wave is high, the wavelength will be short; if the frequency is low, the wavelength will have to be long (Fig. 1.10).

The relationship among velocity, frequency, and wavelength can be expressed in the following formula.

$$c = \lambda\nu \ (\text{lambda} \times \text{nu})$$

where c = velocity of light (3×10^8 m/sec)
λ = wavelength in meters
ν = frequency in hertz (cycles per second)

PARTICLE CONCEPT OF ELECTROMAGNETIC RADIATION

Short electromagnetic waves, such as x-rays, may react with matter as if they were particles rather than waves. These particles are actually discrete bundles of energy

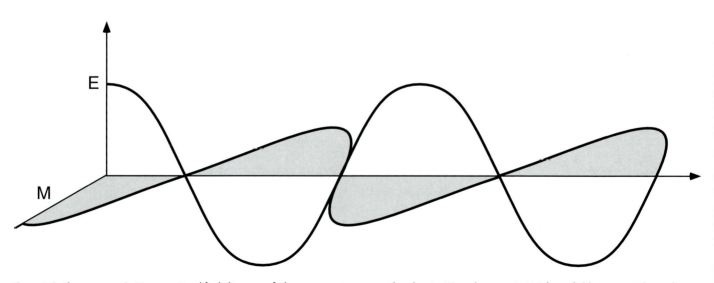

Figure 1.8. Electromagnetic Waves. Simplified diagram of electromagnetic waves. The electric (*E*) and magnetic (*M*) force fields are at right angles to each other and perpendicular to the direction of the wave propagations (movement).

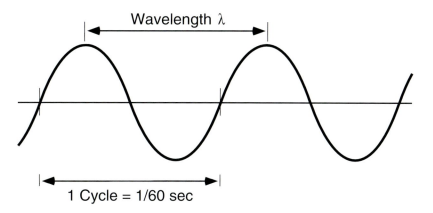

Figure 1.9. Wave Concept of Electromagnetic Radiation. Wave diagram illustrating wavelength and frequency.

having no mass, and each of these bundles of energy is called a **quantum** or **photon**. These photons travel at the speed of light. The dual natures (waves and particles) are inseparable. For instance, the amount of energy carried by each quantum or photon depends on the frequency (ν) of the radiation. If the frequency (vibrations per second) is doubled, the energy of the photon is doubled. The unit used to measure the energy of photons is the electron-volt

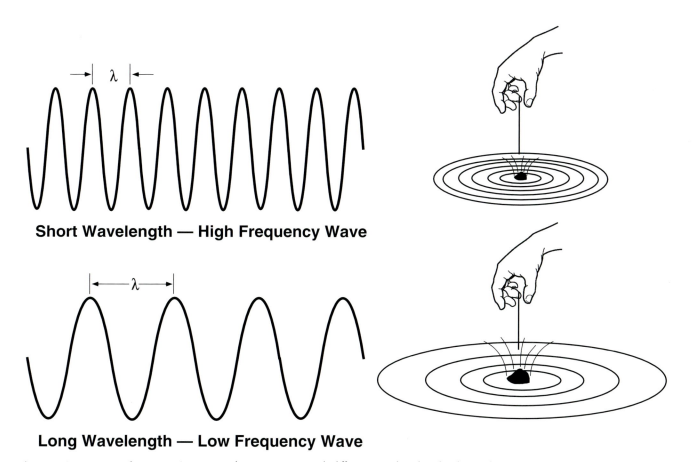

Figure 1.10. Frequency of Wave Motion. Note the two energies with different wavelengths. The shorter the wavelength, the higher the frequency.

(eV), as mentioned previously. If a photon has 15 eV or more of energy, it is capable of ionizing atoms and molecules and is called "ionizing radiation." An atom is ionized when it loses an orbital electron. Gamma rays, x-rays, and some ultraviolet rays are all types of ionizing radiation.

ELECTROMAGNETIC SPECTRUM

Electromagnetic energy is all around us. X-rays, gamma rays, radio waves, and light waves are forms of electromagnetic energy within the spectrum that we encounter every day. The only fundamental differences among them are their wavelengths (or frequency) and the energy of their photons. All these forms of electromagnetic radiation are grouped according to their wavelengths or energy of their photons in what is called the *electromagnetic spectrum* (Fig. 1.11). Figure 1.11 shows their location in the spectrum and some of their common uses. When the wavelengths (or frequency) and the energy of the photons change, so do the properties of the different types of radiation. The wavelength of a radio wave may be 100 yards long, whereas the typical x-ray is only one billionth of an inch in length. For example, the length of electromagnetic waves generated by 60 Hz (cycles/sec) alternating electrical current is approximately the distance from coast to coast of the United States. The wavelengths of the standard broadcast portion of radio waves are as long as a football field and have a frequency of 3 million Hz. The wavelengths used in television are about equal to the height of an average man and have a frequency of 300 million Hz. The wavelength of diagnostic x-rays is extremely short and is usually expressed in nanometers (nm), one of which

is equal to one millionth of a millimeter. The useful range of x-rays in medical and dental radiography is approximately 0.01–0.05 nm. In the earlier literature, wavelengths of electromagnetic radiation were often given in angstrom units (Å). One angstrom unit is equal to one tenth of a nanometer. The wavelength of light in the center of the visible spectrum is about 550 nm, whereas the x-rays used for radiography—those near the center of the medical and dental x-ray spectrum—have a wavelength of approximately 0.05 nm or approximately 1/10,000 that of visible light. Short wavelengths correspond to high energies and frequency. X-rays generated by a 100 keV current will be very short (0.05 nm) and have frequencies of 2.42×10^{19} Hz (cycles/sec).

WHAT ARE X-RAYS?

X-rays are weightless packages of pure energy (photons) that have no electrical charge and travel in waves with specific frequency at a speed of 3×10^8 m/sec. Their energies depend on the frequency of their wavelengths. The greater the frequency of the wavelength, the greater the energy of the photon. The greater the energy of the photon, the more readily it will penetrate matter.

PROPERTIES OF X-RAYS

To gain more understanding of x-rays, it is necessary to know a little more about how they act and what they do. Fundamentally, x-rays obey all the laws of light, but among their special properties some of the following are of interest to the student of dental radiology.

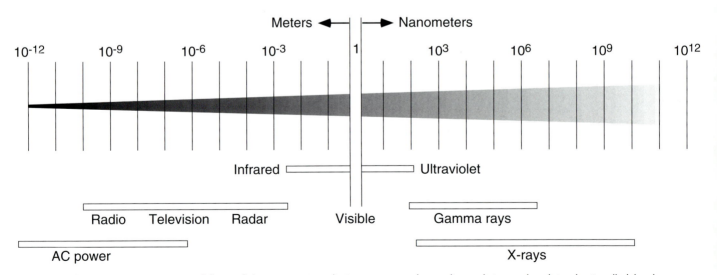

Figure 1.11. Electromagnetic Spectrum. All forms of electromagnetic radiation are grouped according to their wavelength in what is called the electromagnetic spectrum.

PROPERTIES OF X-RAYS

1. X-rays are invisible and weightless; they cannot be seen, heard, felt, or smelled.
2. X-rays travel in straight lines; they can be deflected from their original direction, but the new trajectory is linear.
3. X-rays travel at the speed of light (3×10^8 m/sec).
4. X-rays have a wide range of wavelengths, 0.01–0.05 nm, in length.
5. X-rays cannot be focused to a point; over distance the beam diverges much like a beam of light.
6. Because of their extremely short wavelengths, they are able to penetrate materials that absorb or reflect visible light.
7. X-rays are differentially absorbed by matter; this absorption depends on the atomic structure of the matter and the wavelength of the x-rays. It is this property that produces an image on a photographic film, which in turn can be made visible by chemical development.
8. X-rays cause certain substances to fluoresce, that is, to emit radiation of longer wavelength (for example, visible and ultraviolet radiation). It is this property that makes it possible to use intensifying screens in radiography.
9. X-rays produce biologic changes that are valuable in radiation therapy but necessitate caution when used for diagnostic purposes.
10. X-rays can ionize gases, that is, remove electrons from atoms to form ions, which can be used for measuring and controlling exposure (ionization chambers).

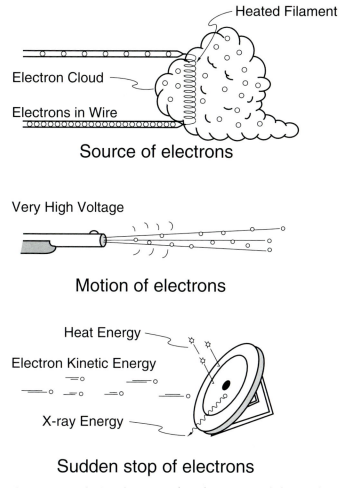

Figure 1.12. Production of X-Rays. Three things are needed to produce x-rays: (1) source of electrons, (2) motion—high-voltage potential to move electrons, and (3) sudden stop. Electrons striking an anode target of high atomic number causes sudden deceleration or stoppage of rapidly moving electrons, which produces heat energy and x-ray energy.

These special properties have applications in dental, medical, and industrial radiography, radiation therapy, and research.

PRODUCTION OF X-RAYS

X-rays are generated when fast-moving electrons (small particles, each bearing a negative electrical charge) collide with matter in any form (Fig. 1.12). X-ray production is a process of energy conversion when electrons are suddenly decelerated (speed is reduced) in the target of the x-ray tube.

X-RAY TUBE

The x-ray tube is only a few inches long. It is contained within the tubehead of the x-ray machine, which is the much larger outer housing to which the beam indicating device (BID) is attached. The most efficient means of generating x-rays is an x-ray tube, and the simplest form of an x-ray tube is a sealed leaded glass envelope from which air has been evacuated. The x-ray tube is made of Pyrex and contains two electrodes in a vacuum. The electrodes are designed so that electrons produced at the **cathode** (negative electrode or filament) can be accelerated to a high potential difference (voltage) toward the **anode** (positive or target electrode) (Fig. 1.13).

Cathode

The cathode of the x-ray tube is the negative terminal of the tube and consists of a tungsten wire (filament) wound in the form of a spiral set in a molybdenum cup-shaped holder (called a focusing cup) and positioned ap-

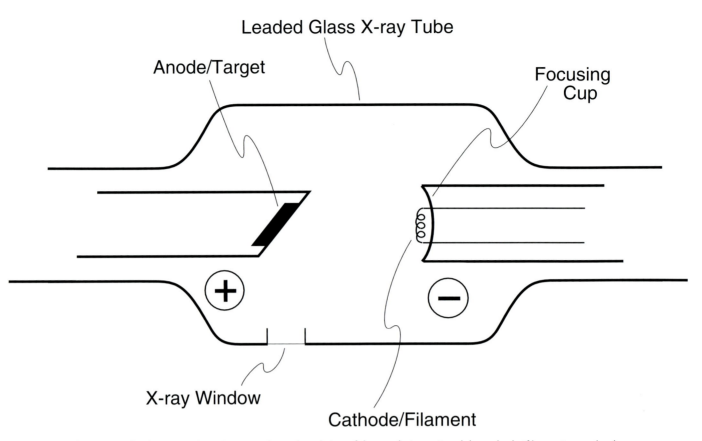

Figure 1.13. Simple X-Ray Tube. Diagram shows the relation of the anode (target) and the cathode (filament) to each other.

proximately 1 inch away from the anode (positive terminal). Tungsten is used for the filament because it has a high melting point (3370°C) and can be drawn into a thin wire (0.2 mm in diameter) and still remain quite strong. The filament electrical circuit (low-voltage circuit) provides a source of electrons that are emitted from the hot wire of the filament and forms an electrical "cloud" around it.

Anode

The anode (positively charged to attract electrons) is usually made of copper because of its good heat conductivity. A block of tungsten is set in the face of the copper anode at the center of the tube. This block of tungsten is referred to as the **target**. The **focal spot** is an area on the target that electrons strike to generate x-rays. The electrons at the filament are set in motion toward the target by activating the high voltage circuit (kVp) as the timer switch is pressed. As the stream of electrons strikes the target, most of the kinetic energy is converted to heat (99%); however, a small amount of energy is converted to x-rays (1%).

The size of the focal spot has a very important effect on the sharpness of the x-ray film image. The smaller the

focal spot, the sharper the x-ray image. However, the smaller the focal spot becomes, the less heat the focal spot will be able to absorb at one time. Some method had to be found to obtain a practical size of the focal spot that would provide image detail without undue heating of the anode.

Line Focus Principle (Anode) The Benson line focus principle developed in 1918 is a method of reducing the effective focal spot size and is used in dental x-ray tubes. The target face is placed at an angle of 15–20° to the cathode, as shown in Figure 1.14. As the angle of the target face is made larger, the projected focal spot becomes smaller. When the rectangular focal spot is viewed from below—where the film would be located—it appears more nearly square. This is called the "effective focal spot," which is only a fraction of the size of the actual target. By using x-rays that emerge at this angle, radiographic definition is improved while the heat capacity of the anode is increased, because the electron stream is spread over a greater area. The effective focal spot of most dental x-ray tubes measures approximately 0.6–1.2 mm², depending on the manufacturer's specifications. The smaller the effective focal spot, the sharper the x-ray image.

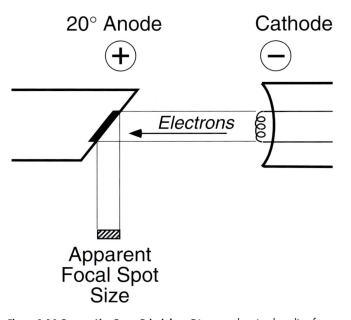

20° Anode (+) Cathode (−)

Electrons ←

Apparent
Focal Spot
Size

Figure 1.14. Benson Line Focus Principle. Diagram showing how line focus principle works. By placing the target/anode at a 20° angle to the cathode, the effective focal spot produced is only a fraction of the size of the actual target. (The smaller the effective focal spot, the sharper the x-ray image.)

CONDITIONS NECESSARY FOR THE PRODUCTION OF X-RAYS

There are four conditions required for the production of x-rays in an x-ray tube. They are as follows:

1. Generation of electrons.
2. Production of high-speed electrons.
3. Focusing of electrons.
4. Stopping of high-speed electrons at the target.

Generation of Electrons

In referring to an x-ray tube, the terms **cathode** and **filament** may be used interchangeably. The *filament* is the *source of electrons* (called cathode electrons) in the x-ray tube. As mentioned previously, the filament is made of tungsten because tungsten has a high melting point of 3370°C and can be drawn into a thin wire 0.2 mm in diameter. Tungsten has orbital electrons circulating around a central nucleus. How can these electrons be liberated from individual atoms within the tungsten filament? The **filament current** (average of 10 V and 3–5 A) that supplies the tungsten filament causes it to become glowing hot, or *incandescent*, in the same way as the filament in an ordinary light bulb. However, the filament is not heated to produce light but to act as a source of electrons that are emitted from the hot wire. When the tungsten is heated, its atoms absorb thermal energy, and some of the outer orbit electrons in the metal acquire enough energy to allow them to move a small distance from the surface of the metal. Their escape from the metal is referred to as the process of **thermionic emission** (boiling off electrons), which is the emission of electrons resulting from the absorption of thermal energy. The separation of electrons from the tungsten filament will form a small cloud of electrons in the immediate vicinity of the filament. The temperature of the filament (at least 2200°C) controls the quantity of electrons emitted from it. As the temperature is raised by increasing the milliamperes (mA), more electrons are emitted, and the flow of electrical current through the x-ray tube (mA) increases. The x-ray tube current, measured in milliamperes (1 mA = 0.001 ampere), refers to the number of electrons flowing per second from the filament to the target of the anode. For example, in a given unit of time, the x-ray tube current of 15 mA is produced by 1.5 times as many electrons as a current of 10 mA. The number and the quantity of x-rays produced in a unit of time depends entirely on the number of electrons that flow from the filament to the target (anode) of the tube. The number of electrons can be varied by altering the exposure time, the mA, or both. Dental x-ray machines use a 7-mA, 10-mA, or 15-mA current. The higher the mA, the more electrons that will be available, and of course the more x-rays produced, in a unit of time.

Production of High-Speed Electrons

When a large potential difference (for example, 90 kVp) is applied across the tube electrodes, it causes the electrons at the cathode filament to accelerate at very high speeds (approximately half the speed of light) across the 1- to 3-cm gap from the filament to the target. The electric current across an x-ray tube is always in one direction only (cathode to anode). The higher the potential (voltage), the greater the speed of these cathode electrons as they strike the target. This produces more energetic x-ray photons that have shorter wavelengths, higher frequencies, and greater penetrating power.

Focusing of Electrons

The electron stream always crosses the x-ray tube in one direction, from cathode (-) to anode (+). Because of the forces of mutual repulsion and the larger number of electrons, the electron stream tends to spread out and bombard an unacceptably large area on the anode tungsten target of the x-ray tube. This is prevented by a structure called the cathode **focusing cup**, which surrounds the filament. The focusing cup is designed so that its electrical forces cause the electron stream to converge onto the target or anode in the required size and shape. The small area of the target that the electrons strike is called the **focal spot** and is the source of the x-radiation. The smaller the focal spot, the sharper the image produced on the radiograph.

Stopping High-Speed Electrons in the Target

When the fast cathode electrons enter the target of the x-ray tube, their **kinetic energy** (energy in motion) changes to other forms of energy.

> The efficiency of ordinary radiographic equipment is such that **at 90 kVp, only approximately 0.6% of this energy is converted to x-rays while the remaining 99.4% is converted to infrared radiation or what we simply report as heat.**

This interaction, responsible for the generation of heat, is primarily an **excitation** rather than ionization interaction. In **excitation**, the projectile electrons interact with the outer-shell electrons of the tungsten target but do not transfer sufficient energy to these outer-shell electrons to ionize them. Rather, the outer-shell electrons are simply raised to an excited or higher energy level. When the outer-shell electrons drop back to their normal state, there is an emission of infrared (heat) radiation. In fact, only about one part in a thousand of the kinetic energy of the electrons eventually results in radiologically useful x-rays! X-rays from the target are emitted in *all* directions, but only those leaving the window of the x-ray tube comprise the **useful beam.**

> The student will have noted that one must avoid confusing the cathode electrons flowing in the tube with the x-rays emerging from the tube. Imagine throwing stones at and hitting the side of a barn. The stones are analogous to the electron beam that hits the target in the x-ray tube, whereas the emerging sound waves are analogous to the x-rays that come from the target when struck by cathode electrons.

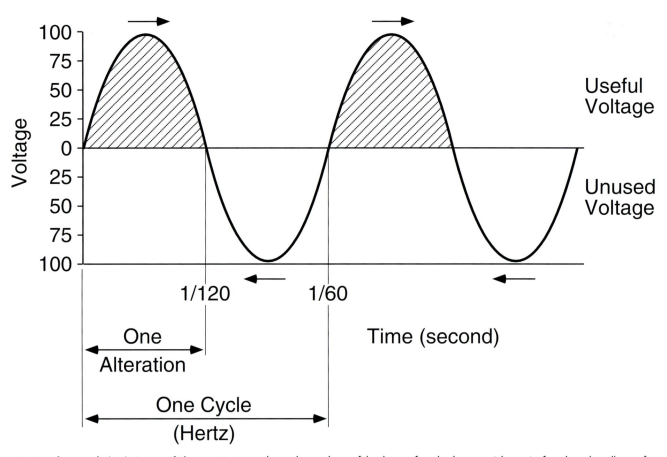

Figure 1.15. Voltage and Kinetic Energy of Electrons Vary. Voltage during the useful voltage of each alteration (change) of each cycle will vary from a low value (0) to a peak value (100). The kinetic energy of the impinging (hitting) electrons will vary according to the voltage applied at the instant the electrons are projected toward the anode target.

Kinetic Energy of High-Speed Electrons

To review, x-rays are produced by kinetic energy conversions when fast-moving electrons from the cathode filament of the x-ray tube (cathode electrons) interact with the anode (target). The kinetic energy (energy in motion) of a cathode electron will depend on the voltage being applied to the tube at that moment. The higher the speed of the electrons, the higher penetrating power of the x-rays produced at the anode.

kVp and keV

First, we must clearly distinguish between *kVp* (*kilovoltage peak*) and *keV* (*kiloelectron volts*). The expression 100 kVp means that the maximum voltage across the tube causing acceleration of electrons is 100,000 volts. The expression keV denotes the energy of any individual cathode electron in the beam (100 keV = 100,000 electronvolts). When the dental x-ray tube is operated at 100 kVp, few cathode electrons acquire a kinetic energy of 100 keV. This is because in the dental x-ray machine generator, the useful voltage of the single phase, half-wave, self-rectified circuit will pulsate from 0 to a maximum 100 kVp and back to 0 at the rate of 60 times/sec (Fig. 1.15). Each cathode electron will acquire a certain kinetic energy (eV), depending on the applied voltage across the tube at that particular instant. Therefore, the high-speed cathode electrons striking the target do not all have the same kinetic energies, because the voltage (v) across the tube that provides the potential to accelerate the cathode electrons is variable by nature. In other words, the energy (eV) of the individual cathode electrons that encounter the target (anode) covers a broad range of kinetic energies.

TWO PROCESSES OF X-RAY PRODUCTION

When the fast-moving cathode electron stream strikes the tube target, the cathode electrons interact with target atoms producing x-rays by the following two processes: general radiation and characteristic radiation.

General Radiation (Bremsstrahlung)

Most of the x-rays produced by dental x-ray machines are called *bremsstrahlung*, *brems*, *white*, or *general radiation*. Bremsstrahlung is derived from two German words: **bremse** meaning "brake" and **strahl** meaning "ray." It is called "braking radiation" because the radiation is produced by "braking" or decelerating of high-speed electrons. A cathode electron that completely avoids the orbital electrons of an atom of the tungsten target may come sufficiently close to the nucleus to come under its influence. Because the cathode electron is negatively charged and the nucleus is positively charged, there is an electrostatic attraction between them. As the cathode electron approaches the tungsten atom's nucleus, it is influenced by

a nuclear force, which is stronger than the electrostatic attraction between the electron and the nucleus. As a result, the projected electron slows down and is deflected from its original course, thereby losing some of its kinetic energy (energy in motion). The kinetic energy lost by the electron is emitted directly in the form of photons of radiation (x-radiation) (Fig. 1.16). Most of the cathode electrons that strike the target will give up their kinetic energy by interactions with many atoms before coming to rest. Each time a cathode electron is decelerated, it gives off only a small part of its energy; the projected electron will penetrate many layers of atoms of the target material before giving up all its energy. Therefore, not all the x-ray photons are produced on the surface of the target; a

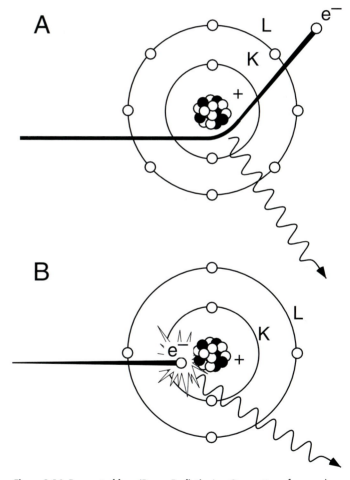

Figure 1.16. Bremsstrahlung (Brems Radiation). *Generation of general or white radiation (Bremsstrahlung) produced by interaction of a cathode electron with a tungsten atom nucleus of the target (anode). (**A**) Cathode electron deflected and decelerated by the nucleus of a tungsten atom producing an x-ray photon. (**B**) Occasionally, the total kinetic energy of a cathode electron is converted into x-ray photon energy by a direct collision with the nucleus of the tungsten atoms of the target (anode).*

fraction of the projected electrons approach the nucleus head-on and are completely stopped by the electrostatic field. In this collision, all the energy of the electron is converted to a single x-ray photon. The cathode electrons are those from the electron stream striking the target, whereas the orbital electrons are those in each atom of tungsten within the target.

Characteristic Radiation

The other process by which x-rays can be produced in an x-ray tube is when a cathode electron has sufficient energy to ionize a tungsten atom within the target (focal spot) by ejecting an inner orbital electron (for example, in K or L shell) from the tungsten atom. To eject a K-shell electron, work has to be done to overcome the attractive force of the nucleus of an atom of tungsten. The binding energy of an orbiting electron in the K shell of tungsten is about 70 keV. Therefore, the cathode electron must have energy of more than 70 keV to eject a K-shell electron. When such an event occurs, both the K-shell electron and the cathode electron leave the atom. (A 60 keV electron beam will not contain any electrons that will eject a K-shell electron from tungsten.) The tungsten atom is now unstable because it is now **ionized** (an electron missing from an atom) and in an **excited state** (an electron vacancy in a shell). For the atom of tungsten to return to a normal state again, the ionized atom of tungsten must get rid of its excess energy. Immediately, the space or "hole" vacated by the ejected electron in the K shell is filled by an electron from one of the outer shells, usually from the adjacent L shell. When an L electron drops down into the K shell, the L electron must give up its excess energy. This energy given off by the L-shell electron is a single photon of x-radiation of 59 keV. This is the difference between the binding energies of the K shell (about 70 keV) and the L shell (about 11 keV). The x-ray photon of 59 keV is the *characteristic radiation* of the K shell of the tungsten atom. The energy emitted is termed a characteristic x-ray because its energy is characteristic of the target element (tungsten) involved (Fig. 1.17). What contribution does the characteristics radiation make to the total x-ray production by a standard x-ray tube? Below 70 kVp, there is no K-shell characteristic radiation. With 80 kVp, characteristic radiation (K-shell characteristic)

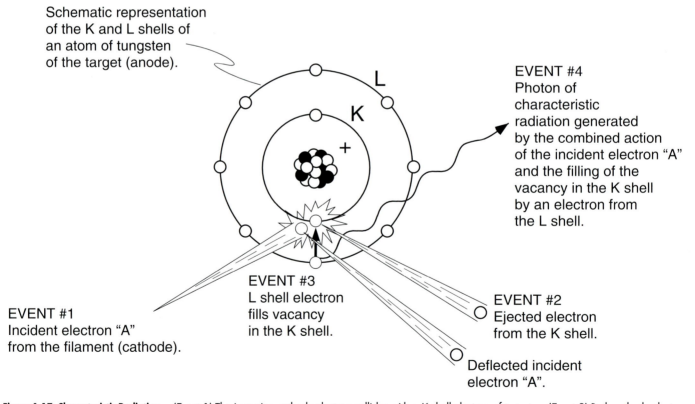

Schematic representation of the K and L shells of an atom of tungsten of the target (anode).

EVENT #4
Photon of characteristic radiation generated by the combined action of the incident electron "A" and the filling of the vacancy in the K shell by an electron from the L shell.

EVENT #3
L shell electron fills vacancy in the K shell.

EVENT #1
Incident electron "A" from the filament (cathode).

EVENT #2
Ejected electron from the K shell.

Deflected incident electron "A".

Figure 1.17. Characteristic Radiation. (Event 1) The incoming cathode electron collides with a K-shell electron of tungsten. (Event 2) Both cathode electron and K-shell electron leave the atom. The atom now is in an excited state. (Event 3) An electron from the L shell jumps into the K shell, giving off K-characteristic radiation with photon energy of 59 keV. (Event 4) The L-shell electron space is filled by the M-shell electron, and L-characteristic radiation with photon energy of 9 keV is emitted.

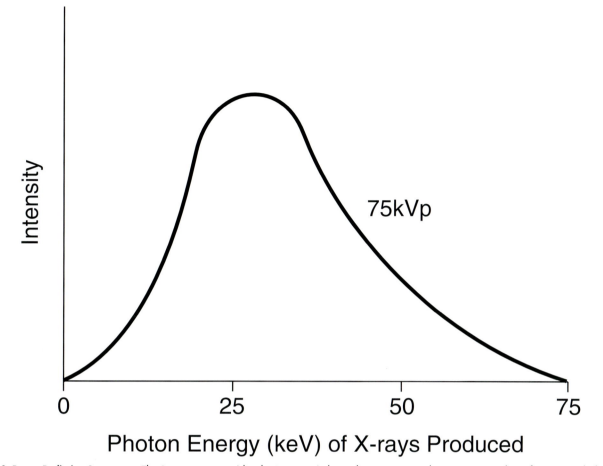

Figure 1.18. Brems Radiation Spectrum. The Brems spectrum (distribution curve) shown here compares the intensity (number of x-rays) with the photon energy of the x-rays produced at a particular kVp. The maximum number of x-rays produced is at approximately the 25 keV level, as shown on this continuous spectrum of Brems Radiation at 75 kVp.

contributes approximately 10% of the useful x-ray beam. It is important to understand the differences between **cathode electrons** striking the target, **orbital electrons** of individual tungsten atoms within the target, and **ejected electrons** from individual orbital shells of tungsten atoms.

HETEROGENEOUS AND HOMOGENEOUS X-RADIATION

X-Radiation used in dentistry can be heterogeneous or homogeneous, depending on the varying wavelengths in the x-ray beam.

Heterogeneous Radiation

Brems radiation is heterogeneous or polyenergetic; that is, it is **not** uniform in energy and wavelength (Fig. 1.18). There are two factors that produce this wide varia-

tion in the energy of radiation produced by the braking phenomenon. *First*, the cathode electrons will undergo many reactions before coming to rest in the majority of cases. With each deceleration of a cathode electron, a corresponding amount of kinetic energy (energy in motion) is converted to x-ray photons of equivalent energy. As the deceleration or braking varies, so does the energy of the x-ray photons produced. *Second*, the cathode electrons have widely different kinetic energies (speed). As the applied kVp varies, so will the kinetic energy of the cathode electrons. In general, the highest-energy x-ray (short wavelengths) photons are determined by the selected kilovoltage peak (kVp) used (i.e., 90 kVp). The lowest-energy x-ray (long wavelength) photons produced will probably *never* reach the patient because they will be filtered out either within the x-ray tubehead (target material, glass, and oil insulation) or by the added aluminum filter placed outside the tubehead exit window. Nevertheless, the x-

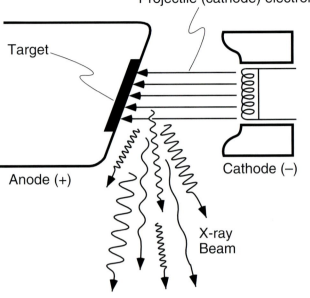

Projectile (cathode) electrons

Target

Anode (+)

Cathode (−)

X-ray Beam

Heterogenous Beam

Figure 1.19. Brems Radiation Is Heterogeneous. Brems radiation is heterogeneous or polyenergetic, that is, it is not uniform in energy and wavelengths. In this diagram, projectile (cathode) electrons of widely different kinetic energies (keV) produce an x-ray beam of x-ray photons of various energies (wavelengths).

radiation that does emerge from the x-ray machine is still, in most instances, heterogeneous; that is, the x-ray beam will contain photons of varying wavelengths (Fig. 1.19).

Homogeneous Radiation

In some x-ray machines, the alternating current (AC) is converted to direct current (DC). When a DC current is applied to an x-ray generator, the kilovoltage rapidly rises to its peak and remains there throughout the x-ray exposure. Thus, all the cathode (projected) electrons will have the same keV, and the resulting radiation is more homogeneous. (That is, the x-ray photons all have the same wavelength.) Thus, the emerging x-ray beam will not contain any low-energy (longer wavelength) x-ray photons that are not sufficiently penetrating; in the heterogeneous beam, these long-wave photons are absorbed by the patient's soft tissues. Thus, they do not penetrate the teeth and bone and do not contribute to the image. In DC machines, most of the x-ray photons penetrate the patient's soft tissues to eventually create the image. Thus, when a DC-type machine is used, the same quality image can be produced with 20% less radiation dose to the patient.

WORKSHOP/LABORATORY EXERCISES

EXERCISE 1.1. PROPERTIES OF X-RAYS DEMONSTRATED WITH A RARE EARTH SCREEN

Materials and Equipment Needed

1. Intraoral x-ray machine.
2. Preferably rare earth screen (Kodak Lanex Regular; Eastman Kodak, Rochester, NY) or older calcium tungstate screen.
3. Small piece of pine board.
4. Small piece of Sheetrock.

Note: Number 2 can be obtained from a dental supply house. Numbers 3 and 4 can be obtained as waste from most construction sites or contractors, a plumber, or a construction supply store.

Instructions

Step 1: Set up the fluorescent screen as follows: place an opened cephalometric or panoramic cassette vertically on a counter top near the intraoral x-ray machine.

Step 2: Set up the x-ray machine as follows: turn it on and set the exposure time at 60 impulses or 1 second, depending on the machine. If there is a kVp dial, set it at 90 kVp. If there is an mA switch, set it at 15 mA or the highest mA setting.

Step 3: Align the x-ray machine and fluorescent screen. Grasp the tubehead and move it toward the screen so that the tip of the BID is about 1 inch away from the screen and perpendicular to it (i.e., aim the BID directly at the screen).

Step 4: Observe the fluorescence of the screen. Turn off the lights in the room and stand behind either a shield or door with a leaded glass panel or stand at least 6 feet away from the tubehead and in the safe quadrant. (The instructor will explain). Depress and hold down the timer or exposure switch (note the sound while x-rays are being emitted).

Now look at the green or blue light being emitted by the screen. Note the size of the fluorescent spot being just a bit bigger than the size of the BID opening.

Step 5: Back the BID tip away from the screen. Grasp the tubehead and move the tubehead and BID back so it is about 6 inches away from the screen, but still pointing directly at it.

Step 6: Repeat Step 4. Do this with the lights on and also with the lights off. Now the fluorescent spot will be somewhat larger than before and not as bright or as intense as during the first exposure when the lights were off. When the lights are on, it is harder to see the fluorescent light. When the lights are on or off, the beam of x-rays cannot be seen.

Step 7: Place a piece of wood between the BID tip and the screen. Obtain a small length of 3/4-inch pine board and tape it to the BID tip, so that the BID tip is completely covered. Place the BID tip about 1 or 2 inches away from the screen as before. Depress and hold down the timer or exposure switch. Observe the green or blue light being emitted by the screen. Note the presence or absence of the fluorescent spot and its relative brightness.

Step 8: Place a piece of Sheetrock between the BID tip and the screen. Obtain a small piece of 3/4-inch or 5/8-inch Sheetrock. Remove the piece of wood from the BID tip and replace it with the piece of Sheetrock. Using the Sheetrock only, repeat Step 7.

CASE-BASED QUESTIONS FOR LABORATORY EXERCISE

1. Name as many properties of x-rays you were able to observe by performing this experiment.

2. What did you learn about the x-ray machine?

3. What did you learn about radiation safety?

CASE-BASED PROBLEM-SOLVING

You need to go home and explain to a boyfriend, girlfriend, spouse, or parent how:

1. X-rays are similar to light.

2. X-rays are different from light.

3. Easy it is to protect one's self from radiation exposure.

Clue: Use a **small** pocket-sized flashlight, a piece of clear plastic or glass, and a piece of cardboard from a note pad.

REVIEW QUESTIONS

1. In the x-ray tube, x-rays originate from the:

   A. Filament.
   B. Cathode.
   C. Anode.
   D. Focusing cup.

2. The electrons that revolve in shells around the nucleus:

   A. Have a positive charge.
   B. Have no charge, either positive or negative.
   C. Have a negative charge.
   D. Have either a positive or negative charge.

3. X-rays belong to which of the following radiation categories?

   A. Particulate radiations.
   B. Hygroscopic radiations.
   C. Alpha radiations.
   D. Corpuscular radiations.
   E. Electromagnetic radiations.

4. An x-ray photon is:

   A. A small particle able to penetrate matter.
   B. A small bundle of pure energy with wave-like properties.
   C. An electron that has been accelerated to 186,000 miles/sec.
   D. An electrical current that has been magnified by 1000 V or 1 kV.

5. X-rays are actually produced in the x-ray tube by:

   A. Radioactive decay of particulate matter.
   B. Electrical current passing through a mixture of oil and gases, creating minute explosions.
   C. High-speed electrons colliding with the electrons in the target, giving off radiation.
   D. High-speed photons colliding with the electrons in the oil mixture and target area.

6. The target material (in the anode) for diagnostic tubes is:

   A. Copper.
   B. Tungsten.
   C. Lead.
   D. Samarium.

7. At diagnostic levels, what percentage of the electron energy is converted to x-radiation at the anode?

   A. Less than 1%.
   B. 2%.
   C. 10%.
   D. More than 99%.

8. Increasing the kVp of an x-ray machine increases the:

   A. Number and energy of photons generated.
   B. Mean wavelength of the photons generated.
   C. Focal spot size of target.
   D. Filament temperature.

9. The dental x-ray beam consists of photons of many different wavelengths, with the shortest wavelength photons determined by:

   A. Milliamperage (mA).
   B. Kilovoltage peak (kVp).
   C. Filtration.
   D. Coefficiency of attenuation.

10. Which of the following statements most adequately describes the radiation produced by high kilovoltage?

    A. Short wavelengths of low frequency.
    B. Long wavelengths of high frequency.
    C. Short wavelengths of high frequency.
    D. High penetrating waves of low frequency.

11. In a standard dental x-ray unit, the *quality* of x-radiation produced during exposure energization is controlled primarily by:

    A. Exposure time.
    B. Kilovoltage (kV).
    C. Milliamperage (mA).
    D. Inherent filtration.

12. In a standard dental x-ray unit, the *quantity* of x-radiation produced during exposure energization is controlled primarily by:

    A. Exposure time and kilovoltage (kV).
    B. Exposure time and milliamperage (mA).
    C. Exposure time and inherent filtration.
    D. kV and mA.

13. Ionization occurs:

    A. When atoms lose electrons; they become deficient in negative charges and therefore behave as positively charged atoms.
    B. When atoms gain electrons; they become positively charged.
    C. When an atom loses its nucleus.
    D. Only when a K-orbit electron is ejected and replaced by an L-orbit electron.

14. Which electron has the greatest binding energy to the nucleus?

    A. J-shell electron.
    B. K-shell electron.
    C. L-shell electron.
    D. Q-shell electron.

15. Select the correct statement:

    A. X-rays cannot be focused to a point.
    B. X-rays can be focused to a point.
    C. X-rays cannot increase the electrical conductivity of a gas.
    D. X-rays do not always travel in a straight line.

16. The mean penetrability of an x-ray beam is **not** related to which of the following?

    A. kVp.
    B. Filtration.
    C. Wavelength.
    D. Frequency.
    E. mA.

BIBLIOGRAPHY

Alpen E. Radiation biophysics. Englewood Cliffs, NJ: Prentice Hall, 1990.

Bushberg JT, Seibert JA, Leidholdt EM Jr, Boone JM. The essential physics of medical imaging. Baltimore: Williams & Wilkins, 1994.

Bushong SC. Radiologic science for technologists: physics, biology, and protection. 5th ed. St. Louis: Mosby-Year Book, 1993.

Cember, H. Introduction to health physics. New York: McGraw-Hill, 1996.

Curry TS III, Dowdey JE, Murry RC Jr. Christensen's physics of diagnostic radiology. 4th ed. Philadelphia: Lea & Febiger, 1990.

Glasser O. The science of radiology. Springfield: Charles C. Thomas, 1933:1–14.

Hendee W, Ritenour RE. Medical imaging physics. 3rd ed. St. Louis: Mosby-Year Book, 1992.

Langlais RP, Kasle MJ. Basic principles of oral radiography. Philadelphia: WB Saunders, 1981.

Langland OE, Sippy FH, Langlais RP. Textbook of dental radiology. 2nd ed. Springfield: Charles C. Thomas, 1984.

Rezai RF, Walkhoff O. Renaissance man of dentistry. Bull Hist Dent 1986;34:115–121.

Roentgen WC. On a new kind of rays. Nature 1896;53:274–276.

Rohrmeir G, Walkhoff FO. Leben und werk. Wurzburg, Germany: Wurzburg University, January 1895. Dissertation.

Sellman J. The fundamentals of X-ray and radium physics. 7th ed. Springfield: Charles C. Thomas, 1985.

Sprawls P Jr. Physical principles of medical imaging. 2nd ed. Gaithersburg: Aspen, 1993.

Squire LF, Novelline RA. Fundamentals of radiology. 4th ed. Cambridge: Harvard University Press, 1988.

Ter-Pogossian MM. The physical aspects of diagnostic radiology. New York: Harper & Row, Hoeber Medical Division, 1967.

Wolbarst AT. Physics of radiology. East Norwalk, CT: Appleton-Lange, 1993.

The X-Ray Machine, Attenuation, and Recording of Radiographic Images

2

OBJECTIVES

Upon successful completion of this unit, the student will be able to:

1. *Identify two types of electric current.*

2. *Describe and discuss the purpose of transformers.*

3. *Define the half-value layer.*

4. *Define self-rectification and half-wave.*

5. *Define milliampere second.*

6. *Identify the effect mAs has on the x-ray beam.*

7. *Define leakage and scattered radiation.*

8. *Identify the types of interactions that occur when matter is exposed to radiation.*

9. *Discuss the inverse square law.*

10. *Recognize radiographic film sizes and the appropriate uses for each of the sizes.*

11. *List the four components of the radiographic film and discuss the purpose of each component.*

12. *Discuss the relevance of film speed to radiation safety.*

13. *Define latent image.*

14. *Observe the differential absorption of x-rays by matter through the Workshop/Laboratory Exercises.*

15. *Observe the components of the intraoral film packet through the Workshop/Laboratory Exercises.*

16. *Learn the essentials of x-ray processing through the Workshop/Laboratory Exercises.*

17. *Apply the Workshop/Laboratory Exercises knowledge to solve three common problems occurring with bitewing radiography.*

18. *Test his or her knowledge by answering the Review Questions.*

KEY WORDS/PHRASES

alternating current	emulsion	rectification
autotransformer	filament	remnant x-rays
characteristic radiation	filament circuit	resistance
coherent scattering	film sensitivity	scattered radiation
Compton scattering	half-value layer	screen type film
control panel	high-voltage circuit	sensitivity speck
current	intensity	silver halide
direct current	inverse square law	step-down transformer
direct exposure film	mAs rule	step-up transformer
electricity	potential difference	x-ray generator

THE X-RAY MACHINE

X-rays used in dental radiography are electronically produced. The major components of the x-ray system are the wall switch, **control panel**, generator, and x-ray tube. An **x-ray generator** receives standard alternating current from the wall switch. The **control panel** is used to select predetermined settings of x-ray exposure and to initiate the exposure. The generator provides high-voltage waveforms, according to the factors of exposure selected, that will energize the x-ray tube.

X-RAY GENERATOR

The x-ray generator supplies an electrical source of energy (usually 110 or 220 V) and 60 Hz (cycles/sec) alternating current to the x-ray tube and then modifies it to supply the needs of the x-ray tube. The tubehead is the outer housing that is attached to the arm by the yoke. The beam indicating device (BID) is attached to the tubehead. To understand how the generator works, we should first review some basic electrical physics, because x-rays are produced by the use of electricity.

ELECTRICITY

Electric current or electricity is the flow of electrons through an electric conductor very much like water flowing through a pipe. If the electrons are made to flow in one direction along a conductor, the electrical current is called **direct current** or DC (Fig. 2.1). Most applications of electricity in radiology require the electrons to flow first in one direction and then in the opposite direction. Current in which electrons oscillate back and forth is called **alternating current** or AC (Fig. 2.2). The term "cycle" in AC refers to the curve above and below the horizontal line. Each cycle consists of two alternations; that is, the voltage starts at 0, rises gradually to the maximum in one direction called the kV peak, and finally returns to 0. There are 120 alternations/sec with 60-cycle current. However, only 60 alternations/sec are usable in dental self-rectified x-ray tubes. This is because only half of the available cycle is used to produce x-rays (Fig. 2.3). Rectification is a process of changing AC into DC. Dental x-ray tubes are called **self-rectifying tubes**, in that they act as a simple rectifier in changing AC into DC while producing x-rays.

Direct Current

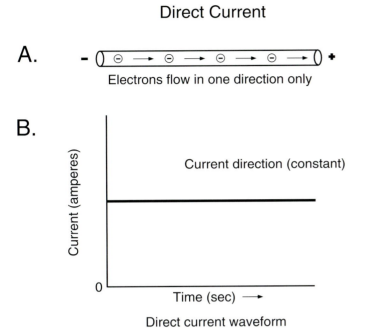

A.

Electrons flow in one direction only

B.

Current direction (constant)

Current (amperes)

0

Time (sec) →

Direct current waveform

Figure 2.1. Direct Current (DC). **(A)** In DC, electrons flow in one direction only. **(B)** Graph of associated wave-form of direct current. The distance between the horizontal line and the time axis represents the magnitude or velocity of the electrons.

ELECTRICAL CIRCUITS

There are three factors that characterize a simple dental x-ray machine electrical circuit. These are **potential difference** (voltage), **current** (amperes [A]), and **resistance** (ohms [Ω]). The first factor is the potential difference, which may be defined as a difference in electrical potential energy between two points in an *electric current* due to excess of electrons at one point relative to the other. The unit of potential difference is the **volt** (V), which is defined as the potential difference that will cause a current of 1 A to flow in a circuit where resistance is 1 Ω. The kilovolt (kV) is equal to 1000 V. The *second factor* in an electrical circuit is *current*, which is defined as the amount of electricity (electrons) flowing per second through a conductor (wire). In a water pipe, this would be the amount of water flowing past a given point in 1 second. The unit of current is the ampere, which may be defined as the quantity of electrons representing 6.3×10^{18} free electrons flowing through a conductor in 1 second. The number of electrons involved is enormous. A milliampere is equal to 11,000th of an ampere. The *third factor* of the electrical circuit is *resistance* and is a property of materials of the circuit itself. Electrical resistance is that property of a circuit

Alternating Current

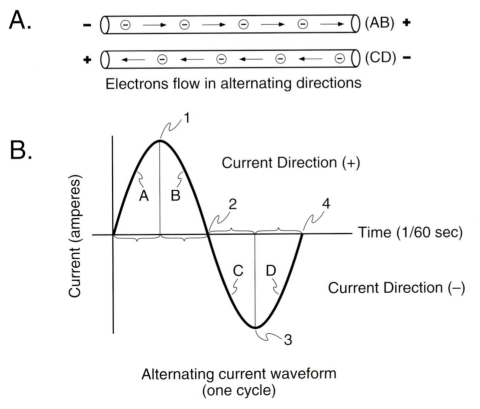

A.

(AB) +

(CD) −

Electrons flow in alternating directions

B.

Current (amperes)

Current Direction (+)

1

A   B

2   4

Time (1/60 sec)

C   D

Current Direction (−)

3

Alternating current waveform
(one cycle)

Figure 2.2. Alternating current (AC). **(A)** In AC, electrons flow in one direction and alternately in the opposite direction, always from the negative to the positive pole. **(B)** Example of a sine wave (represents periodic oscillations) of alternating current. Note that electrons flow first in a positive direction and then in a negative direction (below the 0 axis). At point 0, the electrons are at rest and increase in velocity during segment A. When they reach maximum velocity they are at point 1, where the electrons begin to slow down in segment B. They come to rest again at point 2. They then reverse motion, and the flow of the electrons begins again in a negative direction. At point 4 the cycle ends, which takes 1/60 second in 60 hertz (cycles/sec) current.

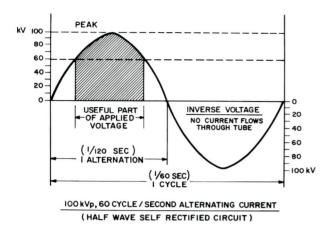

100 kVp, 60 CYCLE / SECOND ALTERNATING CURRENT
(HALF WAVE SELF RECTIFIED CIRCUIT)

Figure 2.3. Dental Self-Rectified X-Ray Tubes. Alternating current used in dental radiography is a 60-cycle current—it flows first in one direction and then flows in the opposite direction, changing directions every $\frac{1}{120}$ second. It makes a complete cycle every $\frac{1}{60}$ second. In the dental x-ray tube, the anode is first positive and then negative with respect to the cathode during each half-cycle ($\frac{1}{120}$ second). When the anode is positive, the electrons flow by attraction to the anode; when the anode is negative, the electrons are not attracted to the anode. Hence, no current flows in the tube. Therefore, the dental x-ray tube in essence changes AC into DC (self-rectification) while producing x-rays.

that opposes or hinders the flow of an electrical current (electrons). The unit of electrical resistance is the **ohm**, defined as the resistance of a standard volume of mercury under standard conditions. The *x-ray tube requires* electrical energy for two purposes: (1) to boil electrons from the x-ray filament and (2) to accelerate and direct these electrons from the cathode to the anode. The *x-ray generator* has a separate current for each of these functions, which will be referred to as (1) the filament circuit and

(2) the high-voltage circuit. The timer mechanism circuit regulates the length of exposure. These three circuits are interrelated.

COMPONENTS OF THE X-RAY GENERATOR

The *x-ray generator* is contained in two separate compartments: the **control panel** and the **tubehead** assembly. The control panel contains the main off-and-on switch, the exposure button, mA selector control, kVp selector control, time selector, x-ray emission light, and pilot light (Fig. 2.4). The tubehead assembly of the x-ray generator (Fig. 2.5) contains a low-voltage transformer, high-voltage transformer, and x-ray tube. Because the potential difference in these circuits may be as high as 100,000 V, the transformers and x-ray tube are immersed in oil (Fig. 2.6). The oil functions as an insulator and prevents sparking from one electrical component to another in the tubehead.

Step-Up and Step-Down Transformers

By definition, a transformer is an electromagnetic device that changes AC from low voltage to high voltage or from high voltage to low voltage without loss of appreciable amount of energy (less than 10%). A transformer is composed of two wire coils wrapped around the opposite ends of an iron core. The first coil circuit is called the primary circuit or input side, and the second coil circuit is called the secondary circuit or output side. When current flows through the primary circuit and coil (transformer), it produces a magnetic field within the magnetic core, and the magnetic field induces a current in the secondary coil and circuit. However, current will not flow in the secondary or output circuit unless the magnetic field is changing (either decreasing or increasing); the current will **not** flow

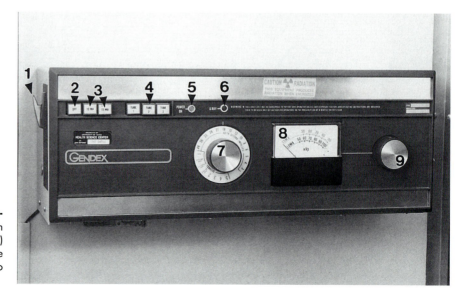

Figure 2.4. Control Panel of Gendex Dental X-Ray Machine. (1) Holder for exposure button, (2) main switch, (3) mA selector, (4) x-ray tube selector, (5) power on light, (6) x-ray/emission light, (7) exposure timer, (8) kVp-mA meter, and (9) kVp selector (auto transformer).

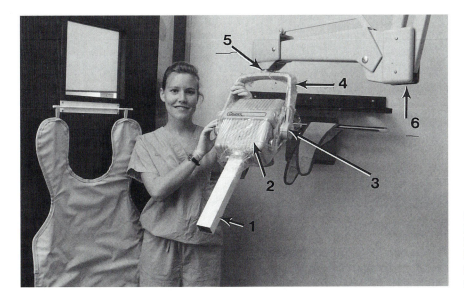

Figure 2.5. Tubehead and Extension Arm of Gendex Dental X-Ray Machine. (1) Long rectangular beam indicating device (BID), (2) tubehead (includes transformers and x-ray tube), (3) vertical rotation, (4) x-ray tube yoke, (5) horizontal rotation, and (6) extension arm.

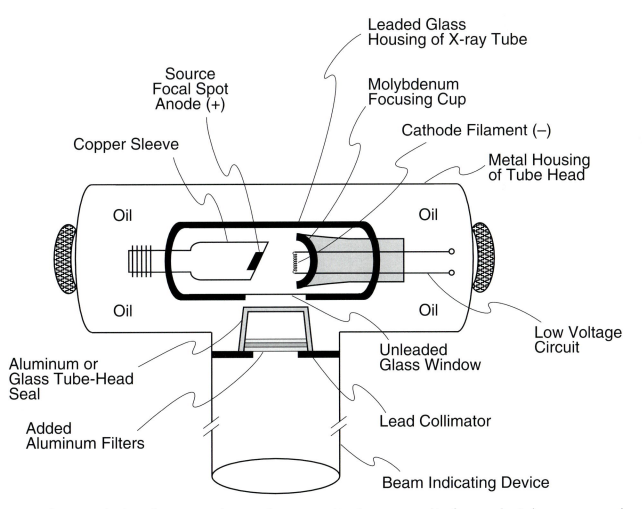

Figure 2.6. Dental X-Ray Head, Tube, and Cone (BID). The x-ray tube is immersed in oil to prevent sparking from one electrical component to another and to disperse the heat from the copper sleeve of the anode.

if the magnetic field is in a stable state, such as with DC. AC is used for transformers because in AC the voltage changes continuously, thus producing a continuously changing magnetic field. Voltage is induced in the secondary coil when AC current is applied to the primary coil. The voltages in the two coils are directly proportional to the number of turns of wire in each, assuming a theoretical 100% efficiency. This means that if the number of turns in the secondary coil is twice the number in the primary coil, then the voltage in the secondary coil will be twice the voltage in the primary. A *step-up transformer* has more turns in the secondary coil than the primary coil (Fig. 2.7). A transformer with fewer turns in the secondary coil than in the primary coil decreases the voltage and is called a *step-down transformer* (Fig. 2.7).

Autotransformer

Although in dental radiography there are x-ray machines with fixed kVp (such as 65 or 70 kVp), it is an advantage to have an x-ray machine in which the kilovolt-

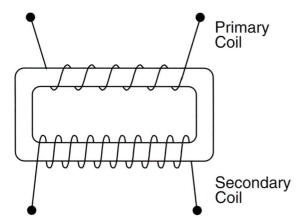

Step-Up Transformer

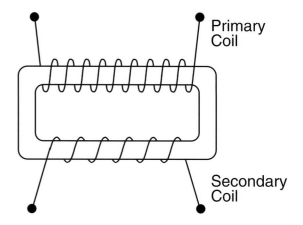

Step-Down Transformer

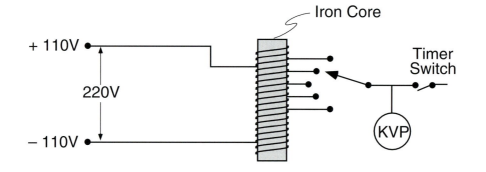

Autotransformer

Figure 2.7. Transformers.   A step-up transformer has more turns in the secondary coil than in the primary coil. In dental x-ray machines, a step-up transformer takes 110- or 220-V current and increases this voltage to 65,000 to 90,000 V (65 to 90 kVp). This provides the high voltage necessary to accelerate the cathode electrons toward the anode at high speeds. **Step-Down Transformer:** In dental x-ray machines, the primary coil of the step-down transformer has more turns than the secondary coil. This decreases the voltage down from 110 or 220 V to 8 to 12 V in the secondary coil, which provides a high current of 3 to 6 A to heat the filament. **Autotransformer (kVp Selector):** The autotransformer varies the voltage input into the primary coil of the step-up transformer, which in turn varies the kVp of the machine.

age can be varied. The kilovoltage can be varied by the use of an autotransformer. The autotransformer has a single coil of insulated wire wound around a large iron core, which serves as both the primary and secondary coil, with the number of turns being adjustable. At regular intervals along the coil, the insulation is interrupted and the bare points connected to metal buttons. By moving a metal conductor to various metal buttons on the wire, the number of turns included in the secondary circuit of the autotransformer is varied, which in turn varies the output voltage. Therefore, where the autotransformer is varied, it in turn varies the output voltage. The autotransformer serves as a kVp selector dial and varies the kVp available to the primary coil of the step-up transformer (Fig. 2.7).

Filament and High-Voltage Circuits

As stated previously, there are two electrical circuits necessary in the x-ray machine to produce x-rays in the x-ray tube. The first is the *filament circuit*, which provides a source of electrons by heating the filament to incandescence to "boil off" the electrons from the filament of the cathode. The second circuit is the *high voltage* necessary to accelerate the cathode electrons from the cathode toward the anode at high speeds.

Filament Circuit The filament circuit regulates the current flow to the filament of the x-ray tube. The **step-down transformer** in the filament circuit reduces the potential difference (110 or 220 V) in the primary coil to 8 to 12 V in the secondary coil, which results in a high current of 3 to 6 A to heat the filament in the x-ray tube. Although the current (amperes) in the filament circuit only heats the filament and does not represent the current (mA) across the x-ray tube, it actually increases the x-ray tube current (cathode to anode electrons) by increasing the filament temperature. A hotter filament emits more electrons, and adds electrons to the current electrons (mA) across the x-ray tube.

High-Voltage Circuit The high-voltage circuit has two transformers: a **step-up transformer** and an **autotransformer**. The **step-up transformer** takes 110- or 120-V current and increases this voltage to 65,000 to 100,000 V (60 to 100 kVp), thereby providing the high voltage necessary to drive the cathode electrons in the x-ray tube at high speed from the cathode to the anode. At the same time it decreases the current to 10 to 15 thousandths of an ampere (10 to 15 mA). As previously stated, although there are x-ray machines with fixed kVp (such as 65 or 70 kVp), it is an advantage to be able to vary the kilovoltage. This is because some conditions, like caries, are best seen in the 65- to 75-kVp range, whereas alveolar bone changes (such as in periodontal and periapical disease) are best seen at 80 to 90 kVp when D speed film is used.

E speed film is generally used at lower kVps than D speed. The kilovoltage can be varied by the use of an **autotransformer**. The autotransformer is an electromagnetic device that operates as a kVp selector because it varies the kVp available to the primary coil of the step-up transformer.

INTENSITY OF THE X-RAY BEAM

Because the x-ray beam is composed of photons with many energies (heterogeneous), it is common to speak of quality and quantity of a beam of photons. **Quality** refers to the energy of particular photons; **quantity** refers to the number of photons in the beam, each with a particular energy. Quality and quantity are described together in a concept known as *intensity*, defined as the total energy contained in the beam (quality times quantity) per unit area per unit time.

$$\text{Intensity} = \frac{(\text{no. of photons in beam}) \times (\text{energy of each photon})}{(\text{area}) \times (\text{exposure rate})}$$

The area referred to is the cross-sectional area of the beam at a particular point in space. Because most photons spread out as they move away from the source, it is important to specify where the intensity is being calculated (distance from source). The intensity of the x-ray beam varies with the target material, the mA (current), exposure time (rate), and distance of film from source (inverse square law). In the use of modern dental x-ray units, the variables that are under the operator's control are the **kVp, mA, exposure time**, and **source-to-film distance**. The target material (usually tungsten) in the anode electrode of the x-ray tube has already been placed in the x-ray machine by the manufacturer before the the practitioner purchases it from the dental supply dealer.

TUNGSTEN AS THE TARGET MATERIAL

Tungsten was chosen for the target of the anode because it has a high atomic number (74), which makes it more efficient in the production of x-rays. This is because the K-shell binding energy is high and there are a large number of planetary electrons. Also, it has a high melting point (3370°C) to withstand the high temperature produced in the production of x-rays. In addition, tungsten is a reasonably good metal for the absorption of heat and the rapid loss of heat from the target area.

X-RAY EMISSION SPECTRUM

Because the ordinary x-ray beam is heterogeneous in wavelength and energy, a particular x-ray beam can be classified with a high degree of precision by sorting out the x-rays by wavelength, or its photons, according to energy. This can be done by a special distribution curve or spectrum of x-rays of various wavelengths or photon energies. Graphically, the general shape of the x-ray emission spectrum is the same for all dental x-ray machines, but the relative position of the axis can change. The farther to the right the spectrum is, the higher the effective energy of the photons or **quality** of the x-ray beam. The greater the area under the curve, the higher the intensity (total energy contained in the beam) of the x-ray beam. The number of x-rays produced naturally depends on the number of electrons emitted by the cathode filament. The number of electrons emitted by the cathode filament depends directly on the tube current or mA used. If the operator changes the mA on the control panel from 10 to 20 while other factors remain constant, twice as many electrons will flow from cathode to anode. A change in the mA will make a proportionate area change in the x-ray emission spectrum (change in intensity of x-ray beam) (Fig. 2.8).

INFLUENCE OF EXPOSURE TIME ON INTENSITY

Exposure time is the interval during which x-rays are being produced. The more exposure time used, naturally the more x-rays produced. In dental radiography, the exposure time is the factor that is most commonly used to compensate for anatomic variables of patients. The most popular exposure technique is the "fixed kVp and mA technique," which varies only the exposure time.

Traditionally, timer intervals in dentistry have been in fractions of a second and whole numbers such as ¼, ½, ¾, 1, and 2. Most of the exposure time designations for less than 1 second are timer impulse intervals of 48, 38, 30, 24, 18, 15, 12, 10, 8, 6, 5, 4, 3, 2, and 1. With a 60 Hz (cycle) AC and a half-wave self-rectified dental x-ray tube, there are 60 impulses/sec of electrical energy. Therefore, 1 impulse equals ⅟₆₀ of a second. Any number greater than 60 is designated in seconds (for example, 120/60 = 2 seconds).

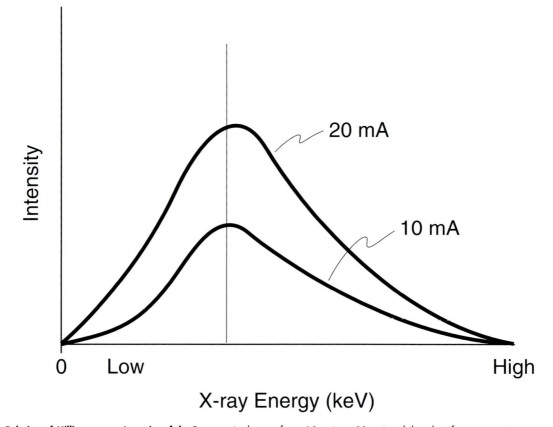

Figure 2.8. The Relation of Milliampere to Intensity of the Beam. A change from 10 mA to 20 mA, while other factors remain constant, will make a proportionate area change in the x-ray emission spectrum shown above. The intensity (total energy of the beam) of the 20 mA x-ray beam is twice that of the 10 mA beam.

Relationship of mA and Exposure Time

The mA and the exposure time have a direct effect on the quantity or number of photons produced in an x-ray beam. When these two factors (mA and seconds) are multiplied together, a common factor, mAs, is formed. When impulses are used instead of seconds for the exposure time, the common factor (mAs) becomes the milliampere impulses (mAi). Milliampere seconds or milliampere impulses determine the total number of x-ray photons produced in the beam, but do not indicate the energy of each photon in the beam. The effective energy of each particular photon in the x-ray beam depends on the kVp applied across the cathode to the anode.

mAs or mAi Rule

> The milliamperage required for a given exposure time is inversely proportional to the exposure time. That is, the higher the milliamperage, the shorter the exposure time. Some examples of mAs and mAi are given to show how the factors may be varied without influencing the quantity of radiation produced.
>
> $$mA \times sec = mAs \qquad mA \times imp = mAi$$
> $$10 \times \tfrac{1}{2} = 5 \qquad\qquad 10 \times 30 = 300$$
> $$15 \times \tfrac{1}{3} = 5 \qquad\qquad 15 \times 20 = 300$$
>
> Because the mAs and mAi in the above examples remain the same, the quantity of the radiation produced remains the same. Note that ½ second is the same as 30 impulses, and ⅓ second equals 20 impulses. There are 60 impulses in 1 second.

INFLUENCE OF TUBE POTENTIAL (kVp) ON INTENSITY

The higher kVp techniques will (1) increase the amount of radiation produced (quantity) and (2) determine the maximum energy (quality) of the x-rays produced. Kilovoltage controls the speed (kinetic energy) of each electron, which in turn has important effects on the photon energy of the x-rays produced. Radiation produced in the higher kilovoltage range (85 to 100 kVp) has more x-rays with greater energy, higher frequency, and shorter wavelengths; such x-rays are much more penetrating and are called "hard" x-rays. Radiation produced in the lower kilovoltage range (60 to 65 kVp) has more x-rays with less energy, lower frequency, and longer wavelengths; such x-rays are less penetrating and are called "soft" x-rays. In addition to controlling the penetrating power (quality) of the x-ray beam, kilovoltage also influences x-ray quantity. If the kVp were doubled from 50 to 100, the x-ray intensity increases by a factor of 4. This will increase the darkness (density) on the film. Actually, to double the x-ray intensity by kVp manipulation alone, one would only have to increase the kVp by 41%. This helps to explain the x-ray "rule of thumb" used by x-ray technologists to make kVp and mAs changes to produce constant density (darkness) on the film. The rule states that, "an increase of 15% in kVp should be accompanied by a reduction of one half in mAs." In dentistry, an increase of 15 kVp usually requires halving the exposure time, and a decrease of 15 kVp necessitates doubling the exposure time to maintain the same density (darkness) on the radiograph.

In summary, because kVp controls the speed of the electrons traveling from the cathode to the anode, more x-ray photons are produced per unit of time. Also, the higher speed of the cathode electrons colliding with the target produces more short wavelength or more penetrating photons of x-radiation (Fig. 2.9). Because of the greater number of photons of x-radiation at higher kVps, the exposure time will always need to be decreased when using higher kVps to avoid overexposing the film.

Varied kVp Technique

Many operators with x-ray machines in which the kVp can be varied use the *varied kVp exposure technique*. In this technique, the mA and exposure times (mAs) are fixed, and the kVp is varied according to differences in the thickness and density of anatomic structures in a particular region of a patient's jaw.

Half-Value Layer

In radiology, the quality or penetrating power of the x-ray beam is controlled by the kVp and is measured by

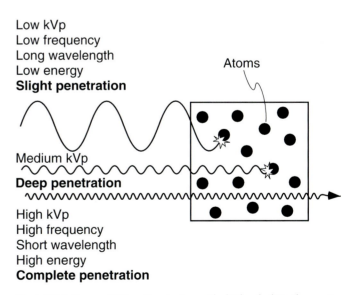

Low kVp
Low frequency
Long wavelength
Low energy
Slight penetration

Atoms

Medium kVp
Deep penetration

High kVp
High frequency
Short wavelength
High energy
Complete penetration

Figure 2.9. Influence of kVp on Penetration. The higher the kVp, the greater the penetration.

its half-value layer (HVL). The HVL of an x-ray beam is the thickness of absorbing material (usually aluminum) necessary to reduce the x-ray intensity to one half its original value. In dentistry, a diagnostic x-ray beam has an HVL of 1.5 mm of aluminum for machines 69 kVp and below; machines capable of 70 to 90 kVp have an HVL of 2.5 mm of aluminum. These thicknesses of aluminum are standards set by the federal government (for more on this, see Chapter 8).

INFLUENCE OF SOURCE-FILM DISTANCE ON INTENSITY

Because they are created at the focal spot of the tungsten target of the anode of the x-ray tube, x-rays act like visible light waves in that they radiate from the source in all directions unless stopped by an absorber. The x-rays of the primary beam emerge from the protective tube housing not as parallel waves but as divergent rays. The primary beam, then, is shaped very much like a cone or a megaphone. Therefore, the intensity of the beam decreases as the distance from the source increases. This can be proven by a simple demonstration. In a darkened room, move a single light source nearer to and farther away from a printed page. As the light source is moved away from the page, the light falling on it is less and less bright. Exactly the same thing happens with x-rays. As the distance from the object to the source of radiation is decreased, the x-ray intensity at the object increases; as the distance is increased, the radiation intensity at the object decreases.

Inverse Square Law

The relationship between distance and intensity of radiation is called the inverse square law because the intensity of radiation varies inversely as the square of the source-film distance (SFD) (Fig. 2.10).

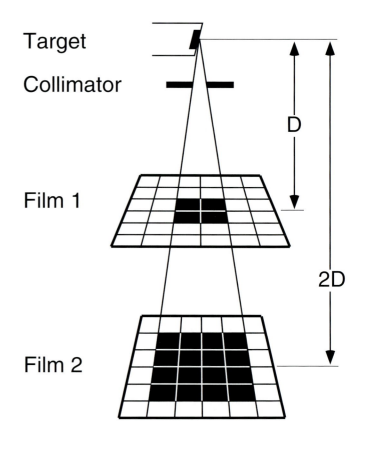

$$\text{Inverse Square Law: } I = \frac{1}{d^2}$$

Figure 2.10. Inverse Square Law. Diagram showing how the x-ray intensity is altered by changing the source-film distance. Increasing the distance by two times decreases the intensity by four times ($1/d^2$).

A practical formula to use in adjusting the exposure factor is as follows:

$$\frac{\text{Original mAs}}{\text{New mAs}} = \frac{\text{Original SFD}^2}{\text{New SFD}^2}$$

where   SFD = source-film distance   and
mAs = milliampere/seconds

Many times the kVp and mA will be fixed in dentistry, and the practitioner may want to change from a short-cone to a long-cone technique, perhaps from 8-inch SFD to 16-inch SFD. This is doubling the SFD distance, so the exposure time will have to be increased by the square of the distance or by a factor of 4 to maintain the same density (blackness) on the film. The intensity of the beam at 16-inch SFD would be one fourth the intensity as that at 8-inch SFD. Because the photons spread out as they move away from the source, the SFD is an important factor in determining the intensity of the beam.

By now, the astute reader would be able to figure out that if the original cone length were 16 inches and the exposure time was 1 second and now an 8-inch cone was going to be used, the exposure time would be cut down to ¼ second to maintain the same intensity of the radiation beam.

INTERACTION OF X-RAYS WITH MATTER

When x-ray photons arrive at the patient with energies produced by dental x-ray machines, three things can happen:

1. Some x-ray photons are merely scattered,
2. Some x-ray photons are absorbed completely in the patient, and
3. Some x-ray photons can pass through the patient without interacting with the tissue atoms.

When the x-ray photons are transmitted through the patient without an interaction, they produce densities (blackness) on the film. The photons that are absorbed are completely or partially removed from the x-ray beam and produce opacities (whites or grays) in the film. When the x-rays are scattered, they are deflected in all directions and therefore contribute no useful information to the film. Scattered radiation that reaches the film is called film fog (unwanted darkness) and can completely obscure the film image (Fig. 2.11).

SCATTERED RADIATION

When x-rays (called incident photons or primary photons) strike any form of matter, such as body tissue, scat-tered x-ray photons are produced that usually possess longer wavelengths than the primary radiation. Because scattered radiation is unfocused and may come from any direction, its action on the film may cover the entire image with a veil or fog unless it is controlled. Radiographically, this fog tends to make the visualization of the image details more difficult. Almost all scatter radiation in dental radiography comes from Compton scattering.

Unmodified (Coherent) Scattering

Coherent or *Thompson scattering* is when low-energy x-rays (below 10 keV) interact with matter and the x-rays undergo a change in direction **without** a change in wavelength. For this reason the name **unmodified** is sometimes used. In this type of interaction between x-rays and matter, no energy is transferred and no ionization occurs. Its only effect is to change the direction of the incident radiation (Fig. 2.12). Most *coherent scattering* is in a forward direction. It is of little importance in dental radiography because it primarily involves low-energy x-rays that contribute little to the radiograph. However, there is some coherent scattering throughout all the ranges of energies in the beam. At 70 kVp, perhaps less than 5% of the radiation undergoes coherent scattering, which contributes only slightly to film fog. It is too small to be of any importance in diagnostic radiology.

Compton (Incoherent) Scattering

An x-ray with relatively moderate to high energy strikes a loosely bound (free) outer-shell electron, ejecting it from its orbit. An electron can be considered free when its

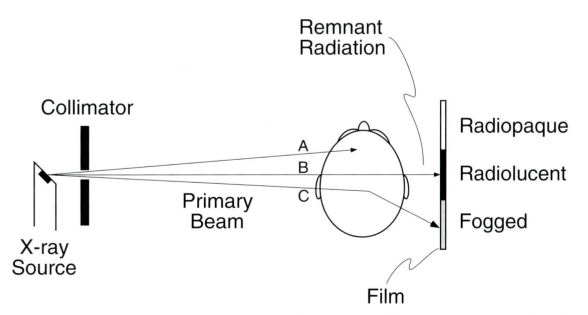

Figure 2.11. Interaction of X-Rays With Matter. (**A**) X-rays absorbed completely by photoelectric effect. (**B**) X-rays transmitted to film without interaction. (**C**) X-rays scattered by Compton interaction.

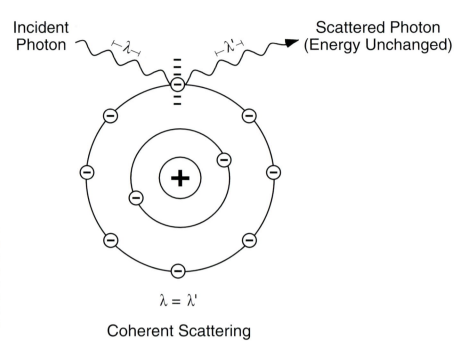

Figure 2.12. Unmodified (Coherent or Thompson) Scattering. An incident photon (usually of low energy) interacts with one of the outermost electrons. They are essentially free because they are so loosely bound. The electron starts to vibrate at the frequency of the incident photon. Because the electron is a charged particle, it emits radiation with the same frequency of the incident radiation and the atom returns to its stable state again.

Incident Photon

Scattered Photon (Energy Unchanged)

$$\lambda = \lambda'$$

Coherent Scattering

binding energy is a great deal less than the incident photon. This reaction ionizes the atom, producing an ion pair—a positive atom and a negative electron—called a **Compton electron** or **recoil electron**. This interaction was first described by A.H. Compton in 1923 (Fig. 2.13). The incident (or primary) x-ray photon is scattered in all directions (including backward) and retains most of its original energy. Both the scattered x-ray photon and the Compton electron may have sufficient energy to undergo many more ionizing interactions before losing all their energy. The original Compton electron will drop into an atomic shell vacant hole created previously by another ionization event and come to rest. Two factors determine the amount of energy the x-ray photon retains: (1) its energy and (2) its

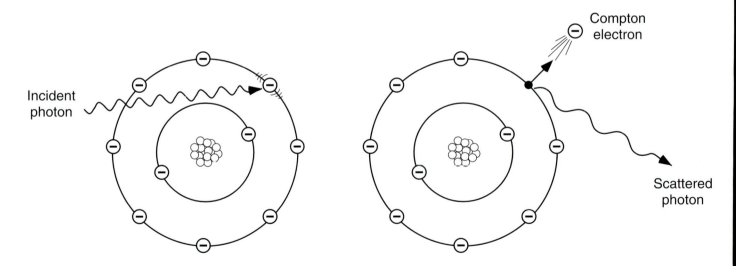

Incident photon

Compton electron

Scattered photon

Compton Scattering

Figure 2.13. Compton Scattering. Compton scattering results in ionization of the atom and change in direction and reduction in energy of the incident x-ray photon.

angle of deflection off the Compton electron. At narrow angles of deflection, scattered photons retain almost all their original energy. This creates a serious problem in diagnostic radiology, because photons that are scattered at narrow angles have an excellent chance of reaching an x-ray film and producing fog. These scattered photons are difficult to remove from the beam by filters because they are so energetic. Because we cannot remove these photons from the beam, they will also cause film fog. At the higher diagnostic energies (60 to 100 keV), Compton scattering is the most common interaction between x-rays and body tissues and is responsible for almost all the scatter radiation. In dental radiology, approximately 62% of the x-ray photons undergo Compton scattering. This can be minimized by using rectangular collimation and shorter exposure times afforded by higher mAs, higher kVps, and faster film speed.

X-RAY BEAM ABSORPTION

X-rays are absorbed in materials and tissues by **photoelectric absorption**. This occurs when an incident x-ray photon, with a little more energy than the binding energy of a K-shell electron of the material or tissue, encounters the electron and ejects it from the orbit. The x-ray photon disappears completely, giving up all its energy to the electron. The ejected electron, called the photoelectron, flies into space and is absorbed by another atom (Fig. 2.14).

The extent that x-rays are absorbed by photoelectron absorption depends on four factors:

1. The wavelength or photon energy of the x-rays (kVp).
2. Thickness of the material.
3. Density (mass/unit volume) of the material.
4. Atomic number of the material.

The wavelength or photon x-ray energy of the x-radiation is indirectly determined by the kilovoltage applied to the x-ray tube. The higher kilovoltages produce more shorter-wavelength x-rays and they penetrate material more readily. The relation of x-ray absorption to thickness is simple, because obviously a thicker piece of any material absorbs more x-radiation than a thinner piece of the same material. Density (wt/vol) of a material can be defined as the compactness of a material and is numerically equal to its specific gravity. The effect is similar to that seen for thickness. For instance, an inch of water (H_2O) will absorb more x-rays than an inch of ice (H_2O). The atomic number (number of protons in nucleus) of an object usually has far more effect on x-ray absorption than thickness or density. The higher the atomic number of the material, the greater the absorption factor of the material. For example, a sheet of aluminum (Z = 13), being of lower atomic number than copper (Z = 29) or lead (Z = 82),

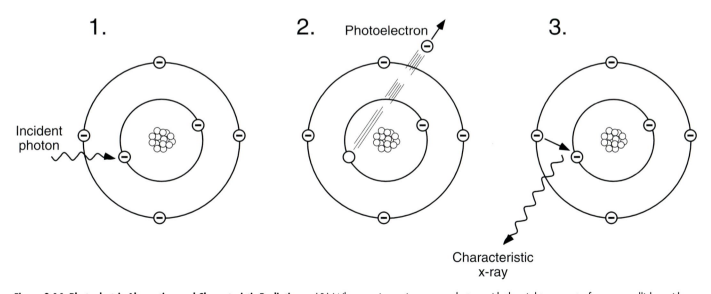

Figure 2.14. Photoelectric Absorption and Characteristic Radiation. (**A**) When an incoming x-ray photon with the right amount of energy collides with an inner K-shell electron of an atom of tissue (for instance, a calcium atom in bone), the K-shell electron is ejected from its orbit. (2) The incoming x-ray photon disappears completely, giving up all its energy to the ejected electron, called a photoelectron. The photoelectron flies into space and is absorbed by another calcium atom. The process of absorbing x-ray photons by matter is called photoelectric absorption. The original calcium atom now is an excited state. (3) An electron from the outer L-shell jumps into the K-shell vacancy, giving off K-characteristic radiation of calcium. (The atom of calcium is now a positive ion because it lacks an electron and will become stable again when it attracts another electron).

absorbs a lesser amount of x-rays than does a sheet of copper or lead of the same area and weight.

X-RAYS PASSING THROUGH A TISSUE WITHOUT INTERACTING WITH TISSUE ATOMS

In dental bitewing x-ray examination, approximately 9% of the primary photons will pass through the tissues of the jaw without interacting with tissue atoms. The remnant radiation collected on the film emulsion from these photons will produce radiolucent, or darker density areas, on radiographs after the films have been chemically processed.

ATTENUATION OF X-RAY BEAM IN DENTISTRY

Attenuation is the reduction in the intensity of an x-ray beam as it transverses dental tissues by either the absorption (photoelectric) or deflection (Compton scattering) of the photons from the x-ray beam. To further simplify our discussion, we can disregard the attenuation of scatter radiation resulting from Compton interactions. Once a photon is deflected from its original course, it will be considered completely attenuated or absorbed; that is, completely removed from the beam, because these scatter reactions add nothing to the diagnostic information of the radiographic image. X-rays that undergo photoelectric absorption produce diagnostic information in a negative sense. Because these x-rays do not reach the film, they represent structures that have high absorption characteristics and result in clear, white areas on the film. These white or bright areas—which usually represent cortical

bone, enamel, or metallic restorations—are called **radiopaque** structures or materials. There are other x-rays that penetrate the jaws and are transmitted with no interaction whatsoever. They result in dark areas on the radiograph. These areas are called **radiolucent** because structures such as soft tissue, pulp, and periodontal ligament are easily penetrated by the x-radiation.

Differential Absorption of the X-Ray Beam in Dentistry

In considering the use of x-rays in dentistry, one must understand that the human jaws are complex structures made up of tissues, not only differing in thicknesses and density, but of tissues and materials with different atomic numbers. These structures absorb x-rays to different degrees (differential absorption). Metallic restorations, such as silver alloy (amalgam) and gold, absorb more x-rays than enamel; enamel absorbs more than dentin; dentin more than cementum; cementum more than cortical bone; cortical bone more than cancellous bone; and cancellous bone more than soft tissue, such as the periodontal ligament, the pulp, gingiva, and oral soft tissues. Teeth and bone contain large amounts of *calcium* and *phosphorus*, with atomic numbers of 20 and 15, respectively; the atomic number of muscle is approximately 7.4. Diseased structures often absorb x-rays differently from normal structures. Even the age of the patient may have a bearing on absorption. For example, in the elderly, the bones of the jaws in most instances have *less calcium* content and hence there is less x-ray absorption.

In review, the variations in absorption (differential absorption) of the jaws depend for the most part on the

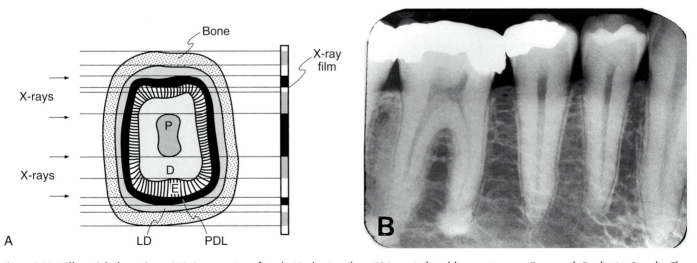

Figure 2.15. Differential Absorption. (**A**) Cross-section of tooth: LD, lamina dura; PDL, periodontal ligament space; E, enamel; D, dentin; P, pulp. The enamel and lamina dura completely absorb radiation, and dentin partially absorbs radiation. Pulp and periodontal ligament transmit most of the radiation because those tissues absorb very little radiation. (**B**) Radiograph of mandibular premolar region. Pulp and periodontal ligament spaces are black (radiolucent); lamina dura and enamel are white (radiopaque). Dentin is gray.

thickness, atomic number, and densities of the tissues of the jaws and, of course, the quality (kVp) of the x-ray beam used (Fig. 2.15).

RECORDING THE LATENT IMAGE AND MAKING IT VISIBLE

After interaction of the x-ray beam with the anatomic structures of the patient, the exit beam or beam of **remnant x-rays** consists of attenuated x-ray photons corresponding to the pattern of thicknesses, atomic numbers, and densities of the tissues and materials through which the beam has passed. We cannot make direct use of this information (an aerial image) unless we transfer it to a recording medium suitable to viewing by the eye. The most important method used to decode this information carried by the attenuated beam is by means of photographic film that can be exposed in one of two ways: First, the film may be exposed by the direct action of the remnant x-rays, as is done in intraoral radiography. Second, the energy of the x-ray beam may be converted into light by intensifying screens, and this light in turn is used to expose the film. This latter method is used in extraoral radiography (panoramic and cephalometric films). The image formed by the exit or remnant radiation exposing the film by either method is called the *latent image*. Chemically processing the exposed film makes the latent image *visible* and permanent.

X-RAY FILM

Radiographic film is composed of a radiation sensitive or photographically active emulsion, usually coated on both sides of a transparent sheet of plastic called the base. The layers of the emulsion are attached to the base by a thin layer of adhesive. The delicate emulsions are covered by a supercoating of gelatin, which protects the emulsion from rough handling before exposure, scratching, pressure, and contamination during processing. The emulsion is applied to both sides of the base (called double-emulsion films) to provide increased speed to the film (Fig. 2.16). This increased speed also means less radiation for the patient because of the shorter exposure times (less radiation) and fewer retakes due to movement during the exposure.

Base

The base is composed of a thin clear plastic, usually either of triacetate or polyester. A blue tint is added, providing a film that is easier to view and that prevents eyestrain. Polyester is more resistant to warping with age and stronger than triacetate. Therefore, polyester bases can be made thinner than triacetate bases but are just as strong.

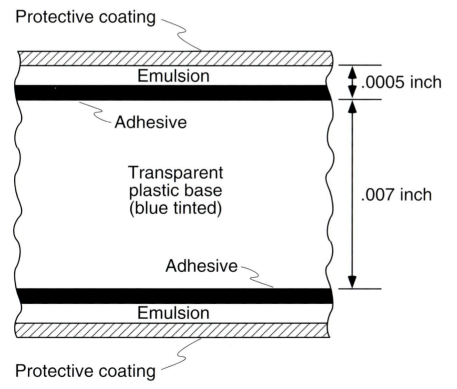

Figure 2.16. Radiographic Film. Cross-section of x-ray film showing its components.

Polyester is the current film base of choice used by almost all manufacturers of radiographic film.

Emulsion

The emulsion consists of a homogeneous mixture of gelatin and silver halide crystals. The gelatin is similar to that used in food preparation but is of much higher quality. It is made from cattle bone. The gelatin is clear, so that it will transmit light, and is sufficiently porous to allow the processing chemicals (developer and fixer) to penetrate it and gain access to the silver halide crystals rapidly without destroying its strength or performance.

Silver Halide

The active ingredient of the radiographic emulsion is the silver halide or silver iodo-bromide crystal. In the typical emulsion, 90 to 99% of the silver halide is silver bromide (AgBr) and approximately 1 to 10% is silver iodide (AgI). The presence of AgI gives the emulsion a higher sensitivity than a pure AgBr emulsion. These atoms have relatively high atomic numbers (I = 53, Br = 35, Ag = 47) compared with the gelatin emulsion and polyester base, both of which are about 7. The interaction of the x-ray photons or light photons with these atoms results in the formation of a latent image that cannot be detected by the naked eye. The astute student will note that x-ray film can be exposed by both x-rays and light. When the exposed film is processed in a solution called the developer, a chemical reaction takes place whereby the exposed silver iodo-bromide crystals are reduced to tiny masses of black metallic silver, leaving the unexposed crystals essentially unaffected. The metallic silver, suspended in the gelatin, produces the visible image on the radiograph.

FORMATION OF THE LATENT IMAGE

The latent image is defined as the invisible image that is produced in the film emulsion by light or x-rays and is converted into a visible image on development (processing). The silver iodo-bromide grain or crystal is flat and triangular, and the arrangement of the atoms in the crystal is cubical. The network or lattice of an individual silver iodo-bromide crystal contains silver, bromine, and iodine ions held together by electrovalence forces (Fig. 2.17). When an x-ray photon interacts with the Ag, Br, and I atoms of the silver iodo-bromide crystal of the emulsion, free photoelectrons are released. These free photoelectrons, while traversing the crystal, will have sufficient energy to dislodge additional electrons from other atoms of the crystal lattice. Therefore, as a result of one x-ray photon interaction, a great number of electrons are released and drift about inside the crystal.

SENSITIVITY SPECK OR TRAP

Eventually, these released electrons are caught by a "sensitivity speck or trap" in the crystal. Such traps can be

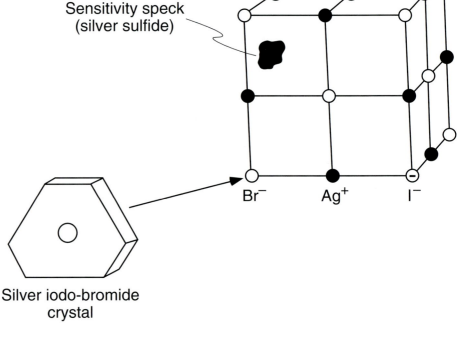

Sensitivity speck (silver sulfide)

Br⁻ Ag⁺ I⁻

Silver iodo-bromide crystal

Figure 2.17. Silver Iodo-Bromide (AgIBr) Crystal (Grain) and Lattice (Network). The AgIBr crystal is triangular, but lattice arrangement of atoms in the crystal is cubical. Lattice diagram of AgIBr crystal is shown on the right. The straight lines joining the circles represent the electrovalence forces holding the ions together in the crystal. Sensitivity Speck (Silver Sulfide) or Trap: The sensitivity speck (silver sulfide) is an imperfection that is usually a result of a sulfur-containing compound (allylthiourea) added to the emulsion by the manufacturer. This makes the crystal very sensitive to x-ray and light photons.

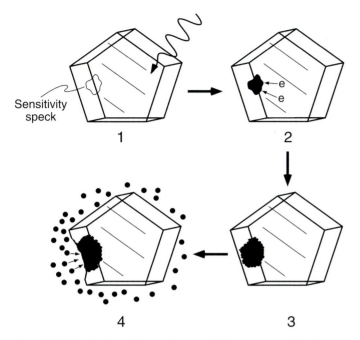

Figure 2.18. Production of Latent Image. (1) An x-ray or light photon interacts with a silver iodo-bromide (AgIBr) crystal to allow an electron to escape from a Br^- or I^- ion. The Br^- or I^- ion, which becomes neutral by loss of an electron, migrates from the crystal and is taken up by the gelatin of the emulsion. (This leaves a remaining Ag^+ ion.) (2) The free electron is captured and temporarily held at the sensitivity speck in the crystal. (3) The trapped electron attracts the remaining Ag^+ ion to the sensitivity speck, forming a neutral Ag atom. (4) The first Ag atom acts as an electron trap for a second Ag^+ ion. The repeated attraction and the neutralizing of silver ions builds up a clump of silver atoms, called the latent image center in the crystal, which must be present before the developing process can cause visual amounts of metallic Ag to be deposited.

imperfections in the crystal structure or chemicals (silver sulfide) in or on the grain (crystal) that may have been introduced during the emulsion-making process by the manufacturer (Fig. 2.17). In any case, the effect (sensitivity trap) is to hold the negatively charged electron at least temporarily in one place. Silver ions (Ag^+), which exist naturally in the crystals, can be thought of as positive ions because they are missing an electron. Positively charged silver ions tend to migrate toward the negatively charged trapped photoelectron at the sensitivity speck, and the positively charged silver ion in turn attracts another negatively charged photoelectron. This process results in the formation of an atom of metallic silver at the trap sight. Because of its effect on the crystal structure, this new silver atom makes the trap still more effective in trapping additional photoelectrons. In turn, these additional electrons attract more ions, forming more silver atoms. When this cluster becomes sufficiently large, it becomes a "development center" on the crystal that is not observable, even microscopically. This unobservable image on the exposed film composed of radiation- or light-activated silver halide crystals and nonactivated silver halide crystals is called the latent image. The development of the exposed film by the developer solution starts at the development center (sensitivity speck) of the radiation or light-activated silver halide crystal. The silver there acts as a catalyst, spreading out from it until the whole grain becomes an irregular mass of black silver producing gray to black areas on the film. Under normal development, the grains that have not absorbed sufficient light or x-ray photons to form development centers will develop into clear, transparent areas on the film (Fig. 2.18).

TYPES OF X-RAY FILM

X-ray films used in dentistry can be of the direct exposure or the indirect exposure type of film. Extraoral film is of the **screen or indirect exposure type film**. Dental x-ray film (intraoral type) is a **direct exposure film** because the film is more sensitive to exposure by x-ray photons than by light photons. The only current use of direct exposure film is for intraoral use where only small areas are exposed and a high definition of the x-ray image is desired.

EXTRAORAL FILM

In the indirect exposure type film (screen film), the energy of the x-ray beam is converted into light by intensifying screens (the film is sandwiched between two screens), and this light is used to expose photographic type film. Extraoral (screen) indirect exposure film is used in dentistry for panoramic, cephalometric, skull, and tomographic x-ray techniques. Extraoral or screen films (indirect exposure) are used with intensifying screens because they decrease the x-ray dose to the patient and still result in a properly exposed x-ray film. Screen-film combinations are discussed in Chapter 11.

DENTAL INTRAORAL X-RAY FILM (DIRECT EXPOSURE FILM)

Dental x-ray film is individually wrapped in packets of white, pebbled, moisture-resistant paper or polyvinyl wrap. Within it, the film is further protected by being wrapped in thin black paper and backed by a thin sheet of lead foil. The lead foil placed in back of the film firstly protects it from radiation that may be back-scattered by the tissues of the oral cavity during exposure. Secondly, it absorbs some of the radiation remaining after the x-ray beam exposes and passes through the film. Thirdly, the lead foil contributes to the rigidity of the packet. The film

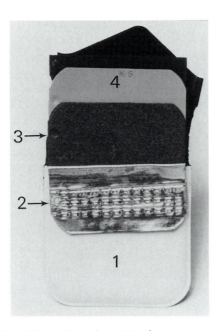

Figure 2.19. Dental X-Ray Film Packet. (1) White, moisture-resistant outer covering, (2) sheet of lead foil to protect the film from radiation backscatter, (3) black interleaving paper, and (4) double-emulsion film.

manufacturer places various geometric patterns in the lead foil backing that will appear in the radiographic image if the back of the film packet is mistakenly placed toward the x-ray tube during exposure (Fig. 2.19). All dental films currently manufactured are double-emulsion coated films. The emulsion is coated on both sides of the base (called double-emulsion films) to provide increased speed to the film. This increased speed means less radiation for both the patient and the operator, because less radiation is required to produce an image. To identify the "tube side" of the film, a raised dot is placed in the corner of the film. The raised portion of the dot is always toward the x-ray tube, and the depressed side of the dot is toward the tongue. An embossed circle on the printed label of the film packet locates the position of the raised dot on the x-ray film. This raised dot is necessary to distinguish films taken on the right and left sides of the patient.

Types of Intraoral Film (Fig. 2.20)

There are three types of intraoral film: periapical film, bitewing film, and occlusal film.

Periapical Film As the name suggests, the objective of using periapical film is to show the apex of the tooth and surrounding bone, but it should also show the entire crown. There are three sizes of periapical film: the no. 0 child film, the no. 1 (narrow) adult anterior film, and the no. 2 (standard) adult film for posterior periapicals and bitewings.

Bitewing Film The bitewing film shows the crowns of teeth of both arches and their interproximal alveolar bone crests on one film. The bitewing packet has a wing, or tab, attached or placed on the side that on which the patient bites. A bite-tab attached to the no. 2 periapical film converts it to a bitewing film. Alternately, an instrument such as the XCP bitewing film-holder can be used. In 9- to 12-year-old children, one no. 2 standard film on each side of the arch is sufficient; in adolescents and adults, two no. 2 periapical films on each side of the arch are usually necessary. A bitewing film can be made for 5- to 9-year-old children by placing a tab on a no. 1 narrow film; one for children younger than 5 years of age can be made by placing a tab on a no. 0 periapical film packet.

Occlusal Film The occlusal film is considerably larger than the periapical film and is so named because the patient bites on the entire film between the occlusal surfaces of the upper and lower teeth. The objective of the occlusal film is to show large segments of the maxillary and mandibular arches, parts of the maxilla, and the floor of the mouth.

Size and Speed of Intraoral Film

Size of Film Dental intraoral film sizes and speed have been standardized by the American Dental Associ-

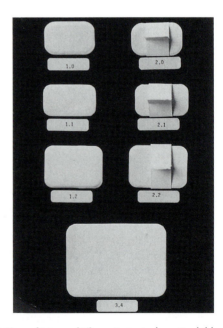

Figure 2.20. Sizes of Intraoral Film. Periapical no. 0, children's film size, 1.0: periapical no. 1, narrow anterior film size, 1.1: periapical no. 2, adult regular film size, 1.2: bitewing no. 0, children's (younger than 5 years of age) film size, 2.0: bitewing no. 1, children's (6 to 9 years) film size, 2.1: bitewing no. 2, adult regular film size, 2.2: occlusal, no. 4, occlusal film size 3.4.

ation. The standard sizes of intraoral film are shown below.

Sizes of Intraoral Film

| Type-Size Number[a] | Dimensions | |
	mm	in
Periapical		
1.00	21 × 32	4/5 × 1¼
1.0	22 × 35	7/8 × 1⅜
1.1	24 × 40	15/16 × 1 9/16
1.2	31 × 41	1¼ × 1⅝
Bitewing (interproximal)		
2.00	21 × 32	4/5 × 1¼
2.0	22 × 35	7/8 × 1⅜
2.1	24 × 40	15/16 × 1 9/16
2.2	31 × 41	1¼ × 1⅝
2.3	27 × 54	1 1/16 × 2
Occlusal		
3.4	57 × 76	2¼ × 3

[a]The digit at the left of the decimal point represents the use of the film (periapical, bitewing, or occlusal). The digits on the right indicate the size of the film (00, 0, 1, 2, 3, or 4).

The comparative sizes of the intraoral films used in dentistry are shown in Figure 2.20.

Speed of Film The efficiency with which a film responds to x-ray exposure is known as *film sensitivity* or, more commonly, "speed." X-ray films that require very little exposure to x-radiation to produce a radiograph are said to be very sensitive, to be very fast, or to possess high speed. Thus, exposure time and film speed vary inversely. In other words, the faster the film, the less radiation exposure needed. Intraoral film speeds have been standardized on an alphabetical basis according to a speed range recorded in "reciprocal roentgens" and is shown below.

Currently, manufacturers of dental film indicate the film speed on the outside of the film box in an alphabetical classification with the expiration date (Fig. 2.21). Also, the back side of the film packet is color coded to indicate film speed. The two speeds currently available are D speed

Speed Classification of Intraoral Film

Speed Group[a]		Speed Range In Reciprocal Roentgens[b]
A	Slowest	1.5–3.0
B		3.0–6.0
C		6.0–12.0
D		12.0–24.0
E		24.0–48.0
F	Fastest	48.0–96.0

[a]No films are sold in speed groups A, B, C, and F. Examples of films sold in groups D and E are Kodak Ultra-Speed in Group D and Kodak Ekta-speed in Group E.
[b]A roentgen is a measure of radiation exposure or quantity. A reciprocal roentgen is 1/R or 1 over the amount of exposure in roentgens to achieve a certain density (blackness) on a film.

and E+ speed. X-ray films are compared by determining their relative sensitivity. This is actually measured by determining the amount of x-radiation necessary to produce a certain density (or "blackness") in the emulsion that has been processed in a rigidly controlled manner. For example, if film E+ requires approximately half as much x-radiation as film D to produce the same blackness in the emulsion, film E is said to be twice as fast as film D.

T-Grain Film

In 1994, Eastman Kodak (Rochester, NY) introduced the newest E speed intraoral film called Ekta Speed Plus (E+) dental x-ray film. The new E+ speed intraoral film uses a flat or tabular grain or T-grain in the emulsion. This gives a greater surface area due to the tabular shape compared with the earlier rounded emulsion grains. These new grains (crystals) effectively eliminate the trade-off between image quality and radiation reduction in selecting intraoral film. E+ film is said to deliver comparable image quality at reduced exposures compared with slower D speed film.

Film Emulsion Sensitivity

The film emulsion is sensitive to a number of conditions. Some of these conditions are heat, light, x-rays, fumes, bending, and pressure. The high-speed emulsions are even more sensitive to these conditions. This means

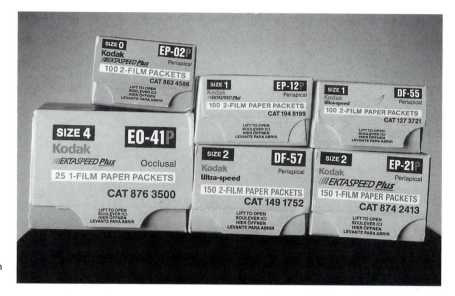

Figure 2.21. Film Box Labels. Speed and size of film are located on film box.

that more care and exactitude are needed when handling, exposing, unwrapping, and processing these films.

Film Storage

All unopened film should be stored in a cool place, such as a refrigerator. It should not be stored beyond the expiration date; thus ordering should be based on use. Open intraoral film should be stored outside of the x-ray room away from any radiation or in the x-ray room in special lead-lined containers that protect the film. Opened boxes of screen film should be stored in a light-tight area in the vicinity of where cassettes are loaded and unloaded.

WORKSHOP/LABORATORY EXERCISES

EXERCISE 2.1. DIFFERENTIAL ABSORPTION AND RECORDING OF IMAGES

Materials and Equipment Needed

1. Wood pencil with attached eraser.
2. Five no. 2 intraoral films.
3. X-ray machine(s).
4. X-ray processing facility.
5. Ball-point pen.
6. X-ray mount and special pencil.

Instructions

Step 1: Turn on the x-ray machine.

Step 2: Set the exposure time at about ¼ second (15 impulses) if you have a short (8-inch) BID or about 1 second (60 impulses) if you have a long BID.

Determine BID length by measuring from the focal spot mark (dot or symbol) on the tubehead to the tip of the BID. Do **not** just measure the length at the BID itself.

Step 3: If the machine has an mA setting, set this at about 7 or 10. If the machine has a kVp setting, set this at about 65 or 70.

Step 4: (Note: Exposure times, mA, and kVp settings may require some further adjustment. Check with the instructor.) Obtain the no. 2 intraoral films and a wooden pencil with a fixed eraser on one end.

Step 5: With a ball-point pen, label the front of one film as no. 1 and write your first name on it. Place this film front side up on the counter top and position the BID tip directly over the film so that the BID tip touches the counter top as it covers the film.

Expose this film and put it in your pocket.

Step 6: Place a second film front side up on the counter top. Place the eraser end of the pencil on top of the film.

Expose this film and put it in your pocket.

Step 7: Place a third film back or tab side up on the counter top. Place the eraser end of the pencil on top of the film.

Expose this film and put it in your pocket.

Step 8: Take a fourth film and unwrap and remove the film; hold the film between your fingers for a few seconds and place this in your pocket. While unwrapping, observe and identify the different parts of the film packet including the outer plastic wrapping, the inner paper wrap, the film itself, and the lead foil.

Place the fifth film, which has had nothing done to it, in your pocket.

Step 9: Now enter the darkroom and place the unwrapped film in the processor. Unwrap and process the other four films. If manual processing only is available, the instructor will demonstrate this.

Step 10: Obtain an x-ray mount with at least five no. 2 film slots or a single sheet of clear acetate or plastic.

Label five areas as follows:

a. Exposed to x-rays and name.
b. Pencil tip image front side up.
c. Pencil tip image back side up.
d. Exposed to light.
e. Unexposed.

Step 11: After the films are processed properly, match the five films with their correct spot on the mount.

CASE-BASED QUESTIONS FOR LABORATORY EXERCISE

Answer the following questions by inserting the correct letter choice(s) (a, b, c, d, or e from Step 10). Each letter may be used more than once and there may be more than one correct answer.

1. Which film(s) demonstrate(s) the differential absorption of x-rays by matter?
2. Which film(s) demonstrate(s) imaging of radiolucent material(s)?
3. Which film(s) demonstrate(s) imaging of radiopaque material(s)?
4. Which film(s) demonstrate(s) exposure of **all** the silver halide crystals?
5. Which film demonstrates exposure of **no** silver halide crystals?

CASE-BASED PROBLEM-SOLVING

You have just taken a set of four bitewing films. Only one image (A) turns out perfect. The others appeared as follows: no image, film looks like a clear piece of plastic (image B); an image **darker** than A with an apparent extra set of teeth (image C); and an image **lighter** than A with the teeth partially obscured by a visible geometric pattern. What went wrong in the taking of images B, C, and D?

REVIEW QUESTIONS

1. The film layer that contains the silver halide crystals is known as the:

   A. Base.
   B. Protective layer.
   C. Top coat.
   D. Emulsion.

2. Films that are all black and white with very few grays are said to be:

   A. Very dense.
   B. High contrast.
   C. Fogged.
   D. Low contrast.

3. A latent image is:

   A. An image that is very late in its formation.
   B. A very light radiographic image.
   C. Produced after exposure but before developing.
   D. A very dark radiographic image.

4. A piece of lead foil is placed in intraoral film packets. Which of the following is true concerning the lead foil?

   A. It filters out back-scattered radiation, as it is in front of the film.
   B. It contributes to the rigidity of the packet.
   C. It may produce a pattern on properly exposed and properly processed film.

D. It is contained in all sizes of intraoral film packets with the exception of occlusal film.

5. The film used with intensifying screens is said to be:

A. More sensitive to radiation.
B. Better when not sandwiched between two intensifying screens.
C. More sensitive to light.
D. Faster because it uses only single emulsions with two screens.

6. The transformer used to heat the filament of the x-ray tube is:

A. The autotransformer.
B. The step-up transformer.
C. The step-down transformer.
D. The high-tension transformer.

7. The step-up transformer is used to:

A. Step up the current to heat the filament.
B. Allow the operator to vary the kVp.
C. Change low-input voltage to high-output voltage with low milliamperage.
D. None of the above.

8. The substance that is the most radiopaque is:

A. Leaded glass.
B. Plastic.
C. Wood.
D. Rubber.

9. A dentist decides to change his or her intraoral exposure technique from 10 mA and 1.5-second exposure to 15 mA; the new exposure time is _____ second(s).

A. 0.35.
B. 1.
C. 2.
D. 6.

10. A 0.5-second exposure would produce how many impulses of x-radiation?

A. 5.
B. 15.
C. 30.
D. 60.

11. Some components of the x-ray tube include:

A. An anode.
B. An aluminum filament.
C. Helium.
D. Cooling oil.
E. A lead collimator.

12. The kilovoltage in an x-ray generating system regulates:

A. The number of electrons produced.
B. Thermionic emission.
C. The velocity of electrons traveling from the filament to the target.
D. The velocity of x-ray photons produced.

13. The interaction in which the entire photon of x-radiation is removed from the beam by atomic interaction is called:

A. The Thomson effect.
B. The photoelectric effect.
C. The Compton effect.
D. Excitation.

14. Which of the following are characteristics of photoelectric absorption?

A. It depends on atomic number.
B. It differentiates between hard and soft tissues.
C. It is more likely to occur in inner orbits.
D. It occurs in dental radiography.
E. All of the above.

15. Sensitization specks:

A. Are defects in calcium tungstate crystals.
B. Are defects in silver bromide crystals.
C. Act as electron traps.
D. A and C.
E. B and C

BIBLIOGRAPHY

Bushong SC. Radiologic science for technologists, physics, biology, and protection. 5th ed. St. Louis: Mosby-Year Book, 1993.

Code of Federal Regulations 21, Subchapter J, Radiological Health, part 1000, Washington DC, 1984. Office of the Federal Register, General Services Administration.

Curry TS III, Dowdey JE, Murry RG Jr. Christensen's physics of diagnostic radiology. 4th ed. Philadelphia: Lea & Febiger, 1990.

Fuchs AW. Principles of radiographic exposure and processing. 2nd ed. Springfield: Charles C. Thomas, 1969.

Goodwin PN, Quimby EH, Morgan R. Physical foundations of radiology. 4th ed. New York: Harper & Row, 1970.

Hendee W, Ritenour RE. Medical imaging physics. 3rd ed. St. Louis: Mosby-Year Book, 1992.

Herz RH. The photographic action of ionizing radiation. New York: Wiley, 1969.

James TH, ed. The theory of the photographic process. New York: Macmillan, 1977.

Jaundrell-Thompson F, Ashworth WJ. X-Ray physics and equipment. 2nd ed. Springfield: Charles C. Thomas, 1970.

Johns HE, Cunningham JR. The physics of radiology. 3rd ed. Springfield: Charles C. Thomas, 1969.

Langlais RP, Kasle MJ. Basic principles of oral radiography. Philadelphia: WB Saunders, 1981.

Langland OE, Sippy FH, Langlais RP. Textbook of dental radiology. 2nd ed. Springfield: Charles C. Thomas, 1984.

Manson-Hing LR. Fundamentals of dental radiography. Philadelphia: Lea & Febiger, 1979.

Meredith WJ, Massey JB. Fundamental physics of radiology. Baltimore: Williams & Wilkins, 1968.

Neblette CB. Photograph, its material and processes: Gurney-Mott hypothesis of latent image formation. 6th ed. New York: Van Nostrand, 1962.

Seeman HE. Physical and photographic principles of medical radiography. New York: Wiley, 1968.

Selman J. The fundamentals of X-ray and radium physics. 6th ed. Springfield: Charles C. Thomas, 1977.

Sensitometric properties of X-ray films. Rochester, NY: Radiography Markets Division, Eastman Kodak.

Sprawls P. The physical principles of diagnostic radiology. Baltimore: The University Park Press, 1977.

The fundamentals of radiography. 12th ed. Rochester, NY: Eastman Kodak, 1980.

Ter-Pogossian MM. The physical aspects of diagnostic radiology. New York: Harper & Row, Hoeber Medical Division, 1967.

X-Rays in dentistry. Rochester, NY: Eastman Kodak, 1985.

Diagnostic Quality of Dental Radiographs

3

OBJECTIVES

Upon successful completion of this unit, the student will be able to:

1.   *Define umbra and penumbra.*

2.   *Define radiopaque and radiolucent.*

3.   *Discuss geometric factors that can be controlled to reduce the amount of magnification and distortion of a radiographic image.*

4.   *Define density and contrast.*

5.   *Discuss the factors that primarily control density.*

6.   *Discuss the factors that primarily control contrast.*

7.   *List the four conditions dependent on a diagnostic quality dental radiograph.*

8.   *Discuss the characteristic curve.*

9.   *Discuss the five rules for accurate image formation.*

10.   *Understand the concept of coverage.*

11.   *Observe accurate image projection through the Workshop/Laboratory Exercises.*

12.   *Observe penumbra, magnification, and distortion through the Workshop/Laboratory Exercises.*

13.   *Explain accurate image projection by shadow casting using the Case-Based Problem-Solving format.*

14.   *Test his or her knowledge by answering the Review Questions.*

KEY WORDS/PHRASES

anatomical accuracy

characteristic curve

contrast

coverage

definition

densitometer

density

distortion

exposure

fog

film contrast

film latitude

film speed

long-scale contrast

magnification

penumbra

scatter radiation

short-scale contrast

unsharpness

INTRODUCTION

Diagnosis is the art of distinguishing one disease from another. The professional education and training of the dentist affords him or her the responsibility of diagnosis and prescription of treatment. To make the most use of the dental radiograph as an aid in the diagnosis of dental disease, it is important that the dentist have a radiograph that provides the maximum possible information concerning a particular anatomical region. In other words, the dentist must have a radiograph that has the highest possible quality. Radiographic quality refers to the fidelity (exactness in detail) with which an anatomical structure is represented on the radiograph and denotes the visibility and definition of the images of structural details. Definition (sharpness) refers to the distinctness and sharp demarcation of all elements in the dental film. Detail is the point-by-point delineation of the minute structural elements of the object in the images formed on the dental film.

The diagnostic quality of a dental radiograph is dependent on four conditions:

1. **Proper Visual Characteristics**
   a. Density.
   b. Contrast.
2. **Minimal Geometric Characteristics**
   a. Radiographic image unsharpness.
      (1) Geometric unsharpness.
      (2) Motion unsharpness.
      (3) Screen unsharpness.
   b. Magnification.
   c. Distortion.
3. **Anatomical Accuracy**
4. **Adequate Coverage of Anatomical Region of Interest**

A clear understanding of the effects and significance of each factor will aid the operator in the routine production of diagnostic quality radiographs.

VISUAL CHARACTERISTICS

The diagnostic quality of the radiograph is directly influenced by two visual characteristics of the radiographic image called **density** and **contrast**.

RADIOGRAPHIC DENSITY

Radiographic density refers to the degree or gradation of "blackness" on a radiographic film. It depends on the amount of radiation reaching a particular area on the film and the resulting mass of metallic silver per unit area. As the reader will recall, the silver halides of the emulsion that have been sensitized by radiation are changed by the developing agents into particles of metallic silver, which appear black because of their finely divided state. The greater the amount of x-ray energy that reaches the film, the greater the degree of blackening on that area of the film. Areas where relatively few or no x-ray photons reach the film will appear gray or translucent on the processed radiograph. After the exposed film is processed, the film is viewed by placing it in front of an illuminator or viewbox. It is the variation in the amount of light passing through the film that identifies the image seen. The heavier the deposit of black silver masses, the greater the quantity of light absorbed (and not transmitted) through the emulsion, and the darker the area appears. The darker areas on the film are regions of the anatomical part of the body that freely let the x-rays pass through to expose the film and are called *radiolucencies*. A high degree of radiographic density produces a **dark film**; a **light film** has a thin or low degree of radiographic density.

Measuring Density

Radiographic density is measured by an instrument called a **densitometer**. This instrument indicates the relationship between the intensity of the light beam of an illuminator as it strikes one side of a given area of a radiograph (called incident light intensity) compared with the light transmitted through the radiograph (transmitted light intensity) (Fig. 3.1).

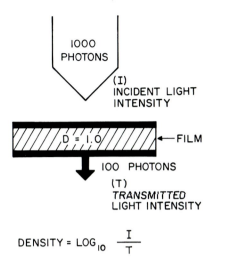

$$\text{DENSITY} = \text{LOG}_{10}\ \frac{I}{T}$$

Figure 3.1. Radiographic Density. The reduction in intensity or the ability of the film to stop light, in this instance, is 1000/100 or 10, or one tenth of the light is transmitted through the film. The log of 10 is 1. Thus, the density of this radiograph is 1.0.

Density is expressed mathematically as a logarithm using the common base 10. It is defined by the following equation:

$$\text{density} = \log(10)\ \frac{\text{incident light intensity (I)}}{\text{transmitted light intensity (T)}}$$

Example: When the silver allows 1/10 of the illuminator or incident light through the radiograph, the ratio is 10:1, which is equal to 10. The common logarithm of 10 is 1; therefore, the density of the film is equal to 1. Again, if the silver allows only 1/100 of the light to pass through the radiograph, the ratio is equal to 100:1 or 100. The common logarithm of 100 is 2, and the density of the film is equal to 2. Actually, one does not have to know logarithms to use a densitometer because it is calibrated to directly read density. In routine radiography, the useful range of film densities is approximately 0.3 (very light) to 2 (very dark). Beyond these extremes, the image is usually too light or too dark to be diagnostically useful.

Importance of Density

Density is extremely important in the diagnostic quality of a radiograph because it carries *information*. Visible detail of the radiographic image is not possible without *density*. However, there must be a correct amount of density to a radiograph because too much density (dark) will conceal information, and not enough density (light) will destroy detail in the lighter areas.

The desirable degree of radiographic density cannot be fixed as permanent, because one dentist may prefer a certain degree of density while another may prefer a greater or lesser density for the same region. The degree of radiographic density may be considered to be largely a matter of individual preference. Of course, one does not want a film that is too dark or too light—the right amount of density is needed to visualize the anatomical structures accurately. In dental radiographs of correct density, the dentist should be able to see a faint outline of the soft tissues in edentulous spaces or distal to the molar teeth when the radiographs are examined in the manner habitually used (Fig. 3.2).

Primary Factors Controlling Density

Listed below are the three important exposure factors that control density of a radiograph. In dental radiography, the first factor mentioned (mAs) is generally the factor of choice.

Milliampere Seconds The density or blackness of the radiograph varies directly and proportionately to the milliamperage (tube current) and the exposure time. Therefore, exposure time and milliamperage are interchangeable and considered as a *single factor* (mAs). For instance, the density of a radiographic image produced by a direct exposure of 1.5 seconds at 10 mA is identical to the density of the image produced by an exposure time of 1 second at 15 mA. The product of mA and exposure time is equal to 15 mAs in each instance. The higher the mAs, the more x-rays that will strike the film and the greater the quantity of metallic silver deposited in the film emulsion. The quantity (or mAs) of the x-ray beam is usually measured by the use of an ionization chamber or **ionization roentgen meter**.

Kilovoltage Kilovoltage is referred to as the "penetrating power" of the x-ray beam and influences density. As the kilovoltage becomes greater and the effective wavelengths of the x-ray beam become shorter, the penetration of the x-ray beam becomes greater. Therefore, a greater amount of x-radiation will strike the film emulsion, which in turn will cause more metallic silver to be deposited in the emulsion. This will result in a higher radiographic density if all other factors remain constant.

Source-Film Distance Because the intensity of an x-ray beam varies *inversely* to the square of the source-film distance (inverse square law), the time of exposure necessary to maintain a constant density in a radiograph varies *directly* to the square of the focal-film distance. The shorter the distance between the focal spot and the film, the more x-rays that strike the film, and therefore the *higher* the density.

Example: Doubling the distance gives one fourth the density; halving the distance gives four times the density.

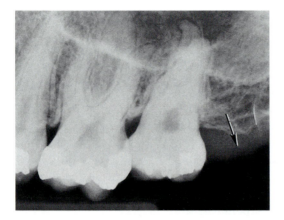

Figure 3.2. The Most Desirable Radiographic Density. Radiograph of maxillary molar region. Note the thin shadow of soft tissue over bone in the tuberosity area distal to the maxillary second molar.

Secondary Factors Controlling Density

Development Conditions The radiograph may be darker or lighter depending on whether the films are underdeveloped or overdeveloped. However, it is difficult to overdevelop a film that has been properly exposed, even when manual processing is used. Underdevelopment frequently occurs and produces a low-density image. This usually occurs as a result of developer solution that is depleted or is too cold.

Type of Film High-speed films, such as ANSI type E+, require less mAs to cause a density change compared with slower-speed films, such as ANSI type D.

Intensifying Screens (Extraoral Radiographs) High-speed screens require less mAs to cause a density change in the radiograph. Intensifying screens are devices used to convert x-ray energy to light energy and are used in panoramic and cephalometric radiography.

Grids The use of grids requires more mAs to keep a constant density. Grids are devices used primarily in extraoral radiography (such as cephalometrics) to prevent scattered radiation from reaching the film. It consists of a series of narrow lead strips separated by spaces of low-density material.

RADIOGRAPHIC CONTRAST

The contrast on a film is the difference in the densities seen on it.

Mathematically, contrast can be expressed as $D_1 - D_2$, where D_1 is the density of an extreme black area of the film and D_2 is the density of an extreme white area.

Contrast is affected primarily by the **kilovoltage**; however, it can be affected by the type of film used, the characteristics of processing solutions, and the type of tissue irradiated (its thickness, density [mass/volume], and atomic number).

Long-Scale and Short-Scale Contrast

The lower the kilovoltage, the greater the short-scale contrast; as the kilovoltage is increased, the long-scale contrast increases. At higher kilovoltages (80 to 90 kV), penetration of the tissues is greater; therefore, the density differences of adjacent areas on the radiograph will be small, and the radiograph is said to have long-scale contrast. If the kilovoltages are low (60 to 65 kV), penetration of the tissue is less, and the density differences between

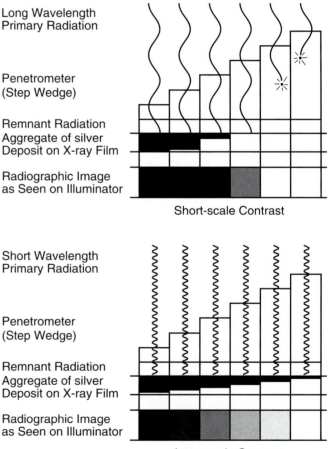

Long Wavelength Primary Radiation

Penetrometer (Step Wedge)

Remnant Radiation Aggregate of silver Deposit on X-ray Film

Radiographic Image as Seen on Illuminator

Short-scale Contrast

Short Wavelength Primary Radiation

Penetrometer (Step Wedge)

Remnant Radiation Aggregate of silver Deposit on X-ray Film

Radiographic Image as Seen on Illuminator

Long-scale Contrast

Figure 3.3. Scale of Contrast. *Short-Scale Contrast:* If the kilovoltage is low (65 kVp), a greater percentage of the wavelengths of the beam will be longer and the amount of penetration will be less. The density differences between adjacent areas will be great, and the film will have short-scale contrast. There will be fewer shades of gray between the lighter and darker areas of the radiographic image. *Long-Scale Contrast:* If the kilovoltage is high (90 kVp), a greater percentage of the wavelengths of beam will be shorter, the penetration of the x-rays through the penetrometer will be greater, the density difference of adjacent areas are small, and the film will have what is called long-scale contrast.

adjacent areas will be great. In this case, the film is said to have short-scale contrast.

Long-scale and short-scale contrast can be illustrated by means of a penetrometer or a step-wedge. A penetrometer is a radiographic testing device made of aluminum and built up in steps of varying thicknesses. Figure 3.3 shows an aluminum penetrometer (step-wedge) being irradiated by x-rays; the exposed x-ray film cross-section is shown beneath each step-wedge or penetrometer. The resulting radiographic image as it appears when viewed on the illuminator is depicted below the film cross-section in both illustrations. The penetrometer demonstrates how long-scale contrast compares with short-scale contrast in Figure 3.4. In general, a compromise between the long-scale and the short-scale contrast is desired. Periapical radiographs should usually manifest long-scale contrast, whereas bite-wing radiographs should have short-scale contrast. A short-scale contrast radiograph is thought to be best for the visualization of dental caries, and the long-scale contrast film is best for visualization of osseous changes such as periodontal and periapical disease in the jaws. However, this concept is debatable; if a dentist uses a darkened room and masks the full-mouth survey of mounted radiographs on a high-illumination viewing box, the long-scale radiographs may be better than short-scale radiographs for reading interproximal caries. It should be remembered that kilovoltage is also a controlling factor in density and contrast. So, if the kilovoltage is increased, the mAs must be decreased to maintain the previous radiographic density.

Relationship among Contrast, Density, and Exposure

When the contrast is changed, the radiographic density of the film will be altered. However, when radiographic density is altered by itself, there will be no obvious change in the contrast. Why is this true? A change in kilovoltage will produce a change in contrast. The higher the kilovoltage, the less will be the contrast. However, because kilovoltage is also a controlling factor in radiographic density, an increase in kilovoltage will also increase the radiographic density.

When the kilovoltage is increased, the milliampere seconds (a controlling factor in radiographic density) must be decreased to maintain the previous radiographic density. Remember that cathode electrons hit the target faster at higher kVps, thus producing more x-ray photons that, in turn, increase the density on the radiograph.

Changing the exposure time is used in most cases when the mA is fixed. To illustrate this concept, the exposure chart below demonstrates the use E speed film and a 16-inch target-film distance for the maxillary molar region. The mAs is 2.5 using the 90-10 technique compared with 7.5 mAs for the 65-10 technique.

Density	Contrast	kVp	mA	Seconds	mAs
Same	Low or long-scale	90	10	.25	2.5
Same	High or short-scale	70	10	.75	7.5

Contrast cannot be varied by a change in milliamperage unless a variation in voltage is made to compensate for the milliamperage variation. If the mA is increased (10 to 15 mA), the kVp must be lowered to maintain the same

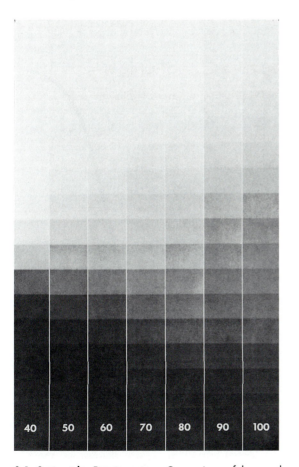

Figure 3.4. Contrast by Penetrometer. Comparison of long-scale and short-scale contrast using penetrometer.

density; by decreasing the kVp, the contrast will increase (short-scale contrast). Density can be altered without changing the contrast. How is this accomplished? Milliampere seconds is the prime factor in controlling radiographic density but it is not a controlling factor in contrast. Therefore, a change in mAs or exposure time will produce a change in radiographic density but not a noticeable change in contrast.

Example: Two radiographs of the same region can be made—one of greater density (higher mAs), and one of lesser density (lower mAs)—with the kVp remaining constant in both radiographs. These two films will have differences in overall blackness (density), but the extreme blackness and whites (contrast) of both films will remain the same.

> In general, it may be said that each increase of 15 kVp will decrease the contrast and increase the density; therefore, the mAs must be decreased by 50% to maintain the same density. With each decrease of 15 kVp, the contrast will increase and the density will decrease; therefore, the mAs must be increased 50% to maintain the same density.

Fog and Scatter

Radiographic contrast will be reduced by the addition of undesirable density from fog and scatter radiation. *Fog* is a darkening (increased density) of the radiograph by sources of energy other than radiation from the primary beam. Film fog can be reduced by proper film storage and film processing. *Scatter radiation* results from Compton interactions with body structures. When the scatter radiation hits the film emulsion, it results in an overall darkening (greater density) of the radiograph, which causes a loss in image contrast.

Characteristic Curve

The characteristic curve was first used in photography by Hunter and Driffield of England in 1890; sometimes the curve is called the H & D curve. Film manufacturers use such curves to monitor film quality and consistency. Characteristic curves are constructed by taking a series of exposures of a certain film type, developing the film, reading the density by use of a **densitometer**, and plotting the density readings against a known exposure. A typical H & D characteristic curve is shown in Figure 3.5. There are great variations in exposure at the high and low levels of exposure, which result in very small changes in density. These low and high levels of the curve are called the toe

(low density) and the shoulder (high density), respectively. In the intermediate straight slope portion of the curve, small changes in exposure result in large changes in density. This is called the straight-line portion of the curve and is the area of proper exposure.

The characteristic curve will give useful information concerning **speed** (sensitivity), **contrast**, and **latitude** of the film (Fig. 3.6).

Film Speed and the Characteristic Curve The characteristic curve of a faster film will be to the left of a characteristic curve of a slower film. This is because less exposure time is required to produce the same level of density even though the films may have similar contrast.

Film Contrast and the Characteristic Curve Film contrast is inherent in the type of film being used. By analysis of the characteristic curve, one can readily determine the degree of contrast for a particular film. The slope of the **characteristic curve** of a film in the useful diagnostic range is a measure of its contrast (Fig. 3.6). There is no simple method to define film contrast. The most often used method is the average gradient or slope of the useful straight line portion of the characteristic curve. The greater the slope of the curve in this region, the **greater**

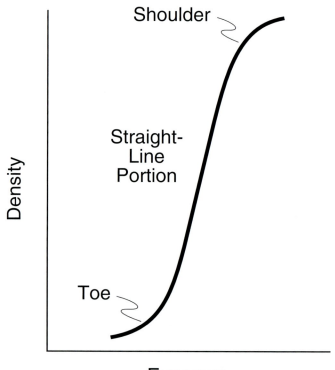

Figure 3.5. Characteristic Curve. Typical characteristic curve of a radiographic film that shows the relationship between exposure and density.

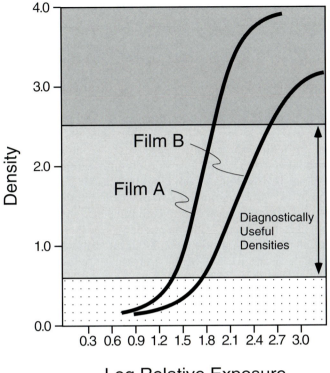

Figure 3.6. Characteristic Curve—Relationships Among Contrast, Speed, and Latitude. Film A has a higher contrast than film B because the slope of the straight portion of the characteristic curve is steeper. Also, the speed of film A is faster than film B because film A requires less exposure to produce any density. Film A has faster speed, higher contrast, and lower latitude than film B. Note that film B has greater latitude (less steepness of the curve) but less film contrast than film A. Generally, the greater the film latitude, the lower the film contrast (long-scale contrast).

the film contrast. In Figure 3.6, film A has a higher contrast than film B. When dental direct-exposure films are considered, the slope of the curve continually increases with increasing exposure. As a result, properly exposed films have more contrast than underexposed (light) films. Film contrast will be maximal when optimum film processing conditions are used. Incomplete or excessive development of films results in decreased film contrast.

Latitude and the Characteristic Curve There are two types of latitude: film latitude and exposure latitude.

Film Latitude Film latitude refers to the range of exposures (mAs) to which an x-ray film will respond with densities within the accepted range for diagnostic radiology (usually considered to be a density range from 0.5 to 2.5). Figure 3.6 shows two films with different latitudes. Film B has a greater latitude (less steepness of the curve) but less film contrast (long-scale) than film A. Generally,

film latitude varies with the reciprocal of film contrast. In other words, the greater the film latitude, the lower the film contrast. Conversely, a film with short-scale (high) contrast (greater slope of curve) will have narrow latitude.

Exposure Latitude Exposure latitude is the range of exposures of an x-ray film permissible for a good diagnostic result. The greater the exposure "error" that can be tolerated, the greater the latitude of the radiographic exposure technique. Exposure latitude improves when the kVp is increased, and the film contrast decreases. In practice, a high kVp technique has more room for error in choice of exposure time (fixed mA) because the exposure latitude is greater. At lower kilovoltage, the latitude is less, and the mAs must be carefully selected.

SUMMARY OF VISUAL CHARACTERISTICS

The mAs (mA and exposure in seconds or impulses) and kVp control **film density** (blackening on film). mAs is the most important factor. When the kVp and mA are fixed, the exposure time is the most important factor in controlling **density**. The kVp controls image **contrast** (density differences on the film). When the kVp is fixed, contrast can only be controlled by the operator's choice of film, screens, and processing solutions. High-contrast (short-scale contrast) radiographs seem to be better for the interpretation of caries. Therefore, a low kVp technique (65 kVp) is usually used for bitewing exposure techniques. Long-scale contrast (low contrast) seems to be the best technique for interpretation of periodontal disease and bony lesions. If long-scale contrast radiographs are used under ideal viewing conditions (darkened room, bright illumination, and masking of films), it is the opinion of many that the long-scale contrast radiograph is even better than a short-scale contrast radiograph for caries interpretation.

> If you're confused . . . think of **density** as the overall **darkness** of a film (controlled by the **amount** of radiation) and **contrast** as a **range of colors**; except in a black and white film, it will be **shades of gray**. If the density is adequate, the image on the radiograph will be neither too dark nor too light. If contrast on the radiograph is the best that can be achieved diagnostically, one can definitely see the enamel, dentin, pulp, alveolar bone, and gingival soft tissue on the radiograph.

GEOMETRIC CHARACTERISTICS

The formation of an accurate radiographic image is dependent on minimizing certain geometric characteristics that are present to a certain degree in every radiograph.

THREE GEOMETRIC CHARACTERISTICS

Image or geometric unsharpness refers to diffusion of detail. **Penumbra** (from the Latin words **pene** for "almost" and **umbra** for "shadow") is a fuzzy, unsharp margin surrounding the radiographic image. Penumbra is often called the **edge gradient**, which is defined as the region of partial illumination that surrounds the *umbra* or complete shadow.

Image magnification is equal enlargement of the radiographic image. It is a form of distortion in which the shape of the object is not substantially altered. However, magnification is rarely uniform because the objects (**buccal cusps**) farther away from the film will always magnify more than objects closer to the film (**lingual cusps**) when the same technique factors are used.

Image shape distortion of the radiographic image is the unequal enlargement or magnification of different parts of the same object.

CAUSES OF IMAGE OR GEOMETRIC UNSHARPNESS, MAGNIFICATION, AND SHAPE DISTORTION

There will always be a certain amount of geometric unsharpness, magnification, and shape distortion of the radiographic image for three reasons:

1. **X-Rays originate from a definite area rather than a point source.** It is impossible to have a point source of x-rays because of the limited heating capacity of x-ray tubes. The source of radiation in modern dental x-ray machines varies from **0.5 to 1.2 mm²**, depending on the mA and kVp capabilities of the machine. The focal spot of the anode acts as if it were composed of many point sources of x-rays, with each point source forming its own image of an object. The edges of each of these images will **not** be in exactly the same point on the film.
2. **X-rays travel in diverging straight lines as they radiate from their source of origin.** This divergent quality of ionizing radiation is an important source of magnification.
3. **Human structures have depth as well as length and width.** Therefore, in dental radiography, a three-dimensional object is recorded on the two-dimensional surface of a film. This results in **unequal** magnification of different parts of an object because of varying distances of these parts from the film.

DEMONSTRATING GEOMETRIC CHARACTERISTICS BY SHADOW CASTING

To understand geometric characteristics of x-rays, we can compare the taking a photograph to the making a radiograph. Proper exposure time and intensity are required for both. After all, x-rays are no more than very short, invisible light waves. Images are recorded in both, because the x-rays and the visible light photons travel in straight lines. In that regard, an x-ray image may be considered analogous to a shadow image. The sharpness of the shadow image from a light source as it is projected on a wall is a function of a number of geometric factors.

To demonstrate shadow formation by light, one needs to obtain a small, clear penlight source (7-W bulb) or small flashlight. The light source should be set up approximately 3 feet from a white wall, turned on, and a hand should be placed an inch or two from the wall. The shadow produced will be nearly the same size as the experimenter's hand, with its edges clear and well-defined. If the hand is moved toward the light source, the shadow will be enlarged or **magnified** and its edges will become fuzzy and indistinct. Next, a large frosted bulb or large flashlight should be substituted for the light source. This time, the hand shadow will have fuzzy edges even with the hand close to the wall. Again, the hand should be moved toward the larger light source; the shadow should enlarge and the fuzziness (blur) increase. The fuzzy portion, or blur, of the shadow around the umbra (shadow) is called the **penumbra** or the *area of unsharpness*. To minimize the *unsharpness* of the light shadow, the *penumbra* must be reduced. The hand image can also be distorted by placing the light source in such a manner that the light waves strike the hand in an oblique direction, rather than perpendicularly. The angle of the hand can also be changed with respect to the wall. This is called **shape distortion**. Nevertheless, the same laws that apply to the fuzziness (blur) at the edge of the object (penumbra) apply to the details of the internal structures of the object.

To avoid confusion in comparing light waves and x-rays, it should be remembered that light waves produce shadows by reflecting light from an opaque object. X-rays will penetrate this same object and will not produce a true shadow, because details of the object will be visible in the processed film. Therefore, x-rays produce x-ray images rather than shadows.

FIVE RULES FOR ACCURATE IMAGE FORMATION

The following five rules for accurate shadow casting by light waves are also applicable to x-rays in the formation of an accurate radiographic image.

1. The x-rays should originate from as small a focal spot as possible. This is determined by the manufacturer. Efforts should be made to minimize voluntary and involuntary motion unsharpness of film or x-ray tube. This will increase the size of the focal spot.
2. The distance between the focal spot (source) and the object to be examined should always be as long as is practical.
3. The film should be as close as possible to the object being radiographed.
4. As far as is practical, the long axis of the object should be parallel to the film.
5. The central ray should be as nearly perpendicular to the film as possible to record the adjacent structures in their true spatial relationships.

By following the above five rules, measures can be taken to minimize the inherent geometric characteristics found in every radiograph.

FACTORS INFLUENCING GEOMETRIC CHARACTERISTICS

Image or Geometric Unsharpness

Radiographic image unsharpness is the fuzzy area or penumbra surrounding the contour lines of the teeth and osseous tissues of the radiograph. Considering the relatively small size of the dental structures and tissues, it is very important to minimize these areas of fuzziness or unsharpness in the dental radiograph. The smaller the size of the focal spot, the smaller the penumbra and consequently the sharper the definition of the radiographic image (Fig. 3.7). When the focal spot is relatively small (0.5 to 1.2 mm), as in dental x-ray tubes, the radiographic image is influenced very little by magnification. The focal spot size cannot be adjusted in dental x-ray machines. It is an important feature to consider when purchasing the x-ray machine. In all situations, sharpness is improved when the source-object distance is increased and the object-film distance is decreased (Fig. 3.7). It should be remembered that the longer the object-film distance, the greater the *unsharpness*. In the dental radiograph, the dental structure farthest from the film will have the greatest unsharpness. Note that the lingual cusp and the lingual root of a tooth will have more sharpness on the radiograph than the buccal cusp and the buccal root or roots on a tooth. The lingual structures are sharper because they are closer to the film.

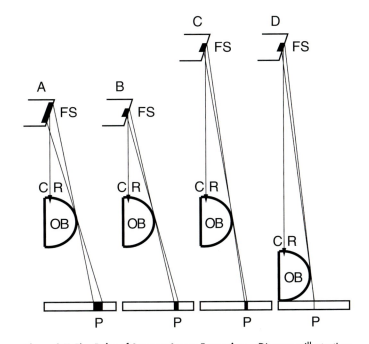

Figure 3.7. Five Rules of Accurate Image Formation. Diagrams illustrating how the accuracy of the radiographic image can be improved by decreasing the size of the penumbra (*P*). The penumbra affects image unsharpness and magnification. Note the changes in size of the penumbra: from *A* to *B* by decreasing the size of a focal spot (*FS*) of the anode; from *B* to *C* by increasing the distance between the focal spot and the film; and from *C* to *D* by decreasing the distance between (*OB*) and the film.

In summary, radiographic image unsharpness can be minimized by **reducing the size of the focal spot, increasing the source-object distance,** and **reducing the object-film distance.**

Magnification

Magnification is the equal enlargement of the actual size of the object as it is projected onto the radiograph. The factors that influence magnification are the same factors that influence radiographic image or geometric unsharpness; however, the distance factors (source-film distance and object-film distance) have more influence than the focal-spot size. It is possible to minimize magnification (equal enlargement) of dental structures by increasing the source-film distance (long cone) and reducing the object-film distances as much as is practical. The relationships among the x-ray beam, the object being radiographed, and the image of the object being projected on the film can be illustrated in a simple drawing (Fig. 3.8).

By using the following formula, the true size of the actual tooth can be calculated. This is helpful in endodontics and orthodontics.

(O) Object size

$$= \frac{d \text{ (source-object distance)} \times I \text{ (image length)}}{D \text{ (source-film distance)}}$$

Example: What is the true size of a tooth when the source-film distance is 16 inches, the source-object distance is 15 inches, and the tooth-image length on the radiograph measures 28 mm?
　Solution:

$$\text{(O) Object size} = \frac{15 \times 28}{16} = 26.25 \text{ mm}$$

In summary, magnification and penumbra size (unsharpness) depend primarily on two factors: **source-film** distance and **object-film distance**. Magnification can be kept at a minimum by keeping the film as close as possible to the object and the source-film distance as long as possible or practical. In Figure 3.9A, the radiograph was taken with a long source-film distance (long cone) and reveals teeth that are less magnified than the teeth in the radiograph in Figure 3.9B, which was taken with a shorter source-film distance (short cone). The width of the staple in Figure 3.9B measured 2 mm longer than the staple in Figure 3.9A.

In a properly exposed radiograph, sharpness and detail are adequate when the lamina dura, periodontal membrane space, and individual bone trabeculae can be seen.

Shape or Dimensional Distortion

Distortion is unequal magnification of different parts of the object. Shape distortion can be minimized by using the radiographic intraoral **paralleling technique**, whereby the film is placed parallel to the long axes of the teeth and the beam of radiation is directed at right angles to the teeth and film. In the **bisecting technique**, the beam of radiation is directed perpendicular to the line bisecting the angle formed by the long axes of the teeth and the film. Inherent shape-distortion problems arise when the bisecting technique is used that are *not* found when the paralleling technique is used (Fig. 3.10). The bisecting "rule of isometry" applies admirably to plane surfaces

that have length and width dimensions, but it has certain shortcomings when objects have depth as well as length and width. If the bisecting principle is even slightly neglected, the resultant image will be foreshortened or elongated. The maxillary molar buccal roots will always be foreshortened in comparison to the lingual root when using the bisecting technique, because the depth dimension is greater in these teeth.

If you're confused . . . think of the **penumbra** as causing the objects in a photograph to appear out of focus, and **magnification** as an enlargement of the objects in a photograph that occurs with a magnifying glass. To minimize **penumbra** and **magnification** on a photograph or a radiograph, it is the *distances* that count in radiography: (1) use a long cone (beam indicating device [BID]) (target-film distance), and (2) get the film as close to the tooth as possible (object-film distance) and still be able to achieve parallelism of film with the teeth.

Think of **distortion** as an altered shape of objects in a photograph that occurs with the use of trick mirrors. To minimize distortion, remember that it is the *angles* that count. The film and the tooth should be parallel to each other, and the flat end of the BID should be parallel to the tooth and the film. Another way to consider the "angles" is to think of the central ray of the x-ray beam (CR) to be perpendicular to the tooth and the film, which are parallel to one another.

If you take into account all the factors to minimize **penumbra, magnification,** and **distortion,** the periodontal ligament space, lamina dura, and individual trabeculae will be easily seen and sharply defined in the x-ray image.

ANATOMICAL ACCURACY

Anatomical accuracy occurs when the anatomical structures are reproduced on the film in the true spatial relationship as they normally appear. Anatomical accuracy is obtained when the film is placed parallel to the long axis of the teeth and the radiation beam directed perpendicular to both.

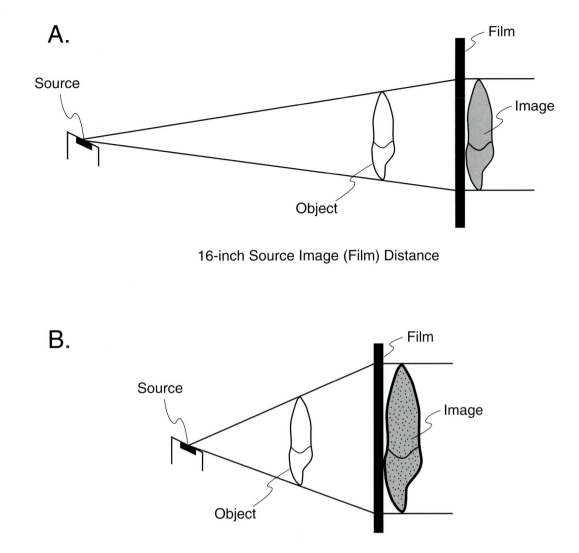

A.

Source

Film

Image

Object

16-inch Source Image (Film) Distance

B.

Source

Film

Image

Object

8-inch Source Image (Film) Distance

Figure 3.8. Magnification and Distance Factors. Note that the magnification of the tooth is less with long source-film distance (**A**) compared with short source-film distance (**B**).

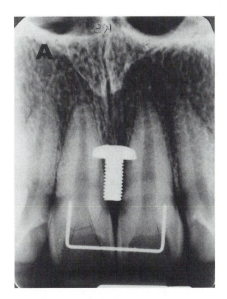
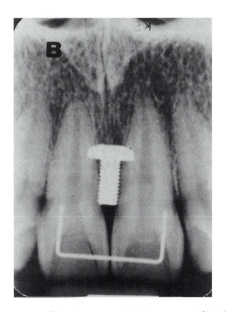

Figure 3.9. Geometric Unsharpness and Distance Factors. Radiographs taken with (**A**) long source-film distance and (**B**) short source-film distance. In both cases, only the source-film distances were different; the object-film distances were the same. Note the sharpness (less penumbra) of outline of the screw in **A** (taken with the longer source-film distance) compared with **B** (taken with a shorter source-film distance). Also, the staple in **B** is 2 mm longer than in **A**.

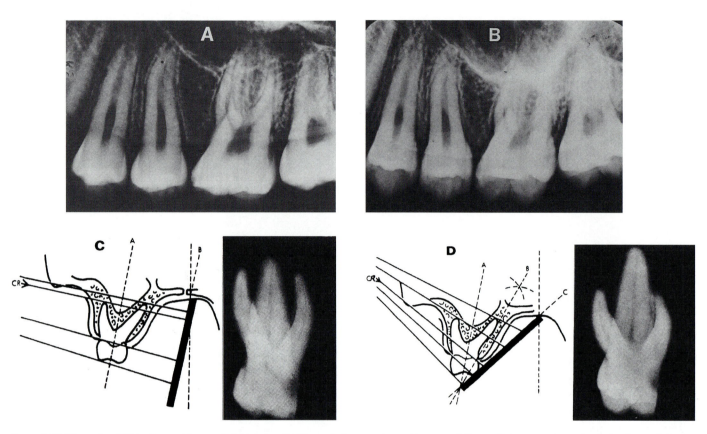

Figure 3.10. Dimensional Distortion and Anatomic Accuracy. Radiograph **A** was taken with a paralleling technique, as shown in **C**. Radiograph **B** was taken with the bisecting technique shown in **D**, which is an oblique angle technique. Note the amount of foreshortening of the buccal roots of the maxillary molar radiograph shown in **D**, when compared with the buccal roots of maxillary molar radiograph shown in **C** (taken with the paralleling technique). Compare **A** with **B** for anatomic accuracy. Both **A** and **B** were taken of the left maxillary first molar region of the same patient.

A properly exposed radiograph is said to have anatomical accuracy when:

1. The labial and lingual cementoenamel junctions of the anterior teeth are superimposed.
2. The buccal and lingual cusps of the posterior teeth (especially the molars) are superimposed.
3. The contacts of the teeth are opened in at least one of the projections of a given area.
4. The buccal portion of the alveolar bone crest is superimposed over the lingual portion of the alveolar bone crest (posterior teeth).
5. There is no superimposition of the zygomatic process of maxilla over the roots of the maxillary molar teeth.

The long-cone paralleling technique radiograph has greater anatomical accuracy than the short-cone bisecting technique radiograph, because the paralleling long-cone technique radiograph reveals the following:

a. Better superimposition of buccal and lingual cusps (better caries detection).
b. Better superimposition of buccal portion of alveolar bone crest over the lingual portion of alveolar bone crest (better interpretation of crestal alveolar bone height).
c. Minimal superimposition of zygomatic bone over roots of maxillary molars (better for interpreting periapical pathology).
d. Better definition and less magnification (better film for overall interpretation).
e. Minimal foreshortening of buccal roots of molars (better for endodontic preoperative and postoperative radiographs).

The reader should compare radiograph A (taken with the long-cone paralleling technique) and radiograph B (taken with the short-cone bisecting technique) in Figure 3.10.

If you're confused . . . think of anatomical accuracy like building a house on a hill; you still want the floors to be horizontal and the walls perpendicular. Here the angles count, so make certain the film is parallel to the tooth and the BID is perpendicular to the film and tooth. The buccal and lingual cusps should be superimposed in the x-ray image.

Explanatory note on cone or BID length: Currently, a long cone or BID is defined as 16 inches. The cone length is measured from the dot or focal spot mark on the tubehead to the tip of the cone. An 8-inch cone or BID is referred to as a short cone; the 12-inch cone is a compromise between the 8- and 16-inch lengths. Both these lengths are measured as previously described. An 8- or 12-inch cone should **never** be used with the paralleling technique, because here the distances between the teeth and film will be quite long, thus breaking one of the five rules for accurate shadow casting or x-ray projection. The long 16-inch BID compensates for this; however, the use of the short 8-inch cone (short target-film distance) breaks a second rule of good x-ray projection (shadow casting) and exacerbates the problem. On the other hand, the bisecting technique calls for the film to be placed as close as possible to the tooth. Therefore, an 8-inch cone can be used, but even then, the longer cone (BID) with the bisecting technique is better.

RADIOGRAPHIC COVERAGE

It is important that the area of interest is well covered in the radiograph. In the periapical radiograph, an adequate amount of bone (at least 2 to 4 mm) surrounding the apices of the teeth should be revealed on the radiograph. Supplemental films, such as occlusal films, may be mandatory at times to completely view the area of suspected abnormality (see Chapter 5). Additional films may have to be taken at right angles to each other to localize the area of interest (Fig. 3.11).

Adequate coverage of the area of interest depends on several factors:

1. Proper alignment of film and the radiation beam to area of interest.
2. Proper selection of film types.
3. Proper selection of film-projection techniques.

SUMMARY OF DIAGNOSTIC QUALITY

The diagnostic quality of the radiographic film is dependent on the proper use of several factors. The functions of these factors are given below:

1. Milliampere seconds (mAs) regulate density (blackness) of the radiograph.
2. Kilovoltage
   a. regulates degree of x-ray penetration of tissues;
   b. influences scatter radiation fog;
   c. regulates contrast scale; and
   d. influences density of the radiograph.
3. Focal-spot size influences unsharpness and magnification of the radiographic image.
4. Source-film and object-film distances influence unsharpness, and magnification of the radiographic image.
5. Alignment of film and beam of radiation influence distortion, anatomical accuracy, and coverage.

Therefore, if all other exposure factors remain constant, the factors listed in Figure 3.12 will influence the x-ray image characteristics of density, contrast, geometric unsharpness, magnification, and shape distortion in various ways.

SUMMARY OF DIAGNOSTIC FEATURES AS VIEWED ON FILM

1. The image will not be too light or too dark overall (density).
2. The five basic tissues can be seen: enamel, dentin, pulp, alveolar bone, and soft tissue (contrast).
3. The apical periodontal membrane space, lamina dura, and individual trabeculae can be seen (detail, sharpness).
4. The buccal and lingual cusp tips are superimposed (distortion, anatomical accuracy).
5. All the needed structures for an accurate diagnosis can be seen (coverage).

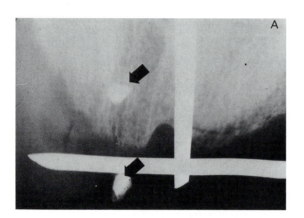
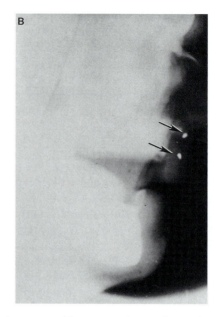

Figure 3.11. Localization of Area of Interest. **(A)** Occlusal radiograph of a patient who seems to have a metal fragment in the maxillary palate and one in the lip. **(B)** Anterior profile radiograph of the same patient locating both metal fragments in the lip.

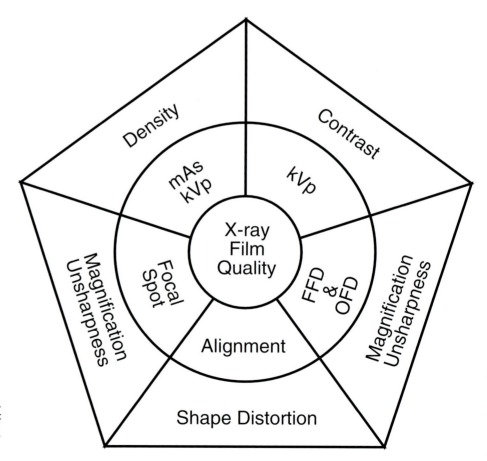

Figure 3.12. Diagnostic Quality Summary. Summary of controlling factors of density, contrast, geometric unsharpness, magnification, and distortion.

WORKSHOP/LABORATORY EXERCISES

EXERCISE 3.1. RULES FOR ACCURATE IMAGE PROJECTION

Materials and Equipment Needed

1. Six no. 2 intraoral films, speed E+.
2. Two small metal paper clips.
3. A small piece of cardboard.
4. X-ray machine and processing facility.

Instructions

Step 1: Turn on the x-ray machine. Set the kVp at about 65 and the mA at 7 or 10, depending on the machine. Twist off the BID. (The instructor will help you.)

Step 2: Obtain intraoral films and two smaller-sized metal paper clips. Separate the two rounded tines of **one** of the paper clips so that they are about ¼ inch apart.

Step 3: For each of the following exposures, place the two paper clips side by side on the plain or front side of the film. With a ball-point pen, label each film number.

Step 4: Exposure no. 1: place film no. 1 on the counter top with the two paper clips side by side along its length. From the focal spot mark on the tube-head, place a distance of 4 inches between it and the film. Direct the x-ray beam perpendicular to the film (90°). Set the exposure time at ⅟₃₂ second (2 impulses) and expose this film. (Exposure values may need adjustment.)

Step 5: For films no. 2 and 3 do exactly as for no. 1, except for film no. 2 use a distance of 8 inches and ⅛ second (7 impulses) exposure time. Expose this film. For film no. 3 use a distance of 16 inches and ½ second (30 impulses) exposure time. Expose this film.

Step 6: For film no. 4 place the cone tip on an angle of 20° off perpendicular (70° or 110°), use a distance of 16 inches, and a 1-second exposure time. Direct the central ray at the center of the film and expose it.

Step 7: Move a little U-shaped spacer or platform made from a piece of cardboard, so that the top of the U is the same size as the no. 2 film and the top stands 1 inch from the counter top. Place film no. 5 on the counter top, the U-shaped spacer on top of the film, and the two paper clips on top of the spacer. Set the focal spot 8 inches from the film. Direct central ray perpendicular to the film and set the exposure time at ⅛ second (7 impulses). Expose this film.

Expose film no. 6 in exactly the same way, except use a focal spot to film distance of 16 inches and an exposure time of ½ second (30 impulses). Expose this film.

Step 8: Process films no. 1 through 6; label and mount the processed films.

CASE-BASED QUESTIONS FOR LABORATORY EXERCISE

1. Explain why the density does not vary among films no. 1, 2, and 3, although the exposure times do.

2. Which films demonstrate the effect of varying BID length?

3. What happens to the images of the paper clips as cone length gets longer?

4. With the distance set at 16 inches, what happens when you vary the perpendicularity of the central ray to the object and film (compare films no. 3 and 4)?

5. What happens when the object-film distance is lengthened when cone length is kept constant (compare films no. 3 and 5)?

6. What happens when the object-film distance is lengthened and then the cone length is changed from 16 inches to 8 inches (compare films no. 5 and 6)?

7. Among the six films, which has the greatest magnification? Why?

8. Among the six films, which has the greatest penumbra? Why?

9. Among the six films, which is the most unsharp? Why?

10. Among the six films, which is the sharpest? Why?

11. Among the six films, which has the greatest distortion? Why?

CASE-BASED PROBLEM-SOLVING

Using a flashlight and a plain wall surface or large piece of white cardboard, show how you could demonstrate the five principles of accurate image formation. Use the wall as the recording surface (film), the flashlight bulb as the focal spot, the beam or cone (BID) of light as the beam of x-rays, and your hand and fingers as the object. Do not forget to demonstrate the geometric factors.

REVIEW QUESTIONS

1. Why is extending the source-film distance to 16 inches or so-called "long cone" or "long BID" a necessary adjunct to the paralleling or right-angle radiographic technique?

   A. To avoid unsharpness of the image.
   B. To avoid shape distortion of the image.
   C. To reduce secondary radiation.
   D. To facilitate correct vertical angulation of the cone.
   E. To avoid superimposition of anatomical structures.

2. How do you change from long-scale contrast film to a short-scale contrast film and still maintain density?

   A. Decrease the kVp and increase the mAs.
   B. Decrease the kVp and decrease the mAs.
   C. Increase the kVp and decrease the mAs.
   D. Increase the kVp and increase the mAs.

3. Which of the following would minimize the size of the penumbra?

   A. Large focal spot.
   B. Long source-film distance.
   C. Short source-film distance.
   D. Long object-film distance.

4. If by mistake you used the exposure time for the short-cone (BID) technique (8-inch source-film distance) while using the long-cone (BID) technique (16-inch source-film distance), what would be the density of the film?

   A. Too light.
   B. No visible change in density.
   C. Too dark.
   D. Altered from long-scale to short-scale.

5. What is the primary factor in controlling density?

   A. kVp.
   B. Source-film distance.
   C. mAs.
   D. Collimation.
   E. Film development.

6. What is the primary factor in controlling contrast?

   A. Film speed.
   B. Source-film distance.
   C. kVp.
   D. Exposure time.
   E. mA.

7. Which of the following properties of x-rays is the basis for the rules of geometric projection?

   A. X-rays travel at the speed of light.
   B. X-rays travel in diverging straight lines from a point source.
   C. The course of an x-ray photon can be diverted with an electromagnetic source.
   D. X-rays can form a latent image on photographic film.

8. Regardless of the target-film distance, incorrect horizontal angulation will cause:

   A. Elongation of the x-ray image.
   B. Foreshortening of the x-ray image.
   C. No significant change in the x-ray image.
   D. Overlapping of teeth in the x-ray image.

9. The size of the x-ray tube focal spot influences radiographic:

   A. Density.
   B. Contrast.
   C. Definition.
   D. Distortion.

10. Which of the following does **not** control magnification of the radiographed object?

    A. Focal spot-film distance.
    B. Alignment of film, objects, and radiation cone.
    C. Object-film distance.
    D. Cathode size.

11. Which of the following does not constitute an advantage of the smallest possible focal spot?

    A. Decreased geometric unsharpness.
    B. Increased magnification.
    C. Increased definition.
    D. Decreased penumbra.

12. The density of an intraoral film indicates the:

    A. Degree of darkness.
    B. Difference between densities.
    C. Speed of the screens.
    D. Kilovoltage used.
    E. None of the above.

13. Fog affects the contrast of an intraoral film because it:

    A. Decreases film density.
    B. Increases film density.
    C. Produces white specks on the film.
    D. Produces phosphorus crystals on the film.

BIBLIOGRAPHY

Bloom WJ, Hollenbach JL, Morgan JA. Medical radiographic technic. 3rd ed. Springfield: Charles C. Thomas, 1969.

Bushong SC. Radiologic science for technologists. 5th ed. St. Louis: Mosby-Year Book, 1993.

Curry TS, Dowdey JE, Murry R. Christensen's introduction to the physics of diagnostic radiology. 4th ed. Philadelphia: Lea & Febiger, 1990.

Fitzgerald GM. Dental roentgenography I: an investigation in adumbration, or the factors that control geometric unsharpness. J Am Dent Assoc 1947;34:1–20.

Fitzgerald GM. Dental roentgenography IV: the voltage factor. J Am Dent Assoc 1950;41:19–28.

Fitzgerald GM. Roentgenography rebuttal. Oral Surg 1960;13:1218.

Fuchs A. Principles of radiographic exposure and processing. 2nd ed. Springfield: Charles C. Thomas, 1971.

Intraoral radiography with Rinn XCP-BAI instruments: Elgin, IL: Rinn, 1986.

Langland OE, Sippy FH. A study of radiographic longitudinal distortion of anterior teeth using the paralleling technique. Oral Surg 1966;22:737–749.

McCormack D. Dental roentgenology: a technical procedure for furthering the advancement toward anatomical accuracy. J Calif State Dent Assoc 1937;May-June, 13:1–28.

McCormack FW. A plea for standardized technique for oral radiography. J Dent Res 1920;11:467–501.

Richards AG. Technical factors that control radiographic density. Dent Clin North Am 1961;July:371–377.

Selman J. The fundamentals of X-ray and radium physics. 6th ed. Springfield: Charles C. Thomas, 1978.

The fundamentals of radiography. Rochester, NY: Eastman Kodak, 1987.

Updegrave W. Simplifying and improving intraoral dental roentgenography. Oral Surg 1959;12:704–716.

Updegrave W. High or low kilovoltage. Dent Radiogr Photogr 1960;33(4): 71–78.

Updegrave W. Higher fidelity in intraoral roentgenography. J Am Dent Assoc 1961;62:3–22.

Waggener DT. The right-angle technique using the extension cone. Dent Clin North Am 1960;November:783–788.

Wuehrmann A, Monacelli CJ. Selection of optimum kilovoltage for dental radiography. Radiology 1951;57:240–247.

Wuehrmann DT. The long cone technic. Pract Dent Monogr 1957;3:30.

SECTION 2:
Radiographic Techniques and Procedures

Radiology Infection Control Procedures

4

OBJECTIVES

Upon successful completion of this unit, the student will be able to:

1. *Discuss his or her general knowledge of the roles of various regulatory agencies in infection control.*

2. *Identify personal protective equipment.*

3. *List Spaulding's classification of inanimate objects.*

4. *List the specific infection control procedures needed in the x-ray room before and during the exposure of an intraoral film.*

5. *Describe how contaminated films are transported to the processing facility.*

6. *Describe how to prevent cross-infection when using a daylight loader or a darkroom to process films.*

7. *List the clean-up procedures required in the darkroom and x-ray room.*

8. *Perform all necessary infection control procedures for the taking of a single intraoral radiograph using the Workshop/Laboratory Exercises format.*

9. *Suggest an alternate radiologic technique with simpler and fewer infection control procedures using the Case-Based Problem-Solving format.*

10. *Test his or her knowledge by answering the Review Questions.*

KEY WORDS/PHRASES

barrier envelopes
contaminated film packets
cross-contamination
cytomegalovirus
daylight loader problems
exposure incident

infection control procedures
infectious organisms
iodophors
panoramic infection control
personal protective equipment
phenolics

regulatory agencies
semicritical
surface barriers
surface disinfection
unit dosing
universal precautions

INTRODUCTION

Dental patients and dental health-care workers (DHCWs) are constantly exposed to many infectious and potentially infectious organisms, whether airborne, salivaborne, waterborne, or bloodborne. Some of these include the common viruses such as the common cold and flu viruses; cytomegalovirus; herpes simplex viruses 1 and 2; hepatitis B, C, and D viruses; Epstein–Barr virus (infectious mononucleosis); and human immunodeficiency virus (HIV). Apart from viruses, bacteria such as staphylococci, diplococci, pneumococci, Mycobacterium, chlamydia, spirochetes, and Pseudomonas may also infect exposed DHCWs or patients. Many apparently healthy ambulatory patients suffer from infectious diseases, including sexually transmitted diseases, involving the oral cavity. Thus, it is necessary to use universal precautions and strict infection control protocols and procedures to protect both DHCWs and patients.

It is postulated that diseases can be spread in three ways:

1. From a patient to a DHCW.
2. From a DHCW to a patient.
3. From a patient to another patient.

Transmission may occur via a common vehicle such as blood, saliva, or airborne particles and through either direct or indirect contact via contaminated instruments or surfaces.

AGENCIES THAT DEVELOP GUIDELINES AND REGULATIONS

Infection control guidelines such as those produced by the Centers for Disease Control and Prevention (CDC) and the American Dental Association (ADA) are meant to break the path of transmission, thus protecting both patients and DHCWs. In 1991, the federal government, through the Occupational Safety and Health Administration (OSHA), published the Bloodborne Pathogens (BBP) Rule, designed to protect the employee who works with bloodborne pathogens; however, the rule does not apply to the employer or patients. DHCWs who take x-rays do not commonly come into contact with blood, although they do come into contact with saliva. OSHA (Bloodborne Pathogens Rule 1991) defines saliva as an "other potentially infectious material" (OPIM) in the transmission of bloodborne pathogens. Therefore, stringent procedures

should be followed in dental radiography to prevent the spread of infectious diseases. This is especially true for intraoral radiography; in panoramic and extraoral radiography, there is little or no potential for contamination. Under normal circumstances, differentiation between the dentally significant body fluid types (saliva and blood) may be difficult or impossible; therefore, all body fluids are considered potentially infectious materials. This is the basic tenet of the principle known as **universal precautions**, which will be discussed later in this section.

Another agency that is important in setting regulations is the Environmental Protection Agency (EPA). Because the EPA is more interested in the environment than people, it regulates surface disinfectant chemicals and the environmental aspects of infectious and other regulated waste disposal. Chemicals used to disinfect and sterilize objects in the radiography area must have an EPA registration number and be approved by the EPA.

Agencies responsible for producing infection control guidelines are the ADA, American Academy of Oral and Maxillofacial Radiology (AAOMR), CDC, and the Office of Sterilization and Asepsis Procedures (OSAP). The ADA plays an important role in coordinating the regulations and recommendations set forth by the various agencies and published their most recent infection control guidelines in April 1996. The CDC played a major role in developing overall guidelines for all forms of medical practice in dentistry. The term **universal precautions** refers to a set of precautions designed to prevent transmission of HIV, hepatitis B, and other salivaborne and bloodborne pathogens in the health-care setting. Universal precautions means that the same infection control measures must be used for all patients for any dental procedure where there is contact with saliva or blood. It also assumes that if there has been an exposure incident, then transmission of disease has occurred until otherwise ruled out by specific medical diagnostic testing procedures and protocols.

Although in most states the CDC and ADA guidelines are adopted by practitioners on a voluntary basis, the BBP rule is enforced by either federal or state OSHA inspectors in a police role. The OSHA inspectors also look for chemical and safety hazards not necessarily covered by the BBP rule but published in other federal regulations. OSHA inspectors may levy fines as low as $25 or $50 for minor infractions and up to $50,000 to $70,000 for repeated or multiple serious violations and/or failure to abate. In most states the State Board of Dental Examiners (BDE) adopts many of the CDC and/or ADA infection control guidelines as regulations. These are actively policed and enforced by inspectors or representatives of the BDE. The difference between state board inspectors and OSHA inspectors is that *state board inspectors* look for infractions of infection control regulations that may affect the spread of disease to and from patients, owner DHCWs, and employee DHCWs. Many state board inspectors are or have been a DHCW. State and federal OSHA inspectors are only concerned with employee DHCWs and may have little knowledge of dentistry per se. Nevertheless, they have been trained to recognize and/or investigate infractions of the bloodborne pathogens, hazard communication, and safety regulations that are applicable to employee DHCWs. The employer DHCW is exempted from the OSHA regulations, as it is the employer who must ensure employee compliance and it is the employer who will pay all fines due to infractions by any employee. DHCWs not exposed to bloodborne pathogens or chemical and safety hazards are not subject to the OSHA rule.

PERSONAL PROTECTIVE EQUIPMENT

Because saliva is considered to be a potentially infectious material in the transmission of bloodborne pathogens, there is a potential for contamination by saliva. During any radiographic procedure, universal precautions must be observed by exposed DHCWs, including the use of adequate personal protective equipment (PPE) such as gloves, the proper handling of contaminated materials, and the decontamination of surfaces and/or instruments exposed to saliva. It is not usually necessary to wear PPE such as impervious gowns, long sleeves, masks, and protective eyewear during routine dental radiology procedures when no aerosols, droplets, or spatter are generated (Fig. 4.1). It is advisable to use gowns, masks, and protective eyewear when treating patients with gagging problems or respiratory infections such as the common cold, if such patients are accepted for treatment.

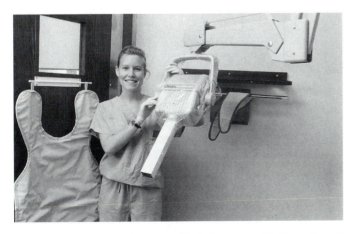

Figure 4.1. Personal Protective Equipment During Intraoral Radiography. If no aerosols are generated, only latex examination gloves are needed. Protective eyewear, masks, long sleeves, and/or gowns are not usually needed.

CONTAMINATION OF DENTAL PROCESSING SOLUTIONS

It is possible to contaminate the processing solutions during the processing of intraoral radiographs. Manipulation of the film packet during processing presents a potential for contamination of the darkroom equipment. Katz et al. (1988) have shown that bacteria, when inoculated in very high concentrations, can survive in the dental radiographic developer and fixer for 2 weeks. Bachman et al. (1990) reported that bacteria inoculated on radiographic film in high doses survive the processing cycles in an automatic processor and contaminate and persist in the processing solutions. Stanczyk et al. (1993) investigated microbiologic contamination of an automatic dental processor and daylight loader during 1 week of simulated clinical use. The results from this study show that microbial contamination on radiographic film can survive the processing cycle. In addition, the films frequently became cross-contaminated within the processor. Cross-contamination within the processor emphasizes the need for strict attention to aseptic film handling before processing. Any lapse in aseptic intraoral film processing may result in contamination of the processor and subsequent processed films that may last for several days.

Because there is no contamination of the hands or film cassette during the taking of panoramic or other extraoral films such as cephalometric radiographs, no particular infection control procedures are needed on a routine basis. The only source of cross-infection is the biteblock used in panoramic radiology. This is usually covered with a plastic barrier or decontaminated between procedures. In either case, the patient is asked to remove the contaminated barrier and throw it in the regular trash or to remove the biteblock and place it in a nearby container for further decontamination and processing. On a routine basis, various parts of the extraoral and panoramic x-ray machines should be disinfected, especially those "high-touch" parts used by patients and DHCWs. A schedule for these disinfection procedures must be available for the OSHA inspector.

SURFACE DISINFECTION AND SURFACE BARRIERS

Based on Spaulding's classification of inanimate objects (1968), surfaces that come into contact with intact mucous membranes but do not enter normally sterile areas of the body are classified as semicritical. Most items that become contaminated in dental radiology are semicritical. Semicritical items require high-level disinfection, but whenever possible it is best to sterilize these. The following table

Spaulding's Classification of Surfaces in Dental Radiology

Spaulding's Categories	Contaminated Items	Level of Decontamination
Critical	Items that penetrate tissue and/or contact blood • None in day-to-day OMR.	Sterilization required OR Disposable instruments
Semicritical	No tissue penetration, but contacts mucous membrane • Most intraoral devices and materials used in OMR. *Examples:* Intraoral films, film holders, position-indicating devices, panoramic bit guides, digital image receptors.	Sterilization, high-level disinfection OR Use of barriers
Noncritical	No tissue penetration, no contact with mucous membrane or saliva by equipment/devices, touches intact skin only • Most extraoral and panoramic OMR devices, especially parts thereof contaminated by the operator. *Examples:* Leaded aprons, thyroid collars, panoramic side and front guides, cones, handles and knobs, yokes, tubeheads, control units, chair seats, handles, and head and arm rests.	Sanitization, intermediate-level disinfection OR Use of barriers
Environmental surfaces	No direct patient contact • Environmental surfaces that do not noramlly touch the patient but may be contaminated by the care provider. *Examples*: High-touch surfaces on which exposed films/instruments are placed, table tops and working surfaces in the operatory, as well as the darkroom and daylight loader.	Sanitization, intermediate-level disinfection OR Use of barriers

enumerates the types of decontamination required for items in Spaulding's categories and provides some examples.

In conjunction with the classification of surfaces and other items, DHCWs should adhere to routines whereby **high-touch** areas/surfaces are delineated. High touch areas/surfaces require sanitation and disinfection using a spray-wipe-spray technique once in the **morning**, once at the **end of the work shift**, and when **visibly contaminated**. The objective of the first step in this technique is sanitization, i.e., removing potentially infectious material. This is followed by disinfection—spraying the decontaminating solution onto the surface and leaving it for 5 to 10 minutes as recommended by the manufacturer. The product selected must have an EPA registration number on the label. Products such as complex phenols, alcohol-phenol sprays, iodophors, and chlorine solutions have all been recommended by the ADA and EPA. Alternately during the day, surface covers or barriers may be used and changed between patients. All products should be EPA-registered, intermediate-level disinfectants that will kill **hydrophilic** and **lipophilic** viruses. Water-based iodophor or dual synthetic phenolic disinfectants are recommended rather than other products such as alcohol-based sprays or aerosols. Iodophors must be mixed daily with distilled water, and a stain remover must be applied to surfaces and equipment routinely to remove iodophor stains. Phenolics have a longer shelf life than iodophors and do not normally stain surfaces. The manufacturers' instructions should be fol-

lowed pertaining to dilution and use of specific products. When disinfectants are used in a secondary container, this container should be labeled to conform with the secondary labeling requirements in the hazard communications part of the **Bloodborne Pathogens Rule**. The secondary label should contain the product name, manufacturer, chemical identity, and appropriate hazardous warnings. In addition, hazard-related PPE such as protective eyewear, mask, gloves, and long sleeves should be worn when diluting concentrates of many of these solutions.

All nondisposable film-holding devices should be properly decontaminated between patients. Sterilization is preferable and should be done with a heat system (steam autoclave, chemical vapor, or dry heat), although ethylene oxide or EPA-registered and ADA-approved chemical sterilants can be used. If routine sterilization of these instruments is not possible, disposable film-holding devices should be substituted. Disposable items, such as Stabe film-holders and bitewing tabs (Dentsply/Rinn, Elgin, IL), should be dispensed in unit doses per patient to minimize contamination of larger supplies of these items. Using barriers or surface covers between patients reduces patient turnaround time and diminishes the need for disinfectants. Preformed covers are commercially available to fit surfaces such as tubeheads or panoramic biteblocks. However, these increase inventory and cost of infection control. An alternative is the use of wide plastic food wrap, which is more economical and as effective as a preformed barrier but may require more time to apply.

ATLAS OF INFECTION CONTROL PROCEDURES IN INTRAORAL RADIOGRAPHY

The infection control procedures for intraoral radiography are more complex than those used in panoramic or extraoral radiography (Fig. 4.2). Standard infection control procedures in intraoral radiography are listed below.

Activities during the Exposure Phase

- Administer a preprocedural mouth rinse with either 0.12% chlorhexidine gluconate or with a phenolic to the patient.
- Disinfect surfaces at the beginning and end of each day (between patients only if contaminated).
- Avoid spraying electrical switches; wipe with disinfectant-moistened paper towel.
- Apply surface covers to the yoke, tubehead, cone, control unit, head rest, arm rest, and any hand-held switches.
- Place a paper towel/surface cover on a work area to hold film packets, sterilized film-holding devices, biteblocks, paper cups, and overgloves.
- Wear latex or vinyl unpowdered examination gloves.
- Place the sanitized lead apron and collar on the patient after seating the patient.
- Set the required mA, kVp, and exposure time on the control unit and reset as required.
- Open the sterile pack containing the film-holding devices; affix the film and position in the patient's mouth.
- Position the tubehead and cone by touching areas with barrier.

- Use a foot switch or a wrapped hand-held switch to trigger the unit.
- Drop exposed films into a paper cup without touching the outer surface of the cup.
- *If films are pouched, disinfect the envelope and remove the noncontaminated film packets. These can now be processed without further infection control considerations as outlined below.*

Activities during the Transportation Phase

- Don overgloves over the vinyl or latex gloves before transportation or remove gloves in two-glove method.
- Pick up the cup with exposed films and the extra empty cup.
- Carry the two paper cups to the processing area.

Activities during the Film Processing Phase

Daylight Loader

- Open lid of the processor with overgloved hands or with clean, bare hands in two-glove method.
- Place a paper napkin/plastic wrap on the floor of the loader's open chamber.
- Place the empty cup and the one with the films in the chamber, keeping the clean/empty paper cup on the right side (for right-handed DHCWs).

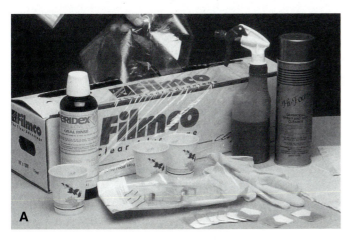
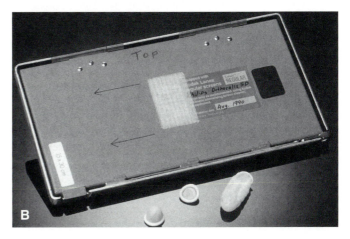

Figure 4.2. Infection Control Materials. **(A)** Numerous infection control materials are needed for intraoral radiography, and the infection control procedures involve many steps. **(B)** Only one biteblock cover or a disposable biteblock is needed for infection control in panoramic radiography, and the infection control procedures are very simple.

- Close the lid of the chamber. With two-glove method, wash hands and don new gloves.
- Insert overgloved hands through sleeves in overgloved method and newly gloved hands in two-glove method.
- Take off overgloves and place them on the left side of the paper napkin.
- Open film packet by pulling gently on outer tab, revealing the inner black paper tab.
- Hold paper tab carefully and tease it out of packaging, shaking it gently until the film drops into clean paper cup.
- Discard paper, lead foil, and plastic wrap on the left side.
- Once all wrappings have been removed and films dropped into cup, discard powder-free latex gloves on the left side.
- With clean, bare hands pick up films by the edges and feed them into processor.
- Remove hands through sleeves.
- Wear nitrile gloves to remove waste from loader chamber; remove surface covers from radiographic equipment, chair, and control unit and discard them into a regular waste bin.
- Wash hands with a liquid soap and water.
- Remove films from processor and mount them.

Darkroom Processing

- Place two paper napkins/plastic wraps on a work surface near processing area.
- Place cup with exposed films on one paper napkin.
- Discard overgloves. With two-glove method, wash hands and don new gloves.
- Open each film packet by pulling gently on outer tab and evert it, revealing the inner black paper tab.
- Carefully hold paper tab and tease it out of packaging, shaking it gently until the film drops onto clean paper napkin.
- Once all wrappers have been removed and the films dropped onto paper napkin, discard powder-free latex gloves.
- With clean, bare hands pick up films by the edges and feed them into processor or attach to processing racks.
- Wear nitrile gloves to remove waste; remove surface covers from radiographic equipment, chair, and control unit and discard them into a regular waste bin.

Unit dosing of the materials is needed before the start of any radiographic procedure and is essential to control cross-contamination. The following is a list of materials that have been unit dosed for infection control procedures used in intraoral radiography.

Unit Dosing of Materials for Intraoral Radiography

Materials during Film Exposure

1. One dose of preprocedural and antibacterial mouthrinse.
2. Paper towel.
3. Disinfectant.
4. Barriers (preformed or a roll of plastic wrap).
5. Powder-free gloves (latex or vinyl).
6. Radiographic films (polysoft type).
7. Sterile film-holders.
8. Two paper cups.
9. Overgloves (food handler's gloves).
10. Leaded thyroid collar and apron

Masks, eyewear, and protective gowns are needed when a patient has a known gag reflex or respiratory infections.

Materials during Transportation
Without barrier envelopes:

1. Empty paper cup.
2. Cup with exposed films.
3. Paper napkin/barrier
4. Overgloved hands.
5. Clean, bare hands (two-glove method).

With barrier envelopes:

1. Noncontaminated exposed film packets.

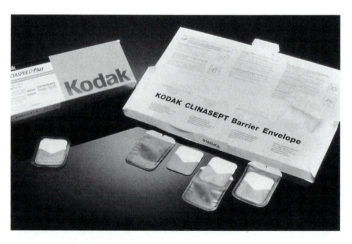

Figure 4.3. Barrier Envelopes. (*Right*) Plastic barrier envelopes. (*Left*) Eastman Kodak has introduced prepackaged intraoral D and E+ speed films sealed in plastic envelopes. Empty polyester envelopes (ClinAsept) may be purchased separately and used to seal and protect conventional film.

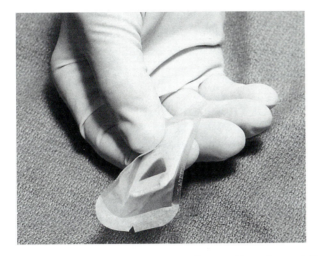

Figure 4.4. Plastic Barrier Envelopes Used With No. 1 Film. The no. 1 film may be placed into these empty barrier envelopes, and the excess plastic folded over the film. Note V-shaped notch.

COMMERCIAL PROTECTIVE BARRIER ENVELOPES (POUCHES)

Eastman Kodak (Rochester, NY) has introduced intraoral D and E+ speed films of all sizes already sealed in plastic barrier envelopes (Kodak dental film with ClinAsept barrier) (Fig. 4.3). This plastic barrier protects the

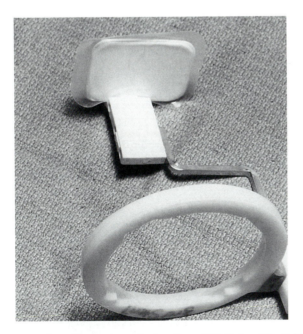

Figure 4.5. Film With Plastic Barrier Envelopes Will Fit Into Film-Holding Instruments. Dentsply/Rinn XCP instrument holding a barrier envelope protecting the film from saliva. The Masel Precision film-holding instrument will also accommodate a film with a plastic barrier envelope.

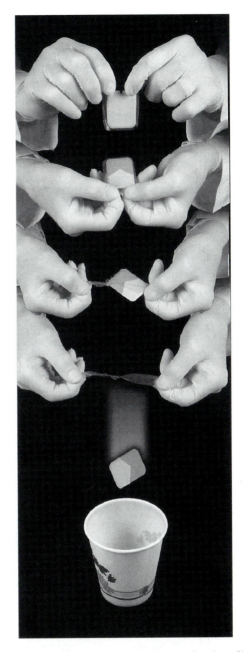

Figure 4.6. Opening the Plastic Barrier Envelope. The clean film can be removed from the plastic envelope and dropped into a container. There is a small "V" cut into the edge of the envelope to facilitate opening.

film from contact with saliva and blood during exposure. These plastic protected films are relatively expensive; however, empty plastic envelopes (ClinAsept barriers) may be purchased separately and used to seal and protect conventionally wrapped film (Fig. 4.3). Although commercial barrier plastic envelopes are large enough to accommodate no. 2 regular film, they do not sell a no. 1 film size plastic barrier. However, a no. 1 film (narrow, anterior film) can be placed in the no. 2 film size plastic envelope and the excess plastic folded over the no. 1 film (Fig. 4.4). The barrier-protected film fits into the Dentsply/Rinn XCP film-holding biteblocks well (Fig. 4.5). If these covers are used on a film, they can be carefully opened and the film packet dropped out (Fig. 4.6). The film packet can then be opened in the conventional manner in the darkroom. The barrier envelope has a small V-shaped notch at the edge (Fig. 4.4) that facilitates opening the envelope. The protective barrier envelopes (pouches) can be conveniently opened in a lighted area, and the film dropped onto a clean paper towel or into a paper cup (Fig. 4.6). The film can then be transported to the daylight loader or darkroom for processing with ungloved, clean hands. Use of these plastic barrier envelopes provides the only uncomplicated method of using a daylight loader and maintaining the integrity of an infection control procedure. They are recommended for use with both paper- or plastic-covered film packets. If barrier envelopes are not used,

refer to the previous section in this chapter, "Atlas of Infection Control Procedures in Intraoral Radiography," for the recommended management of contaminated film packets.

PREPARATION OF THE X-RAY ROOM

Plastic wrap should be used to cover all surfaces that may be touched, including chair arms, headrest, yoke, tubehead, cone (beam indicating device [BID]), and x-ray control panel and switch (Fig. 4.7). These surfaces will then not need to be cleaned and disinfected after dismissal of the patient. Areas that were not covered but were touched and therefore contaminated will require cleaning and disinfection after patient dismissal. The counter top work surface should also be covered with plastic wrap. To avoid unnecessary contamination of patient records, the chart should remain in clean areas of the office only.

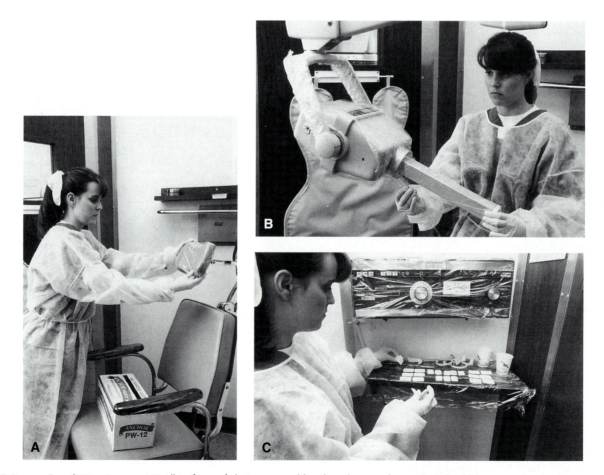

Figure 4.7. Preparation of X-Ray Room. (**A**) All surfaces of chair arms and headrest that may be touched should be covered with plastic wrap. (**B**) The yoke, tubehead, and cone (beam indicating device) should be covered. (**C**) The counter top work surface and control panel should be covered. Sterile x-ray instruments, x-ray film, paper cup, cotton rolls, and latex or vinyl gloves should be placed on the counter top.

EXPOSURE TECHNIQUE

After the patient is seated and the chair adjusted, the disinfected leaded apron and thyroid collar are placed on the patient. Before donning unpowdered latex or vinyl gloves, the operator's hands should be washed with an appropriate antimicrobial soap, such as 4% chlorhexidine gluconate or 3% parachlorometaxylenol (PCMX), or alternately with ordinary liquid hand soap. Although antimicrobial soaps are generally recommended, there is no OSHA requirement specifying that antimicrobial soaps must be used. The patient should be asked to remove partial dentures, dentures, and eyeglasses and store these to avoid cross-contamination. The use of a preprocedural antimicrobial mouth rinse by the patient is a useful and recommended step before inserting any item into the oral cavity. An antimicrobial mouth rinse containing 0.12% chlorhexidine gluconate, a phenolic solution, or a sanguinarine-based active ingredient will reduce intraoral microorganism counts significantly, thereby reducing the quantum of pathogens and minimizing cross-contamination. Before intraoral radiography, the operator should don unpowdered latex or vinyl gloves (Fig. 4.8) and perform a cursory oral examination for complicating factors such as tori, high muscle attachments, ankyloglossia, shallow maxillary palate, malposed teeth, deviations in direction or inclination of interproximal spaces, and the patient's propensity to gag. The operator should then set the x-ray machine control panel for proper mA, kVp, and exposure time settings.

The operator should then open the sterile pack containing the film-holding devices, place the film in the

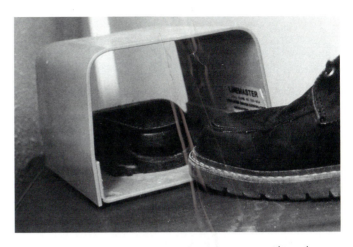

Figure 4.9. Foot Exposure Switch. An x-ray exposure switch can be controlled by a foot pedal to maintain infection control.

biteblock, and position the film and biteblock in the patient's mouth. The tubehead and cone (BID) should be positioned by touching only areas covered with plastic barriers. To avoid contamination, a foot switch can be used to trigger the x-ray unit (Fig. 4.9). If the x-ray machine does not have a foot switch, the exposure button must be covered by a plastic or latex barrier. After exposing the radiograph, excess saliva is wiped from the film packet with a paper towel and then dropped into a clean paper cup without touching the outer surface of the cup. The paper cup should be kept away from the remaining unexposed films. If films are barrier pouched, the operator should remove the plastic envelope from each film (Fig. 4.6) and shake out the films into an empty paper cup after all the films have been exposed. (As an added prevention against contamination, the plastic envelopes can first be disinfected by a spray-wipe-spray procedure; after 10 minutes, the barrier envelope can be removed from the film as described above.)

TRANSPORTATION OF CONTAMINATED FILM PACKETS TO THE DARKROOM

When barrier envelopes are not used, the contaminated film packets require special handling during transportation to the darkroom and the x-ray processor for development. **The first method (overglove method) involves placing overgloves over the contaminated gloves in an aseptic manner before transportation of the exposed films to the darkroom (Fig. 4.10A).** The overgloves should have been placed on the work counter with sleeves folded back toward the palm to facilitate placing overgloves over the contaminated gloves in an aseptic manner. The operator

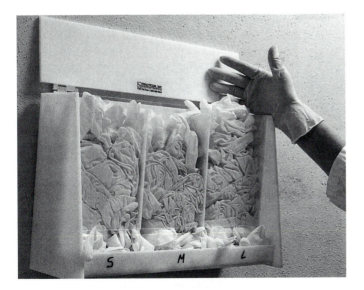

Figure 4.8. Unpowdered Latex or Vinyl Glove Container. Convenient container for three sizes of latex or vinyl gloves.

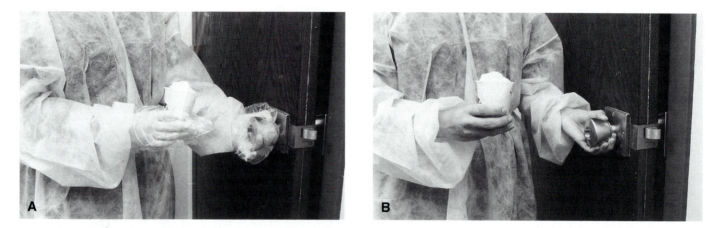

Figure 4.10. Transportation Phase. **(A)** Overglove method of transporting contaminated film to processing area. **(B)** Two-glove method—contaminated gloves are removed for transportation, and new gloves are donned in processing area.

should pick up the paper cup of contaminated exposed films with the overgloved hands. He or she then carries the paper cup to the dark room. Because the overgloves are clean, doors and other items may now be touched (Fig. 4.10A).

The second method (two-glove method) involves the removal of the contaminated gloves in the area of the x-ray machine and transportation of the paper cup of contaminated film to the darkroom or daylight loader with bare, clean hands (Fig. 4.10B). New gloves must be donned over clean, washed hands to unwrap the contaminated film packets in the darkroom or inside the daylight loader. Unpowdered gloves are recommended because glove powders may affect the emulsion and result in artifacts in the image.

DARKROOM PROCESSING OF CONTAMINATED FILM PACKETS

After placing two paper towels on the work surface near the processor, the operator pours the exposed films from the paper cup onto the first (left) paper towel. He or she then discards the overgloves (overglove method) or dons a second set of clean, unpowdered gloves on bare, clean hands (two-glove method of transporting contaminating films). The film is removed from the packet without touching (contaminating) the film (Fig. 4.11). The operator should hold the film packet by color-coded end and grasp the black tab and pull it away from the lead foil and packet (Fig. 4.12). This will pull the black-paper–covered film from the packet. The black-paper–covered film should then be carefully held over the second (right) paper towel and gently shaken until the film drops from the black paper onto the second paper towel (Fig. 4.12).

After all film wrappers have been removed and placed on the first (left) paper towel, the operator should discard these and the contaminated cup while still wearing the contaminated gloves. The contaminated gloves can then be carefully removed and discarded in the normal trash. The operator should wash his or her hands in the darkroom with an antimicrobial or regular hand soap. According to OSHA, hands must always be washed immediately after degloving. With clean, ungloved hands, the exposed films can be held by their edges and fed into the automatic processor slot or be attached to the processing racks used in manual processing. After placing the films into the processor or processing solutions, the authors recommend that hands be washed again. The films should be removed from the processor and dried if necessary. The processed films can now be brought out of the darkroom in a clean paper cup and are ready to be mounted.

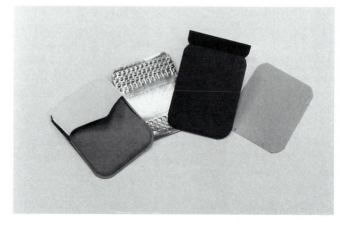

Figure 4.11. Components of Film Packet. From left to right: moisture and light-proof film packet, sheet of lead foil, black light-proof paper, and radiograph film.

placed on the floor of the daylight loader's chamber, and the cup of contaminated, exposed films is positioned on the left side of the floor of the chamber. After closing the lid of the daylight loader, overgloved hands are inserted

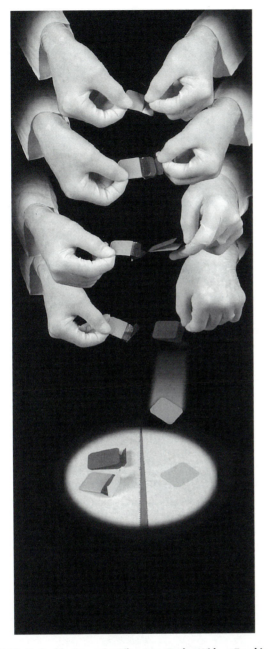

Figure 4.12. Method for Removing Films From Packet Without Touching Them With Contaminated Gloves. From top to bottom: packet tabs are grasped; packet tab is opened; black interleaf paper and film are slid from outer wrapping; and film is dropped onto clean paper towel. Contaminated film packet should be dropped on a separate paper towel.

DAYLIGHT LOADER TECHNIQUE WITH CONTAMINATED FILM PACKETS

OVERGLOVE METHOD

The top lid of the daylight loader should be opened with overgloved hands. A paper towel and clean cup are

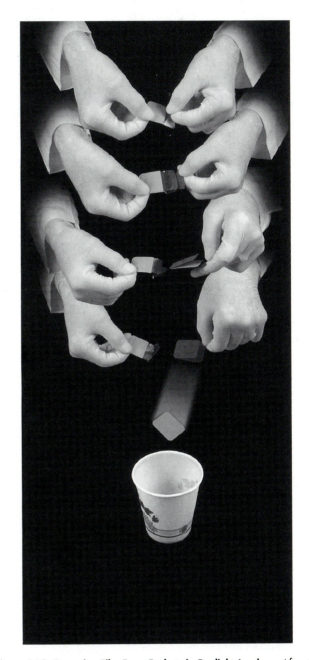

Figure 4.13. Removing Film From Packets in Daylight Loader. After inserting overgloved hands through the sleeves, the overgloves are discarded in daylight loader. With two-glove method, latex or vinyl gloves are placed on clean washed hands outside the daylight loader, and the newly gloved hands are inserted through the sleeves. With latex- or vinyl-gloved hands inside the daylight loader (either method), the polysoft cover should be removed without touching the film. The film is dropped into the paper cup without being touched.

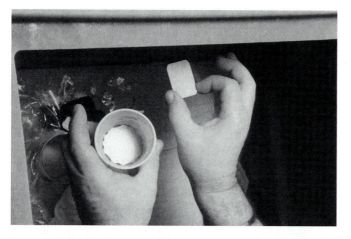

Figure 4.14. Feeding Film In Daylight Loader Slots. After removing film from packets, gloves are discarded. With ungloved, clean hands, the film should be picked up by the edges and fed into processor slots.

through the sleeves (overglove method). The overgloves are removed and placed on the left side paper towel. The film packets are carefully opened with the contaminated gloves by pulling gently on the outer tab. The exposed film should never be touched by the contaminated gloves (Fig. 4.13). The black tab is carefully pulled back; when the black-paper–covered film is out of the white outer packet, the black paper is gently shaken until the films drop into the clean paper cup on the right. As the operator opens each film packet, he or she discards the black paper, lead foil, and plastic white film packet on the left side of the chamber. Once all film wrappings have been removed and the uncontaminated exposed films have been dropped into the clean paper cup on the right, the powder-free gloves are removed aseptically and discarded on the left side of the daylight loader chamber floor. With clean, ungloved hands, the operator picks up the films by the edges and feeds them into the processor (Fig. 4.14). When the last film has been fed into the processor slot, the ungloved hands are pulled through the sleeves. Clean overgloves are worn over bare hands to remove the waste from the daylight loader and to discard this into the regular waste bin. Hands must be washed before processed films are removed from the processor and placed in the film mounts.

TWO-GLOVE METHOD

An alternative two-glove method is for the operator to don new gloves after placing the contaminated films in a cup in the bottom of the daylight loader chamber with bare, clean hands as previously described. Hands are then washed, and new unpowdered gloves are donned. After inserting the gloved hands through the sleeves, the film

unwrapping procedure is the same as previously described, but without overgloves and using a second set of clean gloves instead of the original contaminated gloves Fig. 4.13).

POSTPROCEDURAL DUTIES

According to OSHA, any contaminated film-holders should be placed in a holding solution before further decontamination and sterilization. In the previously used room containing the x-ray machine, operators should wear new overgloves, latex examination gloves, or utility gloves to remove contaminated waste materials and plastic surface covers from radiographic equipment, chair, and control unit. These are discarded into a regular waste bin. Also, any contaminated surfaces or equipment should be disinfected using the three-step spray-wipe-spray method. The apron and/or thyroid collar should be cleaned and disinfected (Fig. 4.15). Soiled disposable items, such as vinyl or latex gloves, paper towels, and x-ray film packets, are not considered as infectious (regulated) medical waste. "Regulated" waste must be "capable of releasing fluids when compressed." Examples include blood or saliva-soaked gauze or cotton rolls.

PANORAMIC RADIOGRAPHS

When taking panoramic radiographs, the operator should come to the panoramic x-ray machine with washed hands and no gloves (Fig. 4.16A). There is no need to wrap anything for this procedure, except to cover the bite guide with a "baggie" or "finger cot" or to use a premanufactured disposable bite guide. The patient

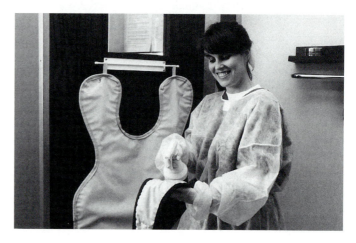

Figure 4.15. Spray-Wipe-Spray. Disinfection by the spray-wipe-spray method of nonwrapped contaminated equipment is necessary on completion of the procedure if contaminated and at the end of the day.

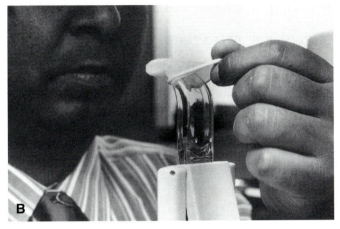

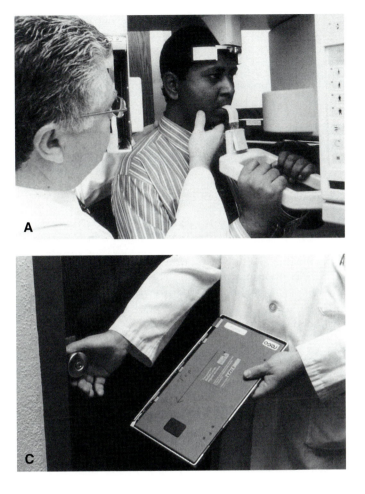

Figure 4.16. Panoramic Radiology. (**A**) No personal protective equipment is required for the operator. (**B**) Patient places and removes latex biteblock sleeve. (**C**) Processing panoramic film requires no infection control procedures.

should be asked to rinse with a preprocedural mouthwash. To prevent contamination of the operator's hands, the patient places and removes the disposable biteblock or cover and discards them after the exposure in a regular waste bin (Fig. 4.16B). The patient chin rest, head positioning guides, and "hand grips" of the panoramic x-ray unit should be sanitized (cleaned) **after** making the exposure. No further infection control procedures are necessary for processing (Fig. 4.16C).

SUMMARY

Although exposure to blood is rare in oral and maxillofacial radiology, contact with saliva occurs, especially with intraoral techniques. Thus, the spread of infectious diseases is possible through cross-contamination, and specific infection control protocols and procedures as well as unit dosing of items are needed. This chapter outlined the rationale for implementing state-of-the-art infection control procedures and explained federal standards and guidelines as they affect infection control and occupational safety in dental radiology procedures.

Proper infection control measures, including the use of disposable gloves, sterilization of reusable instruments, and the use of appropriate environmental cleaning and disinfection procedures, should be practiced at all times during the exposure and processing of dental radiographs. Surfaces that may be contaminated during radiographic techniques should be covered with disposable covers, which is a faster and less-expensive method than routinely using cleaning and disinfecting procedures. When indicated, an excellent alternate to the full-mouth survey is a properly exposed and processed panoramic radiograph. It is a simple radiographic procedure requiring much fewer infection control measures, has greater coverage than the full-mouth survey, and provides diagnostic information regarding periodontal disease, caries, and periapical disease as well as many other diseases affecting the teeth and jaw bones. In panoramic radiology, the radiation dose for the patient is very much lower than in the full-mouth survey.

WORKSHOP/LABORATORY EXERCISES

EXERCISE 4.1. PREPARATION OF X-RAY ROOM

Materials and Equipment Needed

1. One intraoral film.
2. Two paper cups.
3. Food wrap or other barrier material.
4. EPA-registered disinfecting solution.
5. Latex or vinyl examination gloves (powderless).
6. Dentsply/Rinn (or other) biteblocks and film-positioning device.

Instructions

For this exercise, the student must demonstrate the proper infection control preparations of the x-ray unit control and machine parts, chair, and adjacent counter top work areas before taking one periapical radiograph using the paralleling technique. When all preparations have been made, the instructor will check the room before continuing on to exercise 4.2.

EXERCISE 4.2. FOOD DYE DEMONSTRATION

Materials and Equipment Needed

1. Latex or vinyl examination gloves used in exercise 4.1.
2. Vinyl (food handler's) overglove.
3. Cup containing "contaminated" film packet, which has been "whetted" with water or better still, glycerine (available in food and drug stores) solution. The water or glycerine solution should be colored with food dye.

Instructions

Using the overglove method, demonstrate either:

Step 1. Transportation, placement into the daylight loader, unwrapping of the contaminated film packet, and isolation of the clean film therein. Do not process the film. Demonstrate how the contaminated materials are discarded.

Or . . .

Transportation, entry into the darkroom, preparation of the counter top, unwrapping of the contaminated film packet, and isolation of the clean film. Do not process the film. Demonstrate to the instructor how the contaminated materials are discarded.

Step 2. Examine your hands; note if any food dye is on them. Explain the significance of this. Explain the significance of any food dye remaining on the counter top or processing equipment.

EXERCISE 4.3. POSTPROCEDURAL DUTIES

Materials and Equipment Needed

1. Gloves (clean).
2. Waste container(s).
3. Waste materials used in exercise 4.1.
4. Decontaminating solutions.
5. Paper towels or other "wipe" material.

Instructions

Return to the room where the x-ray machine is located. Demonstrate to the instructor all procedures necessary before preparing the room for the next x-ray patient.

Explain why you chose to place all or some discarded materials in either or both the "unregulated" waste container versus the "regulated" waste container.

CASE-BASED PROBLEM-SOLVING

Intraoral radiography is such a hassle, especially when it comes to infection control! For this exercise, and in many other clinical circumstances, we accept that one or several intraoral radiographs will always be needed. However, assuming the information in a full-mouth survey is needed, can you suggest another method whereby all, most, or even more x-ray information about the patient's teeth and jaws can be obtained, but without most of the infection control hassles of the full-mouth survey? Make an infection control comparison chart comparing the full-mouth survey and your proposed alternate method.

Hint: Carefully read "Atlas of Infection Control Procedures in Intraoral Radiography" in this chapter. The answers are mentioned in several areas within the chapter.

REVIEW QUESTIONS

1. In which of the following can diseases be spread as a result of taking an intraoral radiograph?

A. From patient to DHCW.
B. From DHCW to patient.
C. From one patient to another patient.
D. All of the above.
E. None of the above.

2. The components of an infection control protocol in dental radiography include:

A. Operatory.
B. Darkroom.
C. Operator.
D. A and C only.
E. All of the above.

3. Bacterial spores are a problem in sterilizing x-ray instruments and equipment because:

A. They are resistant to antibiotics.
B. They are easy to kill but are usually protected by organic matter.
C. They are very resistant to physical and chemical agents.
D. Most pathogenic bacteria are spore formers.

4. In general, personal protective equipment includes:

A. Gloves.
B. Masks.
C. Gowns.
D. Resuscitation bags, pocket masks, other ventilation devices.
E. All of the above.

5. You are about to perform a full-mouth survey on a patient who has no medical conditions, as indicated by the medical history and interview. For this appointment the dental professional should wear:

A. Gloves only.
B. Glasses and a face mask.
C. Glasses and gloves.
D. Glasses, gloves, and a face mask.

6. Which of the following statements is/are correct?

A. Taking sterilized x-ray instruments out of a package and placing them in clean drawers is recommended.
B. Hands should be washed thoroughly before and after taking intraoral radiographs.
C. The risk of contracting acquired immune deficiency syndrome (AIDS) during x-ray procedures

is greater than the occupational risk for hepatitis B.
D. Both A and C are correct.
E. Both A and B are correct.

7. The most commonly used glove type for x-ray procedures are _____ gloves.

A. Medical grade vinyl.
B. Sterile vinyl.
C. Unsterile latex.
D. Sterile latex.
E. Unsterile polynitrite.

8. The class of chemical that is least effective as a surface disinfecting agent is:

A. Hypochlorite.
B. Iodophor.
C. Complex phenol.
D. Synthetic phenol.
E. 70% isopropyl alcohol.

9. With respect to x-ray instruments, which of the following statements is most appropriate?

A. Sterilize everything.
B. Be certain to sterilize hands before x-ray procedures.
C. Dark drawer sterilization can work under certain conditions.
D. Do not worry about sterilization for most x-ray instruments.
E. Do not disinfect when you can sterilize.

BIBLIOGRAPHY

American Academy of Oral and Maxillofacial Radiology. Infection control guidelines for dental radiographic procedures. Oral Surg Oral Med Oral Pathol 1992;73:248–249.

American Dental Association. Infection control recommendations for the dental office and dental laboratory. J Am Dent Assoc 1992; 123(Suppl 1).

Bachman CE, White JM, Goodis HE, et al. Bacterial adherence and contamination during radiologic processing. Oral Surg Oral Med Oral Pathol 1990;76:112–119.

Bajuscak RE, Hall EH, Giumbarresi LI. Bacterial contamination of dental radiographic film. J Dent Res 1991;70:1439. Abstract.

Bajuscak RE, Hall EH, Weaver T, et al. Sporicidin and chlorine bleach disinfectant of dental radiographic film. J Dent Res 1991;70:1439. Abstract.

Centers for Disease Control and Prevention. Recommended infection control practices for dentistry. MMWR 1993;42:RR-8.

Crawford JJ, Young JM, Stokes L. Proper operatory and instrument recirculation. In: Cottone JA, Terezhalmy GT, Melanuria JA, eds. Practical infection control in dentistry. Philadelphia: Lea & Febiger, 1991:149–160.

Department of Labor (DOL) Occupational Safety and Health Administration (OSHA) 1900.1200. Hazard Communication, Standards and Interpretations. Fed Reg April, 1988;53:15035:806.15–806.31.

Department of Labor (DOL) Occupational Safety and Health Administration (OSHA) 29 CAR, Part 1910.1030. Occupational Exposure to Bloodborne Pathogens: Final Rule. Fed Reg 1991;56:640004–640182.

Favor MS, Bond WE. Chemical disinfection of medical and surgical materials. In: Block SO, ed. Disinfection, sterilization and preservation. 4th ed. Philadelphia: Lea & Febiger, 1991:617–641.

Glass BJ. Infection control in dental radiology. In: Cottone JA, Terezhalmy GT, Melanuria JA, eds. Practical infection control in dentistry. Philadelphia: Lea & Febiger, 1991:167–175.

Goaz PW, White SC. Oral radiology. 3rd ed. St. Louis: CV Mosby, 1994:219–236.

Hubar JS, Oeschger MP, Reiter AT. Effectiveness of radiographic film barrier envelopes. Gen Dent 1994;43:406–408.

Katz JO, Geist JR, Melanuria JA, et al. Potential for bacterial and mycotic growth in developer and fixer solutions. J Dentomaxillofac Radiol 1988;(Suppl 10):52. Abstract.

Katz JO, Cottone JA, Hardman PK, et al. Infection control protocol for dental radiology. Gen Dent 1990;38:261–264.

Langlais RP. OSHA compliance manual. Washington, DC: OSHA, 1995:4–5, 20, 23, 45–46, 55, 64.

Miller CH, Palenik CJ. Sterilization, disinfection and asepsis in dentistry. In: Block SS, ed. Disinfection, sterilization and preservation. 4th ed. Philadelphia: Lea & Febiger, 1991:676–695.

Melanuria JA, Melanuria GE. Is mouth rinsing before dental procedures worthwhile? J Am Dent Assoc 1992;123:75–80.

Neaverth EJ, Pantera EA. Chairside disinfection of radiographs. Oral Surg Oral Med Oral Pathol 1991;71:116–119.

OSAP Research Foundation Infection Control in Dentistry Guide-Lines. May 1993. Available from OSAP, 2150 West 29th Avenue, Suite 310, Denver, CO 80211.

Packota GV, Komiyama K. Surface disinfection of saliva-contaminated dental x-ray film packets. J Can Dent Assoc 1992;58:747–751.

Palenik CJ, Miller CH. Radiologic asepsis. Dent Asepsis Rev 1994;15:1–2. Available from the Sterilization Monitoring Service, Indiana University School of Dentistry, Indianapolis, IN.

Parks ET, Farman AG. Infection control for dental radiographic procedures in US dental hygiene programs. J Dentomaxillofac Radiol 1992;21:16–20.

Puttaiah R, Langlais RP, Katz JO, et al. Infection control in dental radiology. CDA J 1995:12:21–18.

Runnels RR. Infectious diseases important in dentistry. In: Cottone JA, Terezhalmy GT, Melanuria JA, eds. Practical infection control in dentistry. Philadelphia: Lea & Febiger, 1991:1–17.

Spaulding EH. Chemical disinfection of medical and surgical materials. In: Lawrence A, Block SO, eds. Disinfection, preservation and sterilization. Philadelphia: Lea & Febiger, 1968:517–531.

Stanczyk DA, Paunovich ED, Broome JC, et al. Microbiologic contamination during dental radiographic film processing. Oral Med Oral Surg Oral Pathol 1993;76:112–119.

Wolfgang L. Analysis of a new barrier infection control system for dental radiographic film. Compend Contin Educ Dent 1992;8:68–71.

Young JM. Aseptic consideration in dental equipment selection. In: Cottone JA, Terezhalmy GT, Melanuria JA, eds. Practical infection control in dentistry. Philadelphia: Lea & Febiger, 1991:136–147.

Intraoral Radiographic Techniques

5

OBJECTIVES

Upon successful completion of this unit, the student will be able to:

1. *State the three types of intraoral projections.*

2. *Explain the four basic principles of periapical techniques.*

3. *Identify the two types of intraoral periapical techniques.*

4. *Discuss the six rules to follow in using the paralleling technique.*

5. *Demonstrate the Dentsply/Rinn long cone paralleling technique.*

6. *Describe the bisecting angle technique.*

7. *Demonstrate the bitewing technique.*

8. *Describe the three types of occlusal projections.*

9. *Discuss the proper positioning of a patient in the event an aiming device is not used during the exposure.*

10. *Describe how to manage patients with special problems.*

11. *Perform a full-mouth or half-mouth survey on a skull or manikin using the Workshop/Laboratory Exercises format.*

12. *Explain how to handle a common problem with the paralleling technique in the maxilla using the Case-Based Questions format.*

13. *Test his or her knowledge by answering the Review Questions.*

KEY WORDS/PHRASES

ala-tragus line

beam indicating device

bisecting angle technique

biteblock

bitewing radiograph

bitewing tab

film-holders

film placement

gagging patient

glossopharyngeal nerve

horizontal angulation

indicator rod

locator ring

maxillary orientation line

occlusal radiograph

paralleling technique

periapical

periapical radiograph

problematic patients

psychic stimuli

rectangular collimation

rectangular cone

round cone

rule of isometry

sagittal plane

tactile stimuli

topographic

vertical angulation

INTRODUCTION

Intraoral radiographs are made by placing the film packet inside the oral cavity and projecting the x-ray beam at various angles from a position outside the mouth through the anatomical region of interest toward the film. There are three types of intraoral projections: (1) **periapical**, (2) **bitewing**, and (3) **occlusal**.

PERIAPICAL RADIOGRAPHS

Periapical radiographs ("peri" meaning "around," and "apical" meaning "apex" or "end" of tooth root) record images of the outlines, position, and mesiodistal extent of the teeth and surrounding tissues. In a periapical radio-

graph, it is essential to obtain the full length of the tooth and at least 2 mm of the periapical bone (Fig. 5.1). The most universal film size is the no. 2 film size, which can be can be used for the older pediatric patient and for almost all adults.

BITEWING RADIOGRAPHS

Bitewing radiographs record, on a single film, images of the outlines, position, and extent of the crowns and the coronal one third of the interalveolar bone and a portion of roots of the maxillary and mandibular teeth. Much less frequently, vertical bitewings are used to extend the vertical coverage of the interalveolar bone and roots; however, the horizontal coverage is diminished, so more radiographs must be taken. A tab or special bitewing film-holding device is needed to hold the film in place. Bitewing film can be purchased pretabbed in any of the mentioned sizes. Bitewings can also be made by purchasing bitewing tabs that can be centered horizontally or vertically on the film packet. Various sizes of film may be used for bitewings including the type 2, type 1, and type 0 film sizes and a longer version of size 2 called type 3. All film sizes can be purchased in single or double film packets with or without bitewing tabs. They are valuable for detecting interproximal caries, overhangs on restorations, periodontal conditions, calculus deposits, chronic resorption of the interalveolar bone, the pulp chamber shape and size, pulp stones, and the occlusal relationship of the teeth. Bitewings are particularly valuable for the detection of small interproximal carious lesions that are difficult or impossible to find by other clinical methods, including periapical radiographs. This is because the film is very close to and parallel to the teeth, and the x-ray beam is perpendicular to the teeth and film.

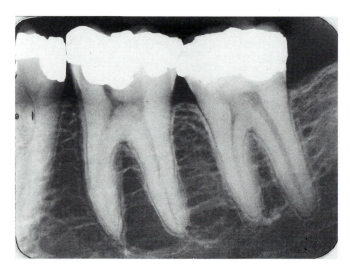

Figure 5.1. Periapical Radiographs. Left mandibular molar view.

OCCLUSAL RADIOGRAPHS

Occlusal radiographs record images of the incisal edges and the occlusal surfaces of the teeth and a cross-section of the dental arches. The maxillary occlusal radiograph depicts images of the hard palate, upper lip, and base of the nose; the mandibular occlusal radiograph records the images of the tongue, floor of the mouth, and lower lip. *Occlusal radiographs* are used to detect the presence and relative positions of impacted or embedded teeth, foreign bodies, fractures, stones in the salivary ducts, and other gross abnormal conditions or lesions of the jaws.

COMPLETE-MOUTH SURVEY/FULL-MOUTH SURVEY

A complete-mouth x-ray survey (CMX) or full-mouth survey (FMX) is composed of a series of individual periapical and bitewing radiographs. This survey should completely cover all the teeth and tooth-bearing alveolar bone of both arches. A complete intraoral radiographic survey may consist of as many as 22 films, whereas another survey may have fewer total films. The number of radiographs needed for a complete radiographic examination of a patient will depend on the technique used, number of teeth present, condition of the teeth, age of the patient, individual anatomical variations, film size used, and diagnostic needs of the dentist. We recommend that an adult dentulous CMX consist of 14 to 16 periapicals and 4 bitewings (Fig. 5.2A). For patients who are partially or totally edentulous (without teeth), the CMX can be streamlined to as many as 10 to 14 periapicals (Fig. 5.2B).

BASIC PRINCIPLES OF PERIAPICAL RADIOGRAPHY

There are certain basic principles that must be considered in the learning and perfecting of periapical intraoral radiographic techniques. They include (1) the anatomy of the teeth and jaws, (2) patient head position, (3) x-ray beam angulation, and (4) point of entry of x-ray beam.

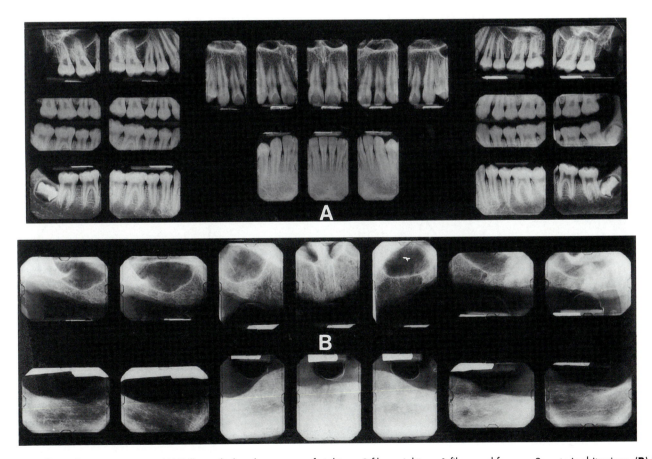

Figure 5.2. Full-Mouth X-Ray Surveys. **(A)** Full-mouth dentulous survey of eight no. 2 films, eight no. 1 films, and four no. 2 posterior bitewings. **(B)** Full-mouth survey of edentulous mouth using 14 no. 2 films.

ANATOMICAL CONSIDERATIONS

There are two anatomical considerations the operator must take into consideration before the placement of the film into the patient's mouth. They are the (1) location of the long axes of the teeth and (2) location of the apices of the teeth.

LOCATION OF THE LONG AXES OF THE TEETH

Excellence in intraoral radiographic technique depends on the operator's knowledge of the approximate positions of the long axes of the teeth in the jaws. Practically all the teeth in the upper jaw are tilted outward (buccally or facially) (Fig. 5.3). The flatter the palatal vault of the maxilla, the greater the tendency for the teeth to tilt outward. In the mandible, the six anterior teeth are usually tilted outward; on occasion, they sometimes are positioned vertically or tilted backward (lingually). The mandibular premolars, on the other hand, are usually positioned more nearly vertical, and the lower molars tilt slightly lingual (Fig. 5.4). Also, the operator should be aware that the crown or apparent axis of the tooth is different from the root or true axis of the tooth (Fig. 5.5). A line drawn through the vertical axis of the crown of the tooth and one drawn through the root forms an angle (crown-root angle) that generally varies from 5° to 20°. Furthermore, the greater the tilt of the tooth, the greater the crown-root angle.

LOCATION OF THE APICES OF THE TEETH

The apical region of the maxillary teeth is located on an imaginary line drawn from the tragus (bump in front of the ear opening) of the ear to the ala (wing) of the nose. To localize each maxillary tooth's apical region, a line is dropped from various landmarks on the face to the ala-tragus line (Fig. 5.6). The apices of the mandibular teeth are 0.5 cm above the lower border of the mandible. The same landmarks used for localizing the maxillary teeth may be used in the mandible, except the vertical lines must be extended further down past the ala-tragus line to the point 0.5 cm above the inferior border of the mandible.

HEAD POSITION

In almost all the intraoral periapical techniques, it is recommended that the patient be placed in an upright position, with the occlusal plane of the teeth to be radiographed parallel to the floor, and the sagittal plane of the head perpendicular to the floor. The **sagittal plane of the**

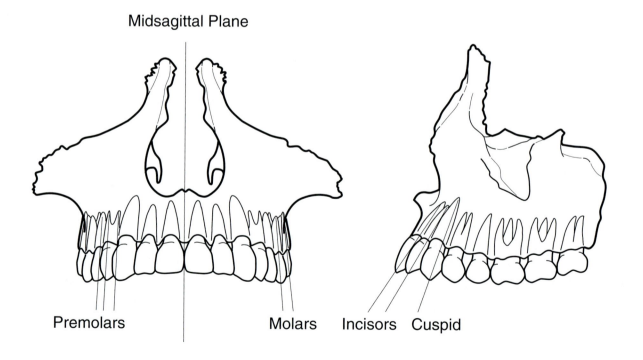

Midsagittal Plane

Premolars   Molars   Incisors   Cuspid

Maxillary Arch

Figure 5.3. Maxillary Teeth Angulations.   Drawing of long axes of teeth in the maxillary arch. Note that all teeth are inclined outward.

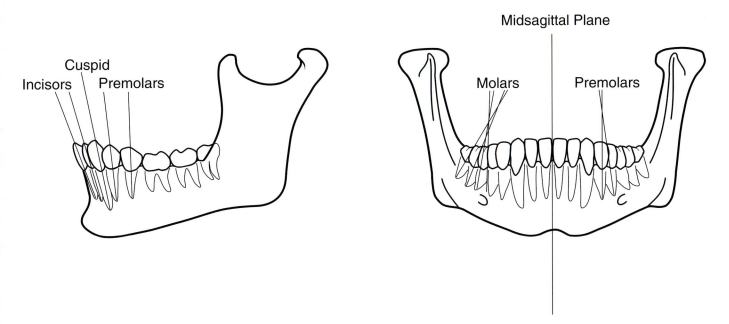

Figure 5.4. Mandibular Teeth Angulations. Drawing of long axes of teeth in mandibular arch. Anterior six teeth are usually tilted outward; the mandibular premolars are usually positioned more nearly vertical. Lower molars tilt slightly inward.

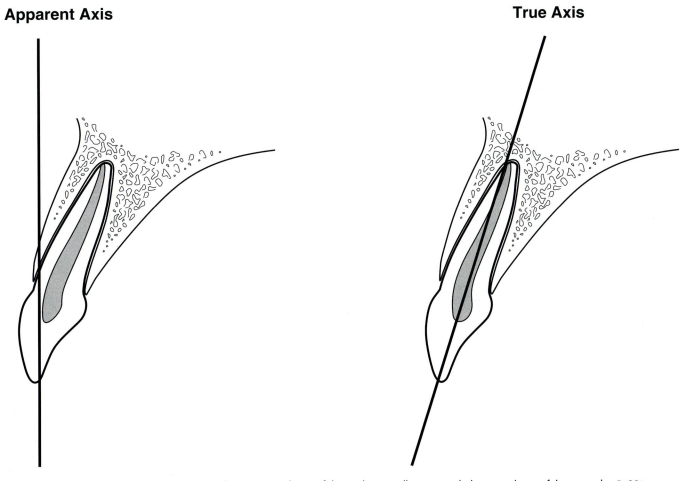

Figure 5.5. True Vertical Axis of Tooth. The true vertical axis of the tooth generally varies with the vertical axis of the crown by 5–20°.

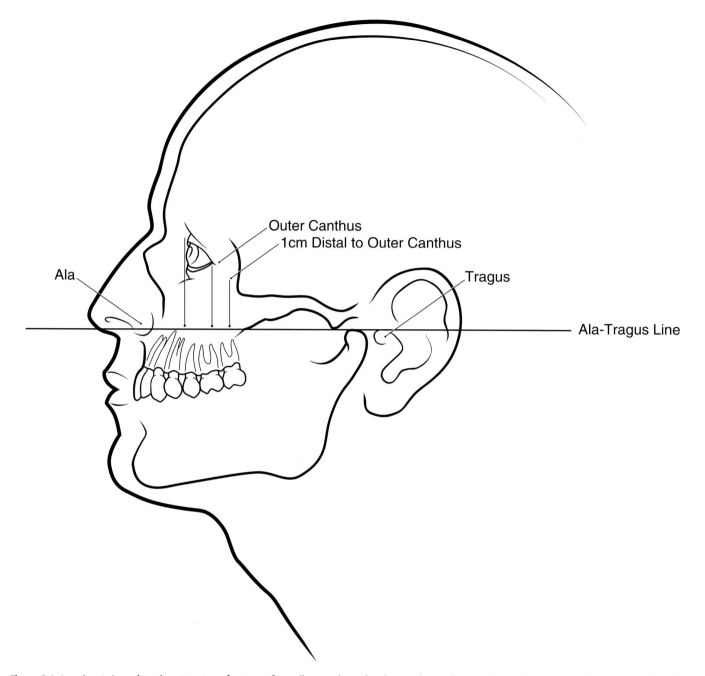

Outer Canthus
1cm Distal to Outer Canthus

Ala

Tragus

Ala-Tragus Line

Figure 5.6. Locating Apices of Teeth. Drawing of apices of maxillary teeth. To localize each maxillary tooth apical region, use the imaginary line from various landmarks on the face to the ala-tragus line. The landmarks for the maxillary second molar, first molar, second premolar, canine, and incisors are shown on the drawing. In the mandible, the root apices can be established by estimating the points of entry from the lower border of the mandible. This is usually the width of the thumb (0.25 inches).

skull divides the skull vertically in the midline into right and left halves. The **maxillary orientation line** is an imaginary line drawn from the tragus of the ear to the ala of the nose and is often referred to as the ala-tragus line. This line should be parallel to the floor when radiographing the maxillary teeth. The **mandibular occlusal plane** changes when the mouth is opened. It is on a line from the corner of the mouth to the tragus of the ear. Therefore, the patient's head should be tilted slightly backward so the occlusal plane of the mandible will be parallel to the floor when the mouth is opened. The operator should make sure that the patient does not open too wide, as this will contract the muscles of the floor of the mouth and make it difficult to place mandibular periapical films down far enough. If the patient tenses the muscles of the floor of the mouth, the film will not go down far enough, and the patient will experience pain when closing down on the biteblock. These muscles can be relaxed by swallowing.

The **sagittal plane of the skull** (midline of the face) should be perpendicular to the floor before placing films into the mouth. The correct head position makes for a good starting point no matter what intraoral radiographic technique is used. Also, for the operator's comfort and to avoid back strain, the chair should be raised or lowered so the patient's mouth is about level with the operator's elbow when he or she stands beside the patient.

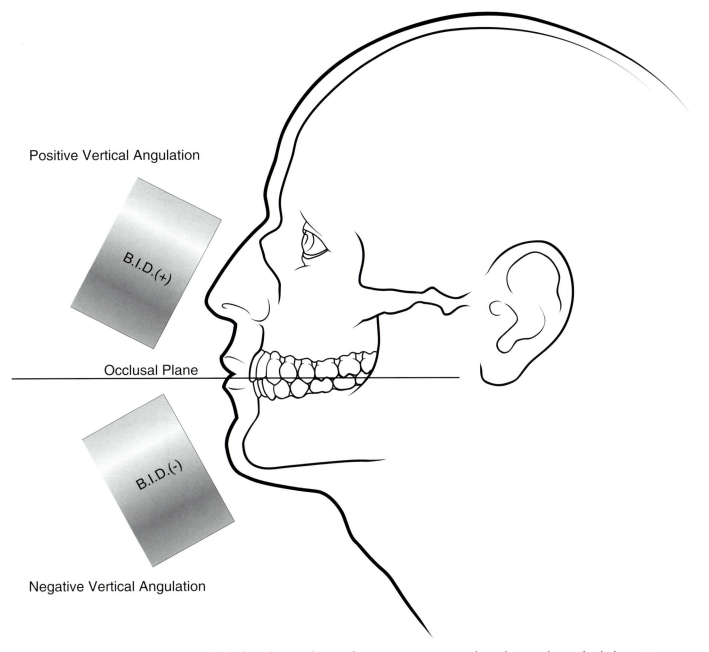

Positive Vertical Angulation

B.I.D.(+)

Occlusal Plane

B.I.D.(-)

Negative Vertical Angulation

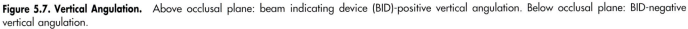

Figure 5.7. Vertical Angulation. Above occlusal plane: beam indicating device (BID)-positive vertical angulation. Below occlusal plane: BID-negative vertical angulation.

X-RAY BEAM ANGULATION

The x-ray tubehead has two directional projections: **vertical** angulation and **horizontal** angulation. **Vertical** angulation is the movement of the tubehead up and down in relation to the occlusal plane, which is parallel to the floor (Fig. 5.7). The changes in vertical angulation are measured in degrees and recorded on a dial located on the side of the x-ray tubehead. A downward angulation of the cone is a positive, or plus (+), angulation; an upward angulation of the cone is a negative, or minus (−), angulation. **Horizontal** angulation is the movement of the x-ray tubehead around the patient's head in relation to the sagittal plane when the patient is in an upright position (Fig. 5.8). Horizontal angulation is the same direction as the horizon. The horizontal angles rotate around the patient's head, or 360°, as if the head were a center of a circle. The horizontal angulation of the x-ray beam should be directed through the contacts of the teeth and perpendicular to the horizontal plane of the film, if possible (Fig. 5.9). There are countless ways that teeth may be rotated or malposed from the normal occlusal pattern. To open the contact areas of teeth on a radiograph, the operator must observe how the teeth contact each other and then project the x-rays through the contact areas of the teeth at a 90° angle to the film. Improper horizontal angulation will cause **overlapping** of the tooth images, which may obscure diagnostic information such as the presence of caries, redecay, calculus, or an open contact (Fig. 5.10).

POINT OF ENTRY

The point of entry of the x-ray beam should be directed through the center of the region being radiographed. The objective is to completely cover the film with the beam of radiation. If this is **not** done, a "cone-cut" or "partial image" will be seen in the resultant radiograph (Fig. 5.11). This area on the film will be clear, as it was not exposed to the x-ray beam.

PERIAPICAL RADIOGRAPHY TECHNIQUES

There are two intraoral periapical techniques that are used in dental radiography to minimize shape distortion of the radiographic image: the **paralleling technique** and

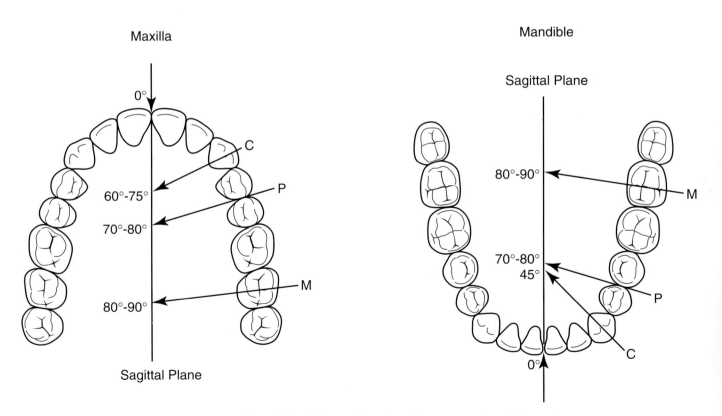

Figure 5.8. Horizontal Angulation.   Horizontal angulation for various regions of the mouth.

Maxilla

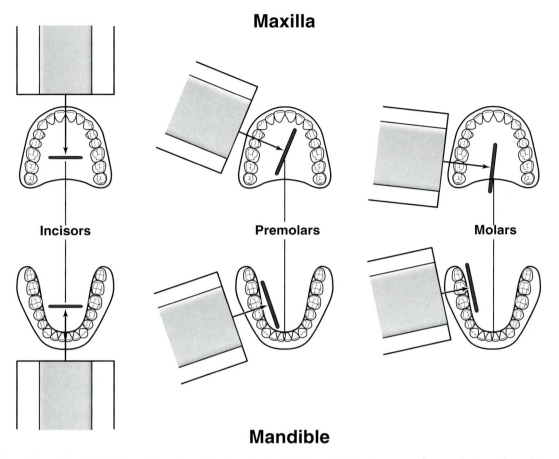

Incisors **Premolars** **Molars**

Mandible

Figure 5.9. Horizontal Angulation (Path of Central Ray Perpendicular to Horizontal Plane of Film). Summary of proper horizontal angulations of BID (cone) and film coverage with x-ray beam for each region of the jaw. Note the size of the smaller rectangular BID (cone) and the size of the larger circular BID (cone).

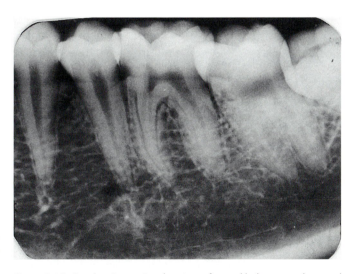

Figure 5.10. Overlapping. Overlapping of mandibular premolars and molars from improper film placement or cone (BID) placement.

the **bisecting angle technique**. The **paralleling technique** is preferred because it produces a more accurate and less distorted radiographic image than the **bisecting angle technique**. However, there are advantages and disadvantages to both techniques, and there are anatomical variations from patient to patient or within the oral cavity of the same patient that present circumstances for modification of the projection technique used.

PARALLELING OR RIGHT ANGLE TECHNIQUE

The paralleling or right angle intraoral radiographic technique is based on the paralleling principle. The paralleling principle, in essence, follows the five rules of accurate image formation (discussed in Chapter 3) to minimize the undesirable image characteristics of **unsharpness, magnification,** and **shape distortion** (Fig. 5.12).

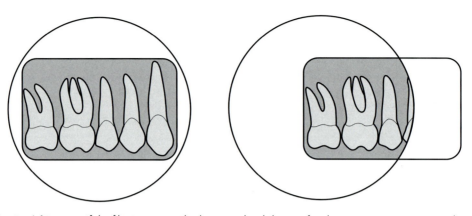

Figure 5.11. "Cone-Cut" or Partial Image.   If the film is not completely covered with beam of radiation, a cone-cut or partial image will be seen on the radiograph. Round cone (BID) in right diagram is positioned too far posteriorly for film placed in premolar region.

The **two** fundamental rules for the paralleling technique are:

1. The film is placed in the mouth in a position that is parallel to the long axes of the teeth.
2. The central ray of the x-ray beam is directed perpendicular or at right angles to both the long axes of the teeth and the plane of the film.

To achieve parallelism between the film and the long axes of the teeth, the object-film distance will have to be increased (especially in the maxillary arch). Of course, this goes against one of the five rules of accurate image formation, which states that the film should be as close as possible to the object being radiographed. Therefore, to compensate for the undesirable image characteristics of geometric unsharpness and magnification caused by this modification, the source-film distance is *increased* as much as possible. This is probably why this technique has been referred to as the "long cone" technique in the past. The source-film distance of *16 inches* is the most practical distance to be used in most dental offices. If the room is small, an x-ray machine with a recessed cone (beam indicating device [BID]) can be obtained. Although the 12-inch source-film distance is a compromise, the authors do not recommend the use of a 12-inch source-film distance or less (8 inches) with the paralleling technique because this goes against the second rule of accurate image

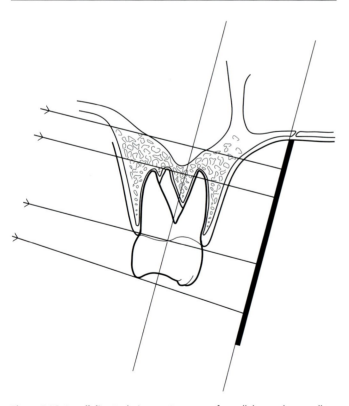

Figure 5.12. Paralleling Technique.   Diagram of paralleling technique illustrating the relationship of the film and teeth in the paralleling (right-angle) technique.

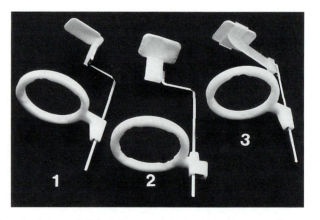

Figure 5.13. Dentsply/Rinn XCP Instruments.   (1) Anterior no. 1 film instrument. (2) Posterior no. 2 film instrument. (3) Bitewing instrument with no. 2 film.

formation, which states that the source-film distance should be as long as possible. A typical FMX using the paralleling technique consists of 16 periapical and 4 bitewing projections, as shown in Fig. 5.2A.

Film-Holders (Paralleling Technique)

According to technique, the film must be placed as nearly parallel to the long axes of the teeth as possible, keeping the film flat at all times and retaining it in position until it is properly exposed.

Various film-holders have been designed to enable the operator to accomplish this and overcome problems associated with film retention and alignment.

1. The Dentsply/Rinn XCP instruments (extension cone paralleling) (Fig. 5.13).
2. The Masel Precision rectangular collimating instruments (Fig. 5.14).
3. The Stabe disposable film-holder (Fig. 5.15).
4. The Snap-A-Ray film-holder (Dunvale Dental Products) and EEZEE Grip Film-Holder (Dentsply/Rinn) (Fig. 5.16).

The first two instruments (Dentsply/Rinn XCP and Masel Precision) have an added benefit in radiation reduction to the patient by **rectangular collimation**. This will be discussed more completely in Chapter 13. The Dentsply/Rinn XCP instruments must be used with a rectangular cone or BID to collimate the beam of radiation rectangularly. However, a stainless steel collimator (Dentsply/Rinn) can be attached to the XCP alignment ring, or a Universal Rectangular Collimator (Dentsply/Rinn) can be

attached to a round cone to provide rectangular collimation when using a round cone (BID) (Fig. 5.17). The Masel Precision instrument collimates the x-ray beam at the skin surface (Fig. 5.14).

Snap-A-Ray or EEZEE Grip Film-Holder

The EEZEE Grip or Snap-A-Ray film-holder is a simple plastic film-holder that can be used in both the posterior and the anterior regions of the mouth. It does **not** use a film backing; therefore, the film may bend and cause image distortion. When the film bends using the Snap-A-Ray (particularly in the maxillary arch), the film position resembles the film position in the bisecting angle technique rather than the paralleling technique, and the BID must be aligned accordingly. In addition, the problem is compounded because the film-holders do **not** have an alignment device to aid in the determination of the vertical and horizontal angulations of the cone (BID). However, it is a useful instrument, particularly in patients who cannot tolerate the use of the film backing part of the biteblock in various regions of the oral cavity (Fig. 5.16).

The **Snap-A-Ray or EEZEE Grip Film-Holder** is particularly useful for the following:

1. Mandibular premolar and molar projections. Because these teeth have almost perpendicular root axes, the film can be positioned parallel to the teeth without increasing the object-film distance.
2. Maxillary and mandibular third molar projections.
3. Patients with hypersensitive gag reflexes.
4. Children.
5. Edentulous projections.
6. Endodontic projections.

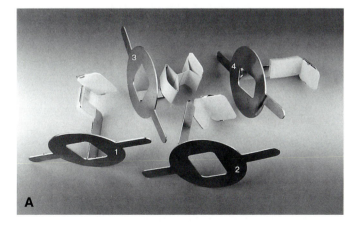 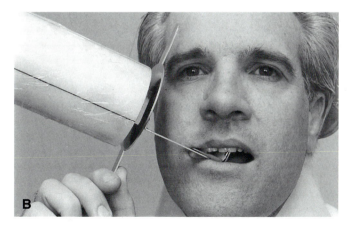

Figure 5.14. Masel Precision Rectangular Collimation Instruments. **(A)** Masel instruments: (1) posterior instrument; (2) posterior instrument; (3) bitewing instrument; (4) anterior instrument. **(B)** Use of Masel Precision Instrument in right maxillary posterior region.

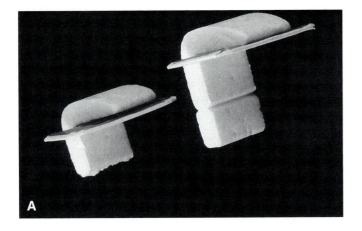

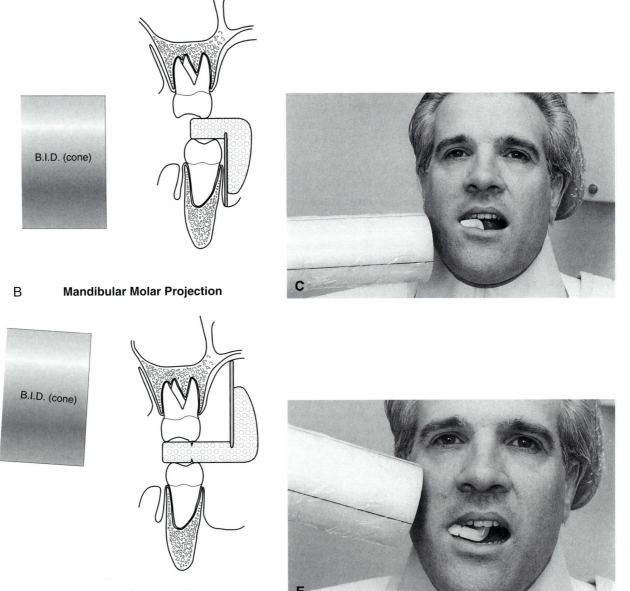

B Mandibular Molar Projection

D Maxillary Molar Projection

Figure 5.15. Stabe Disposable Film-Holder (Dentsply/Rinn) for Paralleling Technique. (**A**) (Left) Bite portion of the Stabe is scored so it may be shortened easily if necessary to avoid the cheek in mandibular projections or when used with children. (Right) Film in Stabe film-holder ready for positioning in the maxillary posterior region. (**B**) Diagram illustrating mandibular molar paralleling projection. (**C**) Film positioned for mandibular molar paralleling projection. (**D**) Diagram illustrating maxillary molar paralleling projection. (**E**) Film positioned for maxillary molar paralleling projection.

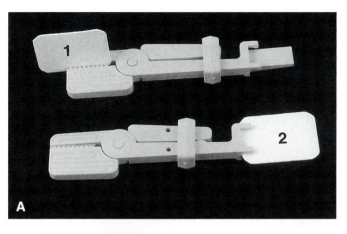

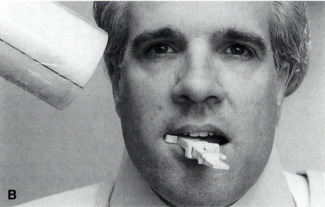

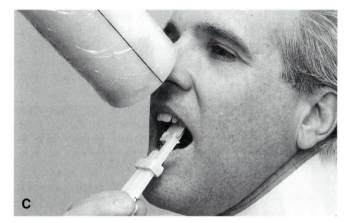

Figure 5.16. Snap-A-Ray (Dunvale) or EEZEE-Grip (Dentsply/Rinn) Film-Holder for Paralleling Technique. (**A**) Dunvale Snap-A-Ray: (1) posterior projection; (2) anterior projection. (**B**) Maxillary posterior projection (Dunvale Snap-A-Ray). (**C**) Maxillary anterior projection (Dunvale Snap-A-Ray).

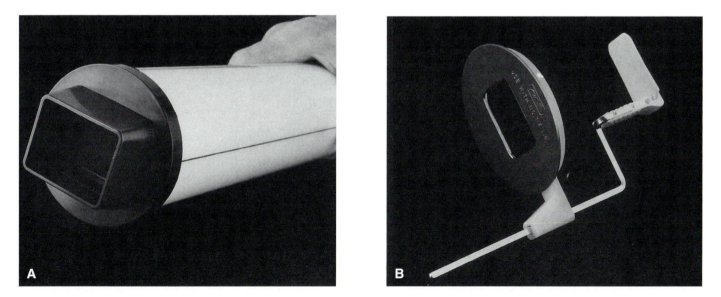

Figure 5.17. Dentsply/Rinn Universal Rectangular Collimator. (**A**) A long, cylindrical cone with a Dentsply/Rinn Universal Collimator attached to provide rectangular collimation to a cylindrical cone (BID). (**B**) Dentsply/Rinn XCP Instrument with stainless steel collimator attachment.

Six Rules of Good Paralleling Technique

The paralleling technique can be accomplished more easily by keeping these six rules in mind. The paralleling radiographic technique requires a film-holder to retain the film in a proper position and guide the placement of the BID. The first three rules deal with **film placement** and the last three rules deal with **BID positioning**.

Rule 1. The film must be placed so that it covers the particular teeth to be examined for each region of the oral cavity. The specific film positions for each area of the oral cavity are shown in Figure 5.2A.

Rule 2. The vertical plane of the film should be positioned parallel to the long axes of the teeth being radiographed. In the maxillary arch, because of the slight facial inclination of the teeth, it will be necessary to increase the tooth-film distance to achieve parallelism.

When the film is positioned parallel to the long axis of the posterior maxillary teeth, the apical or tissue edge of the film packet is at or beyond the median palatal suture line away from the teeth being radiographed (Fig. 5.18) and forces the patient to bite on the outer edge of the biteblock. In the mandibular posterior region, the molars tilt slightly inward toward the sagittal plane while the premolars are nearly parallel to the midsagittal plane. Therefore, the film packet can be positioned closer to the alveolar ridge and still remain parallel to the long axes of the teeth. This permits the patient to bite on the inner part of the biteblock. In the maxillary and mandibular incisor regions, because of the facial inclinations of the teeth, the film must be placed well back into the mouth. The apical or tissue edge of the anterior maxillary film packet will approximate the posterior palatal area (Fig. 5.19), and the apical edge of the mandibular film packet will be placed under the tongue near its anterior base to achieve parallelism of the film and the long axes of the

teeth. In either case, the patient must bite on the outer edge of the biteblock.

Rule 3. The horizontal plane of the film must be parallel to the horizontal planes of the teeth. The correct horizontal position of the film in relation to the teeth differs in various regions of the mouth because the teeth form a curved arch and all teeth will not have the same horizontal position or mean tangent. The mean tangent is defined as the plane joining the most exterior points of the curved facial surfaces in a particular region of the oral cavity. In Figure 5.20, the mean tangents are demonstrated for each film placement. The horizontal placement of the film packet must be parallel to the mean tangent of each region.

Rule 4. The vertical angulation of the cone or BID is such that the open-ended flat surface of the cone (BID) is positioned parallel to the film packet, which will direct the central ray perpendicular to the plane of the film and the long axes of the teeth. Proper vertical angulation of the cone (BID) will help reduce shape distortion of the radiographic image, such as elongation and foreshortening (Fig. 5.21).

Rule 5. The horizontal positioning of the cone or BID directs the x-rays through the embrasures or contacts between the teeth. After correct horizontal placement of the film, the horizontal angulation is easily determined by positioning the open-ended flat surface of the cone parallel to the horizontal plane of the film, thus directing the x-rays perpendicular to the film (Fig. 5.20). Incorrect horizontal angulation results in the overlapping of tooth interproximal surfaces (Fig. 5.10).

Rule 6. The central ray of the x-ray beam must be directed to the center of the film to completely cover the film (Fig. 5.9). Incorrect placement of the central ray results in cone-cutting or a partial exposure of the radiograph (Fig. 5.11).

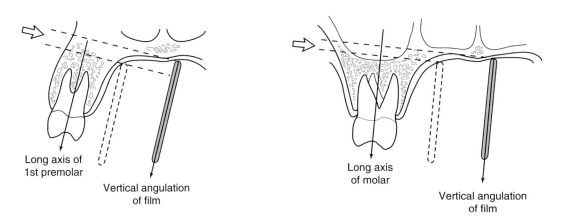

Figure 5.18. Maxillary Premolar/Molar Vertical Angulation of Film. In maxillary premolar and molar film placement, the object-film distance should be increased from the first position (*dashed line*) to the second position (*solid line*). The film can then be positioned vertically to approach parallelism between the long axis of the tooth and the vertical plane of the film. This prevents the apices of the teeth from being cut off.

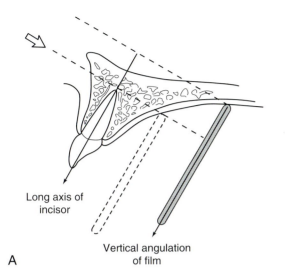

Long axis of
incisor

Vertical angulation
of film

A

Figure 5.19. Placement of Film in Maxillary Incisor Region: Maxillary Incisor Vertical Angulation of Film. (**A**) The tooth apices will not show in the radiograph when the film packet is placed in the first position (*dashed lines*). By increasing the object-film distance, as shown in the second position, it is possible to reveal the apices of the teeth and structures beyond on the radiograph. (**B**) Summary of placing film in incisor region: (1) the film should be positioned horizontally as the operator approaches the patient's mouth; (2) the outer edge of biteblock should make contact with incisal edge of teeth; the film should then be rotated into proper position; (3) patient closes on the biteblock, and the operator slides the locator ring adjacent to patient's skin.

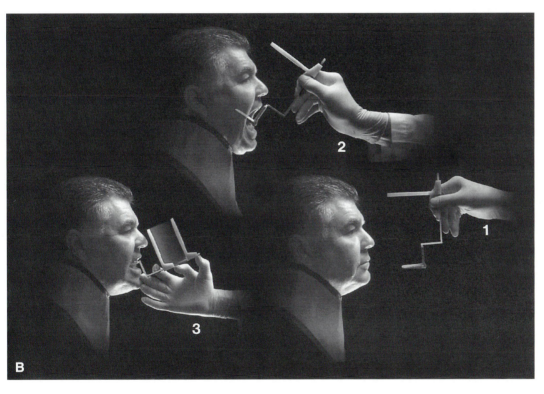

B

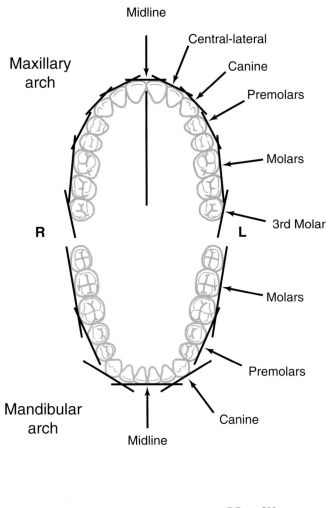

Midline

Central-lateral

Canine

Premolars

Maxillary
arch

Molars

3rd Molar

R   L

Figure 5.20. Mean Tangents: Horizontal Angulation of BID. Proper maxillary and mandibular mean targets and horizontal beam angulation for each region.

Molars

Premolars

Mandibular
arch

Canine

Midline

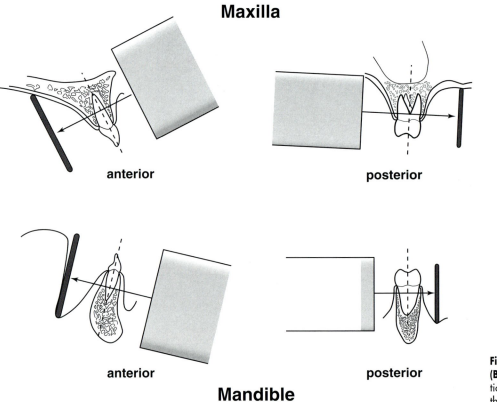

Maxilla

anterior

posterior

anterior   posterior

Mandible

Figure 5.21. Vertical Angulations of Cone (BID). Summary of proper vertical angulation of the cone (BID) for each region of the jaws.

Procedure for Using the Dentsply/Rinn XCP Instruments and Rectangular BID

This procedure should be followed to take a complete radiographic series using the Dentsply/Rinn XCP paralleling instruments. The same principles illustrated may be applied to the other film-holders listed previously. A rectangular cone (BID) is used because it collimates the beam to the size of the film and reduces the absorbed dose to the patient by approximately 60% compared with round cone collimation (see Chapter 13). **If a rectangular cone is not available, the same procedure may be used for the long round cone (BID) by use of the Precision Instrument (Masel) or the Dentsply/Rinn Universal Rectangular Collimator attached to the round, cylindrical cone (BID) (Figs. 5.14 and 5.17).**

A routine sequence of taking radiographs for an FMX should be decided on by the operator. This will save time and make certain that all radiographs are exposed without overlooking some of the projections.

Dentsply/Rinn XCP Instruments (Long Cone Paralleling) Film-holding instruments such as the Dentsply/Rinn XCP instruments provide an external guide for positioning of the BID vertically and horizontally as well as automatically establishing the point of entry of the x-ray beam (Fig. 5.13).

The Dentsply/Rinn XCP instrument consists of three parts:

1. **Anterior and posterior plastic biteblocks.** These are designed to retain the film packet by means of tension created by a semiflexible plastic backing and a groove or slot within which the film is inserted.
2. **Indicator rod.** These are made of stainless steel and are used to align the x-ray cone or BID with the film. There is an anterior offset rod and a posterior right angle rod designed to insert into the receptacle holes of their respective biteblocks for the periapical projections.
3. **Aiming ring.** Aiming rings are made for sliding onto the rods to establish alignment of the cone with the film. This prevents cone-cutting.

The Dentsply/Rinn XCP aiming or locator ring can accept either a round cone or a rectangular cone (BID) (Fig. 5.13). To aid in the alignment of the rectangular BID with the aiming or locator ring, the rectangular BID can be rotated on its own axis. This modification simplifies the use of the rectangular BID and film alignment. The following sections explain the recommended procedures for the long BID paralleling technique using the Dentsply/Rinn XCP instruments and rectangular BID for each region of the oral cavity (Figs. 5.22 to 5.32).

PARALLELING TECHNIQUE

MAXILLARY CENTRAL INCISOR REGION

Dentsply/Rinn XCP Paralleling Procedure (Fig. 5.22)

1. Assemble the anterior instrument and insert a no. 1 film vertically in the anterior biteblock with the plain side of the film facing out.
2. Select the correct exposure factors.
3. Center the film to the maxillary midline and parallel to the long axes of the central incisors. The entire length of the biteblock should be used to position the film back to the palatal region lingual to the first molar.

4. With the biteblock resting on the incisal edges of the teeth to be radiographed, insert a cotton roll between the mandibular incisors and biteblock. Instruct the patient to close firmly to retain the film in the desired position.
5. Slide the aiming ring down the indicator rod to approximate the skin surface and turn the BID vertically. Align the BID with the indicator rod and aiming ring in both the vertical and horizontal planes.
6. Make the exposure.

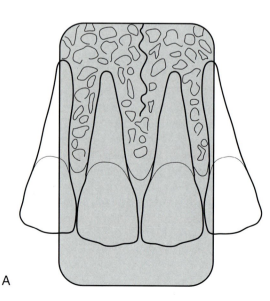

A

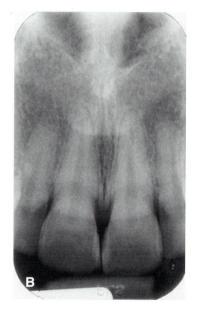

B

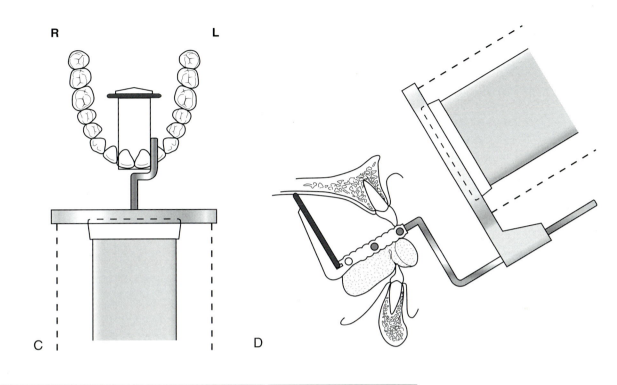

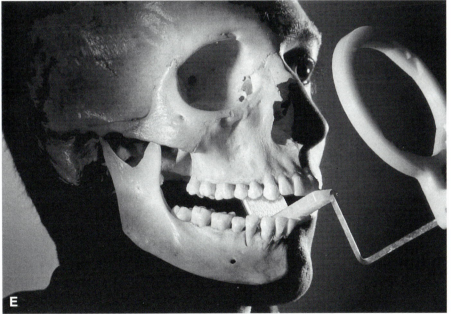

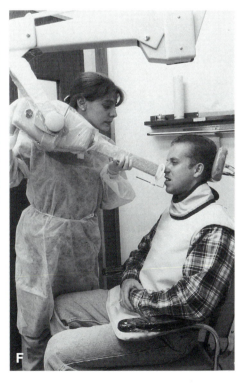

Figure 5.22. Maxillary Central Incisor Region. (**A**) Region coverage. (**B**) Resultant radiograph. (**C**) Horizontal film and BID placement. (**D**) Vertical film and BID placement. (**E**) Proper placement of film. (**F**) Proper alignment of BID with Dentsply/Rinn XCP instrument.

PARALLELING TECHNIQUE

MAXILLARY LATERAL INCISOR REGION

Dentsply/Rinn XCP Paralleling Procedure (Fig. 5.23)

1. Assemble the anterior instrument and insert a no. 1 film vertically in the anterior biteblock with the plain side facing out.
2. Select the correct exposure factors.
3. Center the lateral incisor on the biteblock and position the film parallel to the long axis of the lateral incisor. The entire length of the biteblock should be used to position the film back to the palatal region lingual the first molars.

4. With the biteblock resting on the incisal edges of the teeth to be radiographed, insert a cotton roll between mandibular incisors and biteblock. Instruct patient to close firmly to retain the established position of film.
5. Slide the aiming ring down the indicator rod to approximate the skin surface. Turn the BID vertically and align it with the indicator rod and aiming ring in both the vertical and horizontal planes.
6. Make the exposure.

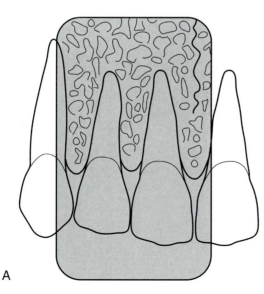

A

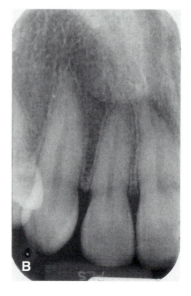

B

R   L

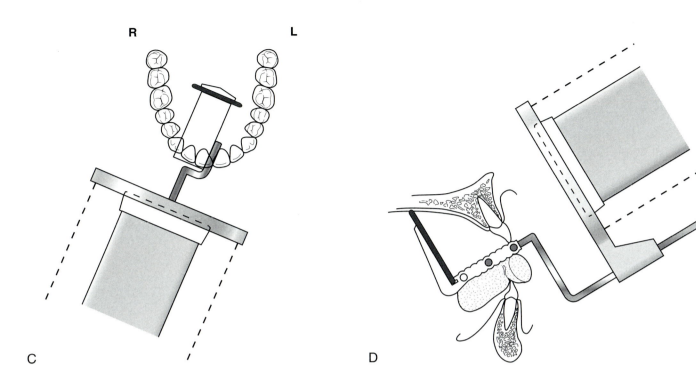

C

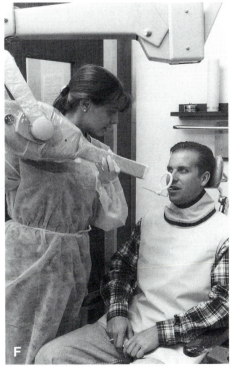

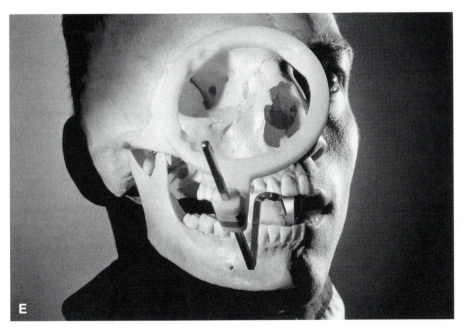

E

Figure 5.23. Maxillary Lateral Incisor Region. (**A**) Region coverage. (**B**) Resultant radiograph. (**C**) Horizontal film and BID placement. (**D**) Vertical film and BID placement. (**E**) Proper placement of film. (**F**) Proper alignment of BID with Dentsply/Rinn XCP instrument.

D

F

PARALLELING TECHNIQUE

MAXILLARY CANINE REGION

Dentsply/Rinn XCP Paralleling Procedure (Fig. 5.24)

1. Assemble the anterior instrument and insert a no. 1 film vertically in the anterior biteblock with the plain side facing out.
2. Select the correct exposure factors.
3. Center the canine on the film, parallel with the long axis of the maxillary canine.

4. With the biteblock resting on the maxillary canine, insert a cotton roll between the mandibular teeth and biteblock. Instruct the patient to close firmly to retain the established position of film.
5. Slide the aiming ring down the indicator rod to approximate the skin surface. Turn the BID vertically and align it with the indicator rod and aiming ring in both the vertical and horizontal planes.
6. Make the exposure.

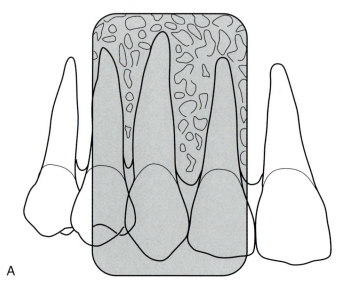

A

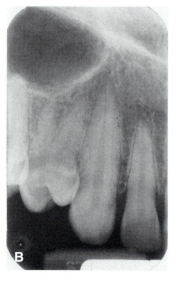

B

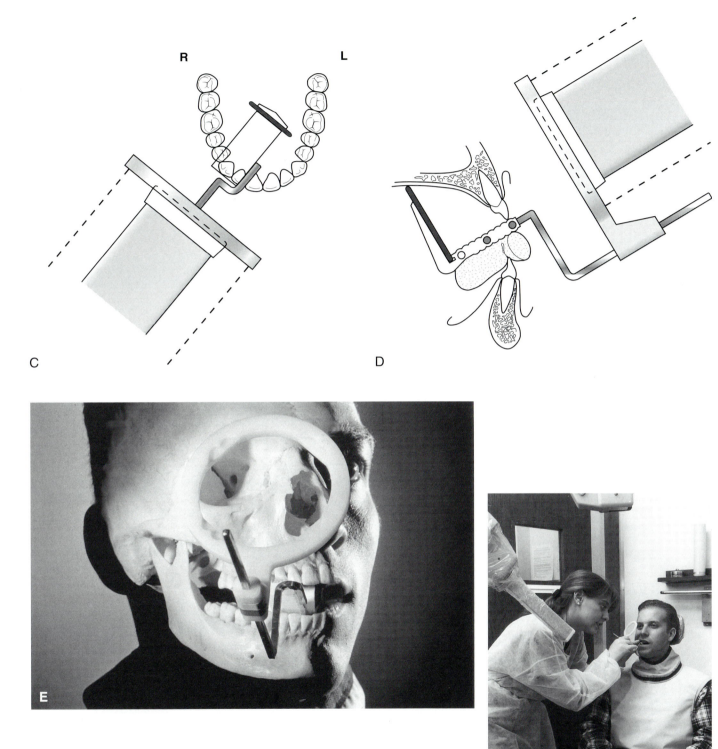

Figure 5.24. Maxillary Canine Region. **(A)** Region coverage. **(B)** Resultant radiograph. **(C)** Horizontal film and BID placement. **(D)** Vertical film and BID placement. **(E)** Proper placement of film. **(F)** Proper alignment of BID with Dentsply/Rinn XCP instrument.

PARALLELING TECHNIQUE

MAXILLARY PREMOLAR REGION

Dentsply/Rinn XCP Paralleling Procedure (Fig. 5.25)

1. Assemble the posterior instrument and insert a no. 2 film horizontally in the posterior biteblock with the plain side facing out.
2. Select the correct exposure factors.
3. Position the film-holder in the mouth with the second premolar centered on the film. The distal of the canine must be seen on this projection. Parallel the film horizontally with the mean tangent of the premolars and vertically with long axis of the premolars.

4. With the biteblock held against the occlusal surfaces of the premolars and first molar, insert a cotton roll between the underside of the biteblock and mandibular teeth. Instruct the patient to close firmly to retain the established position of the film.
5. Slide the aiming ring or locator ring down the indicator rod to approximate the skin surface. Rotate the BID to the horizontal position and align it with both the indicator rod and aiming ring in both the horizontal and vertical planes.
6. Make the exposure.

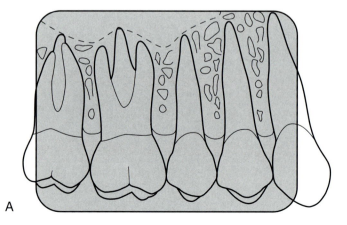

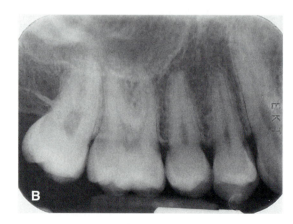

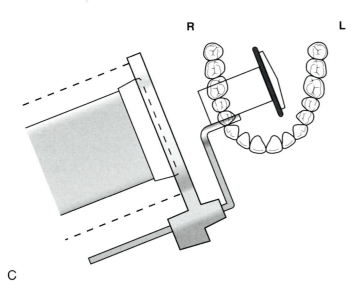

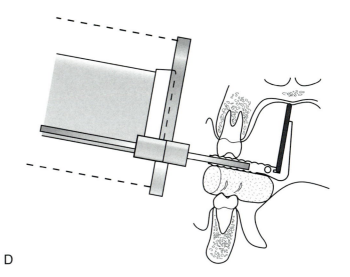

C

D

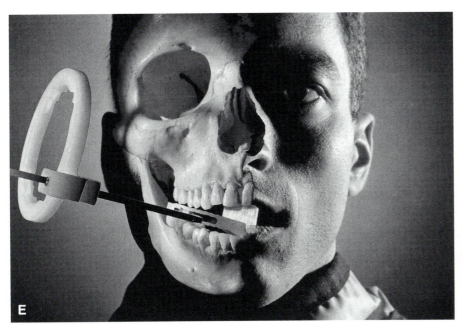

E

Figure 5.25. Maxillary Premolar Region. (**A**) Region coverage. (**B**) Resultant radiograph. (**C**) Horizontal film and BID placement. (**D**) Vertical film and BID placement. (**E**) Proper placement of film. (**F**) Alignment of BID with XCP instrument.

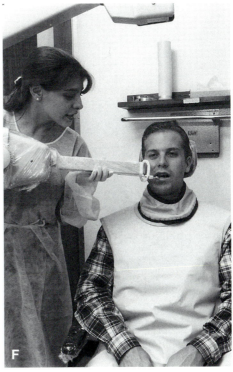

F

PARALLELING TECHNIQUE

MAXILLARY MOLAR REGION

Dentsply/Rinn XCP Paralleling Procedure (Fig. 5.26)

1. Assemble the posterior instrument and insert a no. 2 film horizontally in the posterior biteblock with the plain side of the film facing out.
2. Select the correct exposure factors.
3. Position the film-holder in the mouth with the anterior edge of the film at the middle of the second premolar. If necessary, move the film posteriorly to cover the maxillary third molar or maxillary tuberosity if the third molar is not visible clinically. Position the film at or past the midpalatal suture line and parallel to the mean tangent of the molars. Then make certain that the vertical plane of the film is parallel to the long axes of the molars.
4. With the biteblock held against the occlusal surfaces of the first and second molars, insert a cotton roll between the underside of the biteblock and mandibular teeth. Instruct the patient to close firmly to retain the established position of the film.
5. Slide the aiming ring down the indicator rod to approximate the skin surface. Rotate the BID to the horizontal position and align it with both the indicator rod and aiming ring on the horizontal and vertical planes.
6. Make the exposure.

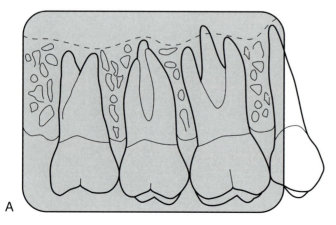

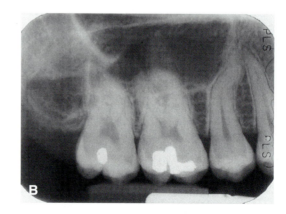

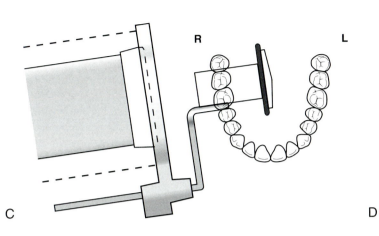

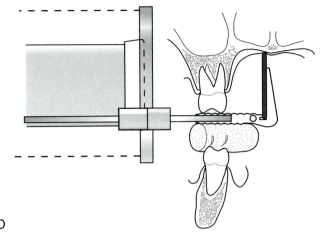

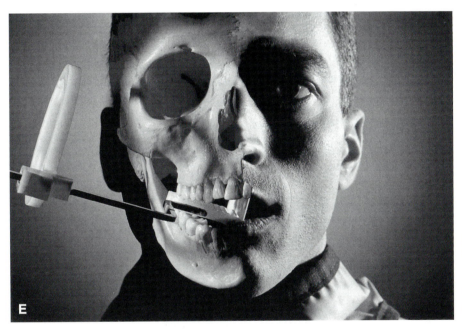

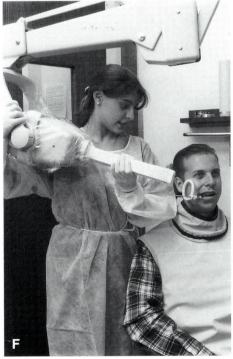

Figure 5.26. Maxillary Molar Region. (**A**) Region coverage. (**B**) Resultant radiograph. (**C**) Horizontal film and BID placement. (**D**) Vertical film and BID placement. (**E**) Proper placement of film. (**F**) Alignment of BID with XCP instrument.

PARALLELING TECHNIQUE

MANDIBULAR INCISOR REGION

Dentsply/Rinn XCP Paralleling Procedure (Fig. 5.27)

1. Assemble the anterior instrument and insert a no. 1 film vertically in the anterior biteblock with the plain side of the film facing out. The procedure is similar to maxillary anterior technique, except for the inversion of the holder to position the film lingual to the mandibular anterior teeth.
2. Select the correct exposure factors.
3. Center the film with the patient's midline parallel to the long axes of the central incisors. The lingual placement of the film packet in the region of the second premolars will accomplish this relationship, and the patient will bite on the outer edge of the biteblock.

4. With the biteblock resting on the incisal edges of the teeth to be radiographed, insert a cotton roll between the top of the biteblock and the maxillary incisors. Instruct the patient to close firmly to retain the established position of the film. Place the film against the floor of the mouth and rotate the film into position as the patient bites on the biteblock. Do not force this procedure. Film placement may be simplified by raising the chair and tilting the patient's head backward.
5. Slide the aiming ring down the indicator rod to approximate the skin surface. Align the BID with the indicator rod and aiming ring on the vertical and horizontal planes. Rotate the BID to the vertical position.
6. Make the exposure.

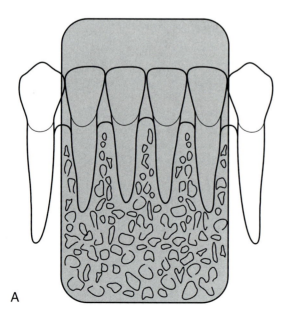

A

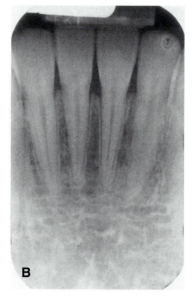

B

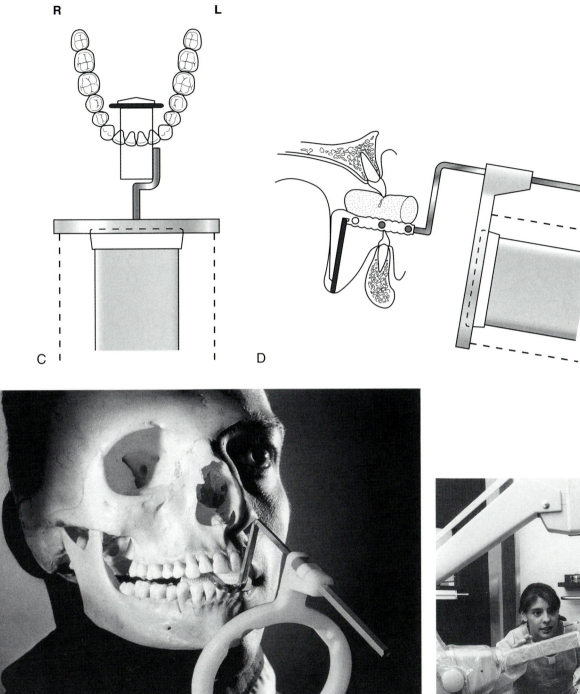

R   L

C   D

E

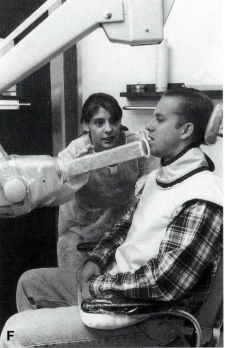

F

Figure 5.27. Mandibular Incisor Region. (**A**) Region coverage. (**B**) Resultant radiograph. (**C**) Horizontal film and BID placement. (**D**) Vertical film and BID placement. (**E**) Proper placement of film. (**F**) Alignment of BID with XCP instrument.

PARALLELING TECHNIQUE

MANDIBULAR CANINE REGION

Dentsply/Rinn XCP Paralleling Procedure (Fig. 5.28)

1. Assemble the anterior instrument and insert a no. 1 film vertically in the anterior biteblock with the plain side facing out.
2. Select the correct exposure factors.
3. Center the canine on the film, parallel to the long axis of the canine.

4. With the biteblock resting on the mandibular canine, insert a cotton roll between the biteblock and the maxillary teeth. Instruct the patient to close firmly to maintain the established position of the film.
5. Slide the aiming ring down indicator rod to approximate the skin surface. Align the BID with the indicator rod and aiming ring on the vertical and horizontal planes. Make certain the BID is rotated vertically.
6. Make the exposure.

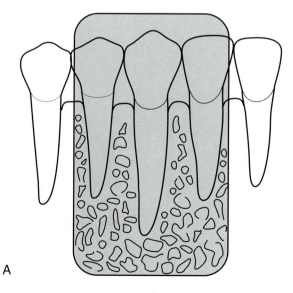

A

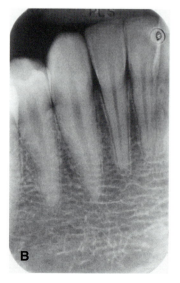

B

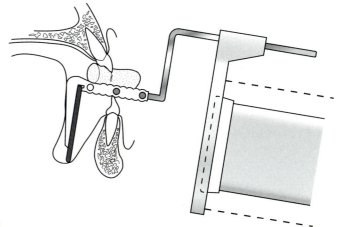

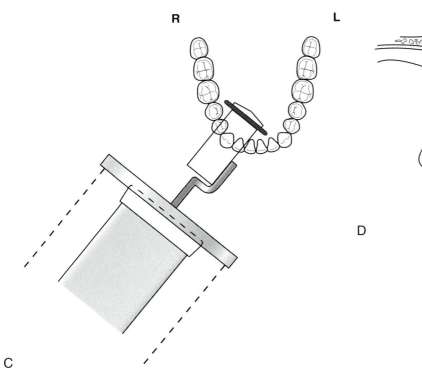

C

D

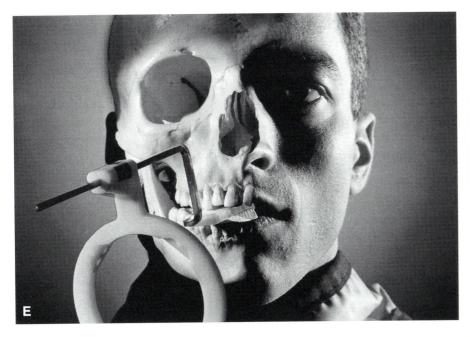

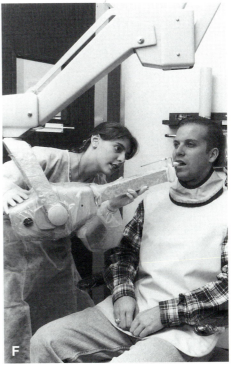

Figure 5.28. Mandibular Canine Region. (**A**) Region coverage. (**B**) Resultant radiograph. (**C**) Horizontal film and BID placement. (**D**) Vertical film and BID placement. (**E**) Proper placement of film. (**F**) Alignment of BID with XCP instrument.

PARALLELING TECHNIQUE

MANDIBULAR PREMOLAR REGION

Dentsply/Rinn XCP Paralleling Procedure (Fig. 5.29)

1. Assemble the posterior instrument and insert a no. 2 film horizontally in the posterior biteblock with the plain side of the film facing out.
2. Select the correct exposure factors.
3. Position the film-holder in the mouth with the second premolar centered on the film. Bending or curving of the lower anterior corner of the film packet will facilitate positioning in some patients, although this procedure is recommended only in extreme circumstances. Parallel the film horizontally to the mean tangent of the premolars and vertically to the long axes of the premolars.
4. With the biteblock held on the occlusal surfaces of the mandibular premolars, insert a cotton roll between the biteblock and the maxillary teeth. Instruct the patient to close firmly to retain the established position of the film.
5. Slide the aiming ring down the indicator rod to approximate the skin surface. Rotate the BID horizontally and align it with both the indicator rod and aiming ring in both the horizontal and vertical planes.
6. Make the exposure.

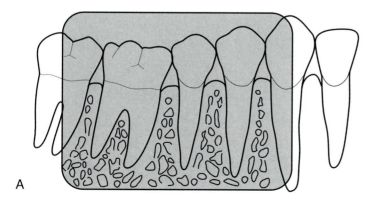

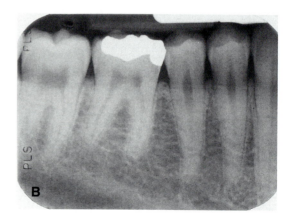

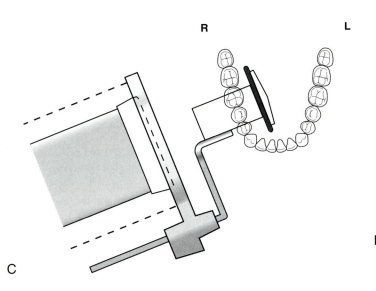

R L

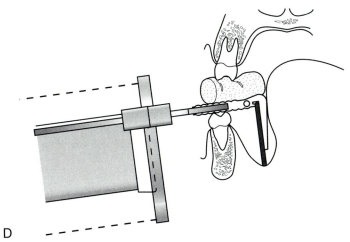

C

D

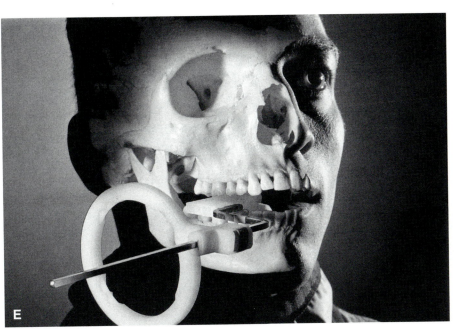

E

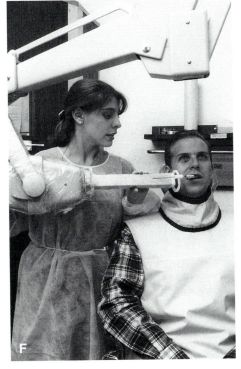

F

Figure 5.29. Mandibular Premolar Region. (**A**) Region coverage. (**B**) Resultant radiograph. (**C**) Horizontal film and BID placement. (**D**) Vertical film and BID placement. (**E**) Proper placement of film. (**F**) Alignment of BID with XCP instrument.

PARALLELING TECHNIQUE

MANDIBULAR MOLAR REGION

Dentsply/Rinn XCP Paralleling Procedure (Fig. 5.30)

1. Assemble the posterior instrument and insert a no. 2 film horizontally in the posterior biteblock with the plain side facing out.
2. Select the correct exposure factors.
3. Position the film-holder in the mouth with the anterior edge of the film in the vicinity of first molar-second premolar embrasure; however, the film must cover all of the third molar. Parallel the film vertically with the long axes of the molars. (The occlusal surfaces of molars are usually at right angles to their long axes. Therefore, if the block is placed flat across the occlusal surfaces, the plane of the film automatically assumes a position parallel to the long axes of the teeth.) Position the film packet in the sulcus between the teeth and tongue.
4. Place a cotton roll between the biteblock and opposing maxillary teeth. Instruct the patient to close firmly to retain the established position of the film.
5. Slide the aiming ring down the indicator rod to approximate skin surface. Rotate the BID to the horizontal position and align it with the indicator rod and aiming ring in both the horizontal and vertical planes.
6. Make the exposure.

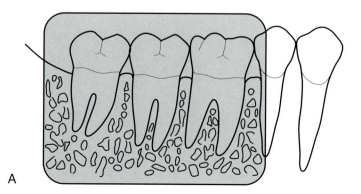

A

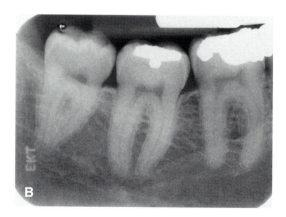

B

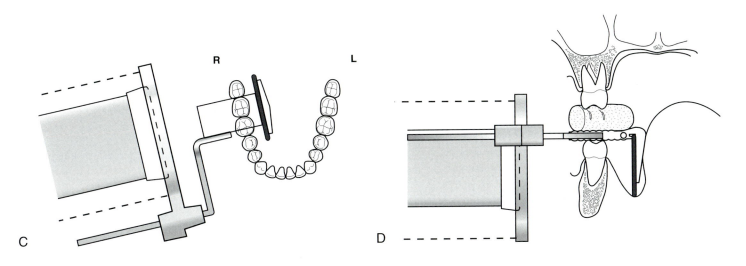

R   L

C   D

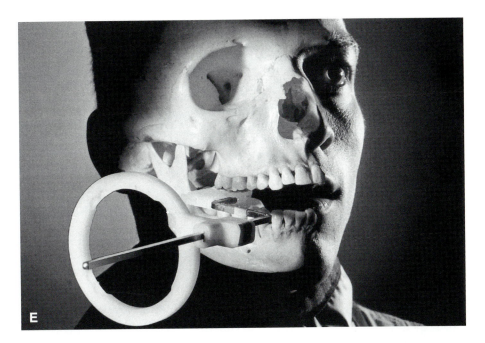

E

F

Figure 5.30. Mandibular Molar Region. (**A**) Region coverage. (**B**) Resultant radiograph. (**C**) Horizontal film and BID placement. (**D**) Vertical film and BID placement. (**E**) Proper placement of film. (**F**) Alignment of BID with XCP instrument.

PARALLELING TECHNIQUE

PREMOLAR BITEWINGS

Dentsply/Rinn XCP Bitewing Procedure (Fig. 5.31)

1. Assemble the bitewing instrument. Center a no. 2 film in the biteblock in the horizontal position. The pebbled or plain side of the film should face outward with the plastic film holder positioned across the face of the film.
2. Select the correct exposure factors.
3. With the biting portion resting on the occlusal surfaces of the mandibular teeth, position the film as shown for premolar bitewings. Instruct the patient to close firmly to retain the film in position.
4. Slide the aiming ring down the indicator rod to approximate the skin surface. Rotate the BID to the horizontal position and align it with the indicator rod and aiming ring in both the horizontal and vertical planes.
5. Make the exposure.

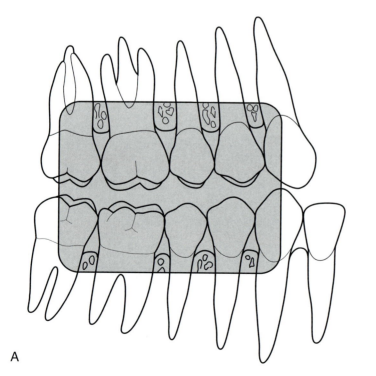

A

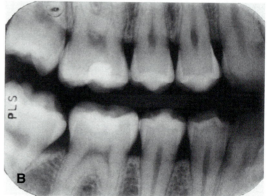

B

R   L

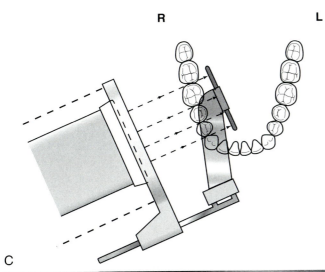

C

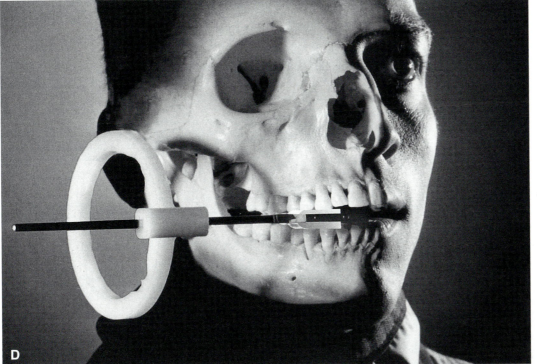

D

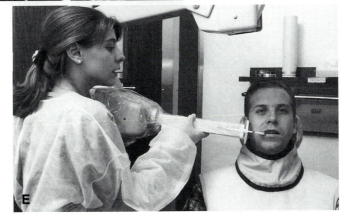

E

Figure 5.31. Premolar Bitewing. (**A**) Region coverage. (**B**) Resultant radiograph. (**C**) Horizontal film and BID placement. (**D**) Proper placement of the film. (**E**) Alignment of BID and XCP instrument.

PARALLELING TECHNIQUE

MOLAR BITEWINGS

Dentsply/Rinn XCP Bitewing Procedure (Fig. 5.32)

1. Assemble the bitewing instrument. Center a no. 2 film in the biteblock in the horizontal position. The pebbled or plain side of the film should face outward with the plastic film holder positioned across the face of the film.
2. Select the correct exposure factors.
3. With the biting portion resting on the occlusal surfaces of the mandibular teeth, position the film as shown for molar bitewings. Instruct the patient to close firmly to retain the film in position.
4. Slide the aiming ring down the indicator rod to approximate the skin surface. Rotate the BID to the horizontal position and align it with the indicator rod and aiming ring in both the horizontal and vertical planes.
5. Make the exposure.

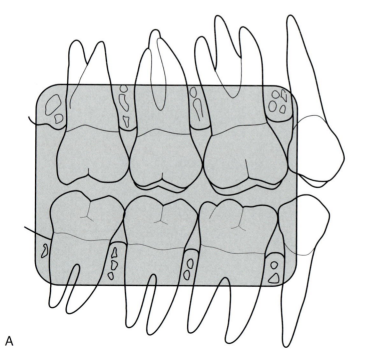

A

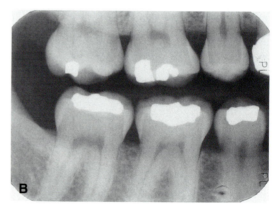

B

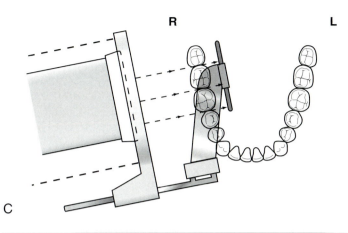

R   L

C

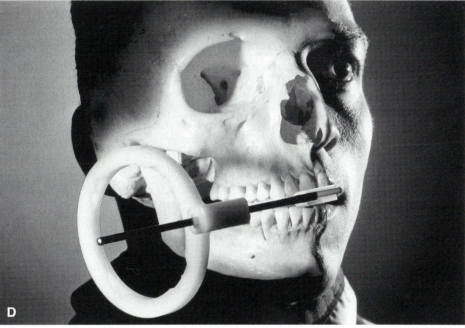

D

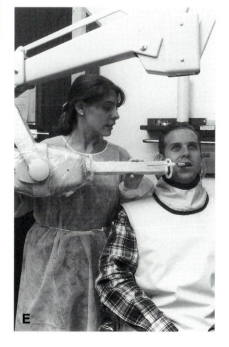

E

Figure 5.32. Molar Bitewing. **(A)** Region coverage. **(B)** Resultant radiograph. **(C)** Horizontal and BID placement. **(D)** Proper placement of film. **(E)** Alignment of BID and XCP instrument.

BITEWING TECHNIQUE

Dentsply/Rinn XCP Bitewing Instrument Technique

The interproximal examination is considered the least difficult of the intraoral techniques, yet the results of incorrect alignment of the film, teeth, and x-ray beam are frequently seen on the finished radiograph. These errors are manifested as cone-cutting, overlapping of crowns of teeth, and occlusal surfaces recorded diagonally on the film. Bitewing instruments such as the Dentsply/Rinn Bitewing Instrument were designed to reduce these errors to a minimum (Fig. 5.33). If vertical bitewings are ordered,

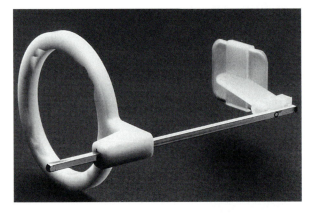

Figure 5.33. Dentsply/Rinn Horizontal Posterior Bitewing Instrument. Bitewing instrument assembled correctly with no. 2 film in horizontal position to take a posterior bitewing radiograph.

the vertical bitewing biteblock must be assembled with the indicator rod and aiming or locator ring as shown in Figure 5.34.

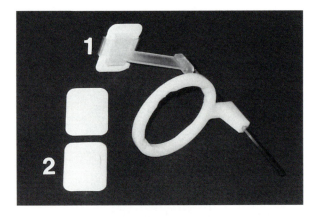

Figure 5.34. Dentsply/Rinn Vertical Bitewing. (1) Dentsply/Rinn XCP bitewing instrument assembled to take a vertical bitewing radiograph using no. 1 size film. A vertical biteblock is also available for no. 2 size film. (2) No. 2 size film with bitewing tab in place to take a vertical bitewing radiograph.

BITEWING TAB TECHNIQUE

Film Size

A bitewing film has a wing or tab attached to the pebbled side of the film. When the tab is placed on the occlusal surfaces of the mandibular posterior teeth and the patient closes on the tab, the film will be held in a lingual position to the maxillary and mandibular crowns.

There are two sizes of adult bitewing films:

1. **Adult or no. 3 (2.3) bitewing film** is designed to record the crowns of all posterior teeth, both maxillary and mandibular. This type of bitewing film is **not** recommended for two reasons. First, there is a slight amount of distortion in the film from conforming to a curved arch. Second, many times this film does not reveal all the interproximal surfaces of all posterior teeth (from the distal of the canines to the mesial of the third molars).
2. **No. 2 (2.2) or standard size bitewing film**, one of which is not long enough to record all posterior crowns in an adult mouth. Thus, in the adult, one no. 2 bitewing film should be used in the molar region and one no. 2 bitewing film should be used in the premolar region, including the distal of the canines.

Head Position

Regardless of the type of cone (BID) being used, the sagittal plane should be perpendicular to the floor, and the ala-tragus line should be parallel to the floor.

Film Placement and Retention

Step 1. The bitewing tab or wing should be placed on the occlusal surface of the mandibular molars or premolars, with the lower edge of the film packet placed in the vestibule between the tongue and the teeth. The anterior edge of the premolar bitewing film should extend to the mesial surface of the mandibular canine, and the anterior edge of the molar bitewing film should be placed at the midline of the mandibular second premolar. To avoid overlapping of the contact points, the film should be positioned perpendicular to invisible lines drawn through the embrasures of the teeth. To do this in the molar bitewing projection, the anterior border of the film packet should be a greater distance from the lingual surfaces of the teeth than the posterior border.

If the patient has a shallow vault, the film should be placed even a greater distance away from the lingual surfaces of the teeth. This will enable the patient to close down on the bitewing tab with less difficulty.

Step 2. Half of the bitewing tab should be folded down over the buccal surface of the teeth. This should be done before the tab is placed on the occlusal surfaces of the teeth. With the index finger of one hand, the operator should press against the lower lingual border of the film to keep it upright. The index finger of the other hand should be used to press the tab against the buccal surface of the mandibular teeth.

Step 3. The operator should remove the finger that is pressing against the back of the film and instruct the patient to close slowly against the bitewing tab in a normal bite. The patient will not close against the index finger because it is pressing against the buccal surfaces of the lower teeth. After the patient has closed against the bitewing tab, the operator can remove the finger from the tab.

Vertical Angulation of the BID or Cone

Short Cone (8-inch source-film distance): +10° vertical angulation.

Long Cone (16-inch source-film distance): +8° for molar region and +6° for premolar region.

If the palate is shallow, the upper border of the film will be forced lingually by the palate on closure. The vertical angle may have to be increased in this case to prevent shape distortion of the maxillary crowns. Usually the maxillary premolars and molars tilt buccally (sometimes as much as 15° from the vertical), while the mandibular premolars and molars slant very little from the vertical. Therefore, to compensate for this discrepancy and to prevent distortion of the crowns, a compromise vertical angulation is used for the bitewing projections (Fig. 5.35).

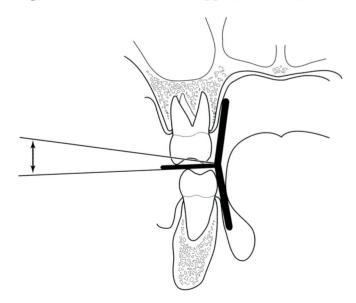

Figure 5.35. Vertical Angulation, Bitewing Tab Technique. Recommended short-cone vertical angulation for posterior bitewing radiograph using a bitewing tab is +10°; for long cone, it is +8° for molar and +6° for premolar projections.

Horizontal Angulation

The ray beam should be directed through the interproximal embrasures of the crowns of the teeth under examination. The flat face of the cone should be horizontally parallel to the film packet.

Point of Entry

The central ray should be directed through the occlusal plane of the teeth toward the center of the film packet. To prevent cone-cutting, the operator should gently pull back the corner of the lips and observe whether the anterior periphery of the cone is covering the anterior border of the film. In the molar projection, the tab should be attached flush with the anterior margin of the film. This will serve as a landmark for the anterior border of the film when the patient's teeth are closed together. In the premolar projection, the anterior margin of the film can be readily seen. To prevent cone-cutting with a bitewing tab, the teeth can be used as landmarks in the following manner.

Molar No. 2 Bitewing Film The anterior margin of the cone should be aligned with the interproximal space between the maxillary first premolar and the maxillary canine. The central ray is directed through the occlusal plane of maxillary and mandibular teeth (Fig. 5.36).

Premolar No. 2 Bitewing Film The anterior margin of the cone should be aligned with the interproximal space between the maxillary lateral and central. The central ray is directed through the occlusal plane of the maxillary and mandibular teeth (Fig. 5.36).

BISECTING ANGLE TECHNIQUE

The bisecting angle technique is based on the geometric principle that states that two triangles are equal if they have two equal angles and a common side. It is called the **rule of isometry.** Isometry is defined as equality of measurement (Fig. 5.37). When the rule of isometry is applied to dental radiography, it is used to determine the *correct vertical angulation* of the cone (BID). Vertical angulation is the up and the down movement of the cone (BID). When applied to intraoral radiography, the bisecting angle rule states that, "The central ray is directed through the median plane of the tooth, perpendicular to a line bisecting the angle formed by the plane of the long axis of the tooth and the plane of the film" (Fig. 5.38). This rule applies admirably to plane surfaces that have only length and width, but it has certain shortcomings when applied to structures such as the teeth that also have depth. If the bisecting angle rule is neglected in the slightest manner, the resulting radiographic image will be distorted. Elongation of the length of the actual image of the tooth will result if the x-ray beam is directed perpendicular to the plane of the long axis of the tooth rather than through

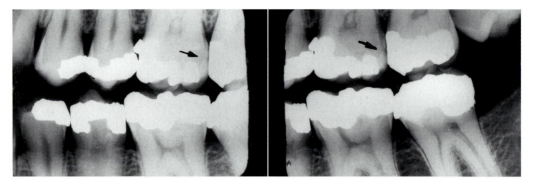

Figure 5.36. Posterior Bitewing Tab Radiographs. Premolar and molar posterior bitewing radiographs using a bitewing tab. (Note that occlusal surfaces of the upper and lower teeth approximate one another.)

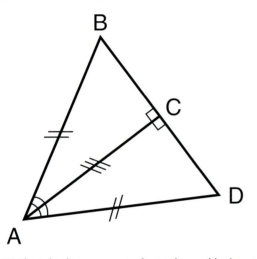

Figure 5.37. The Rule of Isometry. Angle *A* is bisected by line *AC*. Line *AC* is perpendicular to line *BD*. Angle *DAC* is equal to angle *CAB*, and angle *ACD* is equal to *ACB*. If two triangles have two equal angles and a common side, then it can be said that the two triangles are equal. Therefore, triangle *DAC* is equal to triangle *CAB*.

the bisecting line. Foreshortening of the radiographic image will occur when the x-ray beam is directed perpendicular to the plane of the film, rather than the bisecting line (Fig. 5.39). For the most part, the bisecting technique is practiced with the short cone (8-inch source-film distance). If the short cone is used, it should have an open-ended, flat face. The long or extension cone may also be used with the bisecting technique. A source-film distance of 16 inches seems to be the most practical distance to use in most dental offices. The advantage of the extended source-film distance is that it minimizes geometric unsharpness and magnification of the radiographic image.

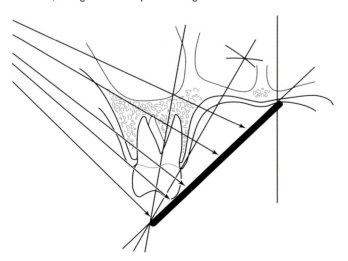

Figure 5.38. Bisecting Angle Technique. The rule of isometry applied to the intraoral radiographic technique commonly called the bisection-of-the-angle technique. The path of central ray is directed perpendicular to a line bisecting the angle formed by the long axis of the tooth and the plane of the film.

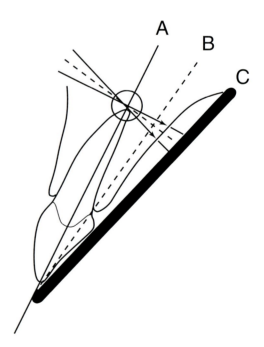

Figure 5.39. Elongation and Foreshortening. In the bisecting angle technique, if the central ray is directed as line (above) perpendicular to the film (*C*), the radiographic image will be foreshortened; if the path of the central ray is directed as line (below) perpendicular to the tooth (*A*), the radiographic image will be elongated.

Bisecting Angle Technique Procedures

To determine the correct alignment of the central beam, the film, and the teeth using the bisecting technique, the following factors must be considered:

1. Head position.
2. Film placement.
3. Vertical angulation of the BID or cone.
4. Horizontal angulation of the BID or cone.
5. The point of entry of the central ray.

Head Position When using the bisecting technique, the head position is important. The rule for head position is as follows: the occlusal plane of the teeth to be radiographed should be parallel to the floor, and the sagittal plane of the head should be perpendicular to the floor for maxillary projections. Here the ala-tragus line is parallel to the floor. In mandibular projections, **the mandibular occlusal plane** changes when the mouth is open. Therefore, the patient's head should be tilted slightly backward so the occlusal plane of the mandible will be parallel to the floor when the mouth is opened. Here the lip commissure (corner of mouth)-tragus line is parallel to the floor.

Film Placement The rule for film placement in the bisecting technique is this: the center of the film is positioned behind the center of the region to be radiographed. The most popular full-mouth periapical examination (often called the complete-mouth survey) using the bisecting technique is the 14-film survey using all no. 2 periapical films (Fig. 5.40). For years when using the bisecting technique, the film packets were held in the mouth by the patient's fingers (digital method). The digital (finger) method of retaining the film in the mouth is the most undesirable method of film retention, because it places the patient's hand (usually unwashed) into the primary beam of radiation. Also, digital pressure on the film usually causes film bending, which usually results in image distortion and an unnecessary retake. In 1970, the National Council of Radiation Protection (NCRP) recommended the use of film-holders for all intraoral examinations to eliminate the need for patients to stabilize films in their mouths with their hands (NCRP no. 35, 1970).

Vertical Angulation of the BID or Cone As stated previously, the rule for vertical angulation in the bisecting technique is to direct the central ray through the center of the field under examination, perpendicular to the line bisecting the angle formed by the planes of the long axes of the tooth and the plane of the film. Due to variations in the arrangement, inclination, and angulation of the teeth in the jaws, the angle formed by the plane of the film and the long axes of the teeth for any given area of the mouth varies from one patient to another. To aid the operator, average vertical angulations have been calculated into which most patients will fall. These average

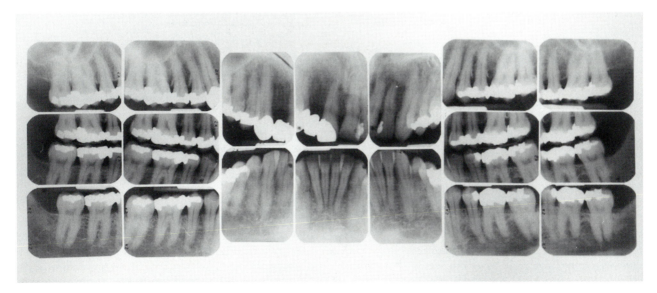

Figure 5.40. Bisecting Angle Full-Mouth Survey. Typical full radiographic survey taken by bisecting angle technique using a short cone (8-inch SFD). (Note that no. 2 regular film is used throughout the survey).

values are used only as a guide by the operator; the exact angle to be used for each region for each patient must be determined after the film in the film-holder has been placed in the mouth. The ranges of prescribed vertical angulations for both the short and the long cone bisecting of the angle techniques are listed below. (A *plus* vertical angulation means the cone is above the horizontal pointed downward, and a *minus* vertical angulation means the cone is below the horizontal pointed upward).

Average Vertical Angles, Short Cone (8-inch Source-to-Film Distance), Bisecting Angle Technique				
Film	Maxillary Range	Maxillary Starting Angle	Mandibular Range	Mandibular Starting Angle
Molar	+25° to 30°	+30°	0°	0°
Premolar	+35° to 40°	+40°	−5° to −10°	−10°
Canine	+45° to 50°	+50°	−15° to −30°	−15°
Incisor	+55° to 65°	+55°	−15° to −30°	−20°
P. Bitewing		+10°		

Average Vertical Angles, Long Cone (16-inch Soruce-to-Film Distance), Bisecting Angle Technique		
Film	Maxilla	Mandible
Molar	+25°	+0° (fixed angle)
Premolar	+35°	−5°
Canine	+45°	−10°
Incisors	+45°	−15°
P. Bitewing	+10°	

Horizontal Angulation of the BID or Cone The rule for horizontal angulation is as follows: as the cone moves around the arch, the x-ray beam is directed perpendicular to the mean tangents of the facial surfaces of the teeth under examination; the flat face of the cone should be placed parallel to the horizontal plane of the film. If there is an error in the horizontal angulation, overlapping of the radiographic images will result in an inadequate image that must be retaken. The mean tangents of the facial surfaces of the teeth will vary from one region to another.

Point of Entry The rule for the point of entry in the bisecting technique is as follows: the x-ray beam is directed through the center of the area to be radiographed. The objective here is to completely cover the film with the cone of radiation. If this is not done, a cone-cut or partial image will be seen in the finished radiograph.

Use of Film-Holders with Bisecting Angle Technique

Film-holders have been devised for use with the bisecting angle technique. Two such film-holders are the Dentsply/Rinn Bisecting Angle Instruments (BAI) film-holders and the Dentsply/Rinn Stabe disposable periapical x-ray film-holders.

Dentsply/Rinn BAI Instruments The Dentsply/Rinn BAI instruments are designed to aid in the determination of horizontal and vertical angulations, minimize distortion from film bending, and prevent cone-cutting. A set of Dentsply/Rinn BAI instruments consists of anterior and posterior periapical biteblocks, indicator rods, and aiming rings (Fig. 5.41). By using the Dentsply/Rinn BAI instruments, the vertical and horizontal BID angulations need not be memorized, and head positioning is not critical. Moreover, correct film placement and retention is accomplished with less strain on the patient. A long or short BID (cone) can be used with the bisecting technique. If a 4-inch or 8-inch short cone (BID) is all that is available for use, the bisecting angle technique is recommended over the paralleling technique. The operator needs to remember how to determine true BID length: locate the focal spot mark on the tubehead housing and measure the distance from this mark to the external tip of the BID.

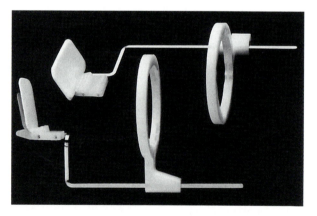

Figure 5.41. Dentsply/Rinn BAI (Bisecting Angle) Instruments. Upper: Posterior BAI instrument. Lower: Anterior BAI instrument. Note that the Dentsply/Rinn BAI instruments differ only from the Dentsply/Rinn XCP instruments in the design of the biteblocks. The instrument avoids the memorization of vertical and horizontal angulation tables and the use of patient-fixed head positions.

Dentsply/Rinn Stabe Film-Holder The Dentsply/Rinn Stabe film-holder is made of an expanded, rigid polystyrene material. It is soft, allowing the patient's teeth to penetrate the biteblock portion of the film-holder, locking it into position. The Dentsply/Rinn Stabe film-holder can be used in the bisecting angle technique by placing the film as shown in Figure 5.42. The removable end of the

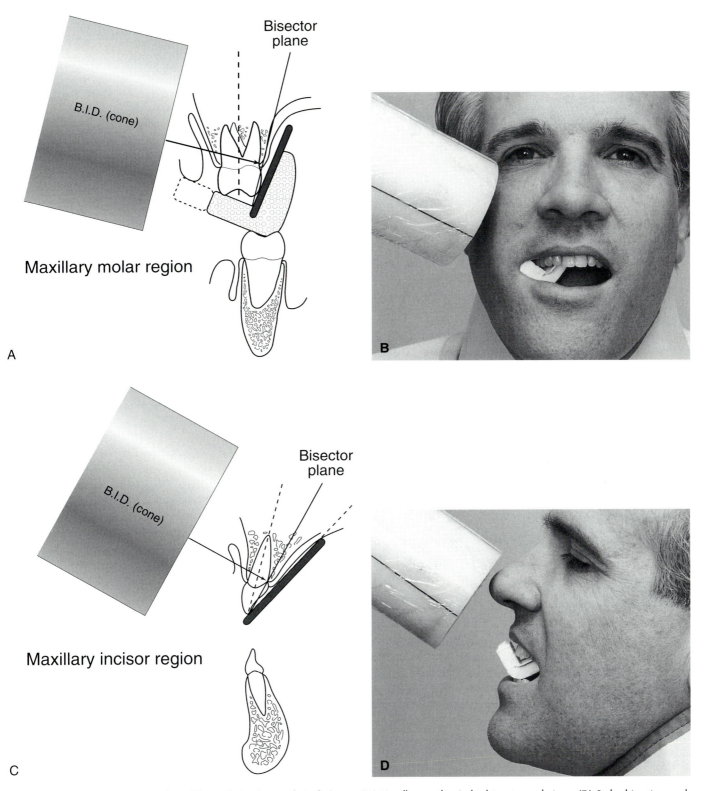

Figure 5.42. Dentsply/Rinn Stabe Film-Holder and Bisecting Angle Technique. (**A**) Maxillary molar Stabe bisecting technique. (**B**) Stabe bisecting-angle technique in maxillary molar region. (**C**) Stabe bisecting-angle technique in maxillary central incisor region (stabe is missing). (**D**) Maxillary incisor Stabe bisecting technique.

Dentsply/Rinn Stabe is taken off for placement of all periapical packets with the bisecting technique. With film in the Dentsply/Rinn Stabe film-holder, the operator places the film as close to the teeth as possible without bending the film. The patient then closes gently on the biteblock portion of the film-holder. The x-ray beam is directed perpendicular to the bisecting plane, bisecting the angle formed by the plane of the film and the long axes of the teeth (Fig. 5.42). **The cone (BID) should be positioned horizontally so the flat portion of the x-ray BID is parallel to mean tangent of the surfaces of the teeth being radiographed.** The use of the bisecting angle method (without an aiming device) requires very careful positioning of the film and cone (BID). (The average bisecting angle vertical angles as shown in the previous boxed section should be used.)

MANAGEMENT OF THE PATIENT DURING RADIOGRAPHIC PROCEDURES

For the procedure to progress smoothly and to avoid retakes, the operator must know how to manage each patient individually. There are certain patient variations that should be considered before beginning any radiographic procedure. After preliminary discussions and removal of intraoral appliances and eyeglasses, the patient's mouth should be examined, and a mental note made about any of the following factors that may have an influence on the procedure.

ANATOMICAL VARIATIONS

Tongue Variations
Large muscular tongues often interfere with placing a film for mandibular projections.

Shallow Maxillary Palates
Absolute parallelism between the film and long axes of the teeth is difficult to accomplish in patients with shallow or low maxillary palatal vaults. However, if the discrepancy of parallelism between the film and the long axis of the tooth does not exceed 20°, the resultant radiograph is usually acceptable. This angle is estimated by observing the angle between the plane of the film in place and the long axis of the teeth being imaged. In those unusual cases in which the patient has a very low or shallow palate, the vertical angulation should be increased by 5° to 15° greater than the Dentsply/Rinn XCP instrument indicates. However, by increasing the vertical angulation, foreshortening of the teeth in the region will result and sometimes a portion of the cusp tips of the teeth may be cut off (Fig. 5.43).

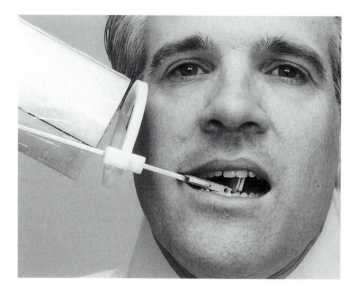

Figure 5.43. Shallow or Low Maxillary Palates. Increasing vertical angulation of cone (BID) in patients with a low or shallow palate to increase periapical coverage.

Torus Palatinus
This is a form of **exostosis** or bony outgrowth in the midline of the hard palate seen quite frequently in the general population (20%). When it becomes sufficiently large, it causes a problem in taking radiographs of the maxillary molars with the Dentsply/Rinn XCP paralleling technic. The film should be placed on the far side of the torus before exposing the film. The film should not be placed on the torus itself (Fig. 5.44).

Torus Mandibularis
This **exostosis** or outgrowth of bone is found on the lingual surface of the mandible, is usually bilateral, and is in the canine-premolar area (Fig. 5.45). The reported incidence in the United States is 6% to 8%, with no difference between sexes. The onset usually is at 30 years of age. It is important **not** to place the apical border of the film on top of a mandibular torus, as it will result in only a partial image of the roots of the teeth. The film should be inserted between the lingual torus and the tongue, away from the torus and teeth, thus increasing the object-film distance (Fig. 5.45).

Sensitive Mucosa in the Mandibular Premolar Region
The preferred method to place films into the sensitive premolar vestibular region using the Dentsply/Rinn XCP

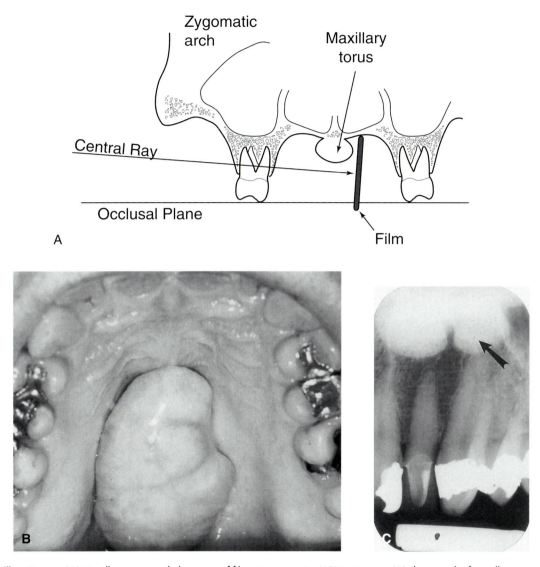

Figure 5.44. Maxillary Torus. (**A**) Maxillary torus and placement of film using posterior XCP instrument. (**B**) Photograph of maxillary torus. (**C**) Radiograph of maxillary torus (*arrow*) taken with anterior XCP instrument.

instrument is as follows. First, the XCP biteblock is brought in firm contact with the teeth to be examined; the apical end of the film packet at this stage should exert very little pressure on the vestibular soft tissues between the tongue and the teeth (Fig. 5.46). The film is brought to its terminal position by a tilting action of the instrument using the biteblock as a fulcrum when the patient closes on the biteblock. The operator coordinates the movement of the film with the patient's jaw movements. As the patient closes, the muscles of the floor of the mouth relax, enabling the film to be brought to place without discomfort. Sometimes moving the tongue or swallowing helps to further relax these muscles. If necessary, topical anesthetic can be used to desensitize these tissues.

High Muscle Attachments in Mandibular Premolar Region

When there are high muscle attachments along with an excessive mandibular occlusal curve and long roots, the conventional Dentsply/Rinn XCP paralleling technique may result in inadequate periapical coverage in the premolar region (Fig. 5.47). One way to overcome this problem is to increase the negative vertical angle of the cone (upward movement of the cone tip) −5° to −15° greater than the instrument indicates (Fig. 5.47). The Snap-A-Ray may be substituted for the Dentsply/Rinn XCP instrument in the mandibular premolar region with some success, because the mandibular premolars are positioned more vertically in the alveolar bone with very little

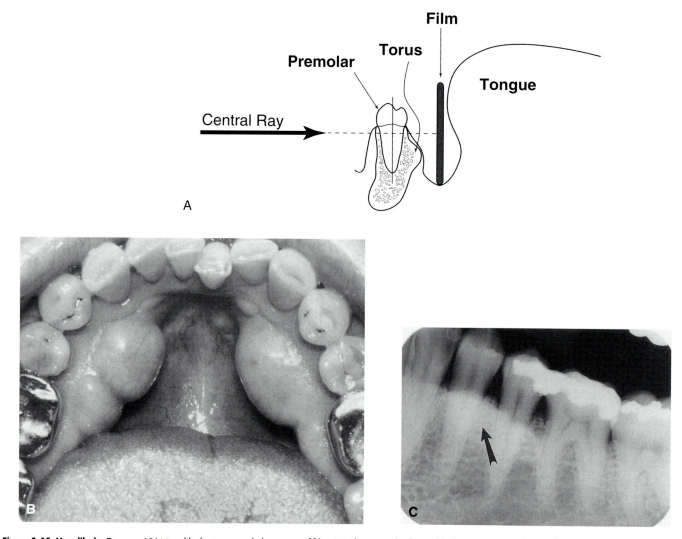

Figure 5.45. Mandibular Torus. (**A**) Mandibular torus and placement of film. (**B**) Photograph of mandibular torus. (**C**) Radiograph of mandibular torus (*arrow*).

lingual inclination. This allows for adequate paralleling of the film with the long axes of the teeth without increasing the object-film distance.

Sensitive Mandibular Incisor Region

Mandibular incisor intraoral radiography using the Dentsply/Rinn XCP instrument can be very sensitive to a patient if the Dentsply/Rinn XCP film-holder is not positioned correctly. The XCP biteblock should first be brought into firm contact with the incisal edge of the mandibular incisor teeth. At this stage, the apical portion of the film packet should exert little or no pressure on the soft tissues of the floor of the mouth (Fig. 5.48). Next, the film is brought into the final position by a rotating movement of the Dentsply/Rinn XCP instrument as the

patient slowly closes the mouth. The film can be placed into position without sensitivity by coordination of the movement of the film with the patient's jaw movement. The muscles of the floor of the mouth relax as the mouth closes and provide adequate room for the film packet (Fig. 5.48).

Edentulous Ridges

Edentulous patients will require less exposure time to produce the radiographic image. Usually, one timer setting lower is a suitable adjustment. When available, the panoramic radiograph is the simplest, quickest, and least uncomfortable radiographic procedure for edentulous patients.

and in any patient a carefully exposed and properly processed panoramic radiograph is an excellent and often desirable substitute for the complete-mouth intraoral periapical radiographic survey.

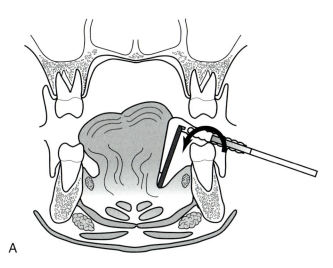

A

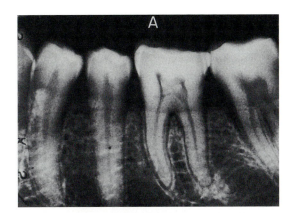

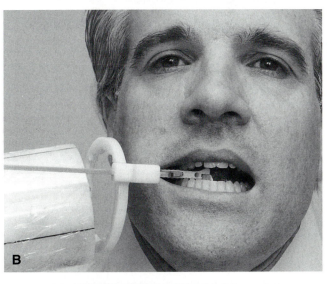

B

Figure 5.46. Sensitive Mucosa Region in Mandibular Premolar Region. (**A**) Initial position. (**B**) Terminal position (a cotton roll between opposing teeth and biteblock may sometimes be used).

SUBSTITUTING THE PANORAMIC RADIOGRAPH FOR DIFFICULT PATIENTS

The panoramic radiograph is an excellent substitute for intraoral radiography. It is quick and easy and usually causes very little problems in difficult-to-manage patients. By alleviating an unpleasant experience and obtaining the needed image information, the patient's confidence can be increased. If further dental hygiene and dental procedures are needed, the anxious patient will be better prepared to undergo these procedures because the preliminary radiographs were well tolerated. Also, at any time

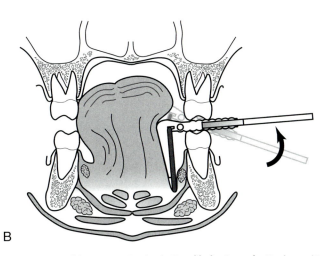

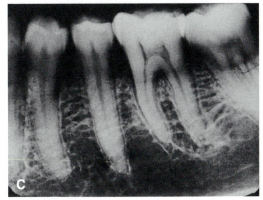

Figure 5.47. High Muscle Attachments in Mandibular Premolar Region. (**A**) Inadequate radiographic periapical coverage in mandibular premolar region because of high muscle attachments. (**B**) Increasing negative vertical angulation of the cone (*BID*). (**C**) Resultant radiograph of patient in A and B.

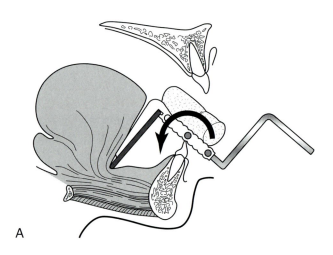

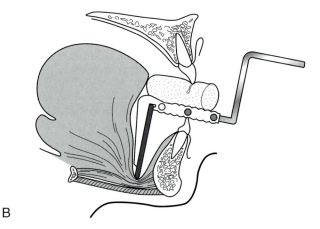

Figure 5.48. Sensitive Mandibular Incisor Region. Positioning anterior Dentsply/Rinn XCP instrument in mandibular incisor region. (**A**) Starting position. (**B**) Terminal position.

MANAGING THE APPREHENSIVE PATIENT

Apprehensive patients are usually nervous or anxious individuals who tend to have a hypersensitive mouth and a low pain threshold. These patients often avoid the dental office and do not have regular check-ups. The first contact with the patient should be a pleasant, reassuring one. It is imperative to be organized for the procedure so that exposures can be made rapidly but accurately. Extreme care must be used in the placement of the films. It is best to begin the procedure in the maxillary anterior region and work progressively posterior. Be encouraging and compliment patient cooperation. Many patients have difficulty maintaining the film in the proper position due to a low pain threshold or nervousness. There are several ways of reducing the level of pain induction, thus accommodating the patient and producing a diagnostic radiograph.

Film Bending

It is preferable not to bend the film. However, conservative bends on certain aspects of the film can make the difference in proper film positioning and patient comfort. The allowable bends are strategically located so that they do not interfere with the teeth of interest on the film. Bent edges should always be unbent, and this edge placed as the trailing edge in the processor. The usual spots are the lower anterior edge of mandibular premolar periapicals and the upper anterior corner of the maxillary canine film.

Edge-Ease Tissue Protectors (Strong Dental Products, Saratoga, CA)

In the lower premolar region, if film feels sharp on closing, the operator should try placing the film further lingual to the teeth, having the patient relax the muscles by moving the tongue, or performing appropriate film bending. If these steps do not diminish the sensitivity, the saliva should be wiped from the film packet and a sponge tissue protector placed on the apical film edge. These tissue sponges have a peel-off backing that exposes a sticky surface, allowing the sponge to adhere to the film packet

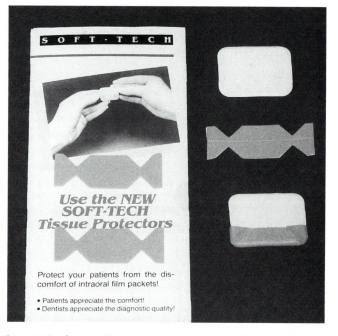

Figure 5.49. Edge-Ease Tissue Protectors (Strong Dental Products, Saratoga, CA). Soft-technique tissue protectors that have been available since 1988 are used to protect patients from discomfort resulting from the inferior border of the periapical film packets encroaching on sensitive intraoral tissues during intraoral radiographic procedures.

(Fig. 5.49). The sponge does not interfere with the image. Use of the tissue protectors should reduce the discomfort experienced by the patient.

Topical Anesthetic

If tissue protectors are not available or are not effective, film placement sensitivity can be reduced by use of a topi-

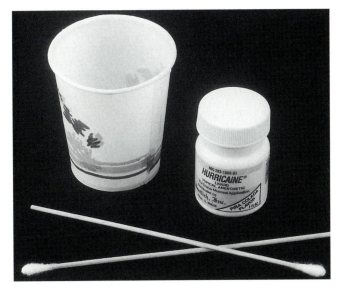

Figure 5.50. Topical Anesthetic Agent for Sensitive Oral Tissues. Liquid Topical Hurricane Anesthetic Agent (Beutlich Co, Waukegan, IL) and cotton-tipped swabs to apply the liquid topical anesthetic.

cal anesthetic agent. It is best to check the patient's medical history before use. The topical solution can be painted on the tissues with a cotton-tipped swab where the film is to be placed (Fig. 5.50). This should reduce the pain sensation long enough to expose the film. The patient should be instructed to rinse and empty the mouth once finished.

Prescribed Anxiolytics

Prescribing tranquilizers, such as Valium or Xanax, can go a long way in reducing patient anxiety and increasing cooperation and tolerance of minor discomfort.

MANAGING THE GAGGING PATIENT

Gagging is the involuntary effort to vomit. It is caused by the gag reflex and is very annoying in intraoral radiography. Some patients have an extremely low threshold for the gag reflex. The receptors for the gag reflex are located in the soft palate, the lateral posterior one third of the tongue, and the region of the retromylohyoid space. The ninth or glossopharyngeal nerve governs the sensitivity of these areas and also controls the reflex movement of swallowing, gagging, and vomiting (Fig. 5.51). The mechanism of the gagging reflex is set off by initial irritation to the soft palate or the posterior third of the tongue and is subsequently conveyed by afferent nerves to the gag center in the medulla oblongata. There is an outflow from this nerve center by way of efferent nerve fibers to the muscles involved in gagging. The gag reflex proceeds by a series of reactions. First there is the cessation of respiration. This is followed by the contraction of the *thoracic-oabdominal* and *oropharyngeal* muscles. (Sometimes food is regurgitated into the larynx, the oropharynx, and the mouth.)

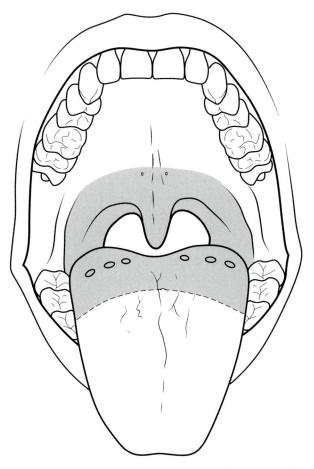

Figure 5.51. Receptors of Ninth or Glossopharyngeal Nerve in Oral Cavity. Areas of the oral pharynx and the posterior one third of the tongue where the receptors of the gag reflex are located. These areas (dark areas) are innervated by the ninth or glossopharyngeal nerve.

The two stimuli that commonly initiate the gag reflex are psychic stimuli and tactile stimuli. To eliminate or diminish the gag reflex, these stimuli must be eliminated or diminished.

Reducing Psychic Stimuli

Persons with an accentuated gag reflex are usually nervous and high-strung individuals with hypersensitive oral tissues.

The following suggestions will aid in the alleviation of psychic stimuli:

1. The first contact should be a pleasant one, and every effort should be made to give the patient confidence in the dental health-care worker's ability to perform the service about to be rendered. The problem should be discussed in a kindly and sympathetic manner. The dental health-care worker should try to gain the patient's confidence, which reduces anxiety.

2. The anterior regions of the oral cavity should be radiographed first, and the most sensitive maxillary molar regions radiographed last. Perhaps by then the patient's fears from psychic stimuli will be forgotten, and these sensitive areas in the oral cavity may be radiographed without incident. The operator should avoid describing where the film will be placed.

3. The health-care worker should try to divert the patient's attention away from the procedure. This can be done in several ways. A running dialogue can be maintained, and the worker can coach the patient through each film. The patient should be encouraged and told to imagine a favorite place or person and focus on that mental picture.

4. The patient should be given a task to perform. For instance, he or she could raise one leg and maintain that position or flex the toes toward the body and hold that position.

5. The patient could be premedicated with the use of anxiolytic agents as prescribed by the dentist.

Reducing Tactile Stimuli

Some persons have an accentuated gag reflex because of hypersensitive pharyngeal areas. Patients suffering from chronic sinus trouble (the well-known postnasal drip) are the worst gaggers. An accumulation of mucus and saliva into the nasopharynx or oropharynx may initiate the gag reflex in these patients.

Methods to alleviate tactile stimuli are as follows:

1. The film should be placed positively and be retained in position without movement. Film-holders like the Rinn EEZEE Grip are very useful in this situation.

2. Exposure of the film should be accomplished as quickly as possible. This can be done by organizing the procedure. The timer, other machine settings, and cone angulation for the approximate anticipated vertical and horizontal angles should be preset. The films should be placed quickly but with precision, and the film exposed with the aid of a helper.

3. If the operator is still experiencing difficulty, use of an agent to desensitize the tissue may be necessary. Ice water, salt placed on the tip of the tongue, or a topical anesthetic applied to the sensitive area often resolves the problem.

4. In cases of an extreme gag reflex, it may be impossible to obtain a complete intraoral survey. The operator should try to obtain as many intraoral projections as possible and then supplement them with extraoral radiographs. Some of the following combinations of films may be suitable alternatives.

a. Maxillary and mandibular topographic occlusals.
b. Bitewings using no. 1 or 0 size film.
c. Panoramic radiograph.

OCCLUSAL RADIOGRAPHY

The occlusal film is much larger than the regular periapical film. It is 3 × 2.25 inches, and its film emulsion speed is the same as the speed of periapical films (E+ speed film). The film is placed between the occlusal surfaces of the teeth and held in place by the patient's teeth. In general, the occlusal radiograph is used to visualize large areas of the maxilla and mandible that cannot be seen on the smaller periapical film. Occlusal radiography is based on the bisecting angle technique theory. Therefore, the central ray will be directed perpendicular to the bisector of the angle formed by the film plane and the long axes of the teeth under examination. Indications for occlusal radiographs have been discussed previously in this chapter. Occlusal radiographs are most often taken to examine the anterior aspects of the maxilla and mandible. The most typical projections will be presented. However, the basics of the technique can be applied to posterior aspects of the mouth by making adjustments in film placement, horizontal angulation, and central ray entry.

MAXILLARY TOPOGRAPHIC PROJECTION

PURPOSE

To observe a much larger area of the maxilla than can be observed with intraoral periapical radiographs (Fig. 5.52).

FILM PLACEMENT

The film is placed in the mouth with the longer axis of the film running laterally from side to side, with the pebbled side against the maxillary teeth and inserted posteriorly as the inner vestibule will permit. The patient bites down gently to hold the film in position. If edentulous, the patient uses the thumbs to hold the film against the edentulous ridges.

HEAD POSITION

The line from the tragus of the ear to the ala of the nose is horizontal and parallel to the floor. The midsagittal plane is perpendicular to the floor.

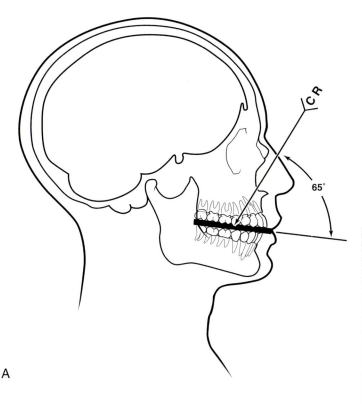

A

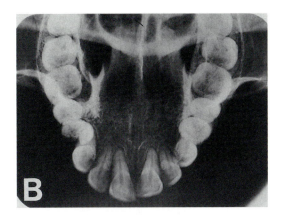

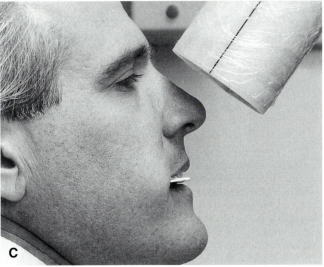

Figure 5.52. Maxillary Occlusal Topographic Radiograph. (**A**) Diagram of maxillary occlusal topographic projection. (**B**) Radiograph of maxillary occlusal topographic projection. (**C**) Side view with the vertical angle of the cone approximately +65° through the point in the midsagittal plane between the nose and the nasal bridge to center of film packet.

PROJECTION OF CENTRAL RAY

The central ray enters perpendicular to the bisector of the angle formed by the film plane and the long axes of the maxillary incisor teeth. The central ray entry point is 0.5 inches above the tip of the nose (Fig. 5.52)

RADIOGRAPHIC FACTORS

Film: Kodak Occlusal Film (E+ speed film) (Rochester, NY).
Source-Film Distance: Long 16-inch cone.
Vertical Angulation (Cone): +65°

EXPOSURE FACTORS

65 kVp and 15 mA
30 impulses—adult.
24 impulses— child.
21 to 24 impulses—edentulous.

Note: For the short 8-inch cone, one quarter of these exposure times can be used.

MANDIBULAR SYMPHYSIS PROJECTION

PURPOSE

This film is used to record a broad area of the mandibular incisor region (Fig. 5.53). It can also be substituted for anterior periapicals when periapical film placement is not possible.

FILM PLACEMENT

The film is inserted into the mouth with the pebbled or plain side of the film facing the mandibular occlusal surfaces. The film is placed with the longer axis of the film placed coincidental with the midsagittal plane. The patient slowly closes down on the film packet with gentle end-to-end bite.

HEAD POSITION

The patient's head is tilted way back until the occlusal plane of the maxillary teeth forms an angle of 45° with

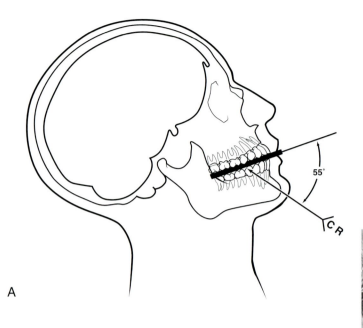

A

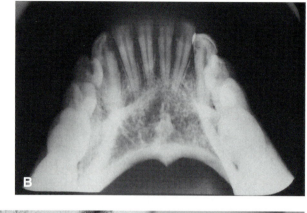

B

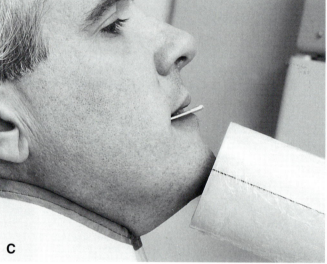

C

Figure 5.53. Mandibular Occlusal Symphysis Radiograph. (**A**) Diagram of occlusal symphysis projection. (**B**) Symphysis radiograph revealing the lower anterior incisors and the lower border of the anterior mandible. (**C**) Cone and film placement. The patient's head should be tilted back until the occlusal plane of the film forms an angle of 45° with the floor. A −20° vertical angulation of cone should be used, and the path of the central ray should be directed through the symphysis of the mandible to the center of the occlusal film.

the floor. The midsagittal plane should be perpendicular to the floor.

PROJECTION OF CENTRAL RAY

A −20° vertical angulation of the cone should be used, and the central ray should be directed parallel to the sagittal plane through the symphysis of the mandible to the approximate center of the packet. The film packet and the central ray should form an approximate angle of 55° (Fig. 5.53).

RADIOGRAPHIC FACTORS

Film: Kodak Occlusal Film (E+ speed film).
Source-Film Distance: Long cone, 16 inches.

EXPOSURE FACTORS

65 kVp and 15 mA
24 impulses—adult.
21 impulses—child.

Note: These exposure times can be reduced to one quarter the exposure time if an 8-inch cone is used.

MANDIBULAR CROSS-SECTIONAL PROJECTION

PURPOSE

This projection shows the relationship of an object to the teeth in the horizontal plane. Thus it provides the information that, when coupled with information obtained from the intraoral periapical survey, accurately localizes the position of an object within the mandible. It is also very important in the diagnosis of sialoliths in the submandibular gland duct (Wharton's) and of calcifications within the gland itself (Fig. 5.54).

FILM PLACEMENT

An occlusal packet is inserted with the pebbled side adjacent to the mandibular occlusal surfaces; the short center axis is coincident with midsagittal plane. The poste-

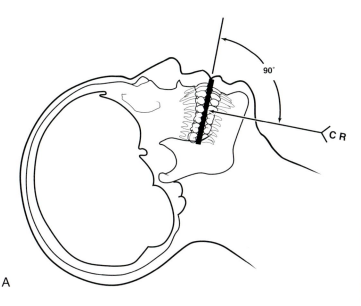

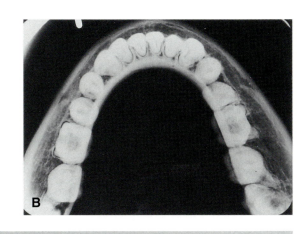

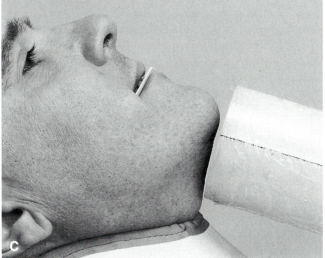

Figure 5.54. Mandibular Cross-Sectional Occlusal Projection. (**A**) Diagram of mandibular cross-sectional occlusal projection. (**B**) Radiograph of the mandibular cross- sectional occlusal projection. (**C**) Cone and film placement. The head is tipped back until the occlusal plane of the maxillary teeth is at a right angle to the floor. The path of the central ray is directed 1 inch posterior to the symphysis and at right angles to the film.

rior edge of packet is against the anterior aspect of the rami bilaterally. The patient slowly closes on the packet with a gentle end-to-end bite. Edentulous patients should hold the film against the ridge with their forefinger.

HEAD POSITION

The head is tipped backward until the occlusal plane of the maxillary teeth is vertical and at a right angle to the floor.

PROJECTION OF THE CENTRAL RAY

The central ray enters beneath the chin approximately 1 inch posterior to the mandibular symphysis at the midline. The central ray is directed perpendicular to the occlusal film (Fig. 5.54).

RADIOGRAPHIC FACTORS

Film: Kodak Occlusal (E+ speed film).

EXPOSURE FACTORS

65 kVp and 15 mA
24 impulses—adult.
21 impulses—child.
21 impulses—edentulous.
Note: If an 8-inch cone is used, the above exposures may be reduced to one quarter of the above settings.

WORKSHOP/LABORATORY EXERCISES

EXERCISE 5.1. THE DENTSPLY/RINN XCP LONG-CONE PARALLELING TECHNIQUE

Materials and Equipment Needed

1. Dentsply/Rinn XCP paralleling instrument set.
2. Twelve no. 2 and eight no. 1 films.

3. Skull or manikin.
4. X-ray machine.
5. Proper exposure chart.

Instructions

Step 1: Using the anterior instrument set up, expose the maxillary centrals, right lateral, and right canine; repeat for the maxillary left lateral and canine. Using the same anterior instrument set up, expose the mandibular incisors and right and left canines.

Step 2: Expose the maxillary right premolars and molars; using the same posterior instrument set up, expose the mandibular left premolars and molars. Repeat for the maxillary left posterior teeth and mandibular right posterior teeth.

Step 3: Using the XCP bitewing instrument, expose the premolar and molar bitewing films on the right side. Repeat this procedure on the left side.
Notes:

1. Use the exposure chart for the proper machine settings for each anatomical region.
   Remember, exposure settings need to be matched with true source-film distance length, and this should be 16 inches. The source-film distance is the distance between the source (marked on the tubehead by a black dot) and the film in the patient's mouth.
2. For each exposure, center the biteblock on the tooth or teeth to be radiographed. Look at the diagrams in this chapter to see which teeth need to be included in each film.
3. Practice the one-two-three motion of placing the film. One, bring the outer edge of the biteblock in contact with the incisal or occlusal edge of the teeth. Two, rotate the film into place with the biteblock still contacting the tooth or teeth. Three, ease the film in place as the patient bites down or the manikin is repositioned for closing and move the ring in.
4. Make small film positioning adjustments once the film is down by asking the patient to open slightly or by opening the manikin's bite slightly and adjust the film forward or backward to obtain the final correct position.
5. Make certain the plane at the end of the BID is parallel to the plane of the positioning ring. Make certain the positioning rod is parallel to the edge of the long BID. Look at the BID tip and rod from

the side and from the top or bottom to check all planes for parallelism.

6. According to your instructor and the time available, expose either half a full-mouth survey (one side only), including maxillary and mandibular central incisors, or expose the full complete-mouth survey.

Step 4. Carefully save these films for a future laboratory exercise.

CASE-BASED QUESTIONS FOR LABORATORY EXERCISE

There are no questions for this session. The objective is to obtain the exposed full-mouth survey of either the half-patient or full-patient.

CASE-BASED PROBLEM-SOLVING

When taking a full-mouth survey using the Dentsply/Rinn XCP long cone paralleling technique, you note that you can get the film very close to the mandibular posterior teeth and, to a slightly lesser degree, in the anterior region. However, you note you cannot maintain film and tooth parallelism in any part of the upper jaw with a close tooth-film distance. First, if a long cone is available, how would you overcome this problem? Second, if only a short 8-inch cone is available, how does this complicate your answer and how would you modify your solution?

REVIEW QUESTIONS

1. Dental radiographic film has a special code number to indicate the film function (purpose) and the size (dimensions) of the film. A box of film with a code designation of 3.4 would indicate films of an appropriate size for:

   A. Periapical radiographs.
   B. Occlusal radiographs.
   C. Interproximal radiographs.
   D. Pedodontic periapical radiographs.

2. What is the main cause of foreshortening in the bisecting angle technique?

   A. Improper placement of the film.
   B. Improper horizontal angulation of the cone.
   C. Vertical angulation of the cone is too flat or obtuse.

D. Vertical angulation of the cone is too acute or sharp.

3. When bitewing x-rays are taken without an alignment instrument, the midsagittal plane of the patient's head should be:

A. Parallel to the floor.
B. Parallel to the tube.
C. Perpendicular to the floor.
D. Perpendicular to the tube.

4. The embossed dot on the film packet should always be placed in which direction from the x-ray source?

A. Away from the source.
B. Toward the source.
C. It does not matter.
D. Away from the source on the mandibular arch and toward the source on the maxillary arch.

5. The standard film size used for adult bitewings and posterior periapicals is number:

A. 1.1.
B. 1.2.
C. 2.2.
D. 3.4.
E. Any of the above size films could be used for bitewings.

6. On a premolar periapical, it is critical to obtain which of the following anatomical structures?

A. Complete view of the premolars and the first molar with an open contact between the premolar and first molar.
B. Complete view of the premolars and at least one third of the canine.
C. Complete view of the premolars plus the first and second molar with an open contact between the two premolars.
D. Complete view of premolars and the canine. Premolars should be centered on the film.

7. The technique that shows the upper and lower crowns on the same radiograph is called the:

A. Bisecting angle technique.
B. Bitewing technique.
C. Paralleling technique.
D. Occlusal technique.

8. If a satisfactory radiograph was produced using a source-film distance of 8 inches and an exposure time of 1 second, what would be the correct exposure time for a source-film distance of 16 inches?

A. 2 seconds.
B. 4 seconds.
C. 6 seconds.
D. 8 seconds.

9. At 90 kVp and 15 mA at a cone (BID) distance of 8 inches, the exposure time for a film is 0.50 seconds. In the same situation, the exposure time at 16 inches would be:

A. 0.25 seconds.
B. 1.00 seconds.
C. 2.00 seconds.
D. 4.00 seconds.

10. A hygienist is currently using 90 kVp, 15 mA, 2.50 mm aluminum filtration, and 0.20-second exposure time. His radiation source-film distance is 8 inches. He decides to change the radiation source-film distance to 12 inches. What should be the new exposure time?

A. 0.30 seconds.
B. 0.45 seconds.
C. 0.60 seconds.
D. 0.80 seconds.

CASE-BASED QUESTIONS

CASE 5.1

The patient is a 35-five-year old woman and a long-standing, usually cooperative patient. This time she complained of discomfort when the film was being placed.

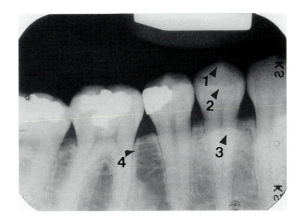

QUESTIONS

1. Forgetting for now that the apices are not showing, mesiodistally the film is:

   A. Poorly placed because part of the canine is missing.
   B. Poorly placed because the second premolar is not centered on the biteblock.
   C. Well placed because the second premolar is in the middle of the film.
   D. Well placed because the distal of the canine and first molar are in the image.

2. With respect to the apices, the problem could be best corrected by:

   A. Increasing the negative vertical angulation, because this will also align the lingual and buccal cusp tips.
   B. Asking the patient to raise the tongue for better film placement.
   C. Asking the patient to bite down more firmly on the biteblock.
   D. Positioning the film more lingually to avoid traumatizing the lingual torus.

3. Match the columns by identifying the following.

Arrow 1 _____	A. Mandibular torus.
Arrow 2 _____	B. Buccal cusp tip.
Arrow 3 _____	C. Lingual cusp tip.
Arrow 4 _____	D. Lamina dura.

CASE 5.2

The patient is a 15-year-old boy who needed to have a radiograph taken of his lower third molar.

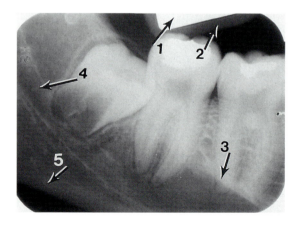

QUESTIONS

1. Most likely, the biteblock is not centered on the film because:

   A. The film was positioned distally in the biteblock for improved film placement.
   B. The film slipped out of the biteblock groove during placement.
   C. The patient pushed the film forward with his tongue.
   D. The patient loosened his bite on the biteblock after film placement.

2. Match the columns by identifying the anatomical structures.

Arrow 1 _____	A. Mylohyoid ridge.
Arrow 2 _____	B. Metallic part of biteblock.
Arrow 3 _____	C. Inferior alveolar canal.
Arrow 4 _____	D. Plastic part of the biteblock.
Arrow 5 _____	E. Inferior cortex.

BIBLIOGRAPHY

Bean LR. Comparison of bisecting angle and paralleling methods of intraoral radiology. J Dent Educ 1969;33:441–445.

Council on Dental Materials, Instruments and Equipment. Recommendations in radiographic practices: an update, 1988. J Am Dent Assoc 1989;118:115–117.

Dempster WT, Adams WJ, Duddles RA. Arrangement in the jaws of the roots of the teeth. J Am Dent Assoc 1963;67:779–797.

Dresen OM. Control of the gagging patient. Texas Dent J 1947;65:332–333.

Ennis LM. The bisecting technique versus paralleling. Dent Clin North Am 1969;November:779–781. (First to actively introduce bisecting technique to dental practice.)

Ennis LM, Berry H. Necessity for routine roentgenographic examination of the edentulous patient. Oral Surg 1949;7:3–19.

Fitzgerald GM. Dental roentgenography. I: an investigation in adumbration, or the factors that control geometric unsharpness. J Am Dent Assoc 1947;34:1–20. (First to introduce paralleling technique to dental practice.)

Fitzgerald GM. Dental roentgenography. II: vertical angulation, film placement and increased object-film distance. J Am Dent Assoc 1947;34:160–170.

Fitzgerald GM. Dental roentgenography. III: the roentgenographic periapical survey of the upper molar region. J Am Dent Assoc 1949;38:293–303.

Fitzgerald GM. Dental roentgenography. IV: the voltage factor. J Am Dent Assoc 1950;41:19–28.

Fitzgerald GM. Roentgenographic rebuttal. Oral Surg 1960;13:1218.

LeMaster CA: A modification of technic for radiographing upper molars. J Natl Dent Assoc 1921;8:328.

Lozier M. Etiology and control of gagging reflex in the practice of intraoral roentgenography. Oral Surg 1949;2:766–769.

Matteson SR, Whaley C, Secrist VC. Dental radiography. 4th ed. Chapel Hill: University of North Carolina Press, 1988.

McCormack D. Dental roentgenology: a technical procedure for furthering the advancement toward anatomical accuracy. J Calif State Dent Assoc 1937;May-June:89.

McCormack DW. Mechanical aids for obtaining accuracy in dental roentgenology. J Am Dent Assoc 1950;40:144–153.

McCormack FW. A plea for a standardized technique for oral radiography, with an illustrated classification of findings and their verified interpretation. Br Dent J 1920;2:467–510. (First to advocate paralleling technique.)

Medwedeff FM, Elcan PD. A precision technic to minimize radiation. Dent Surv 1967;43:45–50. (Inventor of precision film-holder.)

Medwedeff FM, Knox WH, Latimer P. A new device to reduce patient irradiation and improve dental film quality. Oral Surg 1962;15:1079–1088.

National Council on Radiation Protection and Measurements. Report no. 35. Dental X-ray protection. NCRP Publication, March 9, 1970.

Peterson S. Clinical dental hygiene. St. Louis: Mosby-Year Book, 1959.

Price WA. The technique necessary for making good dental skiagraphs. Dental Items of Interest 1904;26:161–171, 1904. (First to advocate bisecting angle technique.)

Raper HR. Uses of bitewing radiographs. Dent Surv 1954;30:763. (Invented bitewing technique.)

Richards A. The control of gagging in dental radiography. J Mich State Dent Soc 1949;31:110–111.

Silha RE. Roentgenographic service for gagging patient. Oral Surg 1962;January:64.

Silha RE. The versatile occlusal dental x-ray film. III: a new pedodontic survey. Dent Radiogr Photogr 1966;39:40–43.

Silha RE. Paralleling long cone technic. Dent Radiogr Photogr 1968;41:3–19.

Silha RE. Paralleling technic with a disposable film-holder. Dent Radiogr Photogr 1975;48:27–35.

Spear LB, Hannah R. Practical and improved periapical technic. Dent Radiogr Photogr 1953;26:212–225.

Stephens DW. Physiological and psychological approach to the problem of gagging. Dent Surg 1949;25:1795–1797.

Updegrave WJ. Paralleling extension cone technique in intraoral dental radiography. Oral Surg 1951;4:1250–1261.

Updegrave WJ. Simplified and standardized bisecting angle technic for dental radiography. J Am Dent Assoc, 1967;75:1361–1368. (Invented Dentsply/Rinn XCP instruments.)

Updegrave WJ. Right-angle dental radiography. Dent Clin North Am 1968;12:571–579.

Updegrave WJ. A plea for a standard intraoral radiography with reduced tissue irradiation. J Am Dent Assoc 1972;85:861–869.

Updegrave WJ. The versatile no. 1 x-ray film. Dent Radiogr Photogr 1975;48:60–62.

Weissman DD, Longhurst GE. Clinical evaluation of a rectangular field collimating device for periapical radiography. J Am Dent Assoc 1971;82:580–582.

Winkler KG: Influence of rectangular collimation and intraoral shielding on radiation dose in dental radiography. J Am Dent Assoc 1968;77:95–101.

Wuehrmann AH. Evaluation criteria for intraoral radiographic film quality. J Am Dent Assoc 1974;89:345–352, 1974. (One of the first to teach paralleling technique in a dental school.)

Processing and Film Mounting Procedures

6

OBJECTIVES

Upon successful completion of this unit, the student will be able to:

1. *Discuss the proper film processing technique and the effect of the processing steps on the radiographic film.*

2. *Identify the components of the processing solutions and the purpose of the components.*

3. *Discuss manual and/or automatic processing of radiographs.*

4. *List the advantages of automatic processing.*

5. *List ways to prevent automatic processor problems.*

6. *Compare manual versus automatic processing procedures.*

7. *Describe the care and maintenance of the darkroom.*

8. *Demonstrate how to mount a full-mouth survey.*

9. *Duplicate a radiograph.*

10. *Process and mount a full-mouth or half-mouth survey using the Workshop/Laboratory Exercises format.*

11. *Explain one method of film duplication using the Case-Based Problem-Solving format.*

12. *Test his or her knowledge by answering the Review Questions.*

KEY WORDS/PHRASES

automatic processing
automatic processor maintenance
automatic processor quick check

automatic processor solution
replenishment
clearing agent

darkroom
duplicating x-rays
emulsion

feeding films
film mounting
glutaraldehyde
halation
manual processing

phenidone
processing solutions
processor problems
roller functions
safelight

safelight check
solarized film
sulfate compounds
water temperature

INTRODUCTION

Even if the finest x-ray equipment is used and the most exacting radiographic technique is employed, the radiograph produced may be of inferior quality if the processing of the exposed x-ray film is carelessly executed. Processing the film completes what the exposure started. It produces a visible, lasting image of the latent image created by the x-rays. When the x-rays or light strike the x-ray or light-sensitive silver salts (AgIBr) in the film emulsion, the energy is stored in the form of a latent image. The latent image becomes visible after the film is immersed in certain chemical solutions that change the exposed silver halide salts into particles of metallic silver. The term for the several operations that collectively produce the visible, permanent images is **processing**. Processing, automatic or manual, consists of the following stages: developing, fixing, washing, and drying. In manual processing, the film is rinsed before fixing. These operations are all performed in a darkroom, unless an automatic processor with a daylight loader is used. Otherwise, the automatic or manual processor must be placed in the darkroom.

DARKROOM

The darkroom or processing room should be clean, efficient, and well equipped. Spots, streaks, fog, and other artifacts on the processed radiograph can be traced to poor darkroom conditions. It is very important that the darkroom be designed to make film processing an efficient, precise, and standardized procedure. Because the processing operations are performed under conditions of reduced visibility, every piece of equipment must be in its specific place. Figure 6.1 illustrates a well-designed darkroom.

PROCESSING METHODS

There are two methods used in processing x-ray film: manual and automatic processing. Most automatic processors use a roller transport or track system to move the film through the developer, fixer, wash, and dry cycles (Fig. 6.2).

MANUAL PROCESSING

Manual processing is the simplest method to develop, rinse, fix, and wash dental films. The most practical processing tank for a dental office consists of a master tank and two removable insert tanks each with a 1-gallon capacity. The master tank holds running water for rinsing, washing, and maintaining the temperature of the insert tanks. The insert tanks are for the developer and fixer solutions (Fig. 6.3).

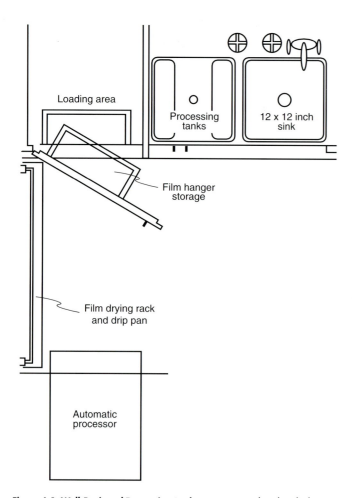

Figure 6.1. Well-Designed Processing Darkroom. Note that this darkroom is designed for manual and automatic processing.

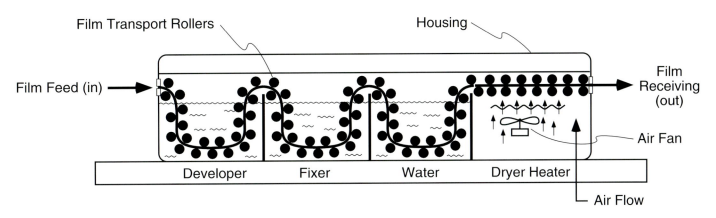

Film Transport Rollers

Housing

Film Feed (in)

Film Receiving (out)

Air Fan

Air Flow

| Developer | Fixer | Water | Dryer Heater |

Figure 6.2. Automatic Processor Diagram. The automatic processor uses a roller system that transports film through the developer, fixer, wash, and dryer cycles.

MANUAL PROCESSING EQUIPMENT

Running Hot and Cold Water

Manual x-ray processing solutions are most effective when used with a comparatively narrow range of temperatures. Below 60°F, some of the chemicals are definitely sluggish in action, which may cause underdevelopment and inadequate fixation. Above 75°F, they work too rapidly and may produce fogging (unwanted density) of the film.

In manual processing, a temperature of 70°F is recommended for three reasons:

1. The optimum quality of the radiograph is attained at this temperature. The contrast and density of the film are more satisfactory, and fog (unwanted density) is kept to an acceptable low level.
2. The processing time is practical.

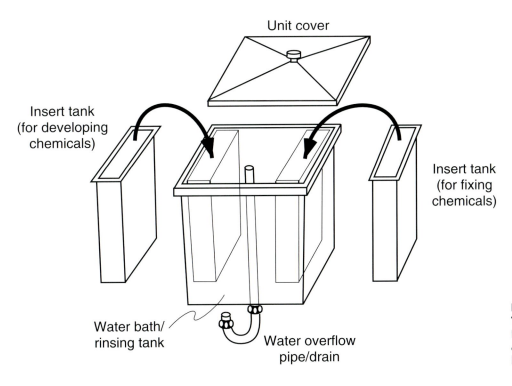

Unit cover

Insert tank (for developing chemicals)

Insert tank (for fixing chemicals)

Water bath/rinsing tank

Water overflow pipe/drain

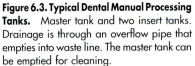

Figure 6.3. Typical Dental Manual Processing Tanks. Master tank and two insert tanks. Drainage is through an overflow pipe that empties into waste line. The master tank can be emptied for cleaning.

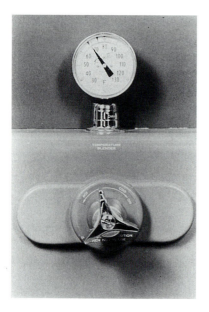

Figure 6.4. Temperature in the Master Tank is Controlled by Mixing Valve. Typical mixing valve to blend incoming hot and cold water to correct temperature is shown. The water is piped into the bottom of the master tank.

3. With contemporary solution-tempering devices, a temperature of 70°F is usually conveniently maintained. The temperature of the water in the master tank is controlled by a thermostatic or manual mixing valve in the water supply (Fig. 6.4). This is the reason hot and cold running water are essential. In turn, the temperature of the water in the master tank controls the temperature of the processing solutions in the insert tanks.

Thermometers and Timer

The processing time is dependent on the temperature of the solutions; thus, proper control of processing time is essential, and a good thermometer is an indispensable item. There are two types: (1) a **tank thermometer** that is plainly marked with both centigrade and Fahrenheit scales and that has a steel clip on the back formed into a hook to hold the thermometer in the tank, and (2) the **floating, stirring rod type of thermometer** that is all glass and can also be used for stirring processing solutions. An **interval timer** is also important to control time of development and fixation (Fig. 6.5).

Safelighting

The function of a safelight is to provide enough illumination in the darkroom so that essential processing activities can be accomplished with a minimum amount of errors but without fogging the film. X-ray film emulsions are primarily sensitive to blue and green light and are less sensitive to light in the opposite region of the spectrum—yellow and red light. Therefore, safelights are safest when made with amber (dark orange-yellow) or red filters. However, most films have some sensitivity to all colors of light transmitted by filters. Therefore, it is necessary to keep **safelight illumination** (wattage of bulb) and **film handling times** under the safelights at a safe, practical, minimum time that should not exceed 5 to 8 minutes. The Kodak (Rochester, NY) Safelight filter GBX-2 (red) is a universal filter that can be used in darkrooms in which both intraoral and extraoral films are used (Fig. 6.6). The GBX-2 filter permits higher levels of illumination than the older Wratten 6B (brown) filter, but lower levels of illumination than the ML-2 (light orange) filter. ML-2 (light orange) filters should be used **only** for intraoral dental film and **never** for panoramic films (screen film),

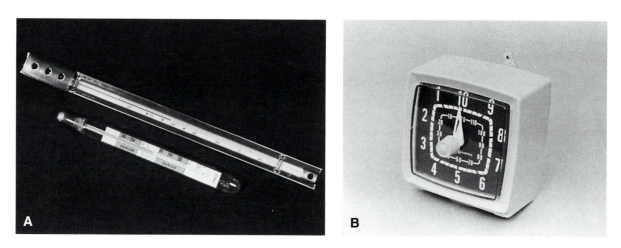

Figure 6.5. Thermometers and Timers. **(A)** Upper: tank thermometer; Lower: floating thermometer. **(B)** Timer.

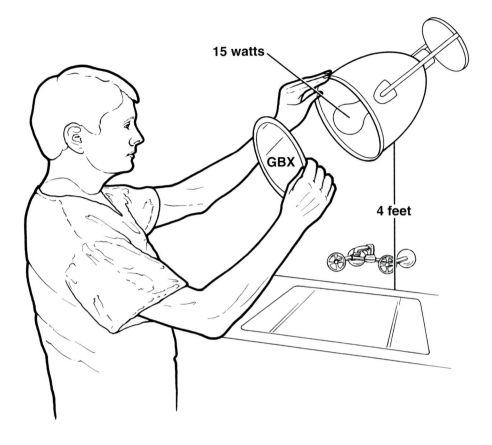

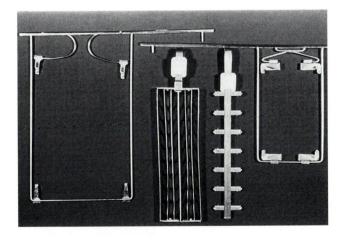

Figure 6.6. Safelighting Specifications. For direct safelighting, use a minimum distance from the workbench of 4 feet, a 7.5- to 15-W bulb, and a GBX-2 filter. Film handling time should not exceed 5 to 8 minutes.

because they transmit light in the color-sensitive range of the screen film emulsions. The Wratten 6B filter is safe for D-speed intraoral film and older extraoral films exposed with calcium tungstate screens.

Safe illumination in the darkroom is also dependent on the **wattage** of the bulb and the **distance** the safelight is from the workbench (Fig. 6.6). Direct-light safelights require a standard 7.5- or 15-watt bulb for most intraoral, panoramic, and extraoral films, whereas a 25-watt bulb may be used for indirect (reflected from ceiling) light. Currently, the GBX-2 filter is recommended for Kodak E+ intraoral film and extraoral films using rare-earth phosphors such as gadolinium. The direct safelight should be placed at a minimum of 4 feet from the workbench. This distance should be not shortened unless absolutely necessary.

Processing Hangers

Processing hangers for manual processing are available in several sizes to accommodate intraoral and extraoral films (Fig. 6.7). The intraoral film hangers are made of stainless steel with white celluloid identification tabs. In most darkrooms, the developer solution will always be in the left-hand tank as one is facing the tank, the water bath will be in the center, and the fixer will be in the

right-hand tank. In unfamiliar darkrooms, the developing solution can be identified by its slippery feeling (alkaline solution), and the fixer by its vinegary odor (acid solution) when fresh.

Figure 6.7. Intraoral and Extraoral Processing Hangers. Assortment of intraoral and extraoral processing hangers. Left to right: 8- to 10-inch screen film hanger, intraoral periapical film hanger without clips, intraoral periapical film hanger with clips, and 5- to 7-inch screen film hanger.

MANUAL PROCESSING PROCEDURE

As previously mentioned, film processing refers to the entire procedure of conversion of the latent image to a visible image (Fig 6.8) and preservation of the visible image. In manual processing, the film processing involves developing, rinsing, fixing, washing, and drying. The sequence of steps in manual processing are outlined below:

Sequence of Steps in Manual Processing

Step	Purpose	Approximate Time (68–70°F)
Wetting	Alkaline developing solution softens and opens up gelatin so developing agents can act on silver halide crystals.	30 sec
Development	Production of visible image from latent image; exposed silver halide crystals are reduced to metallic silver, forming radiographic image.	4.5–5 min
Rinsing	Termination of development and removal of excess chemicals from emulsion.	30 sec
Fixation	Removal of unexposed silver halide crystals from emulsion; hardening of gelatin.	10 min
Washing	Removal of excess chemicals (if fixing agent [ammonium thiosulfate] is left in emulsion, it will eventually change deposited black silver to brown silver sulfide).	15 min
Drying	Removal of water and preparation of radiograph for viewing.	30 min

SEQUENCE OF STEPS IN MANUAL PROCESSING

Steps in Manual Processing

The steps used in the manual processing of x-ray films are summarized in the following paragraphs (Fig. 6.9):

Stir the solutions. The developer and fixer solutions are stirred. A separate paddle is used for each tank to avoid possible contamination. This mixes the chemicals and equalizes the temperature of the solution.

Check the solution level of developer and fixer. If the solution levels are low, the correct level should be maintained by adding fresh solution.

Check the temperature of the solutions. If possible, the temperature should be adjusted to 70°F before development. Ice should never be placed in the solutions to cool them down—this will dilute the solution. One way to cool the solutions in warm weather would be to place ice cubes in a rubber glove and then place the glove in the solutions.

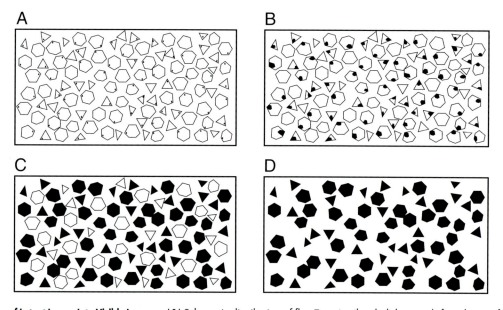

Figure 6.8. Conversion of Latent Image Into Visible Image. **(A)** Schematic distribution of flat, T-grain silver halide crystals found in E+ film. The dots indicate latent image produced by exposure—the silver halide crystals that have been exposed to x-radiation. **(B)** Partial development begins to produce metallic silver black dots in exposed grains. **(C)** Development completed. The greater the action of the x-rays on the film, the greater the amount of metallic silver left. **(D)** Unexposed silver halide crystals have been removed by fixing. The fixing solution dissolves the excess silver salts and fixes the metallic silver on the film by stopping the action of the developer.

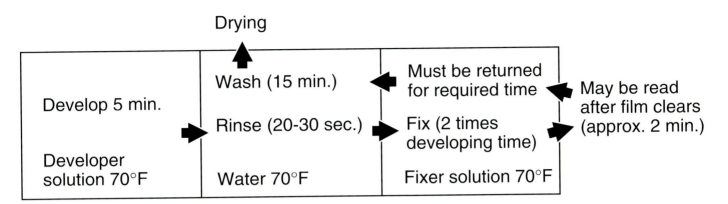

Figure 6.9. Basic Steps in Manual Processing. Developer (5 minutes at 70°F), rinse (30 seconds), fixer (10 minutes), wash (15 minutes), and drying (30 minutes). Total time (dry-to-dry): 1 hour and 30 seconds.

Turn on the safelight(s). All white light should be excluded in the processing room.

Unwrap the exposed film. The operator should carefully remove the exposed film from its packet while wearing gloves. Then, he or she should clip the film into processing hangers with clean, bare hands, carefully holding the film by its edges.

Set the interval timer. The timer is set so it will ring at the end of the desired time of development. The manufacturer's table, which is based on the temperature of the developer, must be consulted. When using manual x-ray developer solutions, the time of development is 5 minutes at 70°F.

Develop the film. The film should be immersed quickly into the **developer solution,** and the timer started. The film hanger is agitated by raising and lowering it vigorously for 5 seconds to break up residual air bubbles and permit the solution to bathe both surfaces of the film. The films should not be agitated during development. The composition of the developer solution is shown below.

Typical Developer Composition: Manual X-Ray Developer (Normally Used at 68–70°F)

General Function	Chemical	Special Function
Reducing agents	Metol	Quickly build up gray tones in the image. The developing agents convert the exposed silver halide crystals into black metallic silver.
	Hydroquinone	Slowly builds up black tones and contrast in the image.
Activator	Sodium carbonate	Swells and softens the emulsion so that the reducing agents may work more effectively.

Activator	Sodium carbonate	Provides required alkalinity for reducing agents.
Restrainer	Potassium bromide	Restrains the reducing agents from developing unexposed silver halide to produce fog.
Preservative	Sodium Sulfite	Prevents rapid oxidation of the developing agents.
Solvent	Water	Liquid for dissolving chemicals.

The main action of the developer is to chemically reduce the silver in the radiation-exposed silver halide crystals into black metallic silver. The unexposed silver halide crystals are not developed.

Rinse the film. The hanger is removed from the developer when the timer rings. Excess developer solution should not be drained back into the developer tank. The film is immersed in the circulating rinse water and agitated continuously for 30 seconds. This will remove most of the adhering developer chemicals. Without thorough rinsing after development, the alkaline developer solution on the film will in time gradually neutralize the acidic fixer. The neutralized fixer will then not act evenly on the emulsion, and the radiograph will become streaked and sometimes stained (brown).

Fix the film. After rinsing, the films are placed in the fixer solution, and the hanger is agitated by raising and lowering it for 5 seconds. The film should be fixed for 8 to 10 minutes, or twice the developing time, or twice the "clearing" time. Fixing, like developing, must be properly timed. Too short a fixing time can result in inadequate hardening, slower drying, and possible loss of permanence of the image. Prolonged fixing (hypofixing) may cause the fixer solution to be bound to the emulsion so it cannot be removed in washing, thereby causing an eventual brown

151

discoloration on the radiograph. If the film is left in the fixer for several days, all the image will be removed. The film should not be exposed to white light until the film has cleared. If one can hold films up to the safelight and see through the white (clear) areas on the film, the emulsion has cleared. It usually takes approximately 2 minutes before the films "clear" in the fixer. At this time, the films can be "wet read" in emergency situations. During fixation, the unexposed silver salts are dissolved out of the emulsion, and the gelatin in the emulsion is hardened to prevent damage from future handling. The fixer is called the clearing agent because it clears out the milky appearance of the film. It changes the unexposed and undeveloped silver halide crystals in the emulsion (milky appearance) to soluble silver salts, which are readily removed by washing the film in water. The composition of the fixer solution is shown below.

Typical Fixer Composition: Manual X-Ray Fixer (Temperature Same as Developer) and Automatic X-Ray Fixer (Fix and Wash 5° below Developer Temperature)

General Function	Chemical	Special Function
Fixing agent	Ammonium thio-sulfate	Clears away the unexposed silver halide crystals.
Acidifier	Acetic or sulfuric acid	Stops development by neutralizing developer. Provides required acidity.
Hardener	Aluminum chloride or sulfide	Shrinks and hardens the emulsion.
Preservative	Sodium Sulfite	Maintains chemical balance of the fixer chemicals.
Solvent	Water	Liquid for dissolving chemicals.

Because exhausted fixer solution contains free silver, the silver can be recovered from the exhausted fixer by silver recovery devices. The recovered silver can help to defray the cost of chemicals and to keep the environment clean.

Wash the film. After completion of fixation, the film hanger should be placed into the water tank between the developer and fixer tanks. Excess fixer should be drained back into the fixer tank before moving it to the water tank. Films are washed in the water tank for 15 minutes in clean running water. A temperature of approximately 70°F is recommended. Prolonged washing tends to make the emulsion soft, especially if left in the wash overnight. The object of washing is to remove residual processing chemicals and silver salts from the radiograph. If these residues are not removed, the radiograph will turn brown with time, impairing its value as a permanent record.

Dry the film. Films should be dried in a dust-free area at room temperature or in a suitable drying oven. In most offices, films are dried by merely placing the film hanger on a rack in the darkroom above a drip tray designed to catch the runoff excess water. Some offices use an ordinary fan to dry films. However, the fan should not blow directly on the films. Cabinet dryers are available and are equipped with a fan and heating elements. The temperature should not exceed 120°F (49°C). Usually, this type of dryer should be vented to the outside to prevent moisture condensation in the darkroom.

Mount the films. The dry radiographs are removed from the hanger by opening the clips. The films should not be pulled from the clips, as it may damage the edges of the films. The hanger clips should be washed because processing chemical residues on the clips will cause marks on the next films developed. Films should be placed into special film mounts (see section on mounting.)

AUTOMATIC PROCESSING

Manual film processing is gradually being replaced by automatic processing. Although there are many advantages to using automatic processors, they are complex mechanisms that must be maintained on a strict basis exactly as recommended by the manufacturer. Without an exacting maintenance schedule, automatic processors are worthless. However, with proper care they eliminate one of the most time-consuming, messy, and cost-ineffective procedures ever known to dentistry—manual processing.

Advantages of Automatic Processors

1. **Processing time** is shortened from 50 to 60 minutes to 1.5 to 5 minutes.
2. Constant **film quality**, due to a fixed cycle.
3. Less floor **space** or counter top space is required.
4. The **darkroom can be eliminated** when the automatic processor is equipped with a daylight loader.
5. **Less equipment is required**, such as film racks, film hangers, film dryers, timer, and thermometer.
6. **Wet reading of films** is eliminated. Wet reading of films drips solutions all over the office; in addition, dry films are much more diagnostic.

How Automatic Processor Rollers Work

The basic mechanism design of automatic processors, as recommended by the author, usually consists of a series of rollers that transport the films through the various solution sections, beginning with the developer, then directly into the fixer, and then the wash and dryer (Fig. 6.2). Note that the film does not go into a wash bath between developing and fixing as in manual processing. The explanation of this is based on the functions of rollers.

The functions of automatic processor rollers are as follows:

1. The rollers **transport the film** through each section of the processor.
2. The rollers **provide a massaging action** that contributes to the uniform distribution of chemicals on the film emulsion in the developer and fixer sections.
3. Special **squeegee rollers remove processing solutions** from the film surfaces, reducing the amount of solution carry-over from one tank to the next.
4. **Squeegee rollers in the wash section** remove most of the water from the emulsion before transport of the film to the drying section, allowing the film to dry uniformly and rapidly.
5. Because the tanks are small, the **motion of the rollers** in the developer and fixer tanks helps to stir the solutions as replenishment occurs frequently.

Automatic Processing Solutions and Replenishment

When using automatic developer solutions, a hardening chemical—glutaraldehyde—is added to the conventional manual processing developer to prevent the emulsion from softening and sticking to the rollers. **Sulfate compounds** are also added to the manual processing developer to minimize the swelling of the emulsion so the films can be transported by the rollers uniformly. If manual processing developer solution is used in an automatic processor, the film emulsion will most likely stick to the rollers and damage the radiographic image. With automatic processors, a rigid schedule of chemical replenishment is necessary to maintain the proper concentrations of the solutions and to neutralize the unwanted by-products of each reaction. To maintain the alkalinity of the developer, the acidity of the fixer, and the chemical strength of both solutions, a replenisher must be added at a constant rate for each film processed. In the drying section, the film is quickly dried by jets of heated air before the film drops into the discharge receptacle.

Because the total processing time is reduced in automatic processing, the chemical concentration and temperature of the solutions must be increased. **Phenidone** is substituted for metol (Elon) as a developing agent because, when combined with hydroquinone, it provides a

rapid synergistic chemical reaction necessary for automatic processing. In the larger extraoral or medical 90-second automatic processors, the temperature is kept at 90 to 94°F in the developer, fixer, and wash sections and 135°F in the dryer section. The dental automatic units regularly process at temperatures of approximately 83°F for a 4.5-minute cycle; however, in some processor models, the processing time can be adjusted to a faster cycle of 1.5 to 2.5 minutes if required (e.g., endodontic and surgical procedures).

Most dental automatic processors now have automatic replenisher systems that are based on the amount and size of film being processed. The replenisher solution is injected into the bottom of the tank while the excess overflows from the top of the tank. Usually 6 ounces must be added to the developer and 3 ounces to the fixer after processing four full-mouth surveys or four panoramic films. If continued satisfactory results are expected, automatic processors must be cleaned routinely (weekly in a busy office), and preventive maintenance procedures must be followed. Experience has shown that the greatest cause of automatic processor problems is failure to keep the rollers clean. A schedule should be established for cleaning the rollers and replenishing and changing solutions. Procedures or products should never be substituted or changed unless recommended by the automatic processor manufacturer.

Automatic Processor Preventive Maintenance Procedures

---

1. **Transport sections should be checked each day to see if they are aligned properly.** The films will fall through to the bottom of the tanks if the transport sections are not aligned.
2. **Moving parts should be lubricated monthly.** Gears, sprockets, idlers, bearings, drive mechanisms, and ring points must be lubricated. Failure to do so will cause excessive wear of moving parts, eventually slow the speed of the rollers, and in turn affect film quality. **No oil should get on the rollers.** Manufacturer's instructions must always be followed.
3. **The solutions should be replenished on a regular basis according to the rate of films processed.** After four panoramic films or full-mouth surveys, approximately 6 ounces of replenisher should be added. Failure to do so will result in low levels of exhausted developer and fixer. This will cause smudgy, low-density (light) films. This is why an automatic replenisher system is recommended.
4. **The temperature of the processing solutions should be checked regularly.** Changes in the temperature of the

---

developer will cause changes in the density of the processed film. (It takes a change in temperature of only a few degrees to affect the density. It is important to be sure that the thermostat on the processor is accurate.)

5. **The cover should be kept open slightly when the processor is not in use.** After each day's operation, the cover should be left open slightly so the chemical fumes can escape. Failure to do so could lead to fogging (blackening) of films.

6. **Solutions should be changed every 1 to 4 weeks, depending on the rate of use of the processor.** Processing solutions especially made for automatic processors should be used. Processing solutions designed for manual processing should never be used.

7. **The manufacturer's instructions should always be followed.** The manual should be referred to as often as needed to assure proper maintenance and to assist in troubleshooting.

How to Feed Films in the Automatic Processor

The following are a few important recommendations for feeding the film into the automatic processor.

1. **Films should be fed slowly and carefully.** Panoramic films should be fed into the processor in a straight line with the roller system. Failure to do so could cause a jam-up in the processor.

2. **If film is bent,** the unbent side of the film should be inserted into the machine first; the bent edge should then be unbended.

3. **Damp or wet films should not be fed into the machine** because they will contaminate the rollers and cause streaking of subsequent films.

4. **Films should not be fed too quickly in succession.** They may stick to each other and jam the machine (allow 5 seconds between films fed into the same slot). Some machines come with a feed light, which comes on when it is okay to feed the next film.

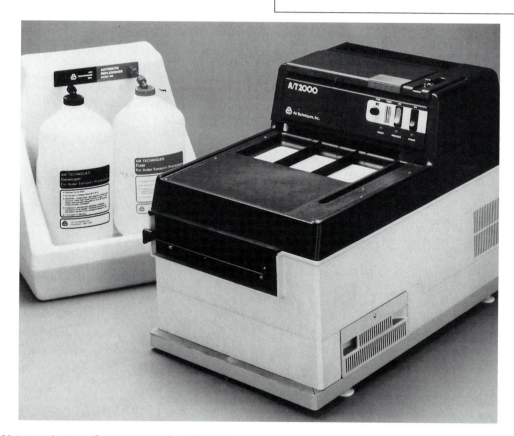

Figure 6.10. A/T 2000 Automatic X-Ray Film Processor. The A/T 2000 Automatic X-ray Film Processor automatically controls time, temperature, chemistry agitation, and chemistry replenishment. It shuts itself off as soon as the last film exits the processor and returns to a stand-by status, which saves water, electricity, and general wear and tear. Normal speed is a 5.5-minute processing cycle for archival quality dental films of all sizes up to 8 X 10 inches. Endo speed is a 2.5-minute processing cycle that provides a "quick look" for nonarchival quality periapical films used in endodontic procedures. (Courtesy of Air Techniques Inc., Hicksville, NY 11801).

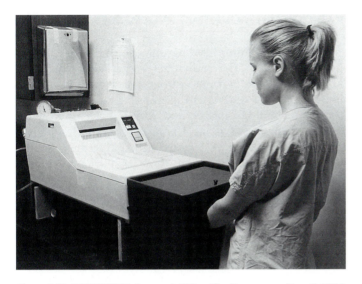

Figure 6.11. DENT-X 9000 Automatic X-Ray Film Processor. Dent-X 9000 with a daylight loader. It features a unique replenishing system that controls all processing chemistry. Infrared sensors measure film size on input and replenish (refresher) developing and fixing solutions based on the amount of film being processed. Develops all sizes of film up to 8 X 10-inch size. Dry films in 4.5 minutes, and endo wet readings in 1 minute. (Courtesy of Dent-X Co., Elmsford, NY 10523).

Which Automatic Processor to Purchase?

Several brands of automatic processors are available. Because they are competitive in performance and price, the decision of which brand to purchase usually rests on the quality and performance of the processor and on the

availability of competent repair service (Figs. 6.10 and 6.11). Other factors to consider include the availability and convenience of use of a daylight loader and counter top space required. The basic features of any automatic processor are cycle time shorter than 5 minutes, a roller transport system, thermostatically controlled solution temperature with digital display, an automatic solution replenishment system, simple-to-follow maintenance instructions and procedures, inexpensive and readily available processing solutions, and reliability of the automatic processor system. No automatic processor is reliable without maintenance.

MOUNTING DENTAL RADIOGRAPHS

REASONS FOR MOUNTING RADIOGRAPHS

The following are reasons dental radiographs should be mounted:

1. **There is less chance for an error in interpretation** because films are mounted in normal anatomical relation to one another.
2. **It prevents finger marks, scratches, and abrasions** because radiographs are not handled as much.
3. **To avoid inefficiency and confusion,** repeated study and comparison of single radiographs with each other is time consuming. It results in inefficiency and confusion.
4. **Mounts exclude illumination around the individual**

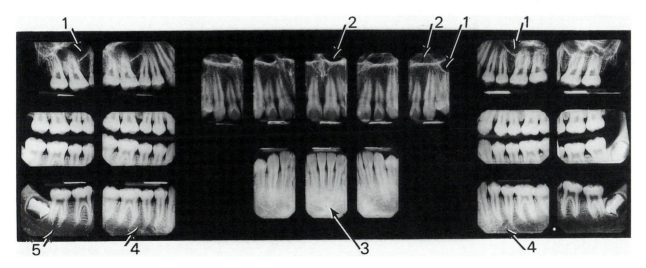

Figure 6.12. Normal Anatomic Landmarks for Mounting. Full mouth radiographic survey (FMX): (1) maxillary sinus, (2) nasal cavities, (3) genial tubercles, (4) mental foramen, and (5) mandibular canal.

radiographs. This is an aid in interpretation because it prevents glare to the interpreter's eyes.

5. **Radiographs in mounts are easy to file.** Therefore, they are instantly available for studying during an operative procedure and consultation.

6. **It has a psychological effect on patients.** The impression and educational value that mounted radiographs have on the patient is in itself sufficient reason for mounting them.

RADIOGRAPH MOUNTING PROCEDURES

Mounting intraoral radiographs is a relatively simple procedure when the individual responsible has some knowledge of the normal radiographic anatomical landmarks for each region of the mouth and can recognize tooth morphology (shape and form). Each anatomical region of the jaws has identifying anatomical landmarks (Fig. 6.12). These landmarks are further described in detail Chapter 14. Before initiation of the mounting procedure,

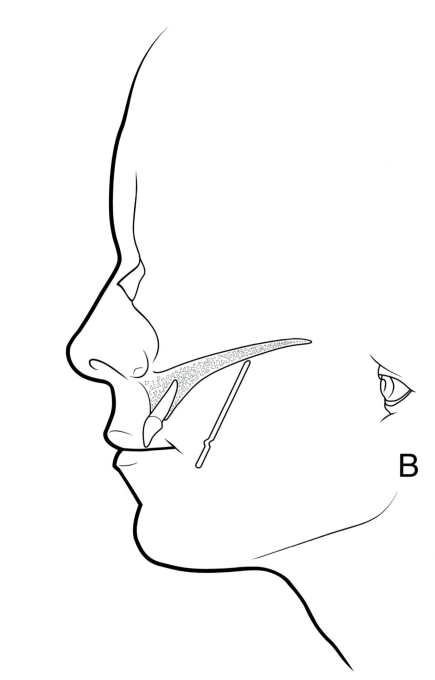

A   B

Figure 6.13. Mounting Films As If Viewer Is Looking Directly At The Patient. The intraoral radiograph is positioned in the mouth with the raised portion of the raised dot positioned toward the x-ray tubehead (**A**) If film is mounted in this manner, it is as though the viewer is looking directly at the patient. (**B**) If mounted with raised dot away from the viewer, it is as if the viewer is in the patient's mouth looking out (mounting procedure not used very often).

it is important to know from what aspect the radiographs will be viewed (Fig. 6.13).

Two Ways of Mounting Radiographs

1. **In the first method of mounting, the radiographs are mounted with the depressed or concave sides of the embossed dots toward the viewer.** The viewer is then observing the radiographs from the lingual aspect, with the tube side of the film toward the back of the mount, as if he or she was inside the patient's mouth looking out. Although still used by many older dentists, this method is less commonly used.

2. **In the second method of mounting, the radiographs are mounted with all the raised or convex sides of the embossed dots toward the viewer.** The viewer is then observing the radiographs from the facial aspect, with the tube side of the film toward the viewer, as if he or she was looking directly at the patient (Fig. 6.13). This is the preferred method because the films are mounted in the same relationship as the teeth are recorded on the examination chart. This makes for less chance of error.

Once the processed radiographs are dry, care must be taken to avoid fingerprinting the radiographs. Consequently, radiographs should be handled only by their edges with clean, dry fingers or by using white cotton cloth gloves (used by photographers) to mount films.

Procedure for Mounting Radiographs

The mounting procedure described is the one in which the radiographs are mounted as though the viewer is looking directly at the patient.

Step 1. Arrange all radiographs of the full-mouth radiographic survey (FMX) on a flat viewbox with the embossed dot or bump upward.

Step 2. Arrange the radiographs on the viewbox in order of anatomical site (e.g., select and arrange in groups all maxillary radiographs according to posterior or anterior regions).

Step 3. Take all maxillary posterior radiographs and arrange them with the crowns of the teeth toward the bottom of the viewbox. With all embossed dots convex side toward you and the crowns of the teeth oriented downward, it will be necessary only to identify mesial or distal anatomical landmarks of teeth to distinguish right from left. Posterior radiographs with the more mesial

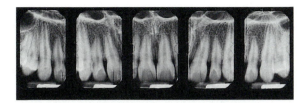

Figure 6.14. Mounting Radiographs of Maxillary Anterior Teeth. The radiographs of maxillary teeth are mounted with their incisal edges downward toward the center of radiographic mount. The maxillary centrals are mounted in the center of the maxillary anterior section. The practitioner should identify the right and left lateral and canine radiographs and mount them with mesial portion of each tooth toward the middle of the mouth.

anatomical structures of jaws and teeth are mounted in the premolar position; those with more distal landmarks are mounted in the molar positions (Fig. 6.12).

Step 4. Identify the maxillary anterior radiographs and rotate the incisal edges of each film down toward the bottom of the viewbox (Fig. 6.14).

Step 5. Identify the maxillary central incisor radiograph and mount it in the center of the anterior section of the mount. Next, identify the right (R) and left (L) lateral and canine radiographs and mount them with mesial anatomical structures always directed toward the middle of the mount.

Step 6. Identify the four posterior mandibular radiographs. Rotate these radiographs until the coronal (crown) portions of the teeth are directed toward the top of the viewbox. Identify mesial and distal structures and arrange in appropriate areas of the mount (Fig. 6.12).

Step 7. Rotate the three mandibular anterior radiographs until their incisal edges are positioned toward the top of the viewbox. Identify the central incisor radiograph and

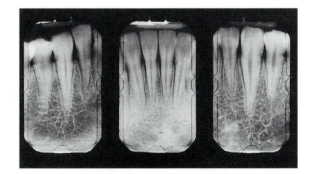

Figure 6.15. Mounting Radiographs of Mandibular Anterior Teeth. The practitioner should mount the three anterior radiographs until their incisal edges are positioned toward the top of the middle of the mount. He or she should identify the central incisor region and mount the radiograph in the center window of the mount. Next, the left and right canine radiographs should be mounted.

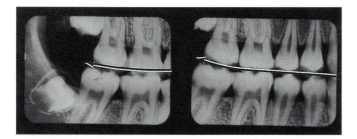

Figure 6.16. Mounting Bitewing Radiographs. The practitioner should orient radiographs with "curve of Spee" directed upward toward the distal. It should be remembered that the mandibular molars have two roots and that the maxillary molars have three roots. Once the maxillary and mandibular arches can be identified, the radiographs can be properly oriented as to whether they are radiographs of the left side or right side of the patient.

mount it in the center window of the mount. Next, mount the left and right canine radiographs (Fig. 6.15).

Step 8. The remaining four films are interproximal (bitewing) radiographs. Orient these radiographs with the curve of Spee (occlusal plane between maxillary and mandibular teeth) directed upward toward the distal. If the occlusal plane is flat, attempt to identify characteristics of the respective crowns; frequently, the bifurcation of the mandibular molar is distinguishable and may serve as a valuable aid in distinguishing mandibular molars from three-rooted maxillary molar teeth. Once the appropriate arch is identified, the radiograph can be properly oriented. The direction of the most mesial structures is used to identify right from left and premolar from molar regions (Fig. 6.16).

COPYING OR DUPLICATING RADIOGRAPHS

Since the discovery of x-rays, persons have been trying to reproduce radiographs. A single radiographic series may seem sufficient at the time taken; however, it may become necessary to refer or transfer a patient to another dentist while keeping the original radiographs. Also, as third-party payments increasingly become a part of every practice, it becomes necessary to find a simple and inexpensive way to copy original radiographs. Radiographs are often duplicated when lawsuits are initiated.

DUPLICATING FILMS

Films can be duplicated by the use of a special duplicating film called direct-reversal films, which have been so-

larized by a chemical treatment of the emulsion. Solarization of a film is exposing the film (chemically or by light) beyond that which produces maximum density until a decrease in density occurs. This coats the latent-image centers with a layer of silver bromide and prevents the action of the developing agent on the emulsion grains. **The important thing to remember about solarized film is that more light exposure produces less density,** which is the opposite of standard radiographic film exposures. Because duplicating film is a direct positive or reversal film, increasing exposure reduces the density produced on a duplicating film. Therefore, a duplicate that is too low in density can be corrected by decreasing the exposure. If the density of the copy is too high, the exposure should be increased to lower the density. Radiographic duplicating film has a **solarized emulsion side** (purple side) on a blue-tinted polyester film base and an **antihalation coating** (shiny side) on the opposite side. Halation is light reflected back from air after it has passed through the duplicating film. This reflected light causes unsharp edges at the boundaries of the duplicated image. **Halation** (reflected light) can be prevented by an antihalation layer on the back side of the duplication film, which contains a dye that absorbs the reflected light before it reaches the light-sensitive emulsion layer. The important thing to remember is that duplicating film has emulsion only on the one (purple) side.

DUPLICATION PROCEDURE

The basis for the duplicating technique is to expose a special duplicating film to a light that has passed through the original film. The duplicating film is designed to be exposed with an ultraviolet light source, such as a BLB ultraviolet fluorescent lamp (Fig. 6.17). The radiograph to be duplicated must be held in close contact with the

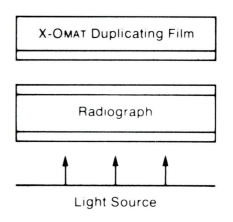

Figure 6.17. Diagram of Technique of Duplicating Film. The duplicating film has emulsion on one side; original radiograph has emulsion on both sides of the film.

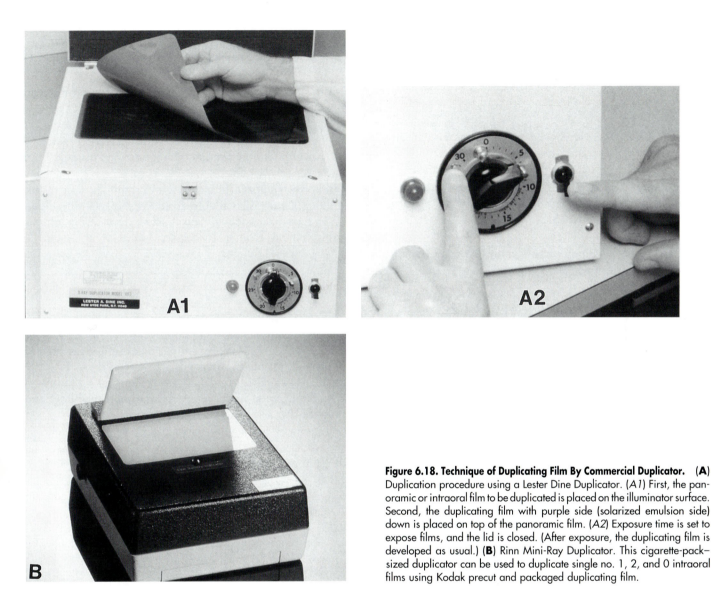

Figure 6.18. Technique of Duplicating Film By Commercial Duplicator. (A) Duplication procedure using a Lester Dine Duplicator. (*A1*) First, the panoramic or intraoral film to be duplicated is placed on the illuminator surface. Second, the duplicating film with purple side (solarized emulsion side) down is placed on top of the panoramic film. (*A2*) Exposure time is set to expose films, and the lid is closed. (After exposure, the duplicating film is developed as usual.) (**B**) Rinn Mini-Ray Duplicator. This cigarette-pack–sized duplicator can be used to duplicate single no. 1, 2, and 0 intraoral films using Kodak precut and packaged duplicating film.

emulsion side of the single-coated duplicating film during exposure to prevent blurring. This may be accomplished by use of one of the commercially available contact printers (Fig. 6.18). Kodak X-Omat duplicating film is available in seven sizes, including the periapical size. Radiographs are duplicated in the darkroom under safelight conditions. The radiographs are placed in full contact with the duplicator top. Film mounts are usually not recommended unless they allow the radiographs to contact the duplicator top. The duplicating film is then placed on top of the radiograph to be duplicated with the emulsion side (usually the lavender or purple side) contacting the radiographs. The lid of the duplicator is closed over the radiographs and duplicating film. The duplicator is then activated for the time specified in the manufacturer's direc-

tions. The duplicating film is removed, and the film is processed in the normal way.

WORKSHOP/LABORATORY EXERCISES

EXERCISE 6.1. FILM PROCESSING AND MOUNTING

Materials and Equipment Needed

1. Exposed full-mouth survey (FMX) or half-mouth survey from previous laboratory exercise.
2. FMX film mount.
3. Darkroom and processing equipment.
4. Viewbox.

Instructions

Step 1: Following the instructions for either manual processing or automatic processing, process all radiographs. Collect the dried films.

Step 2: Using the viewbox, sort the films and mount them in the film mount.

CASE-BASED QUESTIONS FOR LABORATORY EXERCISE

1. Identify any technique errors in the FMX; try to name the error and its cause.

2. Explain how to correct the above errors.

3. Identify any improperly mounted films.

4. What mistake(s) did you make resulting in incorrect mounting?

OPTIONAL EXERCISE 6.2. X-RAY FILM DUPLICATION

Materials and Equipment Needed

1. Film duplicator or contact printer.
2. Original film.
3. Kodak duplicating film.
4. Darkroom.
5. Processing facility.
6. Timer

Instructions

Step 1: In the darkroom, open the top of the film duplicator and place the film to be copied on the plastic surface.

Step 2: Place the duplicating film emulsion side (purple side) down on top of the original film.

Step 3: Close the top tightly so there is good contact between the original film and duplicating film.

Step 4: Set the timer (usually from 5 to 10 seconds, depending on duplicator brand).

Step 5: Remove duplicating film and process.

CASE-BASED QUESTIONS FOR LABORATORY EXERCISE

1. If your original film was too dark, how could you make the duplicate lighter?

2. Explain why it is important to get the correct side of the duplicating film in contact with the original film.

Note to Instructors: An inexpensive, small-sized intraoral film duplicator is available from Dentsply/Rinn, Elgin, IL, and prepackaged intraoral-sized duplicating film is available from Kodak, Rochester, NY.

CASE-BASED PROBLEM-SOLVING

You do not have a film duplicator, but somebody mentioned you can use a simple photographic contact printer (available in photography shops) or even a glass picture frame to duplicate radiographs. How would you do this? Materials available are a darkroom, duplicating film, film to be duplicated, a contact printer or picture frame, and a viewbox.

REVIEW QUESTIONS

1. Which of the following is the clearing agent in the fixer?

   A. Potassium alum.
   B. Ammonium thiosulfate.
   C. Acetic acid.
   D. Potassium bromide.
   E. Hydroquinone.

2. What determines the time an exposed radiograph remains in the developing solution?

   A. The temperature of the solution.
   B. When the unexposed silver bromide is removed.
   C. When the image of the film becomes stabilized.
   D. The time it takes for the image to appear.

3. Which of the following best describes a desirable film mount?

   A. It should be translucent to allow more light to reach the film.
   B. It should be gray and opaque to light transmission.

C. It should be black to block light transmission and prevent glare.

D. It should be purplish because this is the color of the retina of the eye.

4. In correctly mounted radiographs, the curve of Spee:

A. Should curve downward toward the distal.
B. Should curve upward toward the distal.
C. Should curve downward or upward toward the distal, depending on whether the concave or convert side of the embossed dot is used.
D. Indicates correct mounting of the anterior teeth.

5. Placing the film in the fixer first results in:

A. A black film.
B. A clear film.
C. A mottled film.
D. No change.

6. In manual processing, films should be washed in running water for at least:

A. 10 minutes.
B. 15 minutes.
C. 30 minutes.
D. 40 minutes.

7. In manual processing, the optimum time and temperature for developing film is:

A. 3 to 4 minutes at 70°F.
B. 4.5 to 5 minutes at 75°F.
C. 4.5 to 5 minutes at 65°F.
D. 4.5 to 5 minutes at 68° to 70°F.

8. What is the cause of yellow or brown stains appearing on film some months after processing?

A. Aged film.
B. Improper exposure technique.
C. Films stored in a hot place.
D. Incomplete fixing and washing.

9. Radiographs are rinsed in clean running water to:

A. Rid the film of chemicals.
B. Dissolve metallic silver.
C. Shrink the emulsion.
D. Get rid of the latent image.

10. Contrast of radiographic images is slowly enhanced by:

A. Alum.
B. Hydroquinone.
C. Sodium acetate.
D. Sodium sulfate.
E. Sulfuric acid.

11. In manual processing, film gelatin is softened in the developer solution by the addition of:

A. Sodium sulfate.
B. Hydroquinone.
C. Acetic acid.
D. Potassium alum.
E. Sodium carbonate.

12. Chemical fog is controlled in the developer solution by adding:

A. Elon.
B. Acetic acid.
C. Sodium carbonate.
D. Potassium bromide.
E. Sodium sulfite.

13. Unexposed silver crystals dissolve when _____ is added to the fixer solution.

A. Acetate acid.
B. Ammonium thiosulfate.
C. Sodium sulfate.
D. Potassium alum.
E. Sodium carbonate.

14. In the chemistry of processing, potassium bromide:

A. Is an activator for reducing agents.
B. Is an activator for clearing agents.
C. Is a component of the developing solution.
D. Tends to increase radiographic fog.

BIBLIOGRAPHY

Allen MJ, Silha RE. New copiers for dental radiography duplicating film. Dent Radiogr Photogr 1976;49:14–17.

Beideman RW, Johnson ON, Alcox RW. A study to develop a rating system and evaluate dental radiographs submitted to a third party carrier. J Am Dent Assoc 1976;93:1010–1013.

Bureau of Radiological Health. Quality assurance programs for diagnostic radiology facilities, final recommendations. Fed Reg 1979; 44:71728–78740.

Bureau of Radiological Health. Dental exposure normalization technique (DENT). HEW publication (FDA) 76-8042. Rockville, MD: US Department of Health, Education and Welfare, 1981.

Bureau of Radiological Health. Radiographic film processing: a self-teaching workbook. HEQ Publication (FDA) 81-8146, January 1981.

Bushong SC. Radiologic science for technologists, St. Louis: CV Mosby, 1975.

Copying radiographs. Kodak publication no. M3-24. Rochester, NY: Eastman Kodak, 1973.

Erales FA, Manson-Hing LR. A study of the quality of duplicated radiographs. Oral Surg 1979;47:98.

Esworthy S, Fox J. Duplicating dental radiographs. Dent Assist 1968;37:26–30.

Fletcher JC. A comparison of Ektaspeed and Ultraspeed films using manual and automatic processing solutions. Oral Surg 1987;63:94–102.

Fredholm U, Julin P. Rapid developing of Ektaspeed dental film by increase of temperature. Swed Dent J 1987;11:121–126.

Gould RG, Gratt BM. A radiographic quality control system for the dental office. Dentomaxillofac Radiol 1982;11:123–127.

Haist G. Modern photographic processing. New York: John Wiley & Sons, 1979;1.

Hashimoto K, Thunthy KH, Weinberg R. Automatic processing: effects of temperature and time changes on sensitometric properties of Ultraspeed and Ektaspeed films. Oral Surg 1991;71:120–124.

Hedin M. Developing solutions for dental x-ray processors. Swed Dent J 1989;13:261–265.

Hurtgen TP. Safelighting in the dental darkroom. Dent Radiogr Photogr 1979;52:9–15.

Kasle MJ, Langlais RP. Exercises in dental radiology: basic principles of oral radiography. Philadelphia: WB Saunders, 1980;4.

Langland OE, Sippy FH, Langlais RP. A textbook of dental radiology. 2nd ed. Springfield: Charles C. Thomas, 1984.

Langland OE. Radiologic examination. In: Hardin JE, ed. Clark's clinical dentistry. Philadelphia: Lippincott-Raven, 1996.

Management of photographic wastes in the dental office. Kodak dental radiography series. Rochester, NY: Eastman Kodak, 1990.

Mees DEK, James TH. The theory of the photographic process. New York: Macmillan, 1977.

Peterson, S. Clinical dental hygiene. St. Louis: Mosby-Year Book, 1973:239–247.

Sturge JM, ed. Neblette's handbook of photography and reprography—materials, processes, and systems. New York: Van Nostrand Reinhold, 1977.

Simpson CO. The advantages of mounting dental radiographs. Dent Radiogr Photogr 1937;1.

Thunthy KH, Fortier AP, Knapp WB. Automatic film processing in the dental office. Quintessence Int 1977;9:75–79.

Thunthy KH, Fortier AP. Electrolytic recovery of silver from dental radiographic films. J Ala Dent Assoc 1990;74:13–18.

Thunthy KH, Haskimoto K, Weinberg R. Automatic processing: effects of temperature and time changes on the sensitometric properties of light-sensitive films. Oral Surg 1991;72:112–118.

Analysis of Errors and Artifacts

7

OBJECTIVES

Upon successful completion of this unit, the student will be able to:

1. *List the film quality evaluation criteria and the factors that control them.*

2. *State the four areas wherein the majority of errors are produced.*

3. *Recognize and correct technique errors.*

4. *Recognize and correct exposure and processing errors.*

5. *Recognize and correct film-handling errors.*

6. *Purposefully create errors and recognize the errors in the processed images using the Workshop/Laboratory Exercises format.*

7. *Compare and contrast manual versus automatic processing using the Case-Based Problem-Solving format.*

8. *Test his or her knowledge by answering the Review Questions.*

KEY WORDS/PHRASES

apices cut-off	deposits on film	foreshortening
automatic processor film feeding	detail	horizontal angulation
backward film	dimensional distortion	light-density film
bend marks	dot artifact	mean tangent
black artifacts	double image	moisture contamination
blank image	dust and powder artifacts	movement
contrast	elongation	overlapped contacts
dark-density film	film distortion	partial image
definition	fog	"phalangioma"

pressure marks

radiopaque artifacts

retake avoidance

scratched emulsion

stains

static electricity

streaks

technique errors

tongue artifact

torn emulsion

vertical angulation

white artifacts

INTRODUCTION

All dental radiation workers in a dental office or clinic have the responsibility to produce high-quality diagnostic radiographs. These workers must be competent in their techniques and be aware of what constitutes proper handling and correct processing of the film. Strict adherence to the principles of patient management, technique, film handling, film storage, and darkroom procedures will eliminate needless additional radiation exposure to the patient by minimizing the necessity for retaking nondiagnostic radiographs. Each retake doubles the dose of radiation to the patient and doubles the cost of obtaining the image.

EVALUATION CRITERIA

FILM QUALITY EVALUATION CRITERIA

1. **All radiographs must have acceptable image characteristics of detail, definition, density, and contrast.** The operator must control these image characteristics by using the most appropriate techniques available with a minimum of deviations, which will degrade the image. The illumination provided by the viewbox permits differentiation among the various structures of the teeth, the periodontal ligament spaces, the supporting bone, and the normal anatomical landmarks.
   a. **Detail** refers to the point-by-point delineation of the minute elements of the objects in the radiographic images formed on the dental film. Detail is responsible for maximizing the information in an image. **Detail** is controlled by **kVp** and the **developing process.**
   b. **Definition** refers to the distinctness and sharp demarcation of all the detail that makes up the radiographic images of the objects and their structural elements in the dental film. **Definition** is controlled by **distance factors, focal spot size, type of film,** and **motion factors.** Adequate definition is present when the apical lamina dura, periodontal ligament space, and individual trabeculae can be clearly demarcated around a healthy tooth.
   c. **Density** is the general tendency of the film toward a lighter or darker overall appearance. Reasonable density will allow the dental health-care worker to

visualize a faint outline of the soft tissue in the edentulous regions on the radiograph. Density is controlled primarily by the exposure time, mA, kVp, developer solution freshness, and temperature.
   d. **Contrast** refers to the differences in density between adjacent areas in the dental film (Fig. 7.1). When the contrast is too high (short-, gray-scale contrast), minute details in the bone are obliterated; when the contrast is too low (long-, gray-scale contrast), small carious lesions in the interproximal enamel are difficult to read. **Contrast** is controlled primarily by **kVp.** It is also affected by the type of film (D versus E+), processing solutions, and absorption differences in the subject (subject contrast). Each patient has a built-in step-wedge consisting of soft tissue, alveolar bone, enamel, dentin, and pulp. When all these can be clearly seen, optimal contrast is present.
   e. The **radiograph is free from film handling and processing errors** and is not severely creased or stained.
2. **All crowns and roots, including apices, are fully depicted together with interproximal alveolar crests, tooth contact areas, and surrounding apical bone regions.**
   a. All apices of all teeth, together with approximately ⅛ inch of surrounding apical bone, must be seen clearly at least once in a complete radiographic survey.

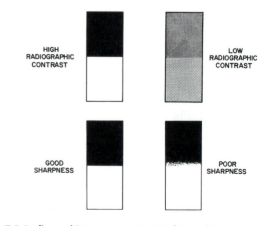

Figure 7.1. Radiographic Contrast. (*Top*) Radiographic contrast is the combination of subject contrast and film contrast that results in density differences between adjacent areas on the radiograph. (*Bottom*) Sharpness is the abrupt change in going from one density to another on a radiograph.

b. Film covers all interproximal, periradicular, and/or retromolar regions of the anatomical region of interest. This includes **distal** of the canine on premolar radiographs, and the **third molar** region is molar radiographs.

c. The radiographs should **not** exhibit "cone-cutting" or "partial images."

d. The embossed (raised) dot should appear at the incisal or the occlusal edge of the radiograph.

3. **Images of all teeth and other structures are shown in proper relative size and contour with minimal distortion and without overlapping images, where anatomically possible.**

a. The interproximal contacts of the two posterior bitewing radiographs should **not** overlap.

b. Images of the teeth and other structures should not be distorted to the extent that radiographic interpretation is impossible. Buccal and lingual cusp tips in posterior periapical radiographs should be superimposed at least to the same degree as is seen in the bitewings.

BITEWING RADIOGRAPH EVALUATION CRITERIA

1. **The interproximal contacts** should **not** be overlapped from the distal surface of the canine to the mesial surface of the third molar, to the extent that interpretation is impossible.

2. **The crowns** of the maxillary and mandibular teeth should be centered in the image from top to bottom.

3. **The crest of the alveolar bone** should be visible with **no** superimposition of the crowns of the adjacent teeth.

4. **The occlusal plane** should be as horizontal as possible.

5. **The buccal and lingual cusps** should not be excessively separated. Slight separation of individual buccal and lingual cusp tips is permissible, as well as in individual teeth, due to malpositioning of a tooth. In general, the cusp tips should be nearly superimposed.

RETAKES

Radiographs that are **nondiagnostic** are almost always retaken. Retakes should be avoided for the following reasons:

1. Retakes **expose the patient** to unnecessary radiation.
2. Retakes **waste the time** of the dental health-care worker and/or his or her coworkers.
3. Retakes **waste film**, which is costly.
4. Retakes **waste infection control** items, supplies, and procedures.

TYPES OF ERRORS

The majority of errors produced can be categorized into three groups:

1. Technique errors.
2. Exposure and processing errors.
3. Film-handling errors.

When errors are made, the dental radiation worker must take the necessary time to troubleshoot the problem and correct it. An error can often be produced in more than one way. Therefore, all possibilities must be taken into account, and the cause identified. For instance, a blank (clear) film with no image may be caused by nonexposure or by placing the film into the fixer solution first. The dental radiation worker needs to check both the exposure technique and the darkroom processing solution sequence. Errors are often the direct result of "shortcuts." Improper attention to technique, film exposure, film processing, and storage procedures almost always compromises film quality and often leads to retakes. Radiographs that are of poor quality also interfere with interpretation of the dental images that, in turn, may influence the diagnosis and treatment planning procedures. In a court of law, radiographs often play a vital role. Poor radiographs may be inadmissible or may be further evidence of sloppiness, negligence, or a lower-than-acceptable standard of dental care.

TECHNIQUE ERRORS

Patient Preparation Errors

Radiopaque Artifacts Dental appliances and eyeglasses left in place will be recorded and appear superimposed over the dental images on the finished radiograph (Figs. 7.2 and 7.3).

Before placing any films in the patient's mouth, the operator should ask the patient to remove dental appliances, such as partial and complete dentures. Sometimes acrylic prostheses may be left in to help with film placement and retention. For extraoral images (such as panoramic radiographs) other items, such as wigs, hairpieces, eyebrow jewelry, necklaces, and napkin chains, must be removed.

Movement Movement of the film, patient, or x-ray tubehead will result in a **blurred** image (Fig. 7.4). Most movement errors are caused by patient (object) movement (Fig. 7.4). The operator, in explaining the procedure to the patient, needs to emphasize and later remind the patient to remain motionless during exposures and **to keep biting** on the biteblock until after the exposure. If the tubehead shakes, it must be stabilized before making the exposure.

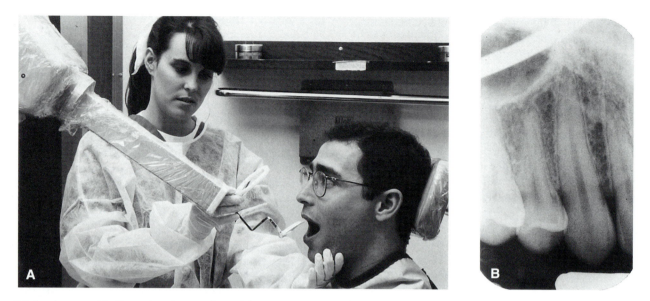

Figure 7.2. Eyeglasses and Radiographs. (**A**) Eyeglasses left on patient. (Patient should be instructed to remove eyeglasses before exposure of film.) (**B**) Radiograph resulting from patient still wearing eyeglasses.

Film Placement Errors

Apices Cut Off This error occurs when the film is not positioned apically enough to record the entire tooth, leaving too much film extending beyond the crowns. The operator can correct this in the paralleling technique by moving the film farther away lingually from the teeth in the maxillary arch and positioning the film more apically in the mandibular arch. Not more than ⅛ inch of film should be seen above or below the crowns of the teeth (Fig. 7.5). Insufficient vertical angulation can project the apices of the teeth off the film.

Specific Region Not Covered This is the result of not placing the film to cover all the teeth in the area of interest (Fig. 7.6). Close inspection of the teeth or area in question,

as well as adherence to specified film placement guidelines, will aid the operator in avoiding this error. Each film is positioned in the mouth to include specific areas of the teeth and related structures. To minimize this positioning error, three guidelines should be followed:

a. The distal surfaces of the canine should be visible in the premolar views.
b. The third molars or retromolar/tuberosity areas of the teeth should be seen in the molar views.
c. The tooth/teeth of specific interest should be centered on the film.

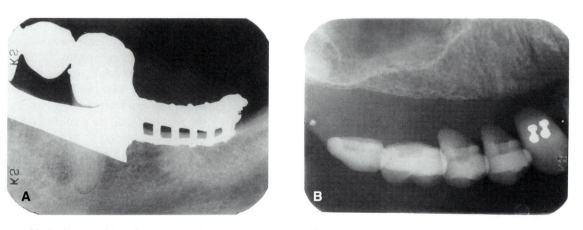

Figure 7.3. Removable Appliance and Complete Denture Left In. (**A**) Lower removable appliance left in. (Patient should be instructed to remove removable appliance [partial denture] before exposure of film.) (**B**) Complete upper denture left in place.

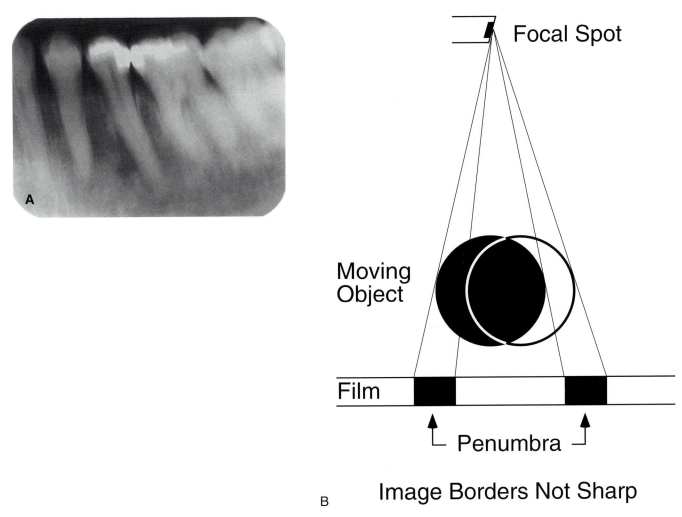

Figure 7.4. Movement of Patient Error. (**A**) Radiograph of patient who moved during exposure. (Patient should be properly instructed not to move.) (**B**) Diagram demonstrates how object movement increases penumbra, producing an unsharp image.

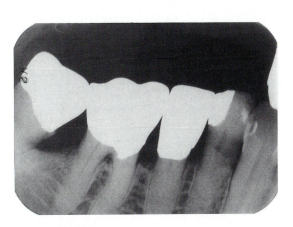

Figure 7.5. Mandibular Molar and Premolar Apices Cut Off. This usually happens when the patient fails to bite down on the biteblock because of discomfort.

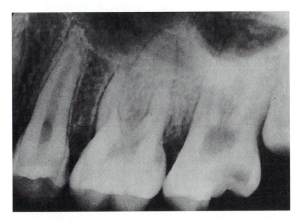

Figure 7.6. Specific Region Not Covered. In this maxillary molar projection, the third molar is not covered properly. The film should be positioned farther back in the mouth.

Backward Film A low-density "herringbone," "tire-track," or "geometric pattern" appearance of a film is the result of directing the x-rays through the lead foil side of the film packet (Fig. 7.7). Current E+ lead foil is embossed with a geometric pattern resembling tightly packed ping-pong balls. When the film is placed backward, the lead foil absorbs much of the radiation, the embossed lead foil pattern superimposes over the dental structures, and the structural orientation is reversed. The raised dot is now reversed! When this happens, the tab or back side of the film packet has been placed toward the source of radiation. Failure to retake this image can result in unneeded procedures on the wrong side of the patient.

Dot Artifact The film identification dot produces a circular radiolucent (dark) artifact on the finished radiograph. This dark dot artifact may interfere with interpretation of the apical areas of the teeth (Fig. 7.8). Therefore, the film identification dot should be placed toward the coronal (occlusal) aspect of the teeth when taking periapical radiographs. Place the dot in the slot.

Double Image When an exposed film is placed in another region and reexposed, the resulting film will have two superimposed images (Fig. 7.9). Use of a film organizer or film receptacle for exposed film will help the operator keep track of the film exposures made and prevent this error, which will result in two retakes. Minimizing interruptions helps to avoid this error. Usually a blank, unexposed film is also found when this error occurs.

Tongue or Finger Artifacts Films must be positioned behind the teeth without interference by the tongue (Fig. 7.10). Otherwise, this structure will be superimposed over the dental images and interfere with interpretation of the radiograph. Digital retention of the film by the patient is sometimes used by older practitioners using the bisecting technique and for some endodontic procedures. This may result in a finger superimposed over the radiographic image (Fig. 7.11). This error has sometimes been referred to as the "phalangioma" error. Digital retention of the film by the patient is not recommended and should be avoided by using film-holding devices.

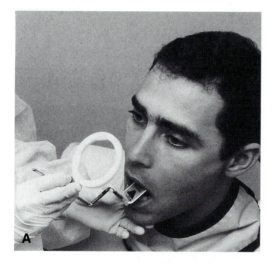

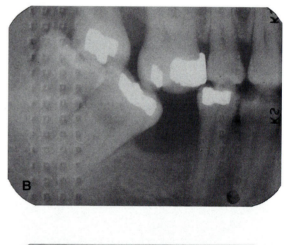

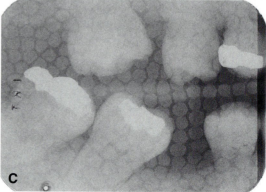

Figure 7.7. Film Placed Backward. **(A)** Photograph of film being placed backward in the mouth. (Note the printed side of the film packet has been placed toward the beam of radiation.) **(B)** Tire track pattern seen in D speed film. **(C)** Geometric pattern seen in E+ speed film.

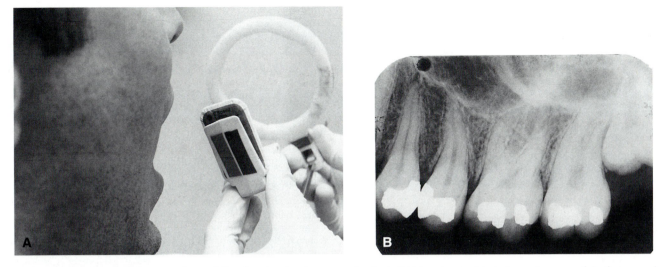

Figure 7.8. Dot in the Apical Region. **(A)** Photo of film placed with "dot **not** in the slot." **(B)** Note that the black dot on the apex of the first premolar is the identification raised dot placed on the film to identify the left and right on the film. It should be remembered that the raised dot should always be placed toward the occlusal surface when taking periapical films, because it could mimic or obscure periapical pathology.

Overlapping Errors

Overlapping is caused by either improper film placement and/or cone (beam indicating device [BID]) angulation.

Film Placement Error (Overlapping)

To prevent overlapping, the flat plane of the surface of the film should be positioned parallel to the mean tangent of the teeth to be radiographed. (The mean tangent is defined as the plane joining the most exterior points of the curved facial surfaces of a specific group of teeth, e.g., premolars or molars.) If this is not done, the contacts and embrasures between the teeth will be **overlapped** (Fig. 7.12).

BID Horizontal Angulation Error (Overlapping)

Overlapped contacts of interproximal surfaces of teeth will superimpose over each other if the direction the x-rays is misdirected in the horizontal plane (Fig. 7.13). The horizontal angle of the x-ray cone (BID) controls the x-ray entry through the interproximal surfaces of the teeth. The BID should be positioned horizontally, so the flat

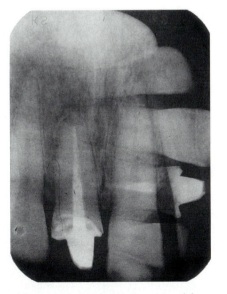

Figure 7.9. Double-Images on Radiograph. Caused by two exposures made on one radiograph before processing. This double exposure was made when two radiographic exposures were made at right angles to each other.

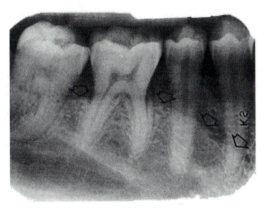

Figure 7.10. Tongue Artifact. Tongue image (*arrows*). Film was improperly placed on top of the tongue.

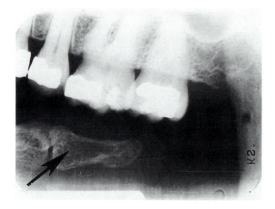

Figure 7.11. Phalangioma or Finger Artifact. Caused by the patient's finger (arrow) being placed between the film and the beam of radiation. This has been jokingly called "phalangioma" (tumor of the finger); in reality, it is only a finger.

plane at the end of the BID is parallel to the film positioned in the mouth. This should direct the x-rays in a proper horizontal angulation to open the interproximal embrasures. Incorrect horizontal angulation not only overlaps contact surfaces, but affects the definition of the total periapical image. By directing the x-rays in an oblique fashion rather than a perpendicular one, the resulting tooth images appear widened and less defined (Fig. 7.14). The overall film density is also reduced because structures are thicker in an oblique plane; consequently, fewer

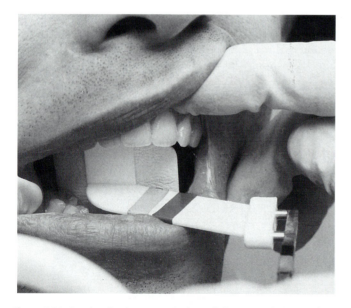

Figure 7.12. Overlapping (Improper Horizontal Placement of Film). Film is **not** positioned horizontally parallel to the mean tangent of the teeth to be radiographed. This will result in the contacts and embrasures of the teeth being overlapped.

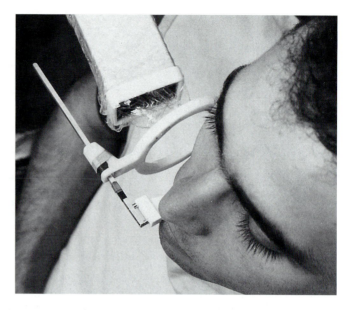

Figure 7.13. Overlapping (Horizontal Angulation Error). Incorrect horizontal angulation of the beam indicating device (BID) that will cause overlapping of contacts of teeth in this posterior bitewing film.

x-rays reach the film. Correction of this error is the same as the correction for overlapped contacts. The x-rays are directed perpendicular to the mean tangent of the teeth being radiographed or to the properly placed film. This is most easily accomplished with the use of an instrument such as the Dentsply/Rinn XCP positioning device (Elgin, IL).

Shape Distortion Error

This error is caused by improper vertical angulation of the cone (BID) and/or placement of the film.

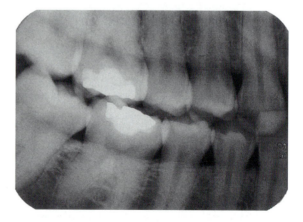

Figure 7.14. Overlapping. Bitewing radiograph showing overlapping of the contacts of upper and lower teeth.

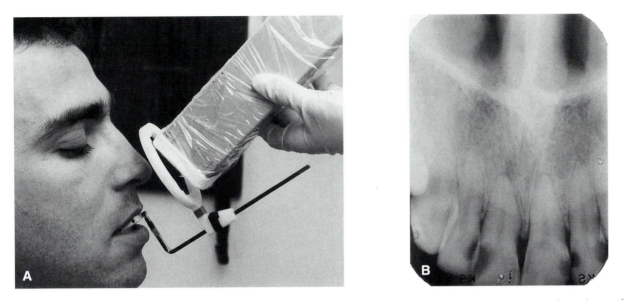

Figure 7.15. Foreshortening. (**A**) Too much vertical angulation of BID. (**B**) Foreshortening of tooth images from too much vertical angulation of BID.

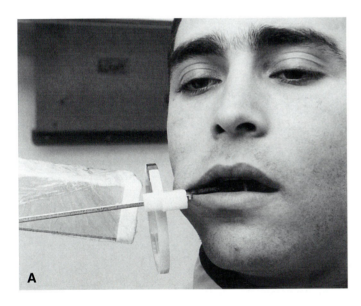

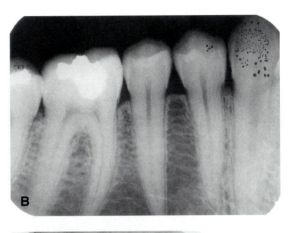

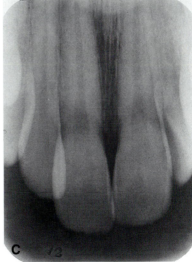

Figure 7.16. Elongation and Apical Ends of Teeth Cut Off. (**A**) Photograph showing "too flat" a vertical angulation of the cone (BID) that results in the apices of the teeth being projected off the film. (Teeth images are longer than their actual lengths and the apices are cut off.) (**B**) Radiograph of elongation of lower premolar teeth with apices cut off. (**C**) Radiograph of elongation of maxillary anterior centrals with apices cut off.

Foreshortening When **too much vertical angulation** is used, the image appears shortened on the radiograph (Fig. 7.15).

Elongation Elongation of tooth lengths occur **when not enough vertical angulation** is used, thus lengthening the teeth images (Fig. 7.16).

Film Distortion Image lengthening and distortion, as shown in Figure 7.17, may occur if the patient exerts too much biting pressure on the biteblock or if the film backing portion of the biteblock is trimmed or removed. This causes the film packet to bulge in the center. The image conforms to the distorted shape of the film surface. This error can be avoided by keeping the film in contact with the biteblock backing for support or instructing the patient to reduce the biting or pressure they are exerting on the biteblock.

Dimensional Distortion This type of image distortion is inherent radiographic distortion in the length of the roots of the maxillary molar teeth when using the bisecting-angle technique. It results in elongation of the palatal root and foreshortening of the two buccal roots. Neither of the roots lie in the bisecting-angle plane (Fig. 7.18). Correction of this distortion necessitates use of a paralleling technique for more accurate recording of the root lengths of the maxillary molars.

Cone-Cutting Errors

A **cone-cut** is the result of partial coverage of the film by the x-ray cone (BID) (Fig. 7.19). The term cone-cutting is a phrase that has stuck with us since the time dentists used a "pointed plastic cone" to direct the x-rays to the film. The plastic cone we speak of today is a **beam indicat-**

Summary of Intraoral Projection and Technique Errors

Error	Cause
Radiopaque artifacts on radiograph	Leaving dental appliance in mouth and/or eyeglasses or jewelry on the patient
Blurred image on radiograph	Movement of film, patient, or tubehead during exposure
Apical ends of teeth cut off	A. Film placed too close to the teeth in the maxillary arch in paralleling technique B. Too flat a vertical angulation, which causes elongation
All of specific region not showing	Faulty film placement (center the film over the area of interest)
Herringbone effect or ping-pong ball and light density	Printed back side of film placed toward beam of radiation (film reversed)
Black dot in apical area	Manufacturer's identifying depression on film placed toward apical area of the teeth (place "dot in slot"—XCP instrument)
Double images on radiographs	Film exposed twice to radiation; "use film cup"
"Phalangioma" (patient's finger in image)	In holding the film (bisecting angle technique), the finger is placed between the film and the teeth
Tongue image	Placing the film on top of the tongue
Overlapping of teeth	A. Plane of the film is not parallel to the lingual surface of the teeth B. Incorrect horizontal angulation of the cone (BID)
Foreshortening of image	Bisecting technique: Vertical angulation of cone (BID) too steep Paralleling technique: Film not parallel with long axes of the teeth Paralleling technique: Long cone (BID) is not positioned correctly
Elongation of image	Bisecting technique: Vertical angulation of cone (BID) is too flat Paralleling technique: Film is not positioned parallel to the long axes of the teeth Paralleling technique: Long cone (BID) not positioned correctly
Dimensional distortion of image	Inherent error in bisecting angle technique produces elongation of palatal roots and foreshortening of buccal roots of molars in the same view
Image distorted severely	Film is bent as patient bites on the film-holder or biteblock
Partial image "cone-cut"	Cone (BID) of radiation not covering the area of interest
Crowns of teeth not showing	Not enough film (⅛") showing below or above the crowns of the teeth Vertical angulation too steep

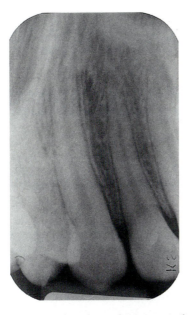

Figure 7.17. Film Distortion and Tooth Lengthening From Film Bending. Improper film placement and film retention causing the film to bend. Note elongation of teeth and "fuzzing-out" of tooth images in the upper left corner where the film has been bent or curved.

ing device (BID), which is an open-ended, lead-lined, circular or rectangular cylinder that helps to position and collimate the beam of radiation.

Crowns of Teeth Not Showing

The cause is not enough film showing below the maxillary teeth or above the crowns of the mandibular teeth.

Another cause is that the vertical angulation of the BID was too steep (Fig. 7.18B).

EXPOSURE AND MANUAL PROCESSING ERRORS

Blank Film, No Image

A film that has received no radiation will have no image and will reveal a clear, blue-tinted film. This may occur in several ways: (1) the x-ray machine was not "turned on" or the control panel was set for another tubehead, (2) the operator had completely failed to align the x-ray cone with the film, or (3) the operator may not have depressed the timer button properly to activate the exposure. Or this film was not exposed at all, while another was used twice to produce a double exposure.

Low-Density Film

A faint or low-density film may be the result of insufficient radiation exposure or a processing error (underdevelopment) (Fig. 7.20). Exposure factors must be checked to make sure the proper kilovoltage, milliamperage, source, film distance (locator ring placed close to skin), and correct timer setting were used. The exposure settings may have been too low or the focal-film distance too long for the exposure settings. A common error is **not** aligning the BID and the ring locators close to the patient's cheek. If the exposure settings are correct, the timer button exposure technique should then be checked. The timer button has a "deadman" switch and must be held down constantly until the audible sound stops, indicating the exposure has been completed. Light-density films may also be the result of a drop in line voltage or insufficient power at the time

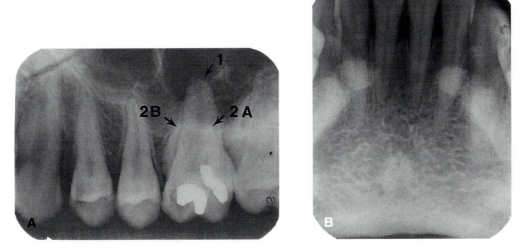

Figure 7.18. Dimensional Distortion and Crowns Cut Off. **(A)** Dimensional distortion on the maxillary first molar (1) elongated palatal (lingual) root, (2A) foreshortened distal buccal root, and (2B) foreshortened mesial buccal root. This is usually caused by using bisecting technique, which is inherent in the technique. **(B)** Crowns cut off due to excessive vertical angulation. Note the mandibular tori that could have caused interference with film placement.

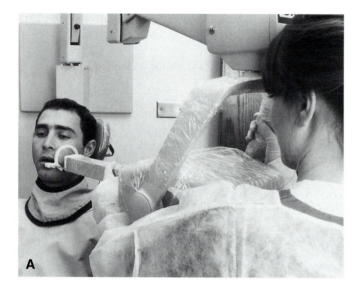

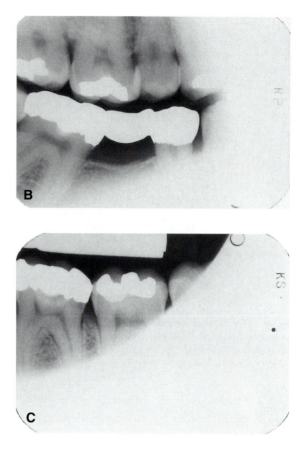

Figure 7.19. Cone-Cutting or Partial Image Error. (**A**) Photograph showing how a "cone-cut" will result from improper alignment of BID. (The central ray of the beam must be directed to the center of the film to completely cover the film.) (**B**) Cone-cut, rectangular BID. (**C**) Cone-cut, circular BID.

of exposure, although this is rare. A separate circuit may be necessary for optimal performance of the x-ray machine. A correctly exposed film may be light or low in density if darkroom factors are not optimal. Low developer solution, low temperature, insufficient developing time, exhausted or contaminated developer chemicals, and

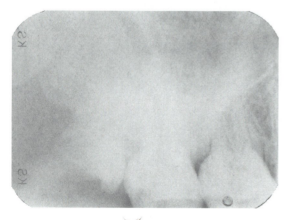

Figure 7.20. Low-Density Film. Low-density film may be the result of insufficient radiation exposure or underdevelopment of the film.

overfixation can be responsible for this problem. Each factor must be thoroughly examined. The most frequent of these is depleted developer solution in the automatic processor. Eventually (2 to 4 weeks), the chemicals will need complete replacement. All processing solutions exhibit reduced chemical activity after a period, no matter how often they are replenished.

High-Density (Dark) Film

A dark or high-density film may be the result of too high a radiation exposure, overdevelopment of film, or unsafe darkroom (Fig. 7.21). Exposure factors such as milliamperage, kilovoltage, source-film distance, and exposure time must be checked for accuracy. These settings may have been too high or the source-film distance too short for the exposure settings. The film speed should also be checked—is D or E+ speed film being used? D speed settings for E+ speed film will result in dark or overexposed images. A correctly exposed film may appear dark in density, if darkroom factors are not optimal. High developer solution temperatures, prolonged developing time for the temperature of the solution, or overstrength developing solutions are all potential causes of overdevelopment of the film. Each factor should be checked thor-

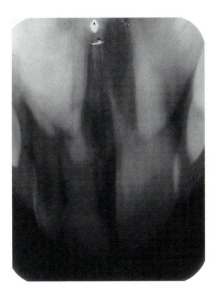

Figure 7.21. High-Density Film. This may be the result of overexposure or overdevelopment of the film.

oughly. Darkroom problems are rarely the cause of dark films. The films are usually overexposed.

Partial Image (Processing Error)

A technically accurate and properly exposed film with a partial image can be due to partial immersion of the film in the developer chemicals in hand processing. Over time, the level of developer solution drops due to evaporation and carry over of the solution into the water bath by the film hangers and films. Replenishment is necessary to maintain proper solution strength and level.

Black Artifacts

Contamination of the radiographic film surface before immersion into the developer solution can result in artifacts on the finished radiograph (Fig. 7.22A). Contaminants that cause black artifacts include developer chemicals, moisture (saliva), stannous fluoride, light leaks in the film packet, and overlapping of films during processing (Fig. 7.22B). The darkroom working surfaces, operator's hands, and film packets must be clean and dry. Careful handling of the film by the edges and orderly spacing of the films on the hangers will prevent unnecessary artifacts such as fingerprints (Fig. 7.22C).

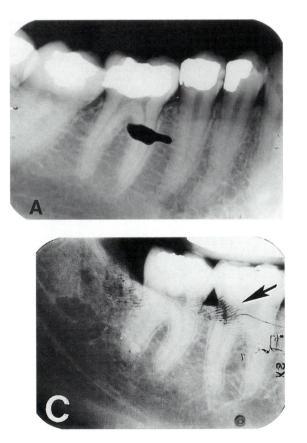

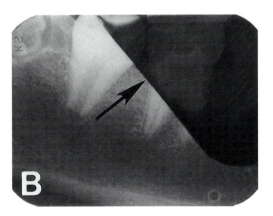

Figure 7.22. Black Artifacts on the Film. Contamination of the film before immersion in the developer solution can result in black artifacts on finished film. A black artifact can also be caused when a film cannot clear because different films are sticking together in the fixer tank. (**A**) Developer chemical black artifact. (**B**) Films that stuck together in the fixer solution. (**C**) Fingerprint black artifacts caused from hands contaminated with processing solutions or stannous fluoride before processing the films.

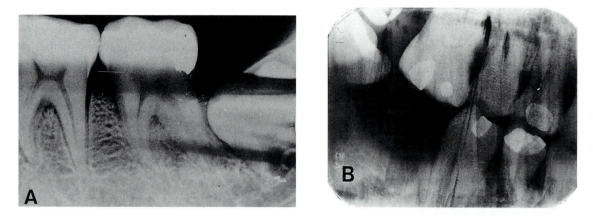

Figure 7.23. Black Streaks on the Film. Black streaks can be caused by many things, such as overinspection during development, lack of agitation of films in the developer, fixer-contaminated hanger clips, and dirty rollers in the automatic processors. **(A)** Developer chemical reaction with fixer residue left on the hanger clips, causing black streaking. **(B)** Black streaking marks caused by dirty rollers in the automatic processor.

Black Streaks

Streaking of the film emulsion may be the result of overinspection of the films during development, lack of proper film agitation when first immersed in processing solutions, fixer-contaminated processing hanger clips, insufficient fixing, or improper rinsing (Fig. 7.23A). Streaks may also be caused by dirty rollers in automatic processors (Fig. 7.23B). Processing "shortcuts" such as those cited above detract from film quality and often result in needless retakes.

White Artifacts

Precontamination of the film surface with droplets of fixer solution, as well as air bubbles that form on the film surface during initial immersion of the film in the developing solution, can cause white teardrop artifacts on the finished radiograph (Fig. 7.24). Also, fixer solutions on the fingers can cause white fingerprints in the image. Clean and dry working surfaces are essential for proper processing. Gentle agitation of the films when first placed in the processing solution will remove air bubbles (Fig. 7.25) and allow complete development of the latent image.

Deposits on Film

Chemical precipitants that adhere to the film and mar its surface are most often due to contaminated, improperly prepared, or exhausted solutions. Unclean film hanger clips may also carry chemical deposits that may be the source of solution contamination. When changing solutions, the operator must thoroughly clean the tanks, not interchange the tanks between the two solutions (the same tanks should always be used for developer and fixer), mix the new chemicals according to manufacturer's instruc-

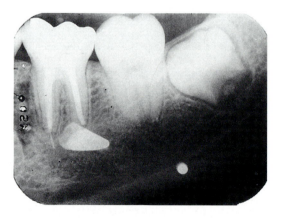

Figure 7.24. White Artifacts on the Film. Contamination of the film emulsion surface with droplets of fixer solution before development. The fixer droplets will clear the film of silver halide in the emulsion during the development phase, forming white artifacts.

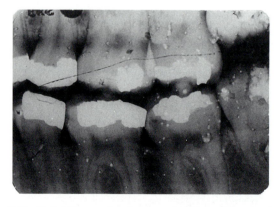

Figure 7.25. Air Bubbles on the Film. Air bubbles (white round areas) forming on the film as the film is first placed into the developer solution can be removed by agitation of the films. The black line running across the film is caused by rough handling of the film during processing.

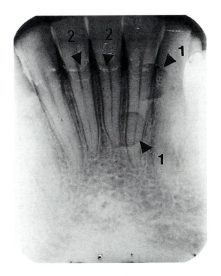

Figure 7.26. Developer Stain. (1) Darker areas are watery developer stains. (2) White areas are deposits of zirconium prophy paste on teeth.

tions, and use separate stirring rods to mix the solutions.

Stains

Most stains that appear on finished radiographs are the result of exhausted solutions or insufficient rinsing (Fig. 7.26). Manual and automatic processing solutions need replenishment and have a limited life span. The maximum life for manual processing solutions is usually 15 to 30 days, depending mainly on the number of films processed. A thorough rinsing of the processed radiographs is necessary not only to remove any remaining chemicals from the film, but also to rinse the film hangers free of chemicals. Films should be rinsed in a running water bath for 15 minutes. The most common stain is brown due to insufficient removal of the fixer solution from the manually processed film (Fig. 7.27). The brown stain occurs with age and is due to the retained hypo (thiosulfate) from the fixer reacting with the metallic silver image to form brown silver sulfide—just as silverware acquires a brown tarnish when exposed to hydrogen sulfide produced by cooking gas.

AUTOMATIC FILM PROCESSING ERRORS

There are several errors in automatic processing that can be made to render the film unreadable. An automatic film processing troubleshooting chart is shown on the next page.

Feeding Film in Automatic Processors

The following are a few important recommendations for feeding the film into the automatic processor to prevent errors.

---

1. Films should be fed slowly and carefully. Panoramic films should be inserted into the processor in a straight line with the roller system. Failure to do so could cause a jam-up in the processor.
2. If film is bent, the unbent side of the film should be inserted into the machine first; the bent corner or edge should be unbent.
3. Damp or wet films should not be fed into the machine because they will contaminate rollers and cause streaking of subsequent films.
4. Films should not be fed too quickly in succession. They may stick to each other and could jam the machine (allow 5 seconds between films fed into the same slot). There will be a dark density area on the film where the films stuck together.

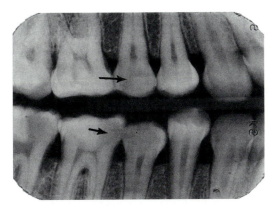

Figure 7.27. Brown Stain on the Film. This is caused by not washing film properly after fixing. If the film is not washed long enough after fixing, the hypo (thiosulfate) retained in the film emulsion will in time react with the metallic silver grains in the radiograph to form a brown-silver sulfide stain.

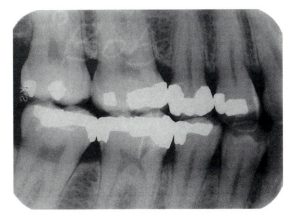

Figure 7.28. Marks From Ball-Point Pen. Writing on the film with a ball-point pen produces white marks. The name "Bob" can be clearly seen.

Automatic Film Processing Trouble Chart

Condition	Cause
Low-density (light) films	A. Solution temperature too low B. Exhausted developer (underreplenishment) C. Improper agitation or massaging action of rollers D. Processing too fast (higher temperature and/or faster roller speed)
High-density (dark) films	A. Solutions overheated B. Light leaks in the processor cover C. Too much replenishment
Wet or tacky films	A. Dryer and developer temperatures too low B. Dryer thermostatic control or heater inoperative C. Dryer air circulation inadequate (high humidity in dryer section) D. Wrong chemistry and/or film E. Processing too fast (higher temperature and/or faster roller speed)
Film discoloration (brown)	A. Contamination of fixer by the developer solution
Film discoloration (greenish yellow)	A. Fixer solution exhausted (underreplenishment) B. Processing too fast (higher temperature and/or faster roller speed) C. Wrong type of film for the processor solution
Fogged films (unwanted density)	A. Incorrect or defective safelight filter or bulb B. Light leaks in the darkroom C. Developer temperature too high D. Improper storage of films
Streaking (uneven density)	A. Underreplenishment B. Rollers encrusted with chemical deposits C. Dirty wash water D. Film not hardened properly by chemicals
Surface marks	A. Foreign materials or irregularities on the surface of the rollers B. Rough handling of the film before processing
Films chalky or dirty	A. No wash water or dirty wash water B. Fixer contaminated
Jams or failure of film to transport	A. Chemicals contaminated or diluted B. Chemical temperature too high C. Films excessively soft and not adequately hardened; when enough gelatin lubricates the rollers, films will jam up with one another D. Dirty rollers E. Racks not seated properly F. Dirty wash water G. Incorrect dryer temperature H. Hesitation in drive assembly, causing film to pause in transit I. Film not tracking though the processor in straight course (improper feeding of films) J. Bent film corners as leading edge

FILM-HANDLING ERRORS

Pressure Marks

Writing on the film packet with a ball-point pen or pressure from the cusps and incisal edges of the teeth (occurring mostly in pediatric occlusal radiography) will produce marks on the finished radiographs (Fig. 7.28).

Bend Marks

Black linear artifacts (Fig. 7.29) on finished radiographs are the result of purposeful bending of the film to reduce patient discomfort. Film bends must be kept to a minimum and be strategically located so that the bends do not interfere with the major images on the film. Black crescent creases (Fig. 7.30) are the result of incidental crimping of

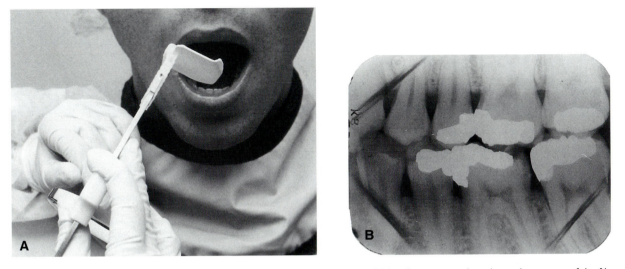

Figure 7.29. Bend Marks (Purposeful Bending). (**A**) Photograph showing purposeful bending. (**B**) Bend marks on the corners of the film.

the film, usually produced by excessive bending and not the fingernail. Films should be handled with care to avoid distracting artifacts.

Moisture Contamination

Saliva contamination of the film packet may cause the inner black paper wrapping to adhere to the film emulsion, producing a black artifact (Fig. 7.31). Film packets (especially paper packets) should be wiped off with a paper towel before inserting them into a film receptacle. Moisture present on the fingers can also produce artifacts on the film. When handling films out of the film packet, hands should be clean, dry, and free from contamination from processing chemicals. Film should be handled only on the edges, without touching the surface.

Static Electricity

A dry indoor environment, such as occurs in winter, combined with rough unwrapping of films or rapid sliding of panoramic films out of the film box or soft cassette may produce a small charge of static electricity that exposes the film at the point of origin. Also, synthetic uniform materials and rubber-soled shoes rubbing against carpet contribute to static electricity production by the film handler (Fig. 7.32). This can be reduced by placing a humidi-

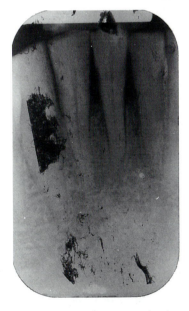

Figure 7.31. Moisture (Saliva) Contamination. Saliva from the patient soaking through the film packet (especially paper packets) and causing the black protective paper to stick to the wet emulsion of the film, causing black areas on the film.

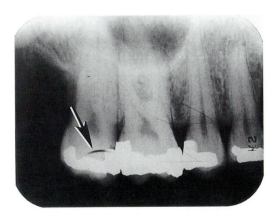

Figure 7.30. Black Crescent Mark (Incidental Crimping). Black crescent artifact caused by excessive crimping and bending of the film packet to make it more comfortable for the patient.

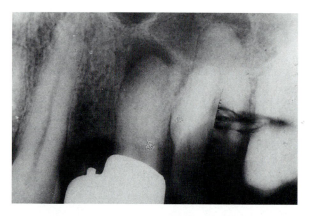

Figure 7.32. Static Electricity Error. Linear form of static electricity marks with lightning-like streaks. This may take several forms, such as small dots or a tree-like configuration.

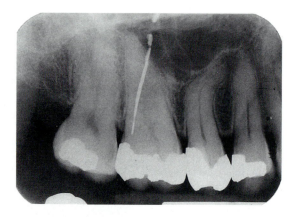

Figure 7.33. Torn Emulsion Error. Emulsion torn due to rough handling in the processing cycle when emulsion was soft.

fier or container of water in the darkroom during cold months when the heating system is working.

Torn Emulsion and Scratches

Careless handling of the film, especially during film processing when the emulsion is soft and swollen, often results in a removal of the emulsion and a visible scratch when the surface of the film is examined in reflected light. If the film surface is scraped against the processing tank, another film hanger, or the operator's fingernail, the emulsion can be easily peeled off (Fig. 7.33).

Dust and Powder Artifacts

Film contact with dust, grit, dirt, or glove powder before film processing can result in pinpoint black artifacts on the film emulsion. It is recommended that nonpowdered gloves be used during radiology infection control procedures. After processing, when films are dry and ready

to mount, contact with the above contaminants should be avoided. These contaminants cause the particles to cling to the film surface.

Film Fog

Film fog, evidenced by a dull-gray low-contrast image, has several possible causes (Fig. 7.34). Films can be fogged by use of outdated film, improper film storage, radiation before and after exposure, improper safelight conditions, above optimum developing solution temperatures, and white light darkroom leaks. Radiographic film must be stored according to expiration date in a cool, dry environment (preferably a refrigerator) and away from radiation and strong chemicals. Radiographic film is also sensitive to white light. Because of this the darkroom should be white-light–tight, with proper safelight lamp distance (4 feet of the working surface), red filter (GBX-2), and bulb (15 watt) to guard against fog. When opening film packets and feeding film in the slots of the automatic processor

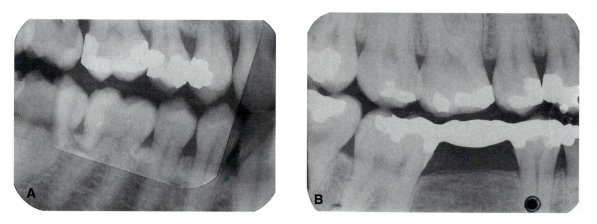

Figure 7.34. Fogged Film. **(A)** Film was superimposed over another film. (Note the difference between the fogged portion of the film and the portion of the film under the superimposed film that is not fogged.) **(B)** Overall gray appearance of film fog (unwanted density) from various causes such as unsafe safelight, light leaks, outdated film, overheated film, and film exposed to scatter radiation.

Summary of Film Handling Errors

Error	Cause
Black pressure marks on film	Teeth marks on film (especially pediatric occlusal film)
Black bend lines on film	From bending film to reduce patient discomfort
Black marks on film	Saliva contamination of black protective paper covering film; caused by failure to blot film packet with paper towel
Black "lightning- or tree-like" marks on film	Static electricity; removing film too rapidly from packet or box in air with dry humidity
Torn emulsion and scratches on film	Careless handling of film during processing when emulsion is soft and swollen
Dust and powder artifacts	Film contact with dust, grit, or glove powder before processing
Fogged film (unwanted density) A. Light fog	1. Light leaks in the darkroom 2. Improper safelight; check bulb wattage, distance, and filter-film compatibility 3. Turning overhead (white) light on too soon; (be certain films have cleared in fixer first)
B. Radiation fog	Improper storage; insufficient protection of film next to x-ray machine
C. Processing (chemical fog)	1. Developer temperatures too high 2. Overstrength developer (check manufacturer's instructions) 3. Prolonged development for temperature 4. Contaminated developer (clean tank routinely)
D. Deterioration of film	1. Temperature of storage area too high (store in refrigerator) 2. Humidity of storage area too high (store in refrigerator) 3. Strong fumes (ammonia, paint)
White ball-point pen marks	Writing on front of film packet with ball-point pen

in the *daylight loader*, the operator's hands should not be removed from the sleeves until the films placed into the slots have moved completely within the machine. *Chemical film fog* may be due to excessive developing temperature, overdevelopment and use of poorly mixed, contaminated, or exhausted developer solution.

WORKSHOP/LABORATORY EXERCISES

EXERCISE 7.1. INTRAORAL TECHNIQUE ERRORS

Materials and Equipment Needed

1. X-ray machine and processing facility.
2. Film-holding device.
3. Eight no. 2 films (intraoral).
4. Manikin or skull.

Instructions

Using the x-ray machine and manikin, **improperly place** each film and expose it to obtain the following errors:

1. Backward or "reversed" image.
2. Dot artifact error.
3. Double image.
4. Overlapped bitewing contacts.
5. Foreshortening of maxillary centrals.
6. Elongation of maxillary centrals.
7. Dimensional distortion of maxillary first molar.
8. Cone cut.

After processing, mount the films and label each error.

EXERCISE 7.2. INTRAORAL EXPOSURE AND/OR PROCESSING ERRORS

Materials and Equipment Needed

1. All equipment items in Exercise 7.1.
2. Seven no. 2 films (intraoral)

Instructions

Using the x-ray machine and manikin, **improperly expose and/or process** a film to obtain the following errors:

1. Blank image.
2. Light image.
3. Dark image.
4. Black fingerprint in image.
5. Fixer stain in image.
6. Fogged film with an image of teeth.
7. Bent corner of film

After processing, mount the films and label each error.

CASE-BASED PROBLEM-SOLVING

You are trying to figure out if you prefer manual processing to automatic processing. Make a chart listing the comparative advantages and disadvantages of each and report what you would do if you had your choice.

Hint: Do not forget potential for errors, cost, maintenance, time for obtaining a dry processed film, infection control, and so forth. You may want to give some factors more weight or importance than others.

REVIEW QUESTIONS

1. Which of the following could explain why your films are coming out too dark?

    A. Unsafe safelight.
    B. Light leaks in the darkroom.
    C. Overexposure.
    D. Overdevelopment.
    E. All of the above.

2. A very light density radiograph may be caused by:

    A. Too long an exposure time.
    B. The leaded side of the film placed toward the tube.
    C. Developing solution that is too warm.
    D. Removing the film from the fixing bath too soon.
    E. The leakage of white light in the darkroom.

3. Tree-like or lightning-like black streaks on a processed film are caused by:

    A. Bending the film packet.
    B. Static electricity.
    C. Films overlapping in the processor.
    D. Automatic processing roller marks.
    E. Scratching the emulsion.

4. Radiographic films that are not properly fixed:

    1. May turn orange-brown.
    2. Emerge wet from the processor.
    3. Lose archival quality.
    4. Show an increase in contrast.
    A. 1, 2, and 3 only.
    B. 1, 2, and 4 only.
    C. 2 and 4.
    D. 1 and 3.

CASE-BASED QUESTIONS

CASE 7.1

Identify the error in this radiograph:

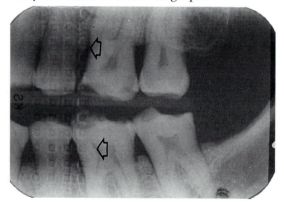

A. Film contaminated by fixer before development.
B. The film packet was reversed.
C. Excessive exposure to thermal changes before development.
D. Improper use of Styrofoam biteblock.
E. Use of outdated film.

CASE 7.2

A 16-year-old girl with a very sensitive palate had this maxillary premolar radiograph taken.

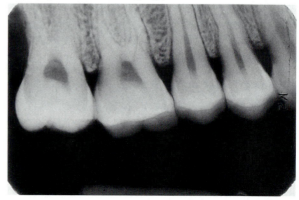

QUESTION

The radiograph has to be retaken. What is the most likely cause of this common radiographic error?

A. The film was placed too far from the teeth.
B. The patient did not bite on the biteblock.
C. Cone was misaligned with the film.
D. Film bending.
E. Film placed too far forward in the mouth.

CASE 7.3

A dental hygiene student was required to take a premolar bitewing of her first patient. She knew it was very important to get the distal of the canines on this projection. This is the resultant bitewing radiograph.

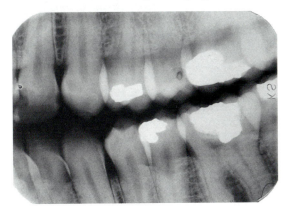

QUESTION

What are the causes of this common error?

1. Improper film placement.
2. Improper exposure time.
3. Improper processing.
4. Improper horizontal angulation of cone (BID).
5. Malposed teeth.
6. Improper vertical angulation of cone (BID).
A. 1 and 6.
B. 2, 3, and 5.
C. 2, 5, and 6.
D. 1 and 4.
E. 3, 4, and 5.

CASE 7.4

A premolar bitewing is taken of an 18-year-old girl in your office. Technically the radiograph is excellent, but it is undiagnostic. The bitewing radiograph is placed on an illuminator in a darkened room, and the light of the illuminator is turned down low. The radiograph is still not satisfactory for your diagnostic needs, and a retake is ordered. The processing solutions are fresh and have been stirred.

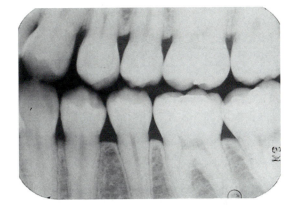

QUESTION

What is the best method to correct for this radiographic error?

A. Decrease kilovoltage.
B. Do not place film backward in the mouth.
C. Decrease developing time.
D. Increase exposure time.
E. Use a slower-speed film.

CASE 7.5

After taking a maxillary premolar radiograph using the Dentsply/Rinn instruments and manual processing, a fellow worker tells you that there were common errors on the radiograph, and you agreed.

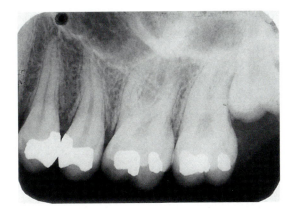

QUESTION

How would you correct for these errors?

1. Leave film in the water bath longer after fixation.
2. Leave film in the developer longer.
3. Decrease vertical angulation.
4. Place dot in the slot of the film-holder.
5. Position the film more mesially.
6. Position the film more distally.
A. 1, 3, and 6.
B. 1, 4, and 5.
C. 3, 4, and 5.
D. 2 and 4.
E. 1, 2, and 6.

CASE 7.6

A loyal patient of your dental clinic comes to you for her 1-year check up and this radiograph was taken.

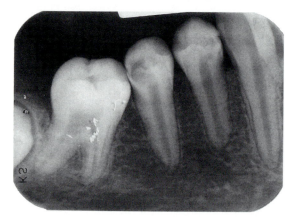

QUESTION

What caused the common errors in this radiograph?

1. Too flat a vertical angulation of the BID.
2. Too steep a vertical angulation of the BID.
3. Fixer artifact.
4. Developer stain.
5. Air on emulsion
6. Rough handling of film.
A. 1 and 3.
B. 2 and 4.

C. 2 and 6.
D. 3 and 6.
E. 1 and 5.

CASE 7.7

Your office has purchased a new automatic processor. The first time you use it, two films come out stuck to each other, with the resultant film.

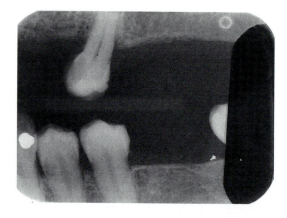

QUESTION

What causes this error?

A. Processing temperatures are too high.
B. The rollers are set too slow.
C. Films were inserted too fast in the same slot.
D. Films have bent edges.
E. Dryer not working properly.

BIBLIOGRAPHY

Bloom WL, Hollenbach JL, Morgan JA. Medical radiographic technic. 3rd ed. Springfield: Charles C. Thomas, 1969:127–128.

Darkroom technique for better radiographs. Wilmington, DE: Photo Products Department, E.I. DuPont de Nemours and Co., 1982.

DuPont guide for dental X-ray darkrooms. Wilmington, DE: Photo Products Department, E.I. DuPont de Nemours and Co., 1982.

Fuchs AW. Principles of radiographic exposures and processing. 2nd ed. Springfield: Charles C. Thomas, 1958:199–258.

Langland OE, Sippy FH, Langlais RP. Textbook of dental radiology. 2nd ed. Springfield: Charles C. Thomas, 1984:322–351.

Matteson SR, Whaley C, Crandell CE. Dental radiology (dental assisting manual V). Chapel Hill: University of North Carolina Press, 1988.

Peterson S. Clinical dental hygiene. St. Louis: CV Mosby, 1959:239–247.

Radiodontic pitfalls. Rochester, NY: Eastman Kodak, X-Ray Division, 1990.

Successful intraoral radiography. Rochester, NY: Eastman Kodak, 1990.

Quality Assurance and Legal Aspects

8

OBJECTIVES

Upon successful completion of this unit, the student will be able to:

1. *Define quality assurance.*

2. *State the two major categories of quality assurance.*

3. *State the three stages of dental radiology facilities.*

4. *Discuss the components of each stage.*

5. *List the two areas of routine testing of the x-ray system.*

6. *Describe the ways to test the x-ray machine.*

7. *Describe the ways to test the darkroom.*

8. *Identify the other areas of quality assurance with regard to radiographic procedures.*

9. *Identify the ownership of dental radiographs.*

10. *Explain the process of billing and loaning of radiographs.*

11. *Discuss the liability for failing to use radiographs and the impact of radiographs as evidence.*

12. *Demonstrate how to make a step-wedge using x-ray packet lead foil through the Workshop/Laboratory Exercises format.*

13. *Simulate and troubleshoot timer failure, darkroom fog, and developer solution failure using the Workshop/Laboratory Exercises format.*

14. *List all possible causes of low-density films using the Case-Based Problem-Solving format.*

15. *Test his or her knowledge by answering the Review Questions.*

KEY WORDS/PHRASES

aluminum filters

"check" films

checking the half-value layer

coin test

collimation test

densitometer

error log

evidence

focal spot checker

fog test

half-value layer

kVp meter

liability

loaning x-rays

mAs reciprocity test

measuring output

pocket dosimeter

quality administration

quality assurance

quality control

quality control staging

resolution

retake log

sensitometer

spinning top

x-ray ownership

INTRODUCTION

As applied to dental radiology, quality assurance refers to those steps that are taken to make sure that a dental office or radiologic facility will produce consistently high-quality radiographs with minimum cost in patient exposure. The common causes of unsatisfactory radiographs were discussed in Chapter 7. Many of these, such as improper angulation and film positioning, result primarily from human error. Others, such as exposure and processing problems, may result from equipment failure. The term **quality assurance** has come into general use to describe the administrative and technical efforts that are made to identify and correct equipment problems before they have become so severe as to affect the diagnostic quality of the radiographs being produced. For instance, if quality assurance principles concerning periodic changes of the developing solutions are not followed in a dental office, the films will begin to be of light or low density because the developer solution has weakened with time. The tendency in this situation is to increase the exposure time when taking radiographs to increase the darkness of the radiograph. This procedure unnecessarily increases the radiation dose to the patient. This one example shows why quality assurance principles are important.

Quality assurance may be divided into two major cate-

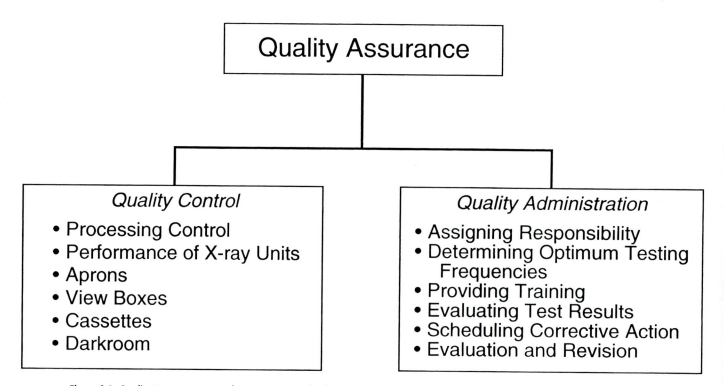

Figure 8.1. Quality Assurance. Quality assurance is divided into two major categories: quality administration and quality control.

gories: quality administration and quality control (Fig. 8.1). Quality administration refers to the management aspect. It includes those organizational steps taken to make sure that testing techniques are properly performed and that the results of tests are used to effectively maintain a consistently high level of image quality. Quality control can be summarized in two ways. First, it comprises the procedures used for the routine physical testing of the x-ray. Second, each testing procedure can be viewed as a method of demonstrating one or several basic principles of dental radiography, thus further clarifying our understanding of the subject.

QUALITY ADMINISTRATION

WHAT IS QUALITY ASSURANCE?

A dental radiology quality assurance program involves periodic evaluation of the x-ray equipment. This includes the entire chain of components from the x-ray machine, through processing, to the viewing of the radiographs. Currently, some states require dental offices to establish written guidelines. Each dental office should establish maintenance and monitoring procedures as summarized below:

Summary of Quality Maintenance and Monitoring Procedures

General	Use reference films Fill out a retake long Check thyroid shields and lead aprons for cracks Use exposure and technique charts Use rectangular collimation Use the fastest film speed and screens available
Daily[a]	Clean the darkroom Perform processor quality control
Monthly[a]	Clean screens and cassettes Check viewing conditions and viewboxes Perform safelight test
Yearly[a]	Check stability of tubehead/arm Check kVp accuracy Check mA accuracy Check timer accuracy Check half-value layer Check focal spot degradation Check collimator efficacy

[a] The frequency of these inspections will vary according to state regulations and manufacturer's directions.

Point System Used to Stage a Dental Facility for Needed Quality Assurance Procedures

	Points
A. **Evaluation of facility, film processing, and workload**	
1. Radiology facilities: equipment and techniques	
Intraoral radiography only (periapical, bitewing, occlusal)	1
Intraoral and panoramic radiography only	3
Intraoral, panoramic, and extraoral skull/cephalometric radiography	7
2. Film processing method	
Manual (time—temperature tanks)	1
Automatic (processing machine)	3
3. Radiograph workload (average)	
Less than 100 films[a] per week	1
100–300 films[a] per week	3
More than 300 films[a] per week	6
B. **Recommended monitoring level of quality assurance program (total point value of 1, 2, and 3 above)**	
Stage I dental practice	<8
Stage II dental practice	8–11
Stage III dental practice	12 or more

[a] One panoramic or cephalometric film equals 20 periapicals.

In 1983 at the request of the American Dental Association, the American Academy of Dental Radiology, now the American Academy of Oral and Maxillofacial Radiology (AAOMR), made recommendations for quality assurance in dental radiology. The AAOMR recommendations were based on the facilities' size and workload, as determined using the point system shown above. Once a facility has been staged, different levels of recommendations apply, as listed in the following outline:

STAGE I DENTAL PRACTICE

It is recommended that facilities qualifying as Stage I use the following program:

1. Reference films.
2. Retake log.

3. Daily visual monitoring of radiographs produced.
4. Monthly check of viewboxes.
5. Monthly darkroom assessment.
6. Annual test of the x-ray machine.

STAGE II DENTAL PRACTICE

It is recommended that facilities qualifying as Stage II use all Stage I recommendations plus the following:

1. Daily assessment of automatic processor/manual processing solutions.
2. Monthly check of cassettes and intensifying screens.

STAGE III DENTAL PRACTICE

It is recommended that facilities qualifying as Stage III use Stage II recommendations plus a sensitometer, a densitometer, and an increased level of effort in administration. A sensitometer is a simple device that exposes an x-ray film to a highly reproducible step pattern of light intensity. After development, the film is studied with a **densitometer.** A densitometer is a device for measuring density, the degree of darkening of exposed and processed x-ray or photographic film.

SETTING UP A QUALITY ASSURANCE PROGRAM

The personnel identified to perform the testing procedures can adapt them to the special requirements of a given facility. For example, a facility is staged to determine the level of quality assurance needed, and specific procedures are then put into place according to the time schedule previously described.

Quality Control Kits

The components of the kit will depend first on the stage of the facility, which identifies what quality control procedures are needed and at what intervals. Second, personnel at each facility will decide which procedures will be used in-house and which ones will be carried out by an outside expert. For the purpose of this chapter, we assume all procedures will be used by personnel within the dental facility. A list of qualified outside experts is generally available from state agencies overseeing the use of ionizing radiation.

The quality control kit usually contains the following:

1. Pocket dosimeter and charger (ionization chamber).
2. kVp test device (kVp meter).

3. Aluminum filters in 0.1- and 0.5-mm thicknesses.
4. Brass spinning top or electronic timer meter.
5. Aluminum or lead foil step-wedge.
6. Lead numbers to mark films.
7. Sensitometer and densitometer (optional).
8. Processing solution thermometer.
9. Resolution test object (focal spot checker).
10. Piece of rare earth screen (collimator checker).

The use of the kit will be explained as if all the procedures are necessary. These radiation testing products can be purchased through Keystone X-Ray (Neptune, NY), Picker X-Ray (Charlotte, NC), Radiation Measurements (Middleton, WI), and Nuclear Associates (Carie Place, NY).

QUALITY CONTROL PROCEDURES IN DENTAL RADIOLOGY (USING QUALITY CONTROL KIT DEVICES)

The routine procedures used for assessing of the x-ray system can be divided into two major parts: the x-ray machine and the darkroom and/or processing.

TESTING THE X-RAY MACHINE

The x-ray machine is tested for the following three factors relating to the x-ray beam: quantity, quality, and collimation. These three factors can be compared to gasoline at the gas pump. The quantity is measured in gallons, the quality is expressed in octane, and the collimation is the rubber collar that prevents the escape of fumes at the pump nozzle that are harmful if inhaled. Although the x-ray beam can be checked for quantity, quality, and collimation by office personnel, most states send inspectors at intervals to inspect and certify the dental x-ray equipment for the above parameters.

Checking the Quantity of the X-Ray Beam (Output)

The purpose of checking the quantity of an x-ray beam is to verify that the output of the x-ray machine has not changed since the last procedure. The quantity of x-ray photons, sometimes referred to as the exposure or output, is affected by the mA circuit (especially if an adjustable mA setting is present) and mainly by the exposure time. The kVp also affects the amount of radiation but is not tested here. To measure for quantity, one needs to set the x-ray machine at a standardized set of exposures, e.g., 15 impulses (0.25 seconds), 7 or 10 mA, and 65 or 70 kVp, and measure the quantity of radiation being generated. A **pocket dosimeter or another type of dosimeter** (ionization

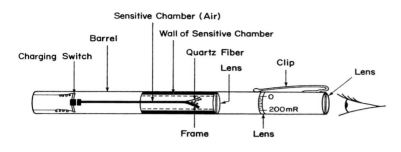

A   Pocket Dosimeter (Fully Charged)

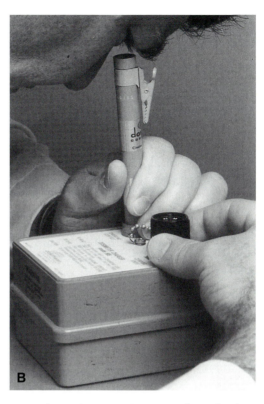

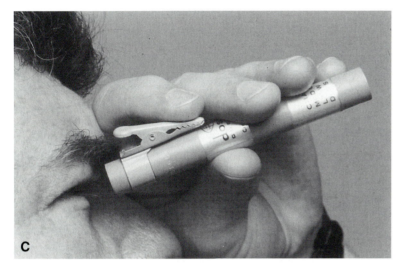

Figure 8.2. Pocket Dosimeter. (**A**) Diagram of a pocket dosimeter for measuring radiation output. (**B**) A pocket dosimeter must be charged before use. (**C**) The pocket dosimeter being read after exposure.

chamber) is used to take this measurement (Fig. 8.2). If the first (baseline) reading has always been 180 milliroentgen (mR), and the current (second) measurement is the same, then no further testing of beam quantity is necessary. This could also be done by using an inexpensive aluminum or lead foil step-wedge (Fig. 8.3) and comparing a baseline step-wedge image (taken some time ago) with a current step-wedge image processed with fresh solutions. Each step in the image of the current step-wedge should be exactly the same shade of gray as in the baseline image (taken some time ago). This test is usually done yearly or as required by local regulations.

Trouble with Quantity If the above dosimeter reading is different (usually less) or if the step-wedge image is different from the reference image (usually lower density), then the timer and the mA circuit are investigated.

Checking the Timer The purpose of checking the timer is to see if it is functioning accurately. This procedure can also be used to visibly demonstrate the principle that

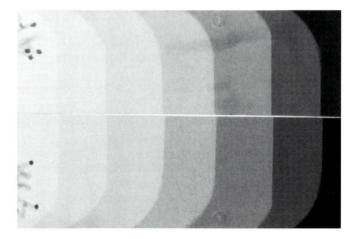

Figure 8.3. Checking Output. If the steps in the baseline image (top) match the densities of the steps in today's image (bottom), then the radiation output reading (top) has not changed between the baseline and today's reading (bottom).

x-rays are generated in impulses in self-rectified dental x-ray machines. Remember, there are 60 impulses in 1 second; therefore, 1/10 second equals 6 impulses. A simple brass spinning top can be obtained for only a few dollars. It is placed on top of an occlusal film or a panoramic film in a cassette (Fig. 8.4). The regular, self-rectifying dental x-ray machine is set at, for example, 15 impulses or 0.25 seconds. The central ray is directed perpendicular to the spinning top, which is in motion. When the timer is activated, one small black dot will be seen on the processed film for each impulse. These dots should be counted and compared with the timer setting. Using this example, one should see 15 dots. Alternately, a more expensive electronic timer meter is recommended for convenience or to check the timer of a high-frequency, constant potential dental x-ray machine; an instant readout is obtained. Remember, constant potential x-ray machines do not put out impulses; the radiation is constant for the selected

exposure time interval. If the timer is inaccurate, the x-ray machine will require servicing.

Checking the mA Circuit The purpose of checking the mA circuit (filament circuit) is to ensure the proper functioning of the 10 and 15 mA settings on some machines. This procedure can also be used to visibly demonstrate the principle of mAs reciprocity. That is to say, "exposure or mAs equals mA times exposure time in seconds." If the x-ray machine has only one mA setting (usually 7 mA), the mA circuit can only be checked by a technician using an **ammeter**. If 10 and 15 mA circuits are available, the "mAs reciprocity" principle is used to test these two circuits. As long as the mAs factor is the same (when using 10 and 15 mA settings) and the output or quantity of radiation measured with the pocket dosimeter remains the same for 10 and 15 mA settings, the mA circuits are said to be operating properly. The other variable in mAs reciprocity is **the timer, which regulates exposure time**

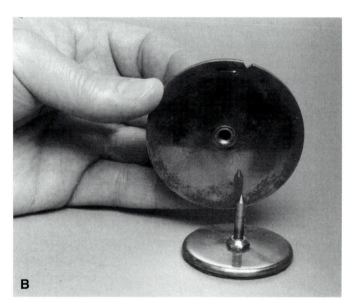

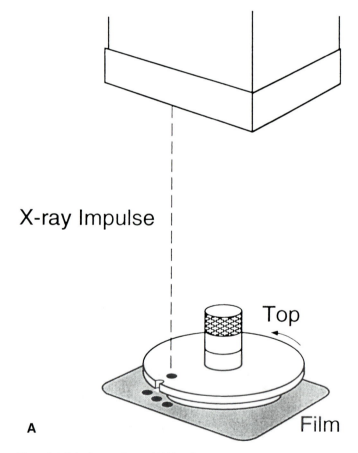

X-ray Impulse

Top

Film

A

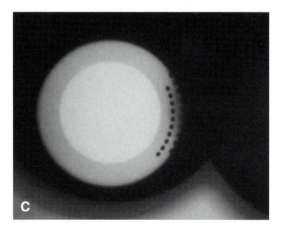

C

Figure 8.4. Spinning Top Test. (**A**) Use of spinning top to measure exposure timer accuracy of self-rectified x-ray machine. The diagram demonstrates that the central ray of the x-ray beam is directed perpendicular to the spinning top, which is in motion, and the film exposed. (**B**) Spinning top. (**C**) A small dot will be seen on the film for each pulse (1/60 second) of the x-ray machine.

and is checked **first** to ensure it is accurate. First, the operator sets the machine at **15 mA** and **1 second or 60 impulses** (i) (15 mA × 1 sec = 15 mAs or 15 mA × 60 imp. = 900 mAi; 15 mAs is the same as 900 mAi) and, for example, 75 kVp. He or she then measures the output in mR with a pocket dosimeter or with a step-wedge film. The x-ray machine should then be set at **10 mA** and **1.5 seconds or 90 impulses** (15 mAs or 900 mAi), and the output is measured with a dosimeter or step-wedge film. While the mA was varied, the mAs remained the same between the two exposures. Given that the timer is accurate, then the output in mR should be the same for the two exposures, if the two mA circuits are operating correctly. This only works because of the principle of mAs reciprocity. If the two readings are different, the x-ray machine will require servicing.

Checking the Quality of the X-Ray Beam

The quality of the x-ray photons is a function of kVp that determines the wavelength or penetrating power of the x-ray beam. However, two other factors control quality of the x-ray beam. They are the accuracy of the kVp setting and the focal spot size. Focal spot size change will usually indicate focal spot degradation that decreases detail and sharpness in the image. X-ray beam quality should be checked yearly or as required by local regulations.

Checking the Penetrating Power of the Beam The purpose of checking the penetrating power of the x-ray beam is to ensure in a general way that the kVp circuit is functioning within safe limits. Also, this procedure can be used to visibly demonstrate the half-value layer (HVL) principle that states: "50% of the x-ray photons should penetrate through a standardized thickness of a given material (usually aluminum) depending on kVp." The quality or penetrating power of the x-ray beam is measured by its **half-value layer.** The standard that is set by the federal government states that if the x-ray machine has a maximum of 69 or less kVp, 50% of the x-ray output must pass through at least 1.5 mm of aluminum; if the machine delivers 70 or more kVp, then 50% of the output must pass through at least 2.5 mm of aluminum. The HVL specification is indicated on the label of every x-ray machine. To test HVL, the operator simply places discs of 1.5 or 2.5 mm of aluminum above a pocket dosimeter (Fig. 8.5). The x-ray machine is set at its maximum kVp setting. The operator then compares output readings in mR with and without the aluminum discs in place. The position of the BID, dosimeter, or any machine settings should not be varied. The readings should be checked to see if the penetrating power of the x-ray machine meets the federal standard. For example, if the machine is set at 65 kVp and the reading without the aluminum is 200 mR, then at least 100 mR of x-radiation must penetrate through the aluminum when 1.5 mm of aluminum is placed between the end of the BID and dosimeter. If the machine fails this test, it must be serviced.

Checking the Accuracy of the kVp Setting The purpose of checking the kVp is to determine the accuracy of the kVp setting on the machine. This procedure of checking

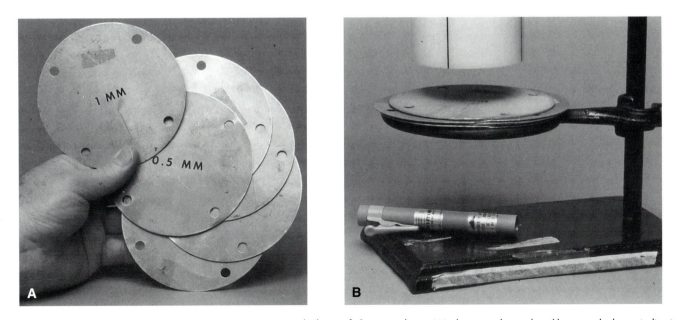

Figure 8.5. Checking the Half-Value Layer of the Beam. (**A**) Various thickness of aluminum sheets. (**B**) Aluminum sheets placed between the beam indicating device (BID) and pocket dosimeter.

the kVp can also be used to visibly demonstrate kVp measurement. It should be remembered that kVp is responsible for wavelength and frequency. If the x-ray machine fails the HVL test, it will require servicing. This is because the quality of the radiation beam is below the federal standard, and the kVp or high-voltage circuit must be checked; kVp inaccuracy and a disturbance in the kVp circuit is the usual cause. A kVp meter (Fig. 8.6) is used to check the kVp or higher-voltage circuit. Some machines have a single preset kVp indicated on the machine label; others have a kVp selector dial, and kVp settings can be adjusted or changed. The machine is set at any kVp setting or the maximum kVp setting and aimed at the target area on the kVp meter. The exposure time should be long enough for the kVp meter to obtain a reading (1 second or 60 impulses). The kVp meter measures the wavelength and frequency of the beam of radiation and gives an accurate read-out of the actual kVp, regardless of the setting of the machine. The measured kVp should be the same as the machine setting. If it is different, the problem is identified as being associated with the machine itself, not the external power supply to the dental office.

Checking the Focal Spot The purpose of checking the focal spot is to evaluate the surface area of the focal spot (target) that becomes pitted over time and enlarges. This procedure can also be used to visibly demonstrate differences in image quality relating to focal spot size. How can a focal spot enlarge over time? One can think of the following example to answer this question. When the focal

spot is new, its surface is smooth like a newly paved roadway. Over time, the focal spot is bombarded by electrons at high speed that results in pitting on its surface, much like a roadway develops potholes. A newly paved road will hold only a thin film of water when wet; a roadway full of potholes will hold much more water. This is because the road's surface area has increased by virtue of all the potholes. So it is with the pits on the surface of the focal spot.

An enlarged focal spot decreases definition (sharpness) and increases magnification. Focal spot size can be checked with relative ease by using a test object containing a number of bar patterns to test the resolution of the image. A small focal spot size provides sharpness that is measured by resolution. Resolution is the ability to visibly separate (or resolve) images of small objects placed close together. It was previously stated that one should be able to distinctly see the periodontal ligament space, lamina dura, and individual trabeculae in the image. When an x-ray machine is new, the target is relatively small, and the eye can separate or resolve about 11 or 12 line pairs per millimeter. However, as the focal spot degrades, the resolution gets down to seven or less line pairs per millimeter, and the image gets fuzzy or unsharp.

Focal Spot Checker The focal spot checker is a relatively simple, inexpensive device consisting of a 6-inch plastic cylinder, which has paired slots in a wafer of lead that are closer and closer together on one end; the other end is open (Fig. 8.7). The slots allow radiation to pass through and expose a film. The open end of this cylinder is centered on a piece of occlusal film, and an exposure is made by placing the end of the BID against the closed end of the cylinder. Because the object (lead wafer test object) is so far (6 inches) from the film, any degradation of the focal spot will show up in the processed radiograph. Excellent resolution is 11 or 12 line pairs; poor resolution is 7 or less line pairs. When the resolution is poor, the focal spot will need to be replaced by rebuilding the tubehead or purchasing a new machine.

Checking the Collimation of the X-Ray Beam

The purpose of checking the collimator is to ensure proper collimation (reduction of size) of the beam. This procedure can also be used to visibly demonstrate the divergent nature of the x-ray beam. The collimator eliminates the peripheral (more divergent) portion of the x-ray beam. What is the function of the collimator? The following example can be used to answer this question. Some better-quality metal flashlights have a focusing ring near the lens of the light. When the ring is turned one way, the beam of light spreads out; when the ring is turned in the opposite way, the beam of light becomes smaller or more focused. According to federal standards, the beam

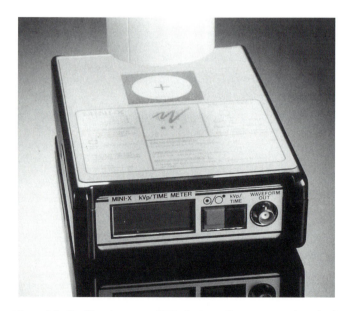

Figure 8.6. Checking Accuracy of kVp Setting. kVp meter used to check kVp setting accuracy; the BID is aimed at the target area on top of the device. This kvp meter also measures exposure time to check the timer switch.

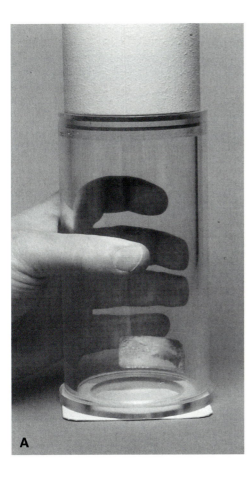

Figure 8.7. Checking Focal Spot. (A) Test arrangement for measuring focal spot size. **(B)** Test pattern on top of focal spot test tool. **(C)** Test films using the focal spot test tool: (1) long cone (BID) and (2) short cone (BID). Note the better resolution and less magnification with the long cone (1).

of radiation must be collimated (focused) to 2.75 inches at the tip of the BID. Any machine failing to comply is considered **illegal.**

Collimation Test To test collimation, the operator simply places the end of the BID of the x-ray machine against a rare earth fluorescent screen or a loaded panoramic cassette (Fig. 8.8). The exposure time is set at about 1 or 2 seconds. The lights in the room are then turned off. The operator looks through the leaded barrier window to see if the fluorescence is limited to the diameter of the BID; he or she could also process the panoramic film to see if the exposed area of the film is limited to the diameter of the BID. Collimation may also be verified by radiographing four no. 2 dental films placed on a piece of paper in the form of a cross-shaped template. The cone (BID) and the location of each film should be traced on

the paper, and the films should be identified with lead numbers or small puncture holes in the film packet made with a pin, so each can be returned to its proper place after exposure. The BID is positioned to cover approximately half of each film packet and to touch the packets. The films are exposed using half the maximum anterior exposure, are processed, and are returned to the proper order (Fig. 8.8). If the exposed area is greater than 2.75 inches in diameter, the lead collimator opening is too large. In some machines, radiation escapes to expose more tissue than the diameter of the BID. Rarely, the beam of radiation will not be centered on the open end of the BID due to faulty positioning of the collimator. When this is the case, unavoidable cone cuts will be the consistent, frustrating problem. Adjusting the collimator by tapping it into place or replacing the cone solves the problem.

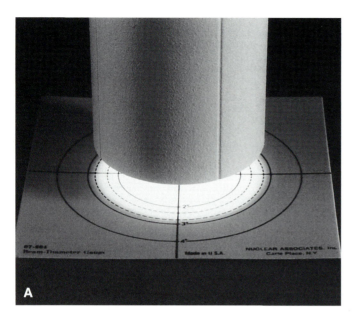

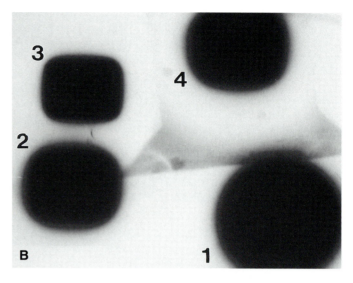

Diameter of Exposed Area
≤ 7 Centimeters or 2.75 Inches

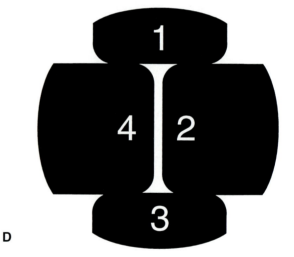

Figure 8.8. Verification of Collimation. (**A**) Collimator checker using a rare earth fluorescent screen. (**B**) Four different collimators checked by exposing a single panoramic film: (1) short round BID; (2) long round BID; (3) long rectangular BID; (4) leakage of radiation from tubehead. (**C**) Arrangement of film for testing collimator. (**D**) The measured diameter of the exposed films should be 7.0 cm, or 2.75 inches, or less.

TESTING THE DARKROOM

The darkroom is tested for the following two factors: fog and processing quality. Fog can be checked monthly, whereas processing quality is a daily check.

Detecting Fog in the Darkroom

Fog consists of unwanted exposed silver halide crystals. This is usually caused by excessive light that degrades the

diagnostic value of the image. A fog check procedure can be used to visibly demonstrate fog (unwanted density) on film and the sources of fog in the darkroom. What does fog look like in an image? The following example can be used to answer this question. On a clear day, one can see for miles; on a foggy day, one may be able to see only a few feet ahead. When driving, fog can obscure a road hazard and endanger lives. Fog from excessive white light in the darkroom obscures the image created by the x-rays. However, unlike a foggy day, film fog is sometimes difficult to see on the radiograph without a proper viewing procedure. First, the darkroom should be inspected for visible white light leaks. The operator can do this by standing in the darkroom with all the lights off, including the safelight(s), for several minutes until his or her eyes become accustomed to the dark. The operator can then look around doors, windows, and at the edges of ceiling tiles. Any white light leaks should be marked and blocked. Processing equipment, radios, or similar devices may be emitting unsafe and unwanted light; these should be checked for glowing lights. Second, the safelight should be tested for causing fog.

Safelight Test One of the tests for a safelight is the coin test (Fig. 8.9). The operator takes the fastest intraoral film in the office (see Chapter 6) and exposes it to approximately 3 impulses of radiation, or 1/20 of a second, or he or she makes an image of a test object like a skull. An exposed radiograph is more sensitive to fog than an unexposed film. The operator then enters the darkroom. On the workbench near the safelight, he or she removes the film from the film packet and places a coin over the center of the film. The film and coin should be left beneath the safelight for varying periods up to about 15 minutes; each film is then processed. As soon as an outline of the coin becomes visible, this is the time beyond which the safelight will not be safe. Most safelights are safe for 5 to 8 minutes. If panoramic or cephalometric film is used in the office, it must be remembered that screen film is faster than intraoral (nonscreen) film and is more subject to fog. A box of panoramic or cephalometric film should be placed on the counter top under the safelight. A film is removed from the box, which is then closed. The panoramic film is then placed under the box. The operator

should then pull out approximately 1 inch of film every minute. After 5 to 8 minutes, a line of darker density will be seen for every minute. The number of inches from the edge of the film to where the first line of density appears is the number of minutes the safelight is safe. Most GBX-2 safelight filters designed for use with panoramic or cephalometric films are safe for 5 to 8 minutes if the wattage of the bulb is 15 or 7.5, the distance from the counter top is no less than 4 feet, and the safelight filter is not cracked or damaged.

Checking the Automatic X-Ray Processor/ Manual Processing Solutions

The purpose of checking processing solutions is to determine the proper freshness of developer solution and developer temperature. This procedure can also be used to visibly demonstrate how a depleted and/or a cold developer solution can result in unacceptable low density (light) films. This is a very common problem. The automatic x-ray processor should be checked daily. The usual problem, more than all others, is depleted developer or cold developer solution due to failure of the heating element or its control. In manual processing, the developer solution becomes depleted with use or by contamination with fixer during wet reading, or there is a failure of the water temperature regulator valve.

Step-Wedge Test The simplest way to check processing is to take a supply of reference films using a step-wedge under the best conditions of exposure and processing. An inexpensive aluminum step-wedge can be purchased or one can be made with varying thicknesses (1, 3, and 6) of lead foil from the film packets (Fig. 8.10). The properly exposed and processed reference films should be stored in the refrigerator. All reference films should be taken from the same box of film using the same x-ray machine and exposure factors. When the solutions are fresh, a baseline film is processed and placed on an illuminator for future daily comparisons. Every day, one of the preexposed reference films is run through the processor or processed manually to see if the density (overall darkness of the image) and contrast (number of visible steps of the wedge) remain constant compared with the baseline film on the illuminator. If not, the solutions should be replenished or changed. The developer solution should be replenished after 4 full-mouth surveys, 4 panoramic films, or 80 intraoral films. Four to six ounces of fresh developer should be added, depending on the size of the tanks or the manufacturer's instructions. Fixer can be replenished at the same time; however, only 2 to 3 ounces of fixer will be needed, as fixer lasts twice as long as developer. If the problem persists, the temperature of the developer solution should be checked. All manual processors require temperature-controlled solutions, usually at 70°F; in auto-

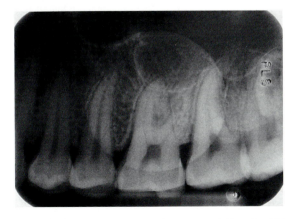

Figure 8.9. Safelight Coin Test. Several preexposed films should be unwrapped and placed on the counter top under the safelight. A coin is placed on top of the unwrapped films. A film is processed every 2 minutes. The interval of time required for the outline of the coin to be seen is the time the safelight is safe.

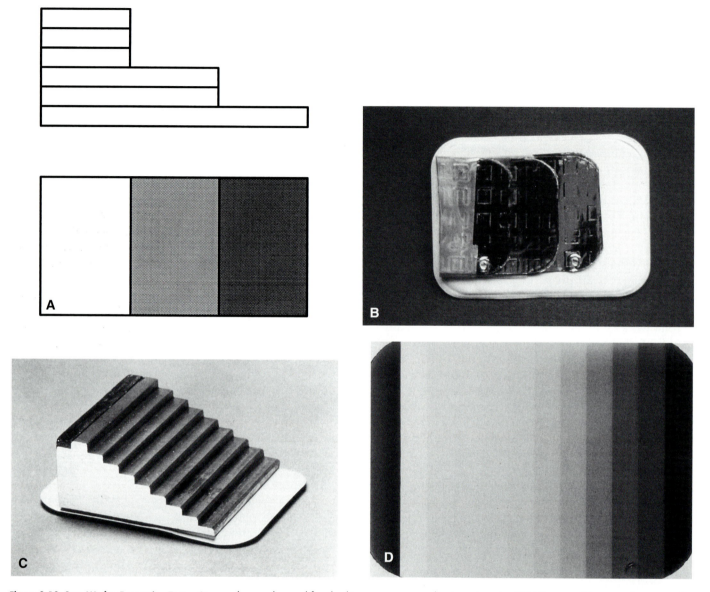

Figure 8.10. Step-Wedge Processing Test. Step-wedge can be used for checking processors and mAs reciprocity. **(A)** Diagram of homemade step-wedge using lead foil and resulting image. **(B)** Lead foil step-wedge. **(C)** Aluminum step-wedge placed on no. 2 film. **(D)** Image of aluminum step-wedge.

matic processors, the developer should be approximately 83°F. Therefore, daily temperature readings of the developer solution should be taken in the morning after the solutions have had a chance to heat up (usually 30 minutes). In manual processing, this can be done with a special floating thermometer that is easily obtainable from a dental supply house or aquarium store. For automatic processors, an inexpensive thermometer for checking automobile air conditioning can be obtained.

Sensitometer and Densitometer Test The purpose of checking processing with the sensitometer and densitometer is to more accurately identify and quantify fog, density

changes, and contrast changes. This procedure can also be used to visibly demonstrate fog and the difference between density and contrast. The goal is to detect processing problems early, before the image is visibly affected. The sensitometer and densitometer (Fig. 8.11) are devices recommended for use in Stage III dental practices. The sensitometer produces three standardized exposures on an x-ray film by light, and then the film is processed. The densitometer measures one of the exposed areas for **density**, the difference between the lightest and darkest exposures for **contrast**, and any other area of the film emulsion (not exposed by the sensitometer) for **fog**.

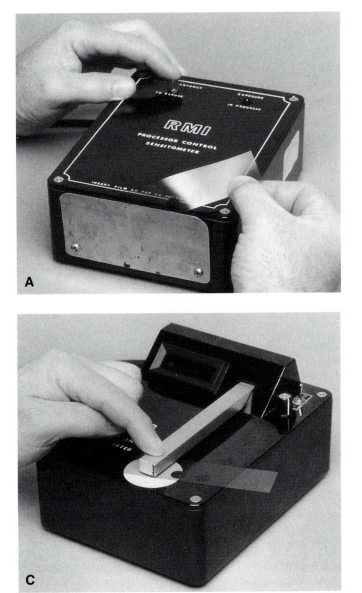

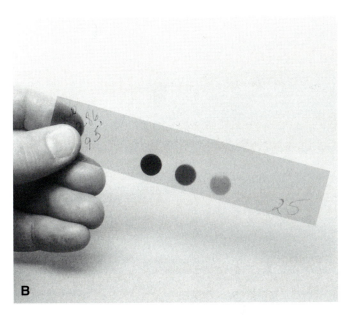

Figure 8.11. Sensitometer and Densitometer. (**A**) Sensitometer and film strip slot. (**B**) Sensitometer exposes x-ray film to a highly reproducible pattern of different light intensities. (**C**) The densitometer measures optical density by using a light source and a photo cell to measure transmitted light.

SIMPLE QUALITY CONTROL DEVICE TO TEST THE X-RAY UNIT AND PROCESSING IN STAGES I AND II DENTAL PRACTICES

A simple and inexpensive method of testing both the x-ray equipment and processing is to use a special reference film produced under ideal conditions of exposure and processing. To achieve this, a dental quality control device called the Dental Radiographic Normalizing and Monitoring Device (Dental Radiographic Devices, Silver Spring, MD) (Fig. 8.12) or the Dental Quality Control Test Tool (Nuclear Associates) can be used to expose reference films that are stored in the refrigerator. The exposure instructions are on the devices. One of the preex-

posed reference films should be developed as a baseline. The density of this baseline film should be compared against one of the numbered film densities provided on a sliding strip in the quality control device (Fig. 8.12). The density step number (each step is numbered) on the sliding strip that matches the baseline reference film density will now be the standard density number for future comparison. The quality control device (Fig. 8.12) should be used to periodically expose monitor films to check radiographic technique. If after processing the monitor film there is a difference of two or more steps between the current monitor film density and the baseline film standard density number previously determined, there is a problem with either the processing technique or the x-ray equipment/

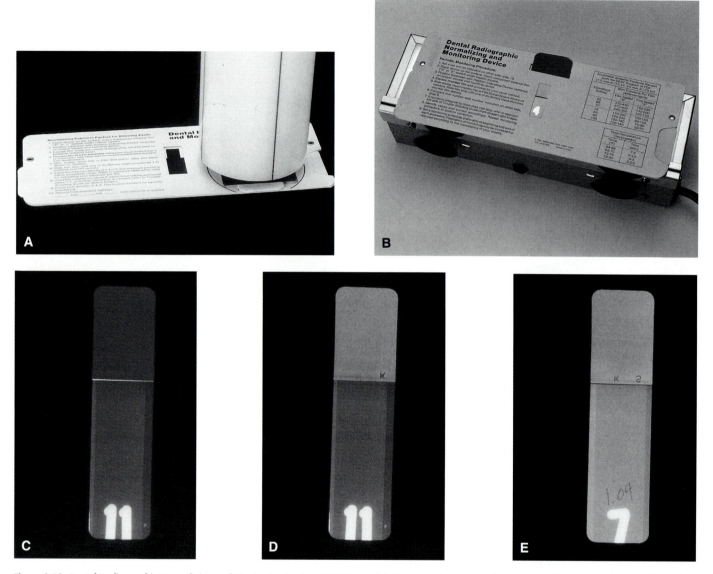

Figure 8.12. Dental Radiographic Normalizing and Monitoring Device. (**A**) Front of device gives instructions for exposing the monitor film. (**B**) The back of the device contains a slot into which the processed film is inserted and matched with the density strip. (**C**) Baseline monitor film measures 11 on the density strip. (**D**) Several days later, a newly exposed monitor film does not match the baseline reading (11). (**E**) By moving the density strip, a new match is found; a problem exists if the density of the monitor film changes by two or more units.

exposure technique. At this point, a previously exposed reference film should be taken from the refrigerator and developed. If the reference film is also off the same number of steps from the standard density number, the problem is in the processing technique. Such a problem is probably in the processing chemistry, because the reference films were previously exposed correctly using the quality control device. If the reference film matches within two steps, the problem is most likely with the x-ray equipment or the exposure technique. However, at this point more specific tests, as previously discussed, will be necessary to trouble-

shoot the x-ray equipment and/or the exposure technique for the specific problem.

OTHER QUALITY CONTROL ITEMS

The office should maintain a common error and retake log so that personnel can be retrained with reference to correcting actual problems. Leaded aprons and thyroid shields, cassettes, and viewboxes should be inspected periodically to ensure proper functioning. Exposure charts should be posted in the vicinity of the x-ray control panel.

Proper settings for varying anatomic areas, bitewings, and film speed (D and/or E+) should be displayed, and stored film should be checked to see if the expiration date has passed. A quality assurance log should be maintained. This log should record the frequency of procedures, results, and any necessary corrective actions.

Benefits of Quality Assurance

The implementation of a quality assurance program will lead to improved diagnostic performance and a substantial savings in cost. Every retake doubles the radiation exposure to the patient, is an additional expense, and wastes valuable time. Quality assurance procedures have been shown to lower the level of radiation to which the patient is exposed by decreasing the number of retakes and by preventing overexposure of the patient in an attempt to compensate for processing deficiencies (increasing exposure time due to low-density films). A well-run quality assurance program also serves to enhance our understanding of many of the concepts in quality image production. Remember the old adage, "What the mind does not know, the eye cannot see."

LEGAL ASPECTS OF DENTAL RADIOGRAPHY

OWNERSHIP OF THE X-RAYS

When the patient pays for a set of radiographs, he or she is paying for the dentist's ability to interpret the radiographs and arrive at a diagnostic opinion based on radiographic and clinical findings. X-rays are a part of the dentist's records and do not rightfully belong to the patient. One of the most important decisions by a higher court concerning ownership of radiographs was handed down by the Supreme Court of Michigan in 1935 (*McGarry vs J. A. Mercier Co.*). In this case, the plaintiff was a physician who was employed by a construction company (J. A. Mercier Co.) to treat their employees in case of injury on the job. J. A. Mercier had refused to pay the physician for services rendered to one of their employees, because the physician failed to deliver to them radiographs taken of the employee during treatment. The court ruled in favor of the physician, stating that the radiographs were the legal property of the physician. The court further declared that, "It is a matter of common knowledge that x-ray negatives are practically meaningless to the ordinary layman. But the retention by the physician or surgeon constitutes an important part of the clinical record in the particular case, and in the aggregate these films may embody and preserve much of value incident to a physician's or surgeon's experience."

CARE IN BILLING

If the radiographs are billed separately from the diagnosis and treatment, the dentist may run the risk that the court may render a verdict in favor of the patient, saying the patient owns the radiographs because they were paid for separately. Thus, radiographs should always be included in services rendered for diagnosis and treatment when billing a patient. A separate charge for radiographs should not be itemized.

PRECAUTIONS IN LOANING RADIOGRAPHS

The dentist should never give radiographs to the patient. The dentist should realize that the radiograph is the greatest protection against a possible claim of negligence. It can be devastating when a dentist is sued for malpractice and the radiographs that would have proved competency have been misplaced or lost.

There are times when the dentist may want to lend the patient's radiographs to another dentist for viewing. When lending radiographs to another dentist, the following suggestions are given:

1. The second dentist should request the radiographs in writing. This letter should be placed in the patient's folder.
2. The original radiographs should be duplicated, and the duplicate set sent by registered or certified mail.
3. Original radiographs should not be sent to the requesting dentist, unless he or she promises in writing to send back original radiographs within 1 week after they have been duplicated. Although the patient may move to another city, the dentist is not legally bound to send the patient's radiographs to a second dentist. The radiographs are still the dentist's legal property. This is a case in which duplicate radiographs are useful. Alternately, an image of the radiographs can be sent by teleradiography, much like a fax.
4. A copy of the cover letter sent with the radiographs and the postal receipt should be kept in the patient's folder.
5. The patient's records should be kept for at least 6 years.

LIABILITY ARISING OUT OF FAILURE TO USE RADIOGRAPHS

The dentist must use professional judgment as to whether taking radiographs should be used as a diagnostic procedure. Certainly, there are instances when radiographs are not necessary to render a diagnosis. However, one of the most common causes for malpractice suits is the failure of the dentist to use radiographs in the diagnosis or in the management of cases involving pain, swelling, or infection.

Consider this case cited by Sarner (1963). A dentist in Kentucky refused to expose a radiograph of a patient's jaws when there was a question as to whether he had left a root tip in the patient's jaws after an extraction. The patient visited a second dentist, who found a root tip in the jaws by means of a radiograph. It is now considered a dental principle that a dentist who fails to expose a radiograph in some circumstances is guilty of malpractice (*Agnew vs City of Los Angeles*, 97 Cal. App. 557, 218 p. 2d 66, 1950). Therefore, if there is any doubt in the mind of the dentist if radiographs should be exposed, then radiographs should be taken. The use of radiographs has been so embedded in the minds of the public that a jury in most cases will find the dentist negligent if there is failure to use x-rays. There are times when a patient will refuse radiographs for some reason. In such a situation, Miller (1970) suggests two alternative procedures for the dentist to take to minimize a malpractice suit.

---

1. The refusal should be recorded in the patient's record, and the patient should sign it.
2. The dentist should offer to take the radiographs at no charge for his or her records.

Either of these procedures would lessen the possibility of a malpractice suit against the dentist for failure to use radiographs. In either instance, the dentist should strongly consider not treating the patient if the patient refuses to have the radiographs taken.

RADIOGRAPHS AS EVIDENCE

In a court of law, one must remember that the best evidence is that which is factual. Radiographs are factual evidence. Of course, the radiographs must be of good diagnostic quality, as they reflect the competency of the dentist. Radiographs of inferior quality should be retaken for two reasons (Miller, 1970):

---

1. These radiographs will be of no use as evidence.
2. They will reflect on the dentist's ability as a practitioner and could cause irreparable harm to the dentist's reputation.

If a dentist retains radiographs of inferior quality in patients' records, they will only prove incompetency if produced as evidence in court. There is no substitute for good radiographs.

WORKSHOP/LABORATORY EXERCISES

EXERCISE 8.1. CHECKING FOR TIMER FAILURE

Materials and Equipment Needed

1. Step-wedge.
2. X-ray machine and processor.
3. Two no. 2 intraoral films.

Instructions

Step 1: Make a step-wedge from film packet lead foil as follows:
1. Cut out a piece of cardboard exactly the size and shape of a no. 2 intraoral film.
2. Using clear tape, **affix one thickness** of lead foil 3 mm from the edge of the cardboard.
3. Follow this with **three thicknesses** 6 mm from the edge, **six thicknesses 9 mm** from the edge, and so on.
4. Trim the extra lead foil at the other end of the cardboard template.

Step 2: Expose reference film using a standardized exposure such as 65 or 70 kVp, 7 or 10 mA, and 20 impulses (1/3 second). (Place the step-wedge on top of the plain side of the film.)

Step 3: Simulate timer failure by taking a shorter exposure of 10 impulses (1/6 second).

Step 4: Process reference film and compare it with the test film.

EXERCISE 8.2. CHECKING FOR DARKROOM FOG

Materials and Equipment Needed

1. Step-wedge.
2. Darkroom and safelight.
3. Coin.
4. One no. 2 intraoral film.

Instructions

Step 1: Expose a reference film as in Step 2 of the previous exercise.

Step 2: Enter the darkroom.

Step 3: Unwrap the preexposed reference film and place it on the counter top beneath the safelight.

Step 4: Place a coin on top of the film.

Step 5: Leave this in place for 15 minutes; process the film.

Step 6: Observe the fogged areas where the coin could not protect the film from fog.

EXERCISE 8.3. CHECKING FOR DEVELOPER SOLUTION FAILURE

Materials and Equipment Needed

1. Two no. 2 intraoral films.
2. Processor(s) or manual processing facility.

Instructions

Step 1: Expose two reference films as in Step 2 of the first exercise.

Step 2: Process one of the preexposed reference films.

Step 3: After the remainder of the class has completed Step 1, now simulate developer solution depletion by diluting it with water (6 to 12 ounces).

Step 4: Process the second reference film.

Step 5: Observe the light or low-density image caused by the depleted developer.

Note: A similar effect can be observed by placing ice cubes in the developer solution. The cold and diluted solution produces a light film.

CASE-BASED PROBLEM-SOLVING

1. You have intraoral radiographs that consistently turn out lighter than expected. You realize there is a problem. List as many causes for a light or low-density image that you can. Any kind of exposure, processing, or other problem you can think of are fair game! Good luck!

2. Design a quality assurance program for a facility that takes less than 100 periapical films per week. The facility uses only intraoral film and manual processing.

REVIEW QUESTIONS

1. In evaluating the timer of a self-rectified x-ray machine, 25 separate densities (dots) were produced by use of a spinning top; the exposure time was set for 0.5 seconds. Does the timer meet the evaluation criteria?

   A. Yes, the reading is 5% off the set time.
   B. No, the reading is 5 dots off the set time.
   C. Yes, the reading is the same as the set time.
   D. No, the reading is 10 dots off the set time.

2. Which x-ray field diameter is acceptable if the source to skin distance is 16 in or more?

   A. 2.60 inches.
   B. 2.75 inches.
   C. 2.50 inches.
   D. Only two of the above.
   E. All of the above.

3. Which parameters should be inspected if a film monitoring strip differs by more than two steps from the standard?

   1. Temperature regulating system.
   2. Rate of replenishment.
   3. Exposure conditions.
   4. Integrity of solutions.
   A. 1, 2, and 3 only.
   B. 2, 3, and 4 only.
   C. 2, 3, and 4 only.
   D. 1, 2, 3, and 4.

4. Which of the following is **not** considered an advantage of keeping a retake log?

   A. Provides clues for the source of most retakes.
   B. Serves as a guide for continuing education topics.
   C. Provides some measure of the operator's competence.
   D. Reduces the amount of paperwork.

5. The half-value layer test is used to evaluate which of the following:

   A. Filtration.
   B. Collimation.
   C. kVp.
   D. mA.
   E. Beam alignment.

6. When using a radiographic normalizing and monitoring device, there is a difference of two or more steps noted for a monitoring film when compared with a baseline density number determined previously under ideal conditions. What should you do?

   1. Take a preexisting reference film from the refrigerator and develop it.
   2. Take a reference film from the refrigerator, expose it with standard exposure factors, and develop it.
   3. If the reference film matches within two steps, the problem is most likely a processing problem.
   4. If the reference film matches within two steps, the problem is most likely in the x-ray equipment or technique.
   5. If the reference film does not match within two steps, the problem is a processing problem.
   A. 1 and 3.
   B. 1 and 5.
   C. 2 and 5.
   D. 2 and 4.
   E. 2 and 3.

7. Which of the following are true statements regarding the legal aspects of dental radiography?

   1. The patient's radiographs rightfully belong to the patient.
   2. The patient's radiographs are legal property of the dentist.
   3. The dentist should not give original radiographs to the patient.
   4. Radiographs should always be taken before and after each tooth extraction.
   5. One of the most common causes of dental malpractice suits is the use of radiographs by the dentist when they are not necessary to render a diagnosis.
   A. 2, 4, and 5.
   B. 1 and 5.
   C. 2, 3, and 5.
   D. 1 and 4.
   E. 2 and 3.

8. A patient is moving to another city. He stops by your dental office before leaving and asks you for the radiographs that you took previously. What is the correct method to handle this situation?

   A. Give the radiographs to the patient. After all, they legally belong to the patient because the patient paid for them.
   B. Give the radiographs to the patient and tell the patient to give them to his dentist in the other city.
   C. Tell the patient he cannot have the radiographs because the radiographs legally belong to the dentist.
   D. Tell the patient that after he has found a new dentist in the other city, the new dentist should send a written request for the radiographs.

9. To perform the coin test for darkroom fog:

   A. Use the slowest film available.
   B. Use an exposed film.
   C. Turn off the safelight.
   D. Use a panoramic or cephalometric film if only intraoral radiographs are taken.

10. Before performing the coin test for safelight fog, you should:

    A. Eliminate all sources of extraneous white light.
    B. Be certain all extraneous sources of white light are "on."
    C. Avoid checking safelight bulb wattage, filter, and distance until later.
    D. B and C only.

11. When two mA settings, such as 10 and 15 mA, are available on a machine, these circuits are checked by:

    A. mAs Reciprocity.
    B. mA Meter (ammeter).
    C. Multiplying the output at 10 mA by 1.5.
    D. A professional technician, as this cannot be done in the office.

BIBLIOGRAPHY

American Association of Physicists in Medicine. Basic quality control in diagnostic radiology. AAPM report no. 3. AAPM, 1978.

Beideman RW, Johnson ON, Alcox, RW. A study to develop a rating system and evaluate dental radiographs submitted to a third party carrier. J Am Dent Assoc 1976;93:1010–1013.

Bureau of Radiological Health. Diagnostic radiology quality assurance catalog. HEW publication (FDA) 77-8028. Rockville, MD: US Department of Health, Education and Welfare, July 1977.

Bureau of Radiological Health. Quality assurance programs for diagnostic radiology facilities, final recommendations. Fed Reg 1979; 44:71728–78740.

Bushong SC. Radiologic science for the technologists. 5th ed. St. Louis: CV Mosby, 1993.

Council on Dental Materials, Instruments and Equipment. Recommendations on radiographic practices: an update, 1988. J Am Dent Assoc 1989;118:115–117.

Gould RG, Gratt BM. A radiographic quality control system for the dental office. Dentomaxillofac Radiol 1982;11:123–127.

Gray JE, Winkler NT, Stears J, et al. Quality control in diagnostic imaging. Baltimore: University Park Press, 1983.

Miller SC. Legal aspects of dentistry: a programmed course in dental jurisprudence. New York: Putnam, 1970.

National Council on Radiation Protection and Measurements. Quality assurance for diagnostic imaging equipment. Report no. 99, Bethesda, MD: NCRPM, 1988.

New Mexico radiation protection regulations. Santa Fe: New Mexico Health and Environment Department (Environmental Improvement Division), 1989.

Platin E, Matteson SR. Quality assurance for dental imaging. Rochester, NY: Eastman Kodak, 1992.

Quality control tests for dental radiography. September 1992 revision. Rochester, NY: Dental Products, Health Sciences Division, Eastman Kodak, 1992.

Sarner H. Dental jurisprudence, Philadelphia: WB Saunders, 1963.

Texas regulations for control of radiation. 1995 revision. Austin: Texas Department of Health, Bureau of Radiation Control, 1989.

SECTION 3:

Special Imaging Techniques

Concepts of Panoramic Radiography

9

OBJECTIVES

Upon successful completion of this unit, the student will be able to:

1. *Relate the basic principles of panoramic image formation.*

2. *Explain the concept of image layer analysis.*

3. *List the seven concepts of panoramic image formation.*

4. *Relate the importance of the seven concepts in recognizing a technically good panoramic image.*

5. *Identify technique-related panoramic anatomic landmarks.*

6. *Test his or her knowledge by answering the Review Questions.*

KEY WORDS/PHRASES

air space	focal layer	layer formation
anatomical structures	focal trough	real images
beam movement patterns	ghost images	single images
double images	horizontal projection	soft tissue
flattening of structures	image layer analysis	vertical projection

INTRODUCTION

A basic understanding of the principles underlying rotational panoramic radiography is necessary for the optimum use of the technique. This chapter examines the process by which the image is formed and the characteristics of the panoramic radiograph that result from this unique process of image formation. The use of the bitewing and periapical radiographs as a diagnostic aid is a major component of this book. However, periapical and bitewing radiographs are somewhat limited in their overall coverage of the mandibulofacial structures. By using panoramic radiography, many of these limitations can be overcome. In panoramic radiology, the dose to the patient is approximately 10 times less than the full-mouth survey using the long, round cone and E+ film; it is 4 times less

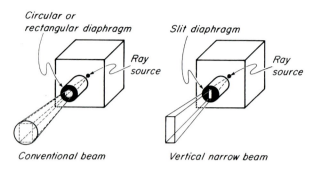

Figure 9.1. Narrow Beam in Panoramic Radiography. A narrow vertical beam is used in rotational panoramic radiography.

than 4 bitewings using the long, round cone and E+ film. The panoramic dose is about equal to that of four bitewings using the long, rectangular cone and E+ film. There are many advantages of panoramic radiography.

Some of the advantages of panoramic radiology are:

1. Increased overall coverage of the dental arches and associated structures.
2. Production of relatively undistorted anatomical images.
3. Significantly reduced radiation dosage to the patient.
4. Simplicity and rapidity of the procedure.
5. Reduced superimposition of anatomical structures.
6. Minimal infection control procedures.
7. Possibility of detecting caries, periodontal disease, and pulp-associated periapical changes earlier and with better reliability in predicting disease.

PRINCIPLES OF PANORAMIC RADIOGRAPHY

Rotational panoramic radiography is accomplished by rotating a narrow beam of radiation in the *horizontal plane* around an invisible rotational axis that is positioned intraorally. In rotational panoramic radiography, a vertical narrow x-ray beam is used compared with the much larger circular or rectangular x-ray beams used in conventional intraoral radiography (Fig. 9.1).

PROJECTION IN THE VERTICAL PLANE

The vertical dimension of the panoramic image is unaffected by the horizontal rotation of the beam, because the vertical dimension of the panoramic image is the result of a conventional radiographic projection. Therefore, the **focal spot in the x-ray tube anode** serves as the functional focal spot for the vertical aspect or dimension of the projection (Fig. 9.2). There is a slight negative angulation of the beam so the x-ray beam will pass beneath the occipital portion (base) of skull. This angle is −4° to −7°.

PROJECTION IN THE HORIZONTAL PLANE

The horizontal dimension of the panoramic image is affected by the horizontal rotation of the beam. Therefore, in the horizontal dimension, the x-rays appear to diverge from an **intraoral source** although they really originate outside the patient at the focal spot of the x-ray tube. This apparent intraoral x-ray source is called the **center of rotation** and is, therefore, called the "effective focal

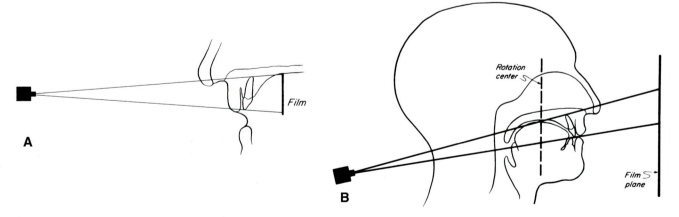

Figure 9.2. Principle of Projection in the Vertical Dimension. (**A**) The conventional projection of an intraoral radiograph is a central projection. In a central projection, the divergent rays have a common origin at a focal spot. The film is perpendicular to the central ray. (**B**) The projection geometry in the vertical plane in rotational panoramic radiography.

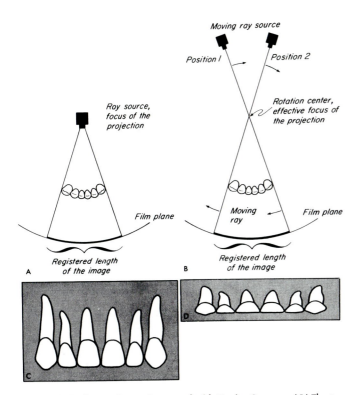

Figure 9.3. Stationary Source Compared with Moving Source. (**A**) The true central projection that results from the use of an intraoral x-ray source. (**B**) A rotating ray will create a true central projection in the rotation plane. The effective focus is at the rotation center. (**C**) With an intraoral x-ray source, the ratio between the focus-to-film and focus-to-object distances is such that the magnification will be uniformly marked in all planes. (**D**) Compare the magnification when a rotating beam projects the object onto a stationary film. It will be equal in the rotation plane but different in the vertical plane.

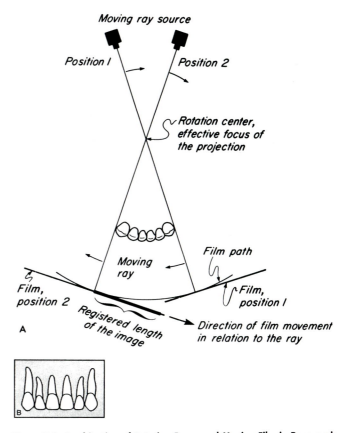

Figure 9.4. Combination of Rotating Beam and Moving Film in Panoramic Radiography. (**A**) The combination of a rotating beam and a moving film changes the horizontal dimensions of the recorded image, but the projection of the object remains the same. (**B**) The resulting image in the rotational panoramic system has its proportions restored.

spot of the projection" for the **horizontal** dimension of the x-ray image (Fig. 9.3).

PRINCIPLE OF IMAGE LAYER FORMATION

If this rotating narrow beam were used to project the object onto a stationary film, the magnification in the horizontal dimension would always be greater than that in the vertical dimension (Fig. 9.3). The discrepancy in horizontal versus vertical magnification can be eliminated by using a moving film to equalize the magnification in the horizontal dimension (Fig. 9.4). The film moves in a direction opposite to the horizontal rotation of the beam.

In some cases, the movement of the film is accomplished by placing the film on a circular drum, which moves by rotating on its own axis. In other cases, the film is placed in a moving flat cassette. By adjusting the speed of the film in respect to projection of the beam, it is possible to

reduce the horizontal magnification to match the vertical magnification. The vertical and horizontal dimensions match only when the object lies within a particular plane called the central plane, or sharply depicted plane of the image layer. Objects outside this sharply depicted plane but still within the image layer will always be somewhat distorted in shape and will appear unsharp or fuzzy.

IMAGE LAYER OR FOCAL TROUGH

The image layer, often referred as the focal trough, is a zone in an object defined as containing those object points depicted with sufficient detail to be distinguished.

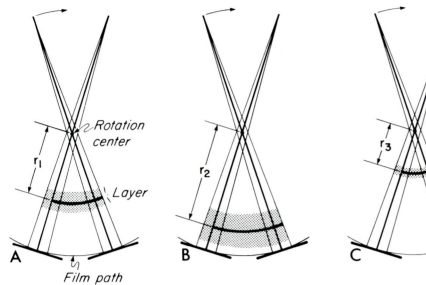

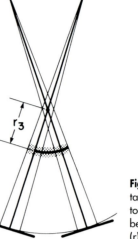

Figure 9.5. Width of Image Layer. The distance from the rotation center of the beam to the central plane of the image layer has been called the effective projection radius (r). The longer the radius, the thicker the layer. Note image layer thicknesses among **A**, **B**, and **C** compared with r1, r2, and r3.

WIDTH OF THE IMAGE LAYER

The width of the image layer is dependent on two important factors:

1. The image layer is directly related to the **distance** from the center of rotation to the central plane of the image, which is called the "effective projection radius." The width of the layer depends on the length of the radius (Fig. 9.5). The longer the radius, the thicker the layer.
2. The layer thickness is inversely proportional to the width of the long, narrow slit beam. The narrower the x-ray beam, the wider the image layer (Fig. 9.1).

Position of Image Layer or Focal Trough

Acceleration of the **film speed** shifts the image layer away from the rotation center, and a wider image layer results (Fig. 9.6A). By decelerating the film speed, the image layer shifts closer to the rotation center and becomes narrower (Fig. 9.6B). In this way, the image layer is shaped to center the jaws and nearby structures within its boundaries. In so doing, the anterior part of the layer is unavoidably narrower than the posterior part of the layer.

Movement Pattern of the X-Ray Beam

The movement pattern of the x-ray beam is chosen to obtain a favorable projection of the jaws. The most popular mechanical movement patterns are those that use a continuously moving rotation center. The x-ray beam is given a sliding movement throughout the total excursion so that the effective projection center or functional focus,

called the "effective center of rotation," is continuously shifted along a defined path. The central ray of the beam is always tangential to a defined curved path of the rotation center at any point (Fig. 9.7). The form of the defined curved path dictates the direction of the x-ray beam (because it is always tangential to the defined curved path) and hence defines the projection of each successive part of the jaws. This results in a continuous radiographic image.

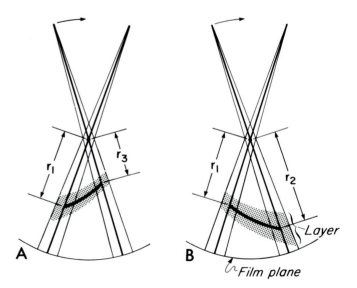

Figure 9.6. Position of Image Layer. The position of the layer depends on the film speed. (**A**) If the speed of the film is increased, the position of the image layer shifts away from the rotation center. (**B**) If the speed of the film is decreased, the position of the image layer shifts toward the rotation center. (Note the simultaneous change in layer thickness.)

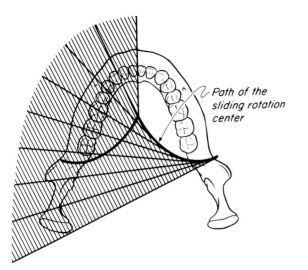

Figure 9.7. Movement Pattern of the X-Ray Beam. The movement pattern of the rotation center is chosen to obtain a favorable projection of the object. The most popular mechanical movement patterns are those that use a continuously sliding rotation center, as shown here. The form of the defined curved path dictates the direction of the x-ray beam, because it is always tangential (touching at a point) to a defined curved path. This results in a continuous radiographic image.

IMAGE LAYER ANALYSIS

Even in a correctly positioned patient, objects that are buccal or toward the film will be narrowed, and objects that are lingual or toward the source will be widened. Additionally, because of the negative projection angle of the beam, buccal objects will be projected lower and lingual objects will be projected higher than objects in the central plane of the layer. For example, if a mandibular premolar has erupted lingually or has been pushed lingually by a tumor, it will be wider than the opposite premolar and higher up in the image than the adjacent teeth in the arch. Conversely, a buccal object, such as the mental foramen in the mandible, would be narrowed and projected downward with respect to another object in the middle of the layer. Also, if a patient is positioned too far forward, the anterior teeth will be narrowed; if a patient is positioned too far back, the anterior teeth will be widened. Overall, objects in the center of the layer are magnified 20 to 30%.

CONCEPTS OF NORMAL PANORAMIC ANATOMY

INTRODUCTION

Certain peculiarities of the panoramic system result in a unique projection of many anatomical structures in the image. This produces several unusual anatomical relationships in the panoramic image that are not found in any other kind of radiographic projection. We have developed a conceptual approach to understanding the panoramic image and have found that most peculiarities of normal structural relationships can be explained by one or more of the following seven concepts.

Concept 1: Structures Are Flattened and Spread-Out

In panoramic radiography, the patient remains stationary as the x-ray tube and film cassette-holder both rotate around the patient during the exposure cycle. The cassette holder has a protective leaded front, and the film is exposed through a long narrow slit opening in the leaded front of the cassette holder. The film that is inside the cassette moves across the narrow slit opening as the x-ray tube rotates. The radiographic image is "laid out" as the film in the cassette passes the slit opening, in the same way that paint is applied to a wall with a roller. The resultant radiograph is a **flattened image of a curved surface**. In the panoramic radiograph, the jaws and structures of the maxillofacial complex as well as the spine are portrayed as if they were split vertically in half down the midsagittal plane with each half folded outward, such that the nose remains in the middle, the right and left sides of the jaws are on each side of the film, and the spine (having been split in half) appears beyond the rami at the extreme right and left edges of the film (Fig. 9.8A). This is much like opening a book with the narrow part of the binding facing the reader; when opened, the front and back covers can be seen.

One of the undesirable effects of the panoramic technique is that if the patient is positioned improperly in the machine, certain structures will also be flattened and spread-out although they normally would not be. For example, when the patient's chin is tipped too low, the hyoid bone is spread-out and projected across the mandible. In the same way, the inferior turbinates and meati of the nose are spread-out and projected across the maxillary sinus when the patient is positioned too far back. This is undesirable, as the image of these flattened and spread-out structures obscures other structures that need to be seen (Fig. 9.8B). To explain why these undesirable effects occur, one needs to understand the **second concept**.

Concept 2: Midline Structures May Project as Single Images or Double Images

In this concept, we refer to the formation of "real" images, as opposed to "ghost" images. Further, we have subdivided **real images** into **single** and **double real images**. We will consider ghost images in the next concept.

Real Image Formation A real, single image is formed when the anatomical structure (object) is located between

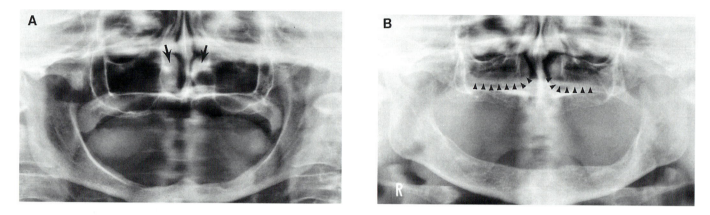

Figure 9.8. Concept 1. Structures Are Flattened and Spread-Out. (**A**) Correct projection of nasal turbinates (arrows) within nasal fossa. (**B**) Nasal turbinates are spread-out across the maxillary sinus due to a patient positioning error (arrowheads).

the rotation center of the beam and the film; that is to say, the object is in front of the rotation center (Fig. 9.9). The anatomical regions where real images are formed are shown in Figure 9.10.

Double real image formation occurs in the central portion of the oral and maxillofacial region in a diamond-shaped zone where objects are intercepted **twice** by the beam (Fig. 9.10).

Double images have the following five characteristics:

1. One image is the mirror image of the other.
2. Both images are real images.
3. Each image will have the same proportions.
4. Each image will have the same location on the opposite side.
5. Double images only occur with midline objects falling in the diamond-shaped zone in the midline.

The diamond-shaped region (Fig. 9.10, shaded pattern) corresponds to the patient's midline from about the middle of the image to the most posterior extent of the radiograph. A double real image is a pair of real images formed by an object lying within this zone. An example of a double real image is shown in Figure 9.11. Here, a single radiopaque tube inserted in the nasal passage appears in two locations (double real images) on the panoramic radiograph. The structural configuration of such double real images may be understood by examining the sequence in which the beam intersects an object during its projection onto the film. Figure 9.12 shows the formation of the double real image of two adjacent points A and B. In the formation of the first image, the beam first intercepts A and then B. On the opposite side of the scan, B is intercepted before A. The result is that double real images are reversed with respect to one another. That is to say, double images are mirror images of each other.

Some examples of structures that normally produce double real images are the **hard and soft palate, palatal torus, body of the hyoid bone, epiglottis,** and **cervical**

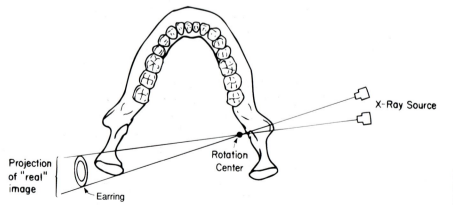

Projection of "real" image

Earring

Rotation Center

X-Ray Source

Figure 9.9. Concept 2. Real Images. Formation of the real image of an earring. The earring is located between the rotation center of the beam and the film.

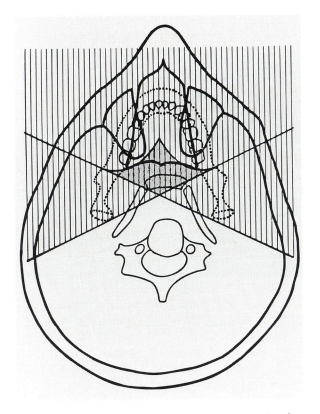

Figure 9.10. Concept 2. Region Where Real Images Are Formed. The zone where real images are formed when a continuous movement pattern is used (vertical hatch marks). Double images are formed in the central diamond-shaped region (shaded area).

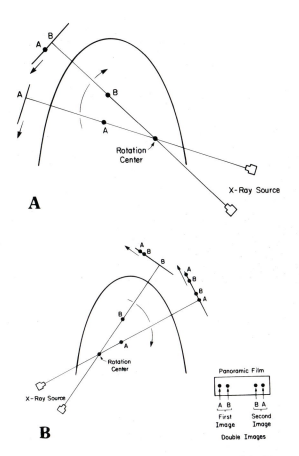

Figure 9.12. Concept 2. Double Real Images. Formation of double images of points *A* and *B*. (**A**) Formation of the first image. (**B**) Formation of the second image.

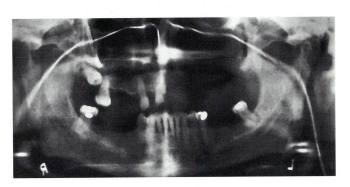

Figure 9.11. Concept 2. Double Real Images. Double image of a single radiopaque tube inserted into the right nasal passage. When tube passes through the central diamond-shaped region, as depicted in Figure 9.10, double real images are formed.

spine (Fig. 9.13). Only midline structures located in the diamond-shaped area can do this. When the patient is malpositioned, the **turbinates of the nose, body of the hyoid, and spine** enter into this diamond-shaped area and produce undesirable double images. However, these undesirable double images help to identify patient positioning errors (see Chapter 10).

Concept 3: Ghost Images Are Formed

A ghost image is formed when the object is located between the x-ray source and the center of rotation (Fig. 9.14). That is to say, anatomically the object is behind the rotation center. The radiograph in Figure 9.16 shows two ghost images of two earrings. Each ghost image corresponds to the earring on the opposite side. The regions satisfying the preceding requirement for the formation of ghost images are shown in Figure 9.15. Structures situated within this region can appear as ghosts (phantoms), whereas structures situated elsewhere cannot.

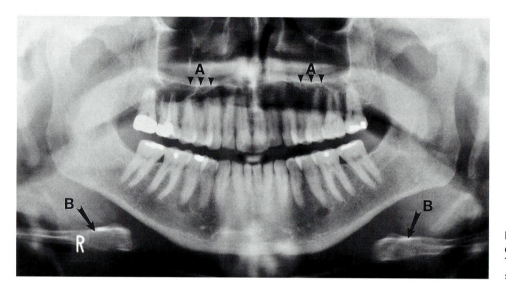

Figure 9.13. Concept 2. Double Real Images. Hard palate (**A**). Hyoid bone (**B**). These structures fall in the diamond-shaped area.

Ghost images have the following six characteristics (Fig. 9.16):

1. The ghost image has the same general shape as its real counterpart (no mirror image formation).
2. The ghost image appears on the opposite side of the radiograph from its real counterpart.
3. The ghost image appears higher up on the radiograph than its real counterpart.
4. The ghost image is more blurred than its real counterpart.
5. The vertical component of a ghost image is more blurred than the horizontal component.
6. The vertical component of a ghost image is always larger than its real counterpart, whereas the horizontal component of a ghost image may or may not be severely magnified.

To understand the differences among the first three concepts, study Figure 9.17, which is a composite diagram showing the zones giving rise to single and double real images and ghost images. Note that two areas in the horizontal plane contain structural details that project only

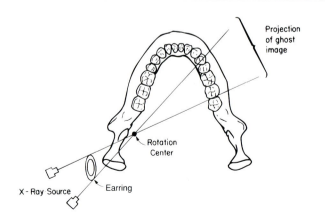

Figure 9.14. Concept 3. Formation of Ghost Images. Formation of the ghost image of an earring. The earring is now located between the x-ray source and the center of rotation. Compare with Figures 9.7 and 9.9.

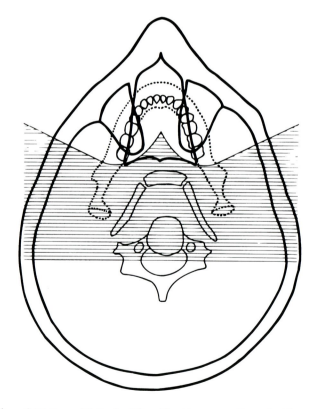

Figure 9.15. Concept 3. Region Where Ghost Images are Formed. The anatomical region where ghost images are formed is marked by horizontal hatch marks and lies behind the rotation center.

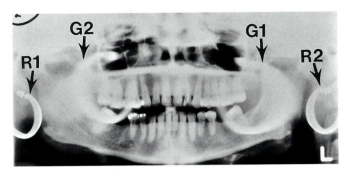

Figure 9.16. Concept 3. Ghost Image Characteristics. *(R1)* Real image of earring. *(G1)* Corresponding ghost image of earring *(R1)*. *(R2)* Real image of earring *(G2)*. Corresponding ghost image of earring *(R2)*. Check ghost image *G1* and *G2* for the six characteristics of ghost images.

real or ghost images, as the case may be. This diagram depicts the properly positioned patient. Where only vertical hatch marks are seen, structures such as the body of the mandible, the teeth, and the antrum (maxillary sinuses) may only produce real images. In the area of the horizontal hatch marks, the spine, neck chains, and horns of the hyoid usually produce only ghost images. The projection geometry of most panoramic machines is such that these ghost-only images are not usually projected onto the film, i.e., they are not seen in an image of a properly positioned patient. In the area where both vertical and horizontal hatch marks are seen, both single real and ghost images of the structures included therein may be produced in the same image. These include the greater horns of the hyoid bone, ramus/condyle of the mandible, earrings, necklaces,

and coat zippers. In the diamond-shaped area, double real and ghost images may be produced. Examples include the body of the hyoid bone and the posterior aspect of the hard palate (Fig. 9.22). Generally, the presence of ghost images are the result of technique errors. Some include ghost images of earrings, necklaces, spine (Fig. 9.23), and rami of the mandible. Recognition of these undesirable ghost images helps to identify and eliminate technique errors.

Concept 4: Soft Tissue Shadows Are Seen

One of the unique advantages of panoramic radiography is that some soft tissue structures attenuate the beam of radiation to a sufficient degree to become visible in the radiograph (Fig. 9.18). This is especially true in the posterior and superior regions, where there are no teeth, and in all regions of edentulous patients. Fluids and cartilaginous tissues such as the ear, nose, and epiglottis are also included in this concept. Other soft tissues include soft palate and uvula, dorsum of the tongue, posterior pharyngeal wall, palatine tonsil, lips, nasolabial fold, and the soft tissues of the nasal turbinates and septum. Additionally, the gingiva, retromolar pad, and operculum of erupting teeth may be seen. Although some soft tissue shadows are normally seen, visualization of the tongue, ears, nose, and nasal turbinates spread-out are an indication of technique errors.

Concept 5: Air Spaces Are Seen

Because areas containing air do not attenuate the x-ray beam as much as soft or hard tissues, air spaces

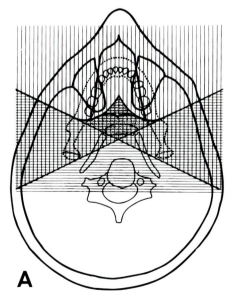

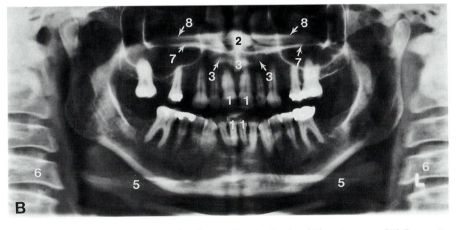

Figure 9.17. Concepts 2 and 3. Composite Diagram Showing Real and Ghost Images. **(A)** Composite diagram showing the zones giving rise to real (single and double) and ghost images in continuous image machines. The zones are marked as in the previous figures. **(B)** Panoramic radiograph depicts structures within these zones mentioned in **A**. Real single images of central incisors (*1*), real single image of nasal septum (*2*), real single image of soft tissue outline of nose (*3*), double real image of hyoid bone (*5*), double real image of spine (*6*), double real images of palate (*7*), and ghost images of palate (*8*).

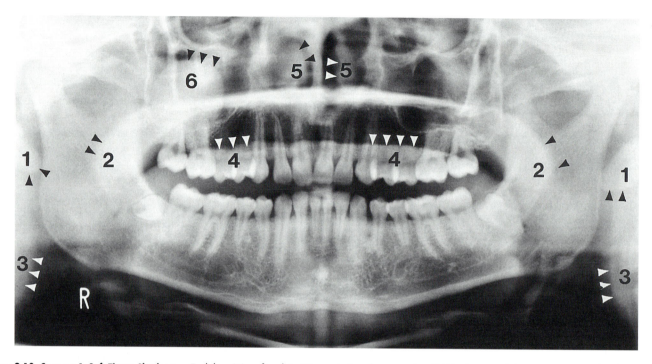

Figure 9.18. Concept 4. Soft Tissue Shadows. Earlobes (*1*), soft palate (*2*), posterior pharyngeal wall (*3*), dorsum of the tongue (*4*), and turbinates (*5*). All these structures can be seen bilaterally. Also note mucous retention cyst in maxillary sinus (*6*).

usually appear black (Fig. 9.19). Some of the air spaces that may be seen include those of the hypopharynx (laryngopharynx), oropharynx, and nasopharynx; the maxillary sinus; and the nasal fossa (meati). These air spaces are normal components of the panoramic image. If an air space is noted above the dorsum of the tongue or in association with the anterior teeth, an error in technique has occurred. Undesirable air spaces help to identify technique errors.

Concept 6: Relative Radiolucencies and Radiopacities Are Seen

In any image, it is important to separate shadows originating from parts of the machine from those coming from the patient. Machine components seen in the image are made of plastic, have a density similar to that of soft tissue, and are usually easy to identify because of their geometric or linear configuration. One may think of the patient as being made of three basic components: hard tissue (teeth and bone), soft tissue (including cartilage and fluid), and air. All these machine and patient components may produce single and/or double real images and/or ghost images. Thus, multiple areas consisting of **relative density changes** are produced (Fig. 9.20).

To understand and separate multiple density changes, the following should be remembered (Fig. 9.21):

1. Air obscures hard tissues.
2. Soft tissue obscures air.
3. Hard tissue obscures soft tissue.
4. Ghost images obscure everything.

This concept ties the previous five together and can allow the dental health-care practitioner to use the panoramic radiograph in a meaningful way to detect disease and to troubleshoot errors. If a pathologic process is present, it will consist of hard tissue, soft tissue, or fluid. In addition, it will affect one or more of the three tissue components in the patient as follows. Conditions producing hard tissue cause all three patient components to become relatively more radiopaque in the region of the disorder. A soft tissue pathologic condition within the mineralized component causes it to become more radiolucent, whereas the soft tissue and air components become more radiopaque when a soft tissue disorder is present. Thus, when a soft tissue lesion encroaches on an air space,

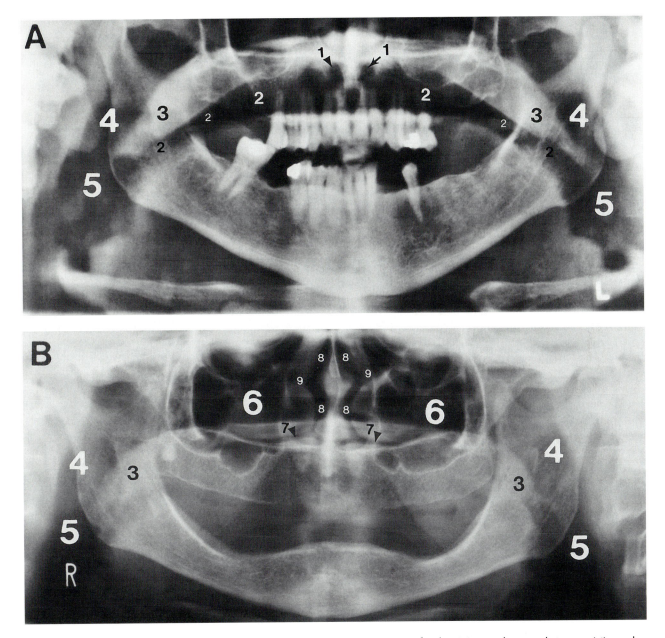

Figure 9.19. Concept 5. Air Spaces. (**A** and **B**) Nares of nose (*1*), glossopalatine air space (*2*), soft palate (*3*), nasopharyngeal air space (*4*), oropharyngeal air space (*5*), maxillary sinus (antrum) (*6*), inferior meatus (*7*), common meatus (*8*), and middle meatus (*9*).

such as the nasopharynx or maxillary sinus, it becomes visible as an opacity superimposed on the air space. When errors are present, further relative radiolucencies and opacities may also appear and affect the three tissue types in the same way. The recognition of these is essential to identify and correct operator errors. Pathology or the absence thereof should only be interpreted from a properly exposed and processed panoramic radiograph.

Concept 7: Panoramic Radiographs Are Unique

The scope of assessment and interpretive potential from panoramic radiographs in many ways exceeds that of the full-mouth intraoral survey. In the study of teeth, angular interrelationships of structures are accurate in panoramic radiographs. Therefore, the relationships of teeth with each other and with other structures may be studied in treatment planning, such as crown and bridge abutment

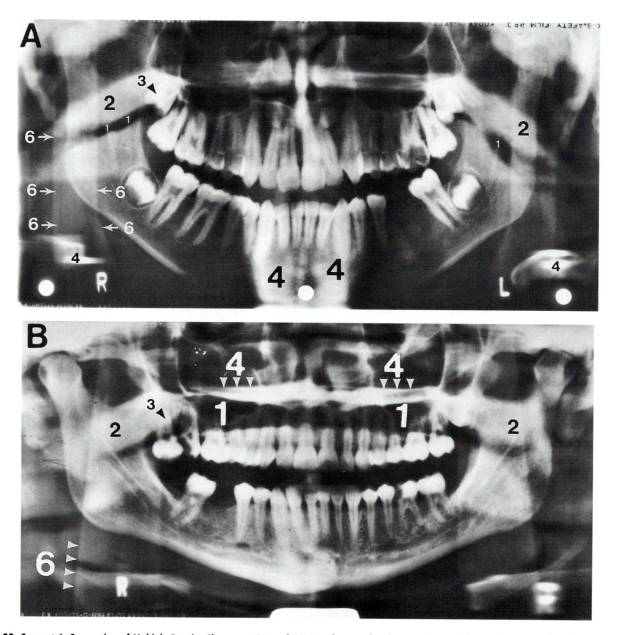

Figure 9.20. Concept 6. Separation of Multiple Density Changes. (**A** and **B**) Air obscures hard tissues (ramus) (*1*), soft tissue (soft palate) obscures air (pharyngeal air space) (*2*), hard tissue (tooth) obscures soft tissue (soft palate) (*3*), ghost images (*R* and *L* markers, spinal column, and hard palate) obscure everything (hyoid bone, mandible, and maxillary sinus) (*4*), external machine components such as the side guides produce relative density changes as shown here (*6*).

tooth parallelism, the path of insertion of partial dentures, the orthodontic tipping of teeth, and the surgical removal of impacted teeth. Because each intraoral film is taken individually, these interrelationships cannot always be studied accurately using full-mouth intraoral surveys. Areas such as the ramus, styloid process, temporomandibular joint, upper portions of the sinus, and tissues below the jaws all give rise to pathologic conditions that are not visualized in intraoral radiographs. The panoramic

radiograph is an excellent imaging modality in patients with trismus or trauma, because such patients cannot open their mouths and this is not needed to take a panoramic film. The uniqueness of the panoramic technique is that it results in an excellent projection of a variety of structures on a single film, which no other imaging system can achieve. Individual structures may be imaged by other methods, once pathologic conditions have been detected using the panoramic radiograph.

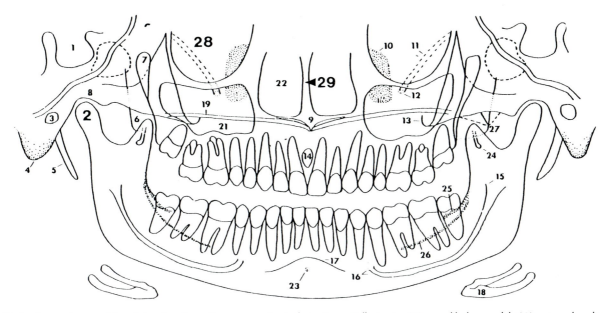

Figure 9.21. Continuous Image of Atomic Landmarks. Common anatomical structures. Sella turcica (*1*), mandibular condyle (*2*), external auditory meatus (*3*), mastoid process (*4*), styloid process (*5*), lateral pterygoid plate (*6*), pterygomaxillary fissure (*7*), articular eminence (*8*), anterior nasal spine (*9*), ethmoid sinuses (*10*), infraorbital canal (*11*), infraorbital foramen (*12*), zygomatic process of the maxilla (*13*), incisive or nasopalatine foramen (*14*), mandibular foramen (*15*), mandibular canal and mental foramen (*16*), mental ridge (*17*), hyoid bone (*18*), hard palate (*19*), maxillary sinus (*21*), nasal fossa (*22*), genial tubercles (*23*), hamular process (*24*), external oblique ridge (*25*), internal oblique or mylohyoid ridge (*26*), zygomatic arch (*27*), orbit (*28*), and nasal septum (*29*).

ATLAS OF ANATOMICAL STRUCTURES

The remainder of this chapter is presented in outline form. The reader should first try to learn the basic bony landmarks needed for technique troubleshooting, then learn the others. It will be impossible to see all anatomical structures on a single panoramic radiograph. It will take various panoramic radiographs to show complete and detailed bony landmarks (Figs. 9.21 and 9.22).

WORKSHOP/LABORATORY EXERCISES

EXERCISE 9.1. PANORAMIC ANATOMY

Materials and Equipment Needed

1. A panoramic radiograph of a patient.
2. Orthodontic tracing sheets and pencil.
3. Viewbox.

Instructions

Trace and use numbered arrows (to the best of your ability) to identify the following key anatomical structures. Use the same numbers as listed below. Some of these structures may not be present in every panoramic radiograph.

1. Mandibular condyles
2. Ramus of mandible
3. Cervical spine
4. Maxillary sinus
5. Nasal fossa
6. Inferior turbinate
7. Real image(s) of hard palate
8. Ghost image(s) of hard palate
9. Soft palate
10. Inferior cortex of the mandible
11. Inferior alveolar canal
12. Mental foramen
13. Hyoid bone
14. Tongue
15. Nasopharyngeal and pharyngeal air spaces

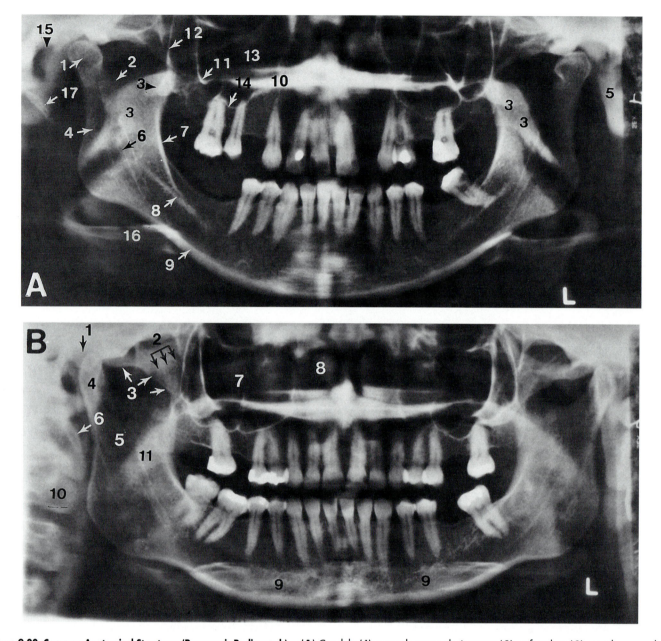

Figure 9.22. Common Anatomical Structures (Panoramic Radiograph). **(A)** Condyle (1), nasopharyngeal air space (2), soft palate (3), oropharyngeal air space (4), soft tissue of ear (5), glossopalatal air space (6), external oblique ridge (7), mylohyoid (internal oblique) ridge (8), lower border of mandible (9), hard palate (10), lower border of zygomatic (malar) bone (11), posterior wall of maxillary sinus (12), maxillary sinus (antrum) (13), lower border (floor) of maxillary sinus (14), external auditory meatus (15), hyoid bone (16), and stylohyoid process (17). **(B)** glenoid fossa (1), nasopharyngeal air space (2), zygomatic arch (3), condyle (4), oropharyngeal air space (5), stylohyoid process (6), maxillary sinus (7), inferior turbinate (8), ghost of hyoid bone (9), and spinal column (10).

NOTE TO INSTRUCTORS:

The authors will supply reasonable numbers of panoramic radiographs of patients for student reuse. Alternatively, specially labeled panoramic radiographs are also available on a very low cost-recovery basis. Please call (210) 567-3340 or fax (210) 567-3334.

REVIEW QUESTIONS

1. In panoramic radiography, the thickness of the image layer increases with:

   1. Widening of the collimator slit.
   2. Narrowing of the collimator slit.
   3. Increased distance between the center of rotation and the layer.
   4. Decreased distance between the center of rotation and the layer.
   A. 1 and 3.
   B. 1 and 4.
   C. 2 and 3.
   D. 2 and 4.

2. In panoramic radiography, the image layer is narrowest in the:

   A. Incisor region.
   B. Premolar region.
   C. Molar region.
   D. Ramus region.

3. In panoramic radiography, when an object is on the buccal or film side of the layer, the image is:

   A. Projected upward and widened.
   B. Projected upward and narrowed.
   C. Projected downward and widened.
   D. Projected downward and narrowed.

4. In panoramic radiography, when an object is on the lingual or tubehead side of the layer, the image is:

   A. Projected upward and widened.
   B. Projected upward and narrowed.
   C. Projected downward and widened.
   D. Projected downward and narrowed.

5. In panoramic radiography, the effective focal spot is:

   A. At the target of the x-ray tube.
   B. At a tangent to the center of rotation.
   C. The center of rotation at any given point.
   D. Within the diamond-shaped area.

6. In panoramic radiography, the central ray of the beam is:

   A. At the target of the x-ray tube.
   B. At a tangent to the center of rotation.

C. The center of rotation at any given point.
D. Within the diamond-shaped area.

7. In panoramic radiography, the radiation dose to the patient is the same as four bitewings with E+ speed film and the:

   A. Long round cone (BID).
   B. Long rectangular cone (BID).
   C. Short round cone (BID).
   D. Short pointed cone (BID).

8. In panoramic radiography, ghost images are produced when structures:

   A. Lie in front of the rotation center.
   B. Fall in the rotation center.
   C. Lie behind the rotation center.
   D. Do not produce real images.

9. If in panoramic radiography the width of the image layer is large:

   A. Patient positioning is more critical.
   B. Patient positioning is less critical.
   C. Objects in the middle of the layer are sharper.
   D. Patient positioning can be compensated by image sharpness.

CASE-BASED QUESTIONS

CASE 9.1

One concept of panoramic radiography is that structures are flattened and spread-out (like taking a horseshoe and straightening it out). In some cases—such as for the mandible, maxilla, and maxillary sinuses—this is desirable because it avoids the superimposition of right- and left-sided structures on top of one another.

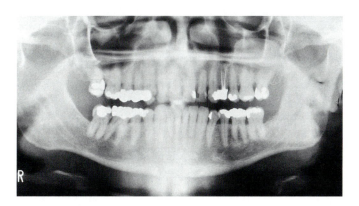

Questions

1. This patient is malpositioned in the machine, and one structure is flattened and spread-out that should **not** be flattened and spread-out. If you recognize this feature, you will know which positioning error has occurred (see Chapter 10). The structure inappropriately flattened and spread-out is the:
   A. Hyoid bone.
   B. Nasal turbinate.
   C. Hard palate.
   D. Occlusal plane.

2. Another concept learned in Chapter 9 is that soft tissues obscure air spaces. Which of the following statements is correct?
   A. When the turbinate is spread-out, it obscures the air space in the upper half of the sinus.
   B. When a mucous retention cyst is seen in an air space (such as the maxillary sinus [left side]), it is because body fluids, like soft tissues, obscure the air space.
   C. A and B.
   D. None of the above.

CASE 9.2

One concept of panoramic radiography is that air can obscure mineralized structures such as teeth and bone. This can occur as a result of the patient malpositioning the tongue.

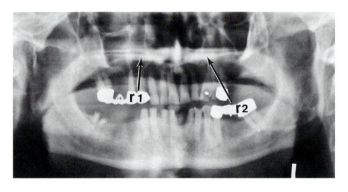

Questions

With respect to an air space located on this panoramic image, indicate which statements are true or false.

1. _____ The air between the dorsum of the tongue and hard palate obscures the root and apical regions of the maxillary teeth.

2. _____ The air of the nasopharynx and oropharynx obscures portions of the ramus bilaterally.

3. _____ The air in the maxillary sinuses is **not** obscured by the turbinates.

Another concept learned is how structures located within the diamond-shaped area can produce **both** double real images and ghost images. Even in a well-positioned patient, this phenomenon is seen with the hard palate. In this case, the two **real images** of the hard palate have been labeled r1 and r2. With respect to images of structures falling in the diamond-shaped area, which statements are true or false?

4. _____ r2 is the mirror image of r1.

5. _____ The ghost image of r1 is the radiopaque line immediately above r1.

6. _____ The ghost image of r2 is the radiopaque line immediately above r1.

7. _____ There are two real (double) images of the hard palate.

8. _____ There are four ghost images of the hard palate.

9. _____ Sometimes only the real images of the hard palate are seen.

10. _____ Air spaces obscure bone or teeth; however, a ghost image of a tooth or bone (this case hard palate) can obscure air.

CASE 9.3

One concept of panoramic radiography is that soft tissues can be seen in the panoramic image, especially cartilaginous tissues or soft tissues at the edge of or within an air space. The recognition of these can be used to identify positioning errors.

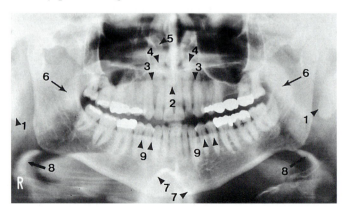

Questions

With respect to the following features seen in this case, indicate which statements are true or false.

1. _____ The ears can be seen bilaterally and indicate an error in patient positioning.

2. _____ The double image of the epiglottis can be seen bilaterally and indicates an error in patient positioning.

3. _____ The nose can be seen in the midline and indicates an error in patient positioning.

4. _____ The soft palate be seen bilaterally and indicates an error in patient positioning.

5. _____ The outline of the dorsum of the tongue can be seen and indicates an error in patient positioning.

6. _____ Mandibular tori can be seen bilaterally and indicate an error in patient positioning.

7. _____ The ghost image of a neck chain can be seen in the midline and indicates an error in patient positioning.

8. _____ The turbinate is spread-out across the upper part of the right maxillary sinus only and indicates an error in patient positioning.

9. _____ The black lines on the lower left second molar are caused by static electricity.

10. _____ This is a good panoramic radiograph.

We have asked you questions about various structures in this image. Now be certain you were looking at the right thing by matching the numbered arrow(s) in Column A with the correct choice in Column B.

Column A		Column B
Arrows 1	_____	A. Ala of nose
Arrow 2	_____	B. Soft palate
Arrows 3	_____	C. Ears
Arrows 4	_____	D. Dorsum of tongue
Arrow 5	_____	E. Epiglottis
Arrows 6	_____	F. Turbinate
Arrows 7	_____	G. Neck chain ghosts
Arrows 8	_____	H. Tip of nose
Arrows 9	_____	I. Mandibular tori

CASE 9.4

This patient was observed to have a round, oval-shaped nodule in the right tonsillar fossa.

Question

1. This soft tissue mass obscures the air space at the:
   A. Mesial of the second molar.
   B. Angle of the mandible.
   C. Midramus area.
   D. Patient's midline.

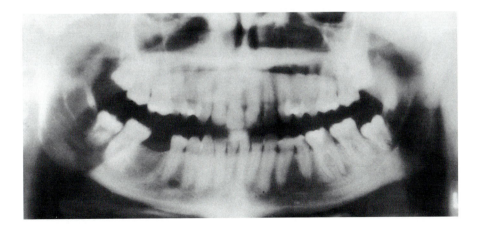

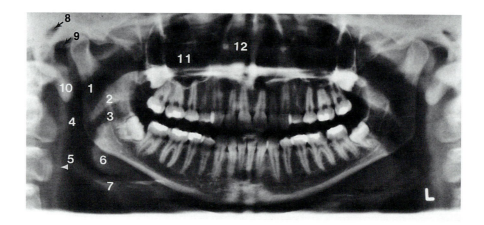

CASE 9.5

Match the numbered anatomical features in Column A with correct answer in Column B.

Column A	Column B
1. _____	A. Internal auditory meatus
2. _____	B. Glossopalatal air space
3. _____	C. Nasal fossa
4. _____	D. Posterior wall of pharynx
5. _____	E. Maxillary sinus
6. _____	F. Nasopharyngeal air space
7. _____	G. Earlobe
8. _____	H. Base of tongue
9. _____	I. Oropharyngeal air space
10. _____	J. Hyoid bone
11. _____	K. External auditory meatus
12. _____	L. Soft palate

BIBLIOGRAPHY

Chiles JL, Gores RJ. Anatomic interpretation of the orthopantomogram. Oral Surg 1973;35:564–570.

Higashi T, Iguchi M. "Ghost images" in panoramic radiograph. Oral Surg 1983;55:221–226.

Katayama H, Ohba T, Ogawa Y. Panoramic innominate line and related roentgen anatomy of the facial bones. Oral Surg 1974;37:131–134.

Knight N. Anatomic structures as visualized on the Panorex radiograph. Oral Surg 1968;26:326–330.

Knight N. Reverse images and ghost of Panorex radiography. J Am Soc Prev Dent 1973;3:53–56.

Langlais RP, Miles DA, Van Dis ML. Elongated and mineralized stylohyoid ligament complex: a proposed classification and report of a case of Eagle's syndrome. Oral Surg 1986;61:527–533.

Langland OE, Sippy FH. Anatomic structures as visualized on the orthopantomogram. Oral Surg 1968;26:475–480.

Langland OE, Sippy FH, Langlais RP. Textbook of dental radiology. 2nd ed. Springfield: Charles C. Thomas, 1985:367–379.

McDavid WD, Langlais RP, Welander U, et al. Real, double and ghost images in rotational panoramic radiography. Dentomaxillofac Radiol 1983;12:122–131.

McDavid WD, Tronje G, Welander U, et al. Imaging characteristics of seven panoramic x-ray units. Dentomaxillofac Radiol 1985; (Suppl 8) 13:1–86.

Nortje CJ, Farman AG, Grotepass FW. Variations in the normal anatomy of the inferior dental (mandibular) canal: a retrospective study of panoramic radiographs from 3,612 routine dental patients. Br J Oral Surg 1977;15:55–60.

O'Carroll MK. Interpretation of Panorex radiographs. J Oral Med 1971;6:86–89.

Pernkopf E. Atlas of topographical and applied human anatomy. Head and neck. Philadelphia: WB Saunders, 1963;1:123–143.

Perrelet LA, Garcia LF. The identification of anatomical structures on orthopantomographs. Dentomaxillofac Radiol 1972;1:11–115.

Smith CJ, Fleming RD. A comprehensive review of normal anatomic landmarks and artifacts as visualized on Panorex radiographs. Oral Surg 1974;37:291–295.

Turk MH, Katzemell J. Panoramic localization. Oral Surg 1970;29:212–219.

Turvey TA, Fonseca RJ. The anatomy of the internal maxillary artery in the pterygopalatine fossa: its relationship to maxillary surgery. J Oral Surg 1980;38:92–95.

Tyndall DA, Matteson SR. Zygomatic air cell defect (ZACD) on panoramic radiographs. Oral Surg 1987;64:373–377.

Updegrave WJ. The role of panoramic radiography in diagnosis. Oral Surg 1966;22:49–56.

Witcher BL, Gratt BM, Sickles EA. A leaded apron for use in panoramic dental radiography. Oral Surg 1980;49:467–471.

Troubleshooting Panoramic Techniques

10

OBJECTIVES

Upon successful completion of this unit, the student will be able to:

1. *Describe the five steps in the generic panoramic technique with mastery.*

2. *Identify panoramic patient positioning errors.*

3. *Recognize panoramic technical errors.*

4. *Test his or her knowledge by answering the Review Questions.*

KEY WORDS/PHRASES

apron	generic panoramic technique	panoramic technique errors
cassette resistance	glove artifact	prostheses
chemical stain	"home base"	split cassette
damaged screen	multiple errors	static electricity
film crimping	no identification	useful errors
fog	panoramic positioning errors	zones of the panoramic film
foreign object in cassette		

INTRODUCTION

In the normal course of events, the perfection of intraoral techniques is part of a dental health-care worker's formal education, whereas panoramic radiography is learned with varying degrees of incompetency on the job from a sales person, another staff member, and/or (heaven help us!) by reading the owner's manual. Most dental health-care workers—including dentists, hygienists, and dental assistants—have little formal training in panoramic radiography. As a result, the quality of the images is poor and the expectations from the panoramic radiograph are often low on the part of both educators and practitioners alike.

GENERIC PANORAMIC TECHNIQUE

All panoramic machines work in essentially the same manner, although they may differ in appearance. Our approach to learning this subject is to present it in conjunction with the generic panoramic technique that works for most machines. Each of the five technique steps will be carefully explained. Then the several errors, which can occur as miscues with each technique step, will be described and analyzed.

GENERAL HINTS IN PANORAMIC TECHNIQUE

Patients have varying amounts of soft tissue, hair on the tops of their heads, and facial hair that may obscure the bony landmarks. Because the hard tissues cannot be seen by the health-care worker (Fig. 10.1), advantage should be taken of positioning lights and other accessory features (such as automatic exposure) to enhance technique. The operator should be certain that wigs, prostheses, jewelry, eyewear, and napkin chains have been removed before placing the patient into the machine. With each of the five steps in the technique, one should go back over the previous step(s) to ensure that an alteration in a previous positioning step has not occurred in achieving the current step. The patient's clothing and build should be inspected to ensure that bulky clothing, short neck, and/or muscular shoulders do not interfere with the motion of the machine. A machine component, such as the biteblock or side guide, should never be removed on a

routine basis; this can only lead to poor imaging and diminished performance unintended by the manufacturer. The fastest film/screen combination should always be used to minimize patient dose; currently, the authors recommend Kodak T-mat G speed film with Kodak Lanex Regular Screens (Rochester, NY) or similar film/screen systems from other manufacturers.

OVERALL ASSESSMENT OF THE PANORAMIC FILM

Too many dental health-care workers are taught to try and identify all positioning errors by looking at the teeth. Although this is useful and encouraged, some patients are missing their anterior teeth or are edentulous, and in these cases another method to identify errors must be used. Therefore, with each error, what happens to the teeth will be described, and then several other undesirable anatomical features that can be used to identify each error will be explained. This allows the recognition of errors even when the teeth look "pretty good" and in persons who have no teeth or missing teeth. In the mind's eye, the operator should divide the panoramic radiograph into six zones (Figs. 10.2–10.5): three are in the midline and three are bilateral on each side (see pp. 228–229).

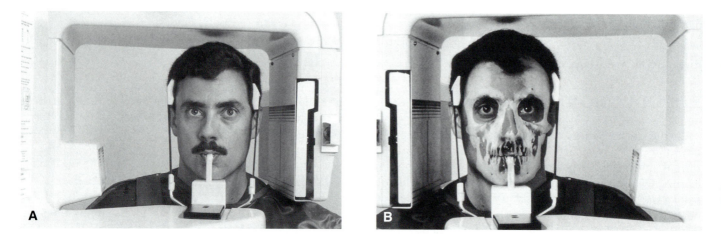

Figure 10.1. Anatomical Features in Patient Positioning.   Because we cannot see the hard tissues (as in B), we must use anatomical structures and machine devices to properly position the patient (as in A).

Zone 1: Dentition (Fig. 10.2)

The teeth should be arranged with a smile-like upward curve posteriorly and be separated from each other. This separation produces an interocclusal space in the radiograph. The anterior teeth should be neither too large or so narrow as to create "pseudospaces" between them. The posterior teeth should not be larger or smaller on one side than the other, nor should there be excessive overlap of the premolars on one side versus the other. The apices of the maxillary or mandibular anterior teeth should not be cut off, nor should the crowns of the anterior teeth appear fractured or obscured.

Zone 2: Nose-Sinus (Fig. 10.3)

The images of the inferior turbinates and their surrounding air spaces (meati) should be contained within the nasal cavity. The soft tissue of the nose cartilage should not be seen. The hard palate shadow (double image) and sometimes the ghost images of the palate must be seen within the maxillary sinuses, well above the apices of the posterior teeth. The tongue should be in contact with the hard palate, with no intervening air between these structures.

Zone 3: Mandibular Body (Fig. 10.3)

The inferior cortex of the mandible should be smooth and continuous. The double image, or ghost image of the body of the hyoid, should be absent in this area. The midline area should not be overly enlarged superiorly-inferiorly.

Zones 4 and 6: Four Corners; Condyles and Hyoid (Fig. 10.4)

Zone 4 contains the condyles bilaterally. The condyles should be more or less centered within the zone and not move off the top or lateral edges of the film. The condyles should be of equal size and on the same horizontal plane, i.e., one condyle should **not** be higher or lower than the other. Zone 6 contains the body of the hyoid bone and sometimes the greater horn. It should appear as a double image equal in size bilaterally; although it may touch the mandible, it should **not** spread across the mandible.

Zone 5: Ramus-Spine (Fig. 10.5)

The ramus of the mandible should be the same width bilaterally. The spine, although usually not seen, may be present so long as it does not superimpose on the ramus. When present, the distance between the spine and ramus should be the same bilaterally.

PURPOSEFUL PATIENT POSITIONING ERRORS

Because in most machines the focal trough or layer cannot be adjusted to the patient or be moved, it is critically important to position the patient in exactly the right place. However, with some errors, patient malpositioning will be done on purpose to better visualize a specific anatomical region. The following table describes useful errors.

Table of Useful Panoramic Errors	
Error	**Region of Improved Imaging**
1. Too far forward	Nasal fossa and sinus
2. Chin too low	Anterior maxilla and teeth
3. Chin too high	Anterior mandible and teeth

TROUBLESHOOTING PANORAMIC POSITIONING ERRORS

As previously mentioned, positioning errors are made in association with the five steps in the panoramic technique. The correct procedure will be described first; then, the several errors occurring with that step will be described. Positioning lights (Fig. 10.6) serve as an aid to assure correct patient positioning before making an exposure. In a properly positioned patient, structures are projected onto the image with specific interrelationships to each other to form a pattern one can recognize as an error-free exposure (Fig. 10.7).

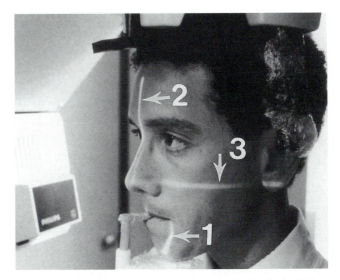

Figure 10.6. Patient Positioning Lights. (1) This vertical light should be at the corner of the mouth. (2) This vertical light is centered on patient's midline. (3) This horizontal light should be on the Frankfort plane. Variations in positioning lights exist in different machines.

ZONE 1: THE DENTITION

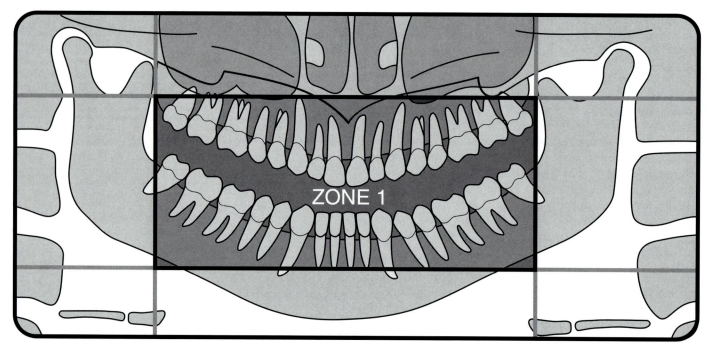

Figure 10.2. Zone 1: The Dentition. The teeth should be separated and arranged with an upward curve posteriorly, producing a smile-like arrangement.

ZONE 2: NOSE AND SINUS
ZONE 3: MANDIBULAR BODY

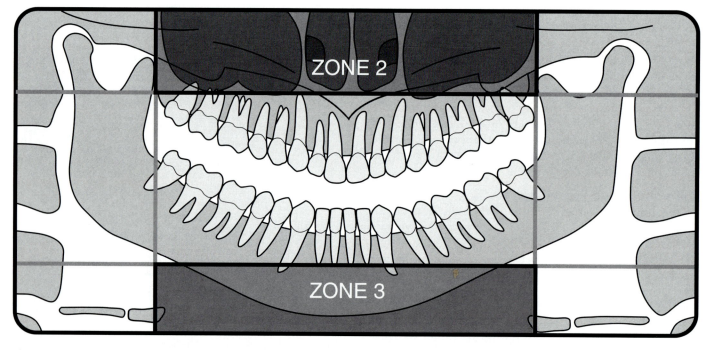

Figure 10.3. Zones 2 and 3: Nose and Sinus and Mandibular Body. Zone 2: The inferior turbinates should be within the nasal fossa, and the hard palate shadows above the root apices. Zone 3: The inferior cortex of the mandibular body should be smooth and uninterrupted.

ZONE 4: TMJ
ZONE 6: HYOID

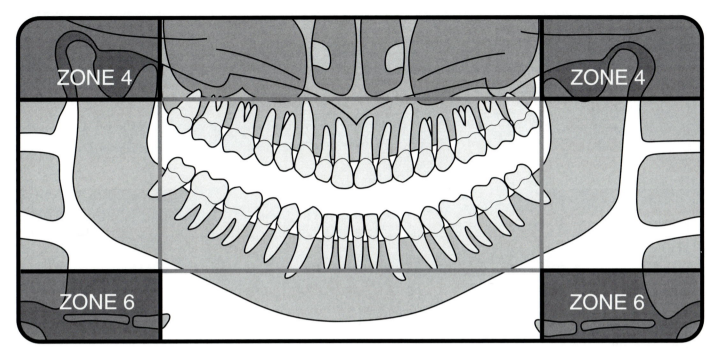

Figure 10.4. Zones 4 and 6: Four Corners. Zone 4: The condyles are centered in this zone and equal in size and position bilaterally. Zone 6: The hyoid bone should remain in this zone.

ZONE 5: RAMUS-SPINE

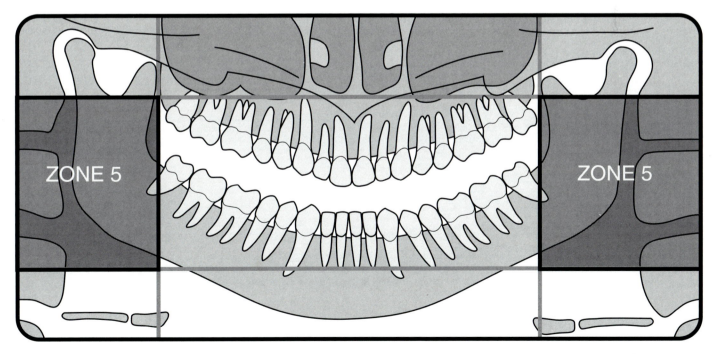

Figure 10.5. Zone 5: Ramus-Spine. The ramus should be equal in width bilaterally, and the spine should not be superimposed on the ramus.

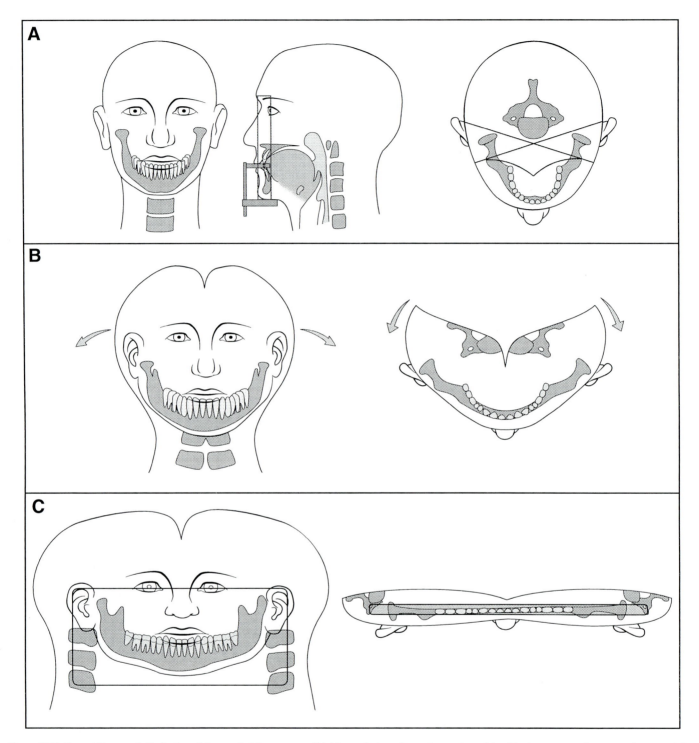

Figure 10.7. Correct Panoramic Projection of Anatomical Structures. (A) Note relation of anterior teeth and biteblock groove to the image layer and the path of the rotation center. (B) The unfolding of anatomical structures in three dimensions much like opening a book with the cover toward you. (C) The relative position of key anatomical structures within the panoramic image (left) and within the image layer (right).

STEPS IN THE GENERIC PANORAMIC TECHNIQUE

Most machines are operated in a similar way. It is easy to learn to operate another machine once one machine has been mastered. Much like driving a car, if you can drive a Chevrolet, you can rent a Ford and adapt quickly to the new automobile.

The following are the five steps in the generic panoramic technique:

Step	Panoramic Technique
1	Bite in the groove.
2	Close the side guides.
3	Position the chin.
4	Stand the patient upright.
5	Have the patient place the tongue on the roof of the mouth, swallow, and hold still; then make the exposure.

Panoramic Technique Step 1: Bite in Groove (Fig. 10.8)

Have the Patient Bite in the Groove in the Biteblock

The purpose of this step is to get the anterior teeth into the middle of the anterior part of the layer, to separate the dentition in the image, and to center the patient in the machine. All current machines have a biteblock; older discontinued Panorex machines do not have a biteblock, but the teeth are separated by placing several cotton rolls between the anterior teeth. Some machines come with a light that should be at the corners of the mouth or in the midcanine region. This helps to avoid errors. One machine has an auto focus beam, whereby the machine will automatically adjust to the patient. If the biteblock is removed or the patient has missing anterior teeth, the upper and lower teeth will not be separated in the image.

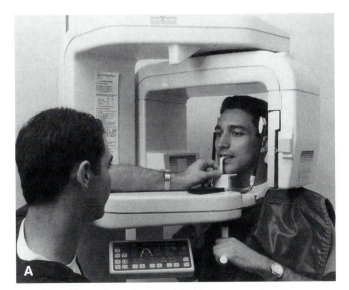
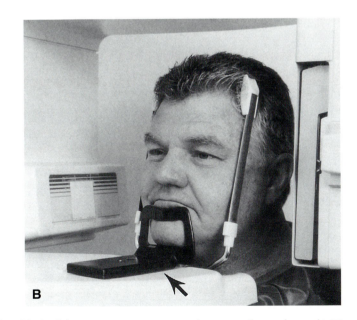

Figure 10.8. Step 1: Bite in Groove of Biteblock. **(A)** Patient biting groove of biteblock. (If there are missing anterior teeth, cotton rolls must be used.) **(B)** A special chin rest (arrow) is available for edentulous patients.

Panoramic Technique Step 2: Close Side Guides (Fig. 10.9)

Close the Side Guides

The purpose of this step is to get the posterior teeth into the middle of the layer on both sides and to fix the head in position to stabilize it during the exposure. The best machine design is one in which the side guides drop down from the top of the machine. These are not usually seen in the image; side guides coming up from the chin rest area are less desirable, as they are usually seen in the image and may interfere with assessment of patient landmarks. Some machines have frontal or temporal guides near the patient's forehead instead of the side guides or in addition to the side guides to further stabilize the patient's head. In machines with a light, the beam should be aligned along the midsagittal plane or midline of the patient's nose and face.

Panoramic Technique Step 3: Position Chin (Fig. 10.10)

Position the Patient's Chin on the Chin Rest

The purpose of this step is to ensure that the chin is tilted downward 4 to 7° to counter the 4- to 7°-upward angle of the x-ray beam. Most chin rests are on a slightly down angle for this reason. Also, the chin rest supports the chin to steady the patient; thus, the chin should rest on the chin rest. Some machines come with a light that is aligned along some anatomical plane, such as the Frankfort plane (lower orbit to tragus) or the ala of the nose to tragus line. This will indicate correct positioning of the chin.

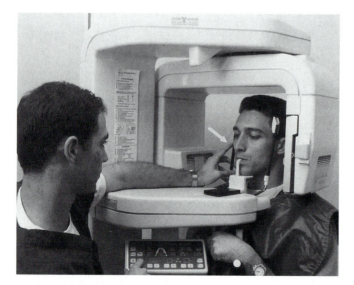

Figure 10.9. Step 2: Close Side Guides. The purpose of this step is to get posterior teeth into middle of layer on both sides.

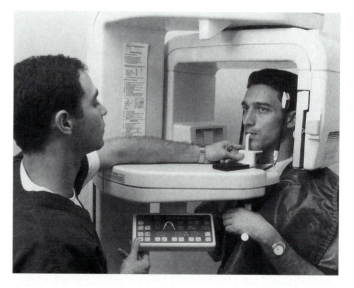

Figure 10.10. Step 3: Position Patient's Chin on the Chin Rest. The chin should be tilted slightly downward to counter the upward projection angle of the x-ray beam.

Panoramic Technique Step 4: Stand Patient Upright (Fig. 10.11)

Stand the Patient Upright or Sit the Patient up Straight

The purpose of this step is to straighten the cervical spine (neck) vertically. Here the patient is asked to advance the feet as far forward as possible and to stand erect; thus, he or she must hold onto the machine handles to avoid falling backward. When positioning the patient in the machine, the operator can guide the patient with gentle hand pressure in the small of the back to encourage the patient to stand erect. In sit-down machines, a similar procedure is followed; cushions may be inserted at the base of the spine to help the patient sit in a more erect position. Some machines have sensors at the film plane that will change the mA and/or kVp automatically to minimize the effects of this error; for example, the kVp is increased to penetrate the broader profile of the spine.

Panoramic Technique Step 5: Swallow, Hold, Expose (Fig. 10.12)

Have the Patient Place the Tongue in the Roof of the Mouth, Swallow, and Hold Still; Then Make the Exposure

The purpose of this step is to be certain that the lips are sealed and the tongue is on the palate. This is done by asking the patient to swallow or suck on their cheeks. Holding still is also important because the exposure time ranges from 14 to 22 seconds, depending on the machine. Patients with uncontrollable tremors are not good candidates for a panoramic radiograph. In most instances of movement, the patient is startled momentarily by the machine, especially if it glances against an item of clothing. Finally, the "exposure" means selecting the appropriate exposure factors for the patient's size and build. The exposure time is fixed and not adjustable. The kVp is adjustable on all machines and is varied for patient size; the mA is adjustable on a few machines and may also need adjustment. Because each brand is a little different, it is necessary to use the specific exposure chart as provided by the manufacturer. Some machines adjust for incorrect exposure values automatically due to the function of a sensor at the film plane.

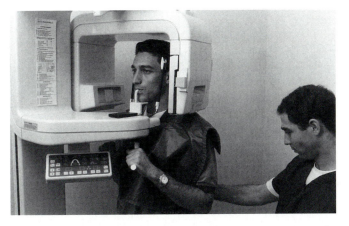

Figure 10.11. Step 4: Stand the Patient Upright. When positioning the patient in the machine, the operator can guide the patient in the machine with gentle hand pressure in the small of the back to encourage the patient to stand erect. The patient should hold onto the machine handles to avoid falling backward.

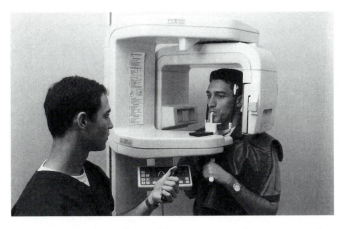

Figure 10.12. Step 5: Swallow, Hold, Expose. Note that the patient's lips are tightly sealed around the biteblock. The kilovolts have been selected at the touch pad, and the operator is ready to stand behind a protective barrier and make the exposure.

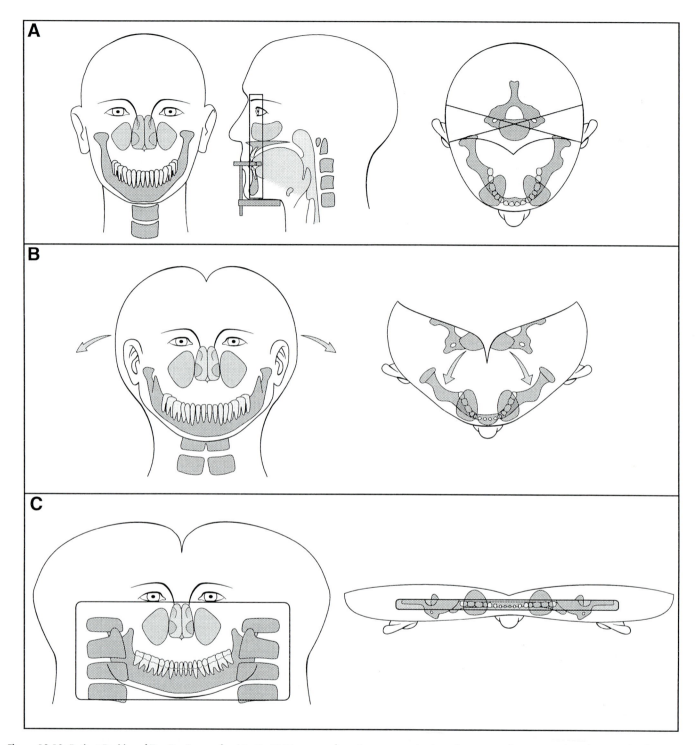

Figure 10.13. Patient Positioned Too Far Forward. **(A, B, C)** Diagrams show incorrect projection of anatomical structures. **(D)** Photograph of a patient biting too far forward. Note positioning light (arrow). **(E, F)** Radiographs depicting typical features of this error. Note improved nasal fossa and sinus regions in the edentulous radiograph.

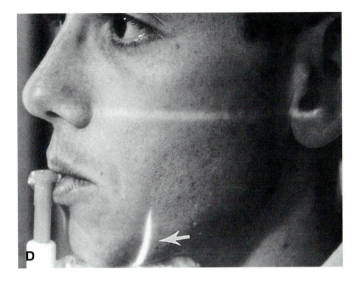

Step 1: Bite in Groove—Error No. 1 (Fig. 10.13)

The Patient Is Positioned Too Far Forward

Zone 1: Dentition. The anterior teeth (especially the lowers) are narrowed, sometimes with pseudospaces between the teeth. Sometimes the crowns of the anterior teeth appear fractured because they are cut out of the image layer.

Zone 5: Ramus-Spine. The cervical spine is superimposed on the ramus and condyles symmetrically on both sides. Overall, the whole patient appears to have been narrowed with respect to the size of the panoramic film.

Too Far Forward Purposeful Error. Here the error results in an improved image of the nasal cavity and maxillary sinus. This radiograph makes it easier to detect sinus disease, extension of sinus disease into the nose and deviated nasal septum.

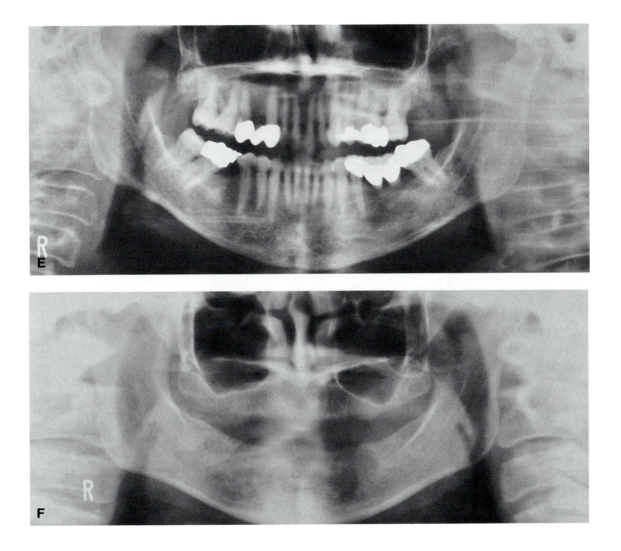

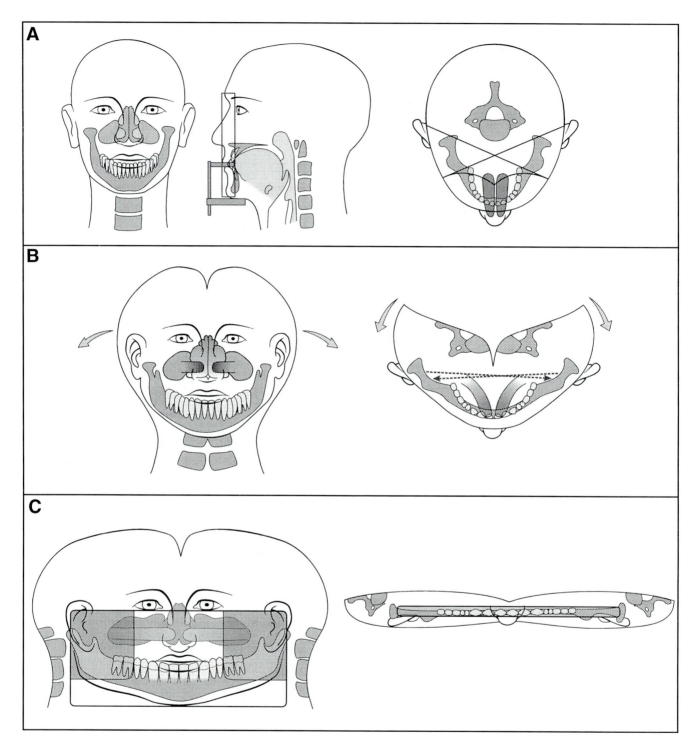

Figure 10.14. Patient Positioned Too Far Back. (**A, B, C**) Diagrams show incorrect projection of anatomical structures. (**D**) Photograph of patient biting too far back. (**E, F**) Radiographs depicting typical features of this error.

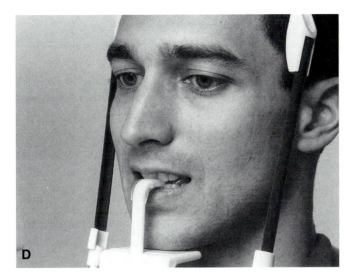

Step 1: Bite in Groove—Error No. 2 (Fig. 10.14)

The Patient Is Positioned Too Far Back

Zone 1: Dentition. The anterior teeth (especially the lowers) are widened. Widening of teeth is sometimes hard to judge.

Zone 2: Nose-Sinus. The soft tissue image of the nose cartilage is seen. The lower turbinate and meati are spread-out across the maxillary sinus bilaterally.

Zone 3: Mandibular Body. The inferior cortex of the mandible should be smooth and continuous. The double image, or ghost image, of the body of the hyoid should be absent in this area.

Zone 4: Condyles. The condyles appear close to or off the lateral edges of the film. The soft tissue outline of the cartilage of the pinna of the ear and earlobe can be seen.

Zone 5: Ramus-Spine. The ghost images of the contralateral rami are superimposed on the posterior molars and rami symmetrically bilaterally. Overall, the patient's image appears too large for the film.

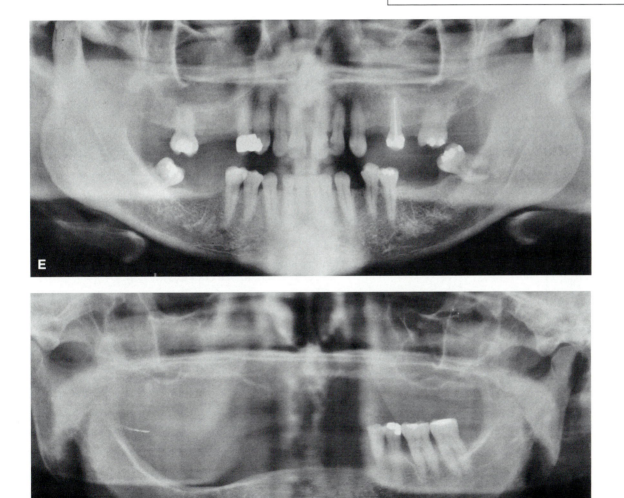

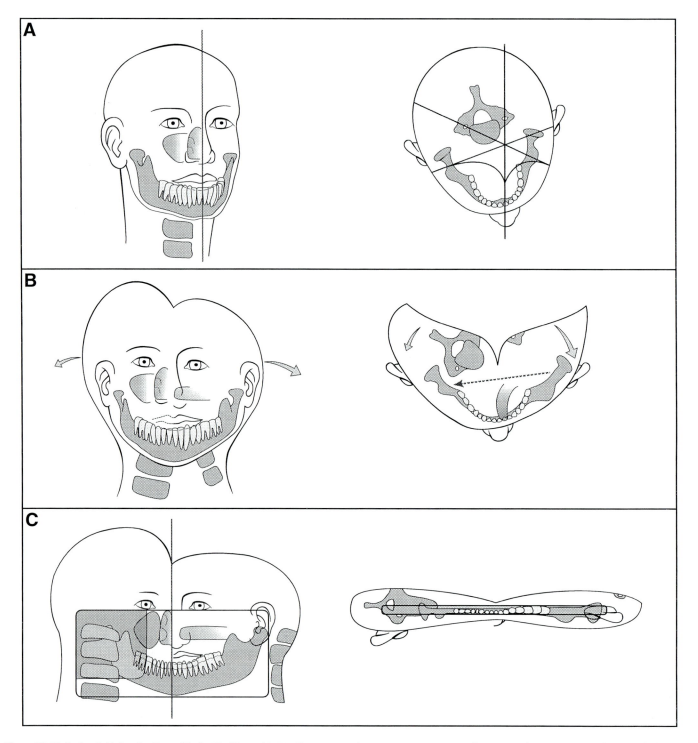

Figure 10.15. Patient Is Twisted or Turned in the Machine. **(A, B, C)** Diagrams show incorrect projection of anatomical structures. **(D)** Photograph showing that the patient is twisted and that the side guides are open. **(E, F)** Radiographs depicting features of this error.

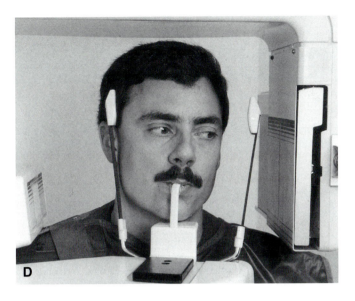

Step 2: Close Side Guides—Error No. 1 (Fig. 10.15)

The Patient Is Twisted or Turned in the Machine

Zone 1: Dentition. The posterior teeth on one side are widened and overlap interproximally. On the other side, the posterior teeth are narrowed.

Zone 2: Nose-Sinus. On the side with the wide ramus, the inferior turbinate and meati are spread-out across the maxillary sinus; the opposite maxillary sinus may have an improved image.

Zone 4: Temporomandibular Joint (TMJ). On the side with the wide ramus, the earlobe can be seen.

Zone 5: Ramus-Spine. On the side with the wide posterior teeth, the ramus is widened; on the other side, the ramus is narrowed and intersected by the ghost image of the contralateral ramus—the spine may approach or superimpose on the ramus on this side.

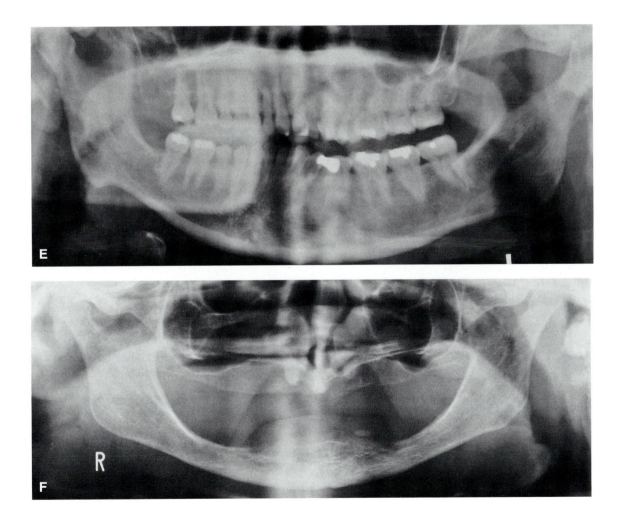

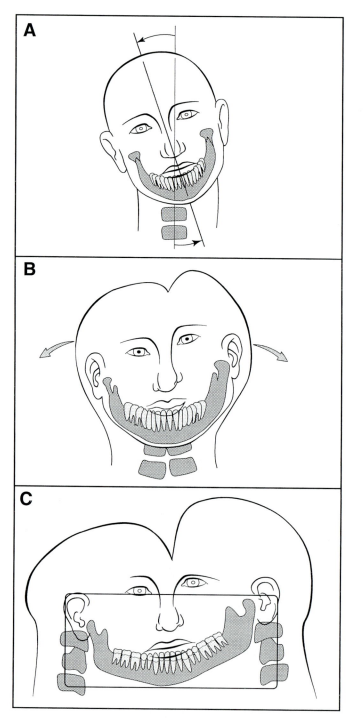

Step 2: Close Side Guides—Error No. 2 (Fig. 10.16)

The Patient Is Tilted in the Machine

Zone 1: Dentition. The posterior teeth may be slightly widened on one side, with a widening gap between the upper and lower teeth in a posterior dentition; on the other side, the interocclusal gap is narrowed.

Zone 3: Mandible Body. The lower edge of the mandible on one side is almost horizontal; on the side with the widened interocclusal gap, the mandible is enlarged and the lower edge appears to be directed upward above the horizontal plane.

Zone 4: TMJ. On the side with the widened interocclusal gap, the condyle is enlarged and above the contralateral condyle, which is smaller and lower in the image.

In general and especially throughout the upper one third of the image (Zones 2 and 4), the bony details appear fuzzy or streaked, rendering them anatomically indistinguishable.

Figure 10.16. Patient Tilted in the Machine. **(A, B, C)** Diagram shows incorrect projection of anatomical structures. **(D, E)** Photographs of patient's head tilted in the machine. Note side guides are open and malalignment of positioning light, as viewed through the machine mirror. **(F)** Radiograph depicting the features of this error.

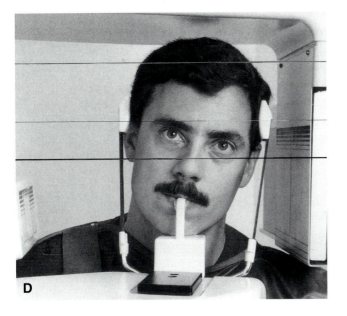

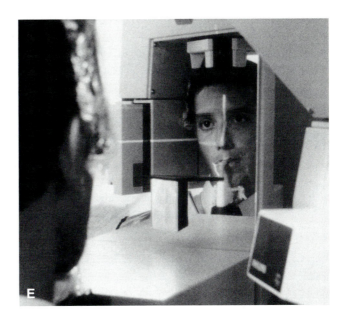

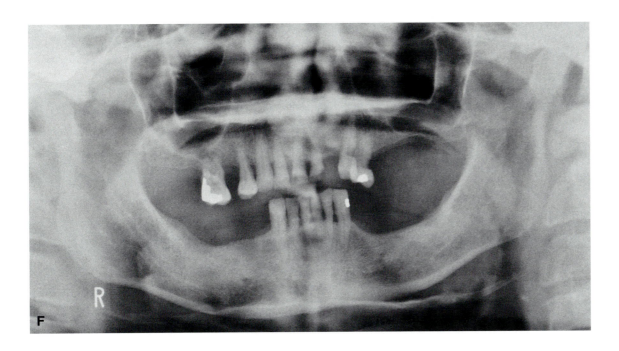

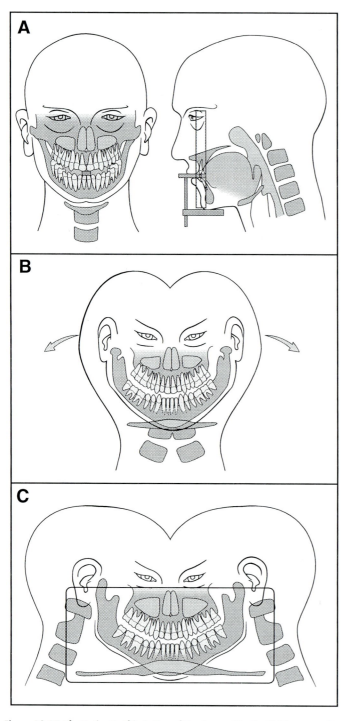

Step 3. Position the Chin—Error No. 1 (Fig. 10.17)

The Chin Is Tipped Too Low

Zone 1: Dentition. The "smile" line created by the interocclusal gap is exaggerated. The apices of the mandibular anterior teeth are "cut-off." The maxillary anterior teeth are better than in the normal projection.

Zone 3: Mandible. The mandible is widened vertically in the anterior region, and there is poor imaging of the trabecular pattern. The mandible is transversed by the elongated double image and/or ghost of the hyoid bone.

Zone 4: TMJ. The condyles approach the upper edge of the film or are cut-off by the upper edge of the film symmetrically bilaterally.

Chin Tipped too Low Purposeful Error. This error is made to improve the image of the maxillary anterior region, especially the teeth and surrounding bone.

Figure 10.17. The Patient's Chin Is Tipped Too Low. (**A, B, C**) Diagrams show incorrect projection of anatomical structures. (**D, E**) Photographs of patients whose chins are tipped too low. Note malalignment of positioning light (*arrow*) in (**E**). (**F**) Radiograph depicting the features of this error.

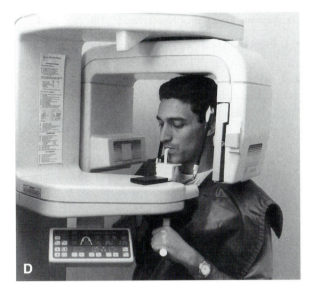

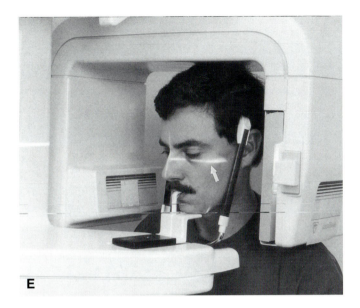

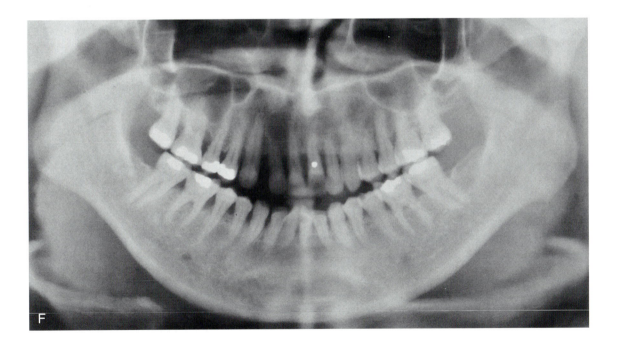

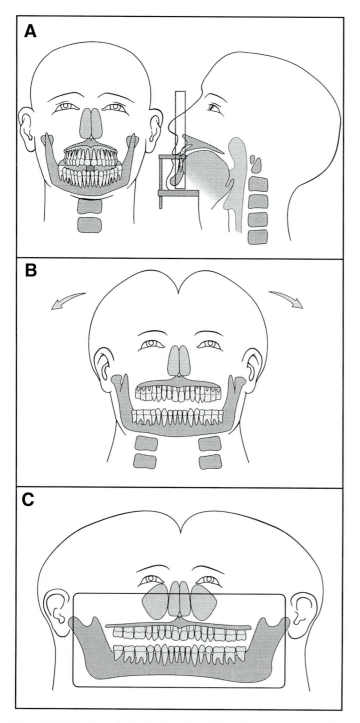

Figure 10.18. The Patient's Chin Is Tipped Too High. (**A, B, C**) Diagrams show incorrect projection of anatomical structures. (**D**) Photograph of patient's chin tipped too high. Note malalignment of positioning light (arrow). (**E, F**) Radiographs depicting the features of this error.

Step 3: Position the Chin—Error No. 2 (Fig. 10.18)

The Chin Is Tipped Too High

Zone 1: Dentition. The "smile" line created by the interocclusal gap is lost entirely; the occlusal plane appears flat or even in a reverse curve or "sad" configuration. The apices of the maxillary anterior teeth are "cut-off." The mandibular anterior teeth are better than in the normal projection.

Zone 2: Nose-Sinus. The real, double and ghost images of the palate form a widened, prominent, radiopaque line which is projected downward to approximate or superimpose on the apices of the maxillary teeth.

Zone 4: TMJ. The condyles approach the lateral edges of the film or are projected off the edges of the film symmetrically bilaterally.

Chin Tipped too High Purposeful Error. This error is made to improve the image of the mandibular anterior region, especially the teeth and surrounding bone.

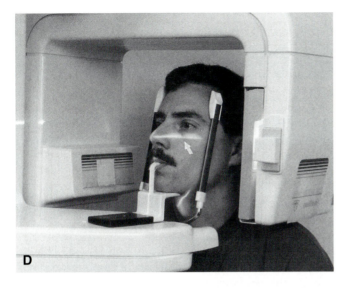

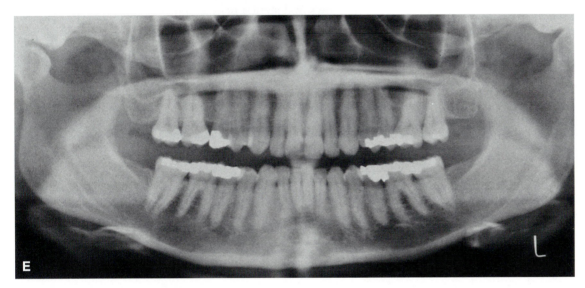

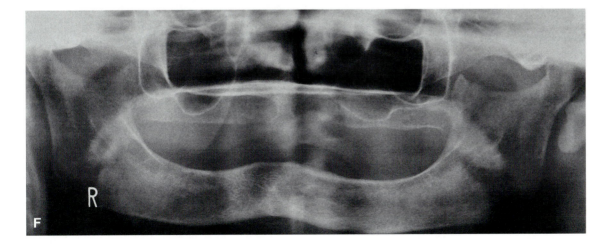

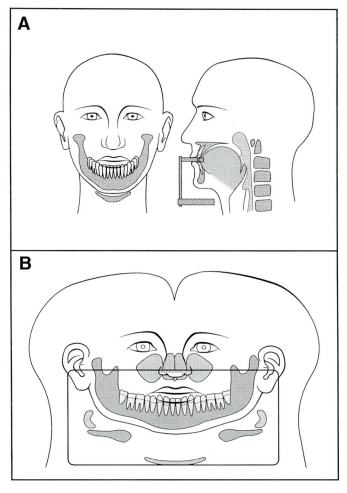

Step 4: Stand the Patient Upright—Error No. 1 (Fig. 10.19)

The Chin Is Not on the Chin Rest

Zone 1: Dentition. This error has no effect on the dentition.

Zones 2 and 4: Nose-Sinus and TMJ. These zones across the upper one third of the film contain structures from lower down that are "cut-off" by the upper edge of the film. The lower edge of the film corresponds with the lower edge of the chin rest; naturally, when the operator asks the patient to stand upright, the chin can come off the chin rest. The machine must now be brought up to meet the chin.

Zones 3 and 6: Mandible Body and Hyoid. These zones across the bottom one third of the film do not contain the structures; instead, only soft tissue shadows and sometimes the unoccupied chin rest is centered at the lower edge of Zone 3.

Figure 10.19. The Chin Is Not on the Chin Rest. (**A, B**) Diagrams show incorrect projection of anatomical structures. (**C**) Photograph of a patient who does not have his chin on the chin rest. (**D, E**) Radiographs depicting features of this error.

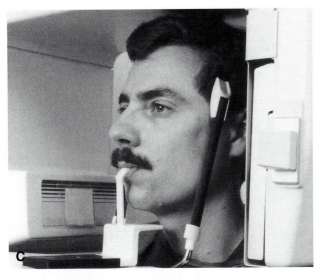

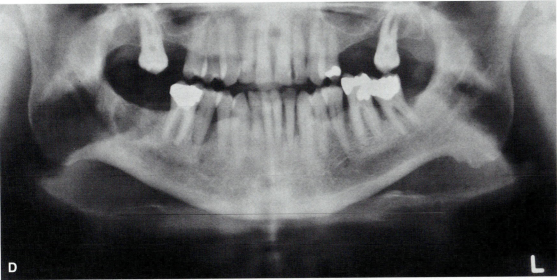

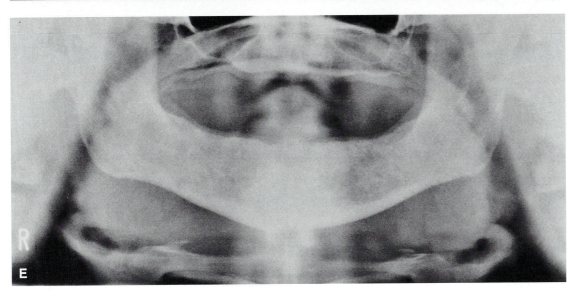

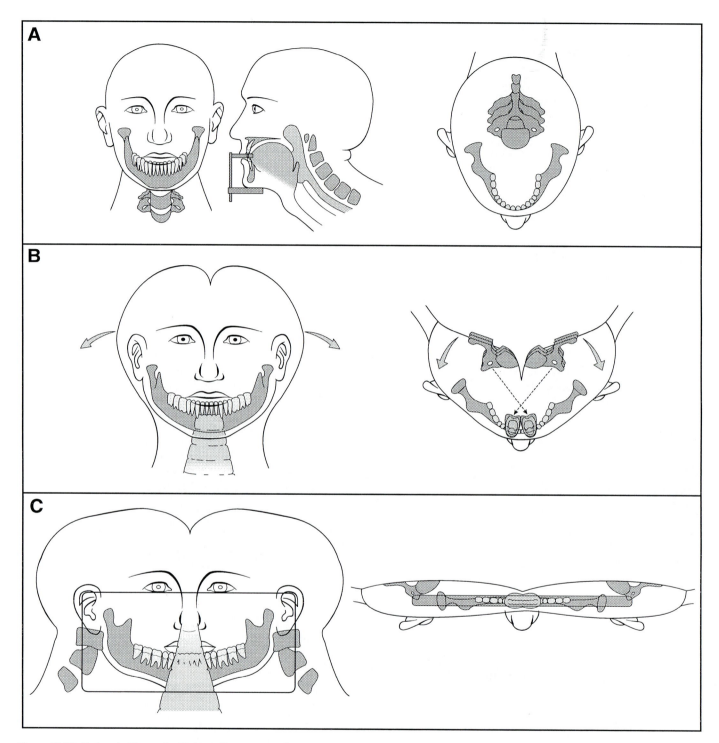

Figure 10.20. Patient Is Slumped. (**A, B, C**) Diagrams show incorrect projection of anatomical structures. (**D**) Photograph of patient slumped in x-ray machine. (**E, F**) Radiographs depicting features of this error.

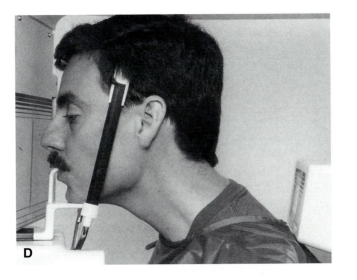

D

Step 4: Stand the Patient Upright—Error No. 2 (Fig. 10.20)

The Patient Is Slumped

Zone 1: Dentition. The anterior teeth are difficult to see, especially the lowers, as the ghost radiopaque image of the spine has superimposed on this area and obliterated it. There are no effects on any other zones with this error. Slumped means the patient's neck is stretched forward on a slant; this causes a ghost image to be produced in the middle of the film.

Zone 3: Mandibular Body. The ghost image of the spine extends downward beyond the mandibular teeth to obscure the midportion of the mandible.

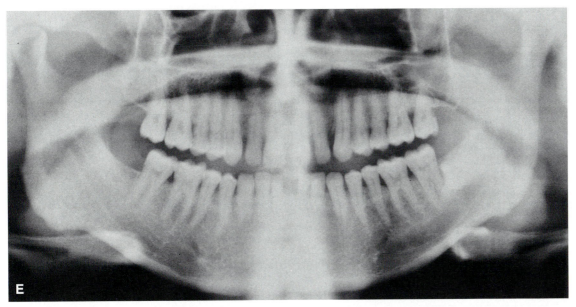

E

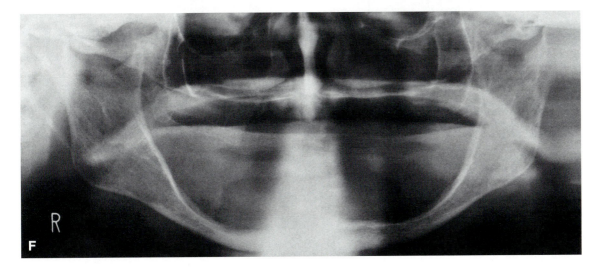

F

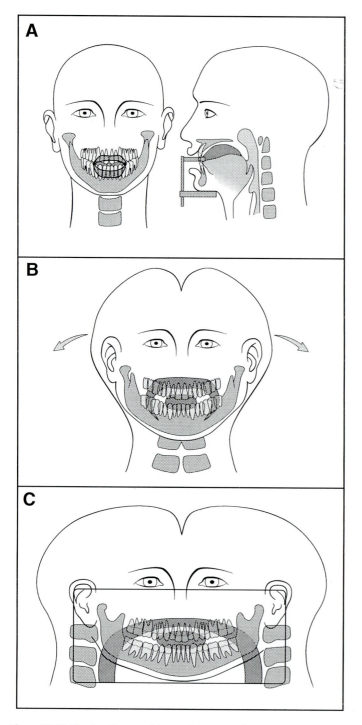

Step 5: Swallow, Hold Still, and Expose—Error No. 1 (Fig. 10.21)

The Lips Are Open and/or the Tongue Is not on the Palate

Zone 1: Dentition. The crowns of the upper and lower anterior teeth are obscured by the air between the parted lips. The apical region of the maxillary teeth is obscured by the dark air space between the dorsum of the tongue as well as the hard and soft palates (palatoglossal air space).

Zone 2: Nose-Sinus. The maxillary apical alveolar bone, which is also in this zone, is obscured by the palatoglossal air space.

Figure 10.21. Lips Are Open and Tongue Is Not on Palate. **(A, B, C)** Diagrams show incorrect projection of anatomical structures. **(D, E)** Photographs of patients with lips open and tongue not on palate. In **D**, the operator is not paying attention to patient's positioning in the machine. **(F)** Radiograph depicts features of this error.

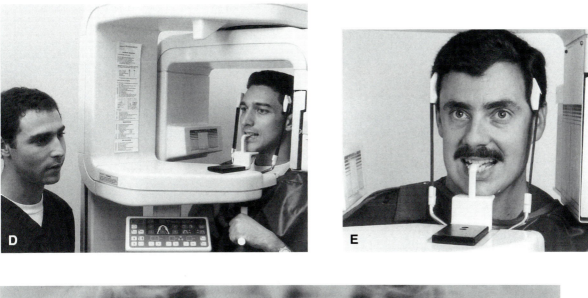

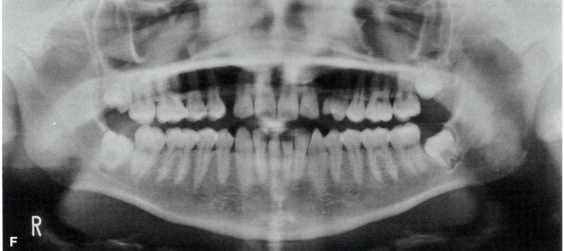

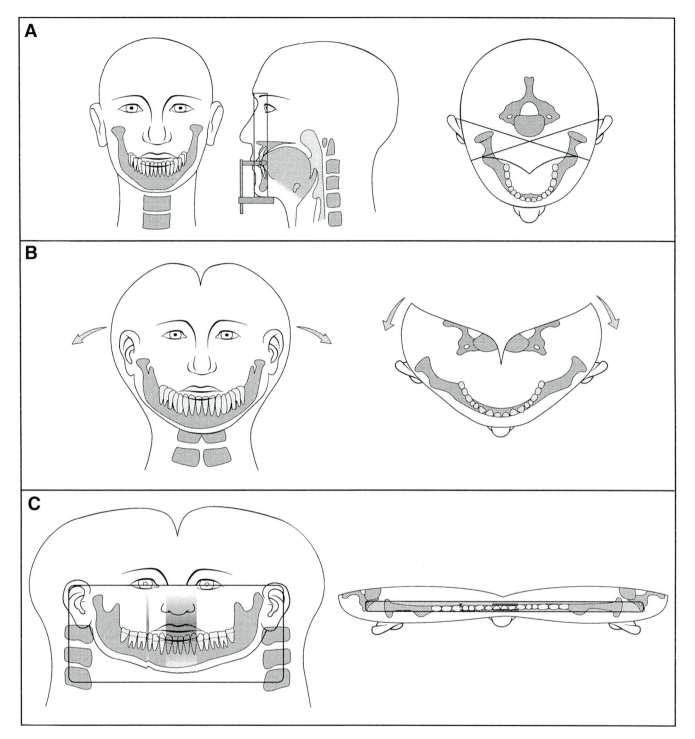

Figure 10.22. The Patient Moved. (**A, B, C**) Diagrams show incorrect projection of anatomical structures. (**D**) Photograph of patient moving during exposure cycle. (**E, F**) Radiograph depicts features of this error (arrows).

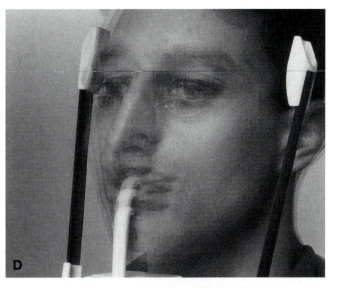

Step 5: Swallow, Hold Still, Expose—Error No. 2 (Fig. 10.22)

The Patient Moved

Zone 1: Dentition. This area is minimally affected by this error.

Zone 3: Mandibular Body. Along the inferior cortex of the mandible, an interruption in its continuity can be seen, especially in the molar area. Also, a wavy image of the inferior cortex is sometimes seen at the inferior cortex of the mandible near the midline. If the observer looks at the other zones above the distorted area of the inferior cortex, unsharpness will be seen throughout the vertical dimension of the image due to the movement.

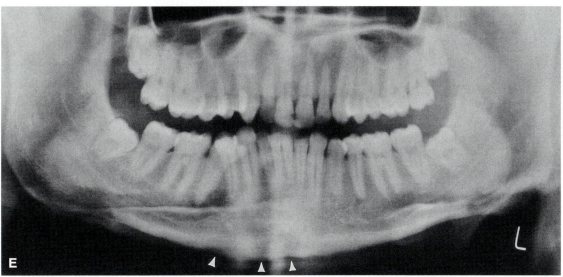

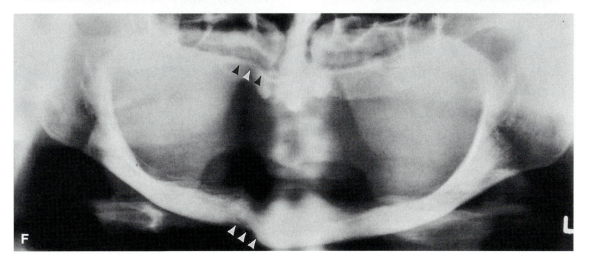

> **Step 5: Swallow, Hold Still, Expose—Error No. 3 (Fig. 10.23)**
>
> **The Film Is Improperly Exposed**
>
> There are a variety of possibilities for this error, including a **double exposure**, in which two sets of teeth are seen; the **film is too light** due to insufficient kVp or **too dark** due to too much kVp; the film is **improperly labeled** with a missing "R" or "L" marker; or the film is **missing the patient identification label.**

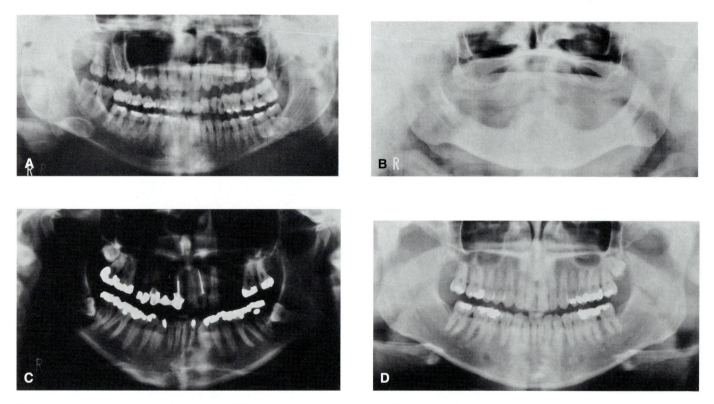

Figure 10.23. Radiographs Improperly Exposed. (**A**) Double exposure of radiograph. (**B**) Radiograph is too light due to insufficient kilovolts. (**C**) Radiograph is too dark due to "too high" kilovolts. (**D**) Radiograph with missing "R" and "L" markers.

Analysis of Panoramic Patient Positioning Errors

Error and Cause	Identifying Features	Correction
Patient too far forward	Narrow blurred anterior teeth with pseudospace Superimposition of spine on ramus Bicuspid overlap bilaterally	Use incisal bite guide Line up incisal edge of teeth with notch Edentulous patients should bite about 5 mm behind notch
Patient too far back	Wide, blurred anterior teeth Ghosting of rami, spread-out turbinates, ears, and nose in image, condyles off lateral edges of film	Use incisal bite guide Line up incisal edge of teeth with notch
Chin tipped too low	Excessive curving of the occlusal plane Loss of image of the roots of the lower anterior teeth Narrowing of the intercondylar distance and loss of head of the condyles at the top of the film	Tip chin down, but ala-tragus line should not exceed −5° to −7° downward Use chin rest
Chin raised too high	Flattening or reverse curvature of occlusal plane Loss of image of the roots of the upper anterior teeth Lengthening of intercondylar distance and loss of head of the condyles at the edges of the film Hard palate shadow wider and superimposed on the apices of the maxillary teeth	Tip chin down −5° to −7° Use chin rest.
Head twisted	Unequal right-left magnification Particularly teeth and ramus Severe overlap of contact points and blurring	Line up patient's midline with middle of incisal bite guide Close side guide
Head tilted	Mandible appears tilted on film Unequal distance between mandible and chin rest at a given point on the right and left sides One condyle is higher and larger than the other	Position the chin firmly on both sides of the chin rest Close side guide
Slumped position	Ghost image of cervical spine superimposed on the anterior region	Stand-up machines: have the patient step forward or place feet on markers All machines: be certain the patient is sitting or standing erect
Chin not on the chin rest	Sinus not visible on the film Top of condyles are cut off Excessive distance between inferior border of the mandible and the lower edge of the film	Position the chin on the chin rest
Bite guide not used	Incisal and occlusal surfaces of the upper and lower teeth overlapped	Use bite guide Compensate for missing anterior teeth with cotton rolls
Tongue not on palate	Relative radiolucency obscuring apices of the maxillary teeth (palatolglossal air space)	Place the tongue firmly against the palate Ask the patient to swallow or suck on his or her cheeks
Lips open	Relative radiolucency on the coronal portion of the upper and lower teeth	Close lips
Patient movement	Wavy outline of cortex of the interior border of the mandible Blurring of the image above wavy cortical outline	Ask the patient to hold still Explain the function of the machine to avoid startling the patient Be certain the patient's clothing will not interfere
Prostheses	Evidence of prostheses in the image Acrylic denture teeth and bases do not show	Remove all complete and partial dentures, eyeglasses, and jewelry

MULTIPLE PATIENT POSITIONING ERRORS

When errors are made, they are not necessarily made in single doses. Operators often make multiple errors during the same exposure. The result is called "hybrid effects," in which several errors compound to produce unique changes in the image. However, most multiple errors can usually be identified in the one image by sorting and separating the undesirable effects of each error. On the good news side of things, it is fortunate that nobody makes all the errors. Because any individual is usually very faithful to their own particular mistakes, these can be corrected easily once they have been identified. The best thing is to learn the technique properly, to be exact with the five patient positioning steps, and to avoid the errors altogether. The machine should never be altered and the manufacturer's instructions should never be modified on a continuing basis.

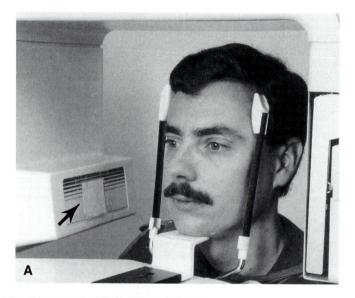

Figure 10.24. Machine Modifications. (**A**) The biteblock has been removed; this should never be done on a routine basis (undesirable). A square piece of rare-earth filter removes 40% of the radiation dose to the patient (*arrow*) (desirable). (**B**) Radiograph with no biteblock. The teeth are not separated. The patient is too far back and twisted, and the chin is too high.

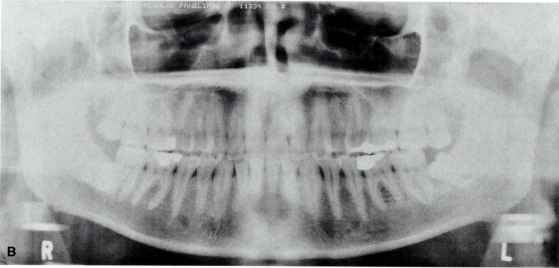

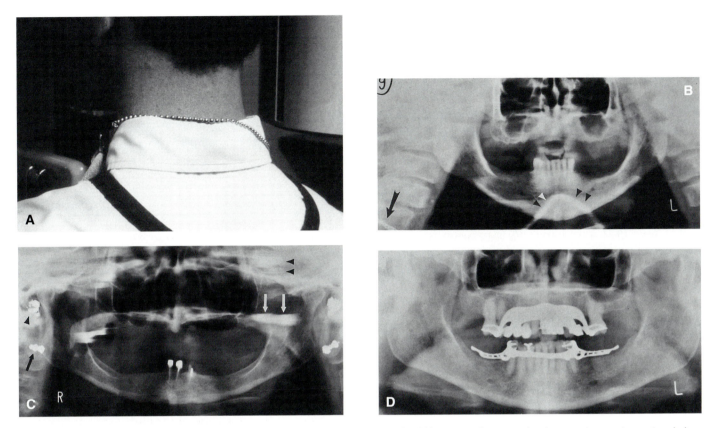

Figure 10.25. Jewelry, Prostheses, and Hearing Aids. (**A**) Napkin and jewelry chain should be removed. (**B**) Jewelry chain; real image (*arrow*) and ghost image (*arrowheads*). (**C**) Bilateral earrings and hearing aids. *Arrows:* Real and corresponding ghost images of earring. *Arrowheads:* Real and corresponding ghost images of hearing aid. (**D**) Prostheses interfere with interpretation.

TROUBLESHOOTING TECHNICAL ERRORS IN PANORAMIC RADIOGRAPHY

ALTERING THE PANORAMIC MACHINE (Fig. 10.24)

Removing essential parts of a panoramic machine such as the biteblock assembly, chin rest, or side guides on a routine basis is an extremely poor practice and does not meet the normal standard of care for routine panoramic radiography. On the other hand, the addition of rare earth screen filtration at the collimator slit and/or conversion to digital imaging can result in significant savings in radiation dose to the patient (see p. 256).

PROSTHESES, JEWELRY, ETC. (Fig. 10.25)

Intraorally, removable items such as complete and partial dentures should be removed before the procedure. Acrylic complete dentures and acrylic partial dentures involving anterior teeth may be left in to better position the patient in the machine, to effect the desired interocclusal

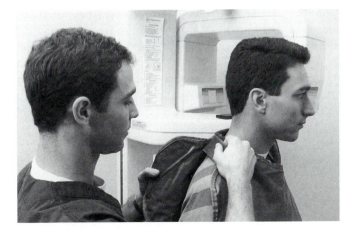

Figure 10.26. Poncho-Style Apron for Panoramic Radiography. The proper type of apron for panoramic radiography is the poncho-style apron shown here that offers radiation protection to the patient's front and back.

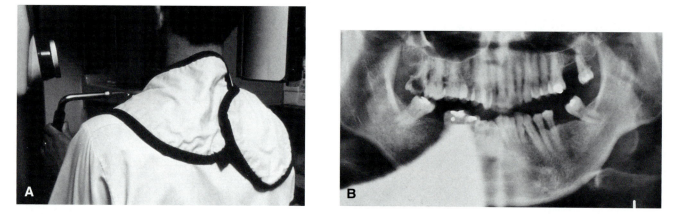

Figure 10.27. Apron Artifact. **(A)** Inappropriate placement of non–poncho-style apron. **(B)** Apron artifact on panoramic radiograph.

gap between the upper and lower teeth, and to help stabilize an otherwise shaky patient. Extraorally, eyeglasses, earrings, nose jewelry, neck chains, and napkin chains must be removed. Normally, eye prostheses, hearing aids, and wigs can be left on during the procedure, although these may also sometimes interfere with the image.

APRON/THYROID SHIELD ARTIFACT

The **proper type** of apron for panoramic radiography is the poncho style that offers particular protection to the back and front of the patient (Fig. 10.26); x-rays come from the sides and back of the patient to expose the film. The intraoral style of apron should not be used in panoramic radiography. When the apron parts extend onto the neck, especially at the sides and back, these are projected onto the film as blank or clear unexposed areas (Fig. 10.27). Thyroid shields are not recommended because they will project onto the film due to the negative projection angle of the beam. In panoramic radiography, there is about 10 times less dose to the thyroid gland without a thyroid shield than for the intraoral full-mouth survey with the long, round cone and E+ speed film with the thyroid shield.

NOT STARTING AT "HOME BASE" (Fig. 10.28)

Most panoramic machine cassette holder assemblies need to be manually aligned with the correct starting point to fully expose the film. When this is not done, a panoramic cone cut results. Only a part of the patient will be imaged, and the remainder of the film is blank or clear because it remains unexposed.

CASSETTE RESISTANCE (Fig. 10.29)

At times, the cassette will hang up on a person with large shoulders and/or a short neck, on an item of the patient's clothing, or on an improperly placed lead apron. This causes the machine to slow down or stop and to overexpose a narrow band of the film over its full vertical breadth. Variants of this problem include several dark bands due to multiple interferences with the machine's progress, or a single dark band followed by an unexposed area where the exposure was aborted and the interfering item repositioned. In such cases, the entire exposure is repeated with a new film. Patient movement is sometimes seen in association with this error.

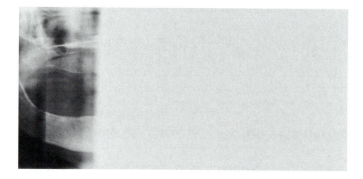

Figure 10.28. Not Starting at "Home Base." Before initiating the exposure, the cassette-drum assembly must be manually aligned to the starting point in some machines; the result of this error is a "panoramic cone-cut."

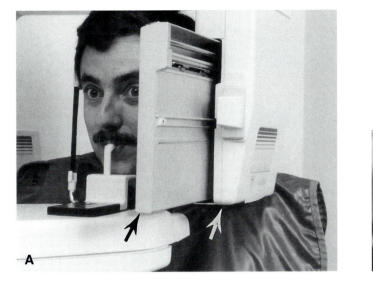

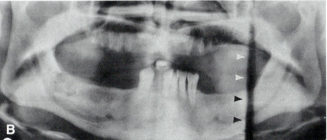

Figure 10.29. Cassette Resistance. (**A**) The cassette assembly (*arrows*) has struck the patient's shoulder, momentarily interrupting the exposure cycle. (**B**) Cassette resistance produces a dark, vertical band in the image representing an overexposed area (*arrowheads*).

FILM CRIMPING (Fig. 10.30)

At one time, the "fingernail artifact" was blamed on the mishandling of the film by persons with long fingernails. The reason for this is that the artifacts are usually curved and resemble fingernail marks. Actually, this artifact is the **result of mishandling the film** by causing the film to crimp as it is pressed firmly between the thumb and index finder, then bent as it is withdrawn from the box or cassette. The crimping causes emulsion damage and can occur anytime before processing. These marks are black in the image. However, the emulsion can still be damaged by scratching it with long fingernails.

DAMAGED SCREEN (Fig. 10.31)

Screens are sometimes improperly manipulated by bending back a portion of the screen to insert or remove a film. Over many repetitions, this causes the screen to crack. This error occurs only with the soft, pliable cassettes for which the **screen should be completely withdrawn**, then folded back to place film. Routine modifications of proper technique can often cause damage to the equipment and degradation of image quality. Another problem is a scratch on the screen that produces a white or clear line on the film, representing an area of nonexposure where the screen did not fluoresce. Dirty, dusty screens will develop

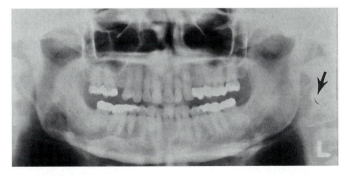

Figure 10.30. Film Crimping. The crimp mark (*arrow*) resembles a fingernail indentation in the film; long fingernails are not the cause.

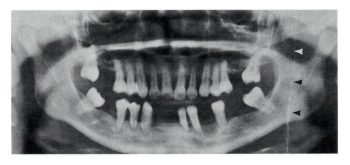

Figure 10.31. Damaged Screen. A crack or scratch in the screen prevents the area from fluorescing, producing a white mark in the image corresponding to the damaged area of the screen (*arrowheads*).

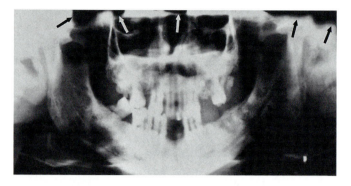

Figure 10.32. Split Cassette. Black, overexposed areas at the edges of a film caused by light leaking into a damaged cassette (*arrows*).

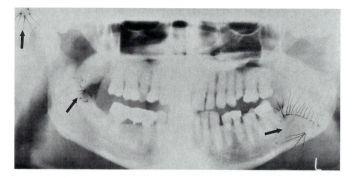

Figure 10.33. Static Electricity. Several patterns of static electricity (*arrows*).

small pits over time, which result in many small, white spots in the image at the site of each pit. These pits represent small pinpoint scratches on the screen surface and will no longer fluoresce; thus, the clear unexposed areas in the image are produced.

SPLIT CASSETTE (Fig. 10.32)

Most flexible vinyl cassettes are so designed because they must be wrapped around a curved drum at the cassette rotation assembly. Over time, the heat-sealed margins of the vinyl material may split and allow light to enter into the cassette and expose the film. Rigid cassettes are not subject to this problem, although light leaks do occur over time. This occurs as the felt wears away at the edges of the cassette back or cover, which ultimately allows light to leak in and expose the film. Exposure to light due to cassette leaks produces black streaks and marks around the edges of the film at the site(s) of the light leak(s). During monthly maintenance inspections, the operator should make certain that the cassette(s) are light-tight by placing a blank film inside and exposing the cassette to a bright light.

NO IDENTIFICATION

All panoramic machines must have the "R" and/or "L" markers to properly orient the right and left sides of the patient in the image. Some manufacturers place these markers on or in the cassette. If these markers are removed or lost, the film should be discarded. Legally, the patient's anatomical features (such as a crown or missing tooth) must not be used to label the film after it has been exposed. It is also recommended that the operator label the patient information by first writing pertinent data—such as the patient name, patient age, and date of procedure—on a card. The card is placed over one edge of the exposed film before processing and further exposed momentarily to

light with a labeling machine. The processed film will now have unalterable patient information as part of the image.

STATIC ELECTRICITY (Fig. 10.33)

Static electricity will cause black lightning-like or starburst artifacts in the film emulsion when the following two circumstances coexist: dry air and friction on the surface of the film. The dry air occurs especially in winter when heating systems dry out the air. The friction occurs when a film is withdrawn rapidly, especially from a new or full box of film or from a flexible cassette. The solution is to humidify the darkroom with a bowl of water, humidifier, or antistatic pad on the floor and to handle the film carefully when withdrawing it from the box or cassette. Static electricity can occur anytime before processing.

FOG (Fig. 10.34)

Panoramic film is exposed by fluorescent light. Thus, the light-sensitive emulsion is subject to degradation by sources of fog in the darkroom, such as white light leaks, improper safelight filter, improper safelight bulb wattage, distance from the counter top, and even the glow from a

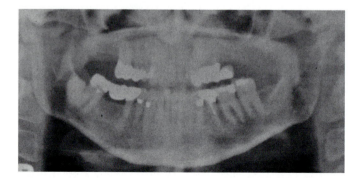

Figure 10.34. Fog. Generalized gray appearance of unwanted density (fog).

Analysis of Panoramic Procedural Errors

Error and Cause	Identifying Features	Correction
Not starting at "home base"	A portion of the film is blank A portion of the anatomy is lost at the edge of the film	Align the machine and/or cassette with starting point
Cassette resistance	One or several dark vertical bands on the film; these represent areas of overexposure as the cassette is stopped, but radiation continues to be emitted until the end of the cycle	Be certain to remove thickly padded items of clothing In stocky patients with a short neck, the cassette may need to be raised slightly above the ideal position
Paper or lint in screen	Radiopacity of unusual shape and location Foreign object prevents complete exposure of film by fluorescent screen	Periodic inspection and cleaning of the screens
"Fingernail" artifact	Crescent-shaped radiolucency	Avoid rough handling of the film when removing from the box or cassette
Static electricity	Lightning-like radiolucency; dot-like radiolucencies Star-burst and other patterns	Dry air in the darkroom can be humidified with a humidifier or large bowl of water. Avoid rapidly pulling the film from envelope-type cassettes or full box of film
White-light exposure	A portion of the film appears overexposed	Avoid smoking near film Check other sources of light leaks in the darkroom, i.e., unsafe safelight or radio Check integrity of cassette
Double exposure	Two images on the same film	Always place exposed films in the same location and where they may not be mistaken for unexposed films
Underexposed	Film too light	Increase kV and/or mA depending on the machine Place film between screens, not to one side only Check developer solution
Overexposed	Film too dark	Decrease kV and/or mA depending on the machine
No name	Patient's name or identification number not on the film	Use film imprinter, special labeling tape, or special pen

radio or cigarette, should smoking be permitted in the darkroom.

REVIEW QUESTIONS

1. If the patient is positioned too far forward, a panoramic radiograph will have:

A. Incisors that appear too large.
B. Incisors that appear too small.
C. Incisors that appear too wide.
D. Incisors that appear too narrow.

2. Which of the following structures can be projected as bilateral structures in continuous image panoramic machines?

1. Hard palate.
2. Epiglottis.
3. Hyoid bone.
4. Vertebral column.
   A. 1, 2, and 4.
   B. 1, 2, and 3.
   C. 2 and 4.
   D. 1 and 3.
   E. 1, 2, 3, and 4.

3. Which of the following are characteristics of "ghost images" on the panoramic x-ray film?

   1. Located opposite side of film from real images.
   2. Below the real image.
   3. Larger than real image.
   4. Smaller than real image.
   5. Vertical component is blurred out, horizontal component is elongated and not blurred out.
      A. 2 and 5.
      B. 1 and 3.
      C. 1, 4, and 5.
      D. 1, 3, and 5.
      E. 1, 2, and 4.

4. In panoramic radiography, spreading-out of the nasal turbinate is seen when the patient is:

   1. Too far forward.
   2. Too far back.
   3. Twisted.
   4. Tilted.
      A. 1 and 3.
      B. 1 and 4.
      C. 2 and 3.
      D. 2 and 4.

5. The ghost image of the spine, seen as a radiopaque band in the center of the panoramic image, is due to positioning the patient:

   A. Too far forward.
   B. Too far back.
   C. In a twisted position.
   D. In a slumped position.

6. Ghost images of the contralateral rami occur due to which panoramic malpositioning problem?

   A. Patient too far forward.
   B. Patient too far back.
   C. Chin tilted upward.
   D. Chin tilted downward.

7. When the double image of the palate in the panoramic radiograph becomes prominent and obscures the apices of the maxillary teeth, the patient is positioned:

   A. Too far forward.
   B. Too far back.
   C. With the chin raised too high.
   D. With the chin depressed too low.

CASE-BASED QUESTIONS

Special Note: When assessing the panoramic image, remember that multiple positioning errors occur and combinations of positioning and technical errors occur in the same image. Select the most correct choice(s).

CASE 10.1

1. The positioning error(s) in this case is (are):

   A. Slumped.
   B. Slumped and twisted.
   C. Too far forward.
   D. Chin down too low.

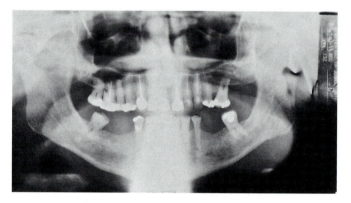

Case 10.1

2. The technical error in this case is:

   A. A light leak.
   B. Fog.
   C. Static electricity.
   D. Chemical (developer) stain.

CASE 10.2

1. The positioning error in this case is:

   A. Too far forward.
   B. Too far back.

C. Chin too low.
D. Chin too high.

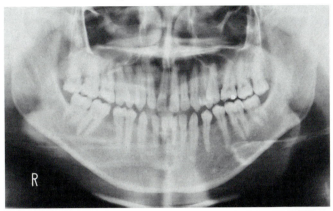

Case 10.2

CASE 10.3

1. The positioning error(s) in this case is (are):

   A. Too far forward.
   B. Too far back.
   C. Chin too low.
   D. Too far forward and no biteblock.

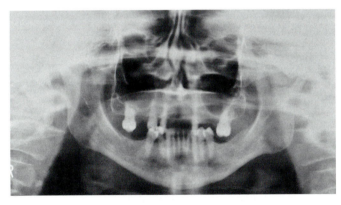

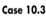

Case 10.3

CASE 10.4

1. The positioning error(s) in this case is (are) (see figure below)

   A. Eyeglasses left on.
   B. Damaged screen.
   C. Foreign object in cassette and damaged screen.
   D. Earrings and eyeglasses left on.

CASE 10.5

1. The error(s) in this case is (are):

   A. Patient slumped and tongue not on palate.
   B. Vinyl cassette light leak.
   C. Chin not on chin rest and patient too far back.
   D. Foreign object in cassette and chin not on chin rest.
   E. Apron artifact and tongue not on palate.

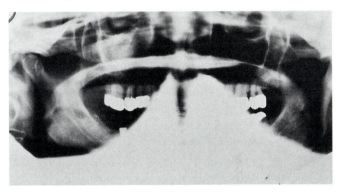

Case 10.5

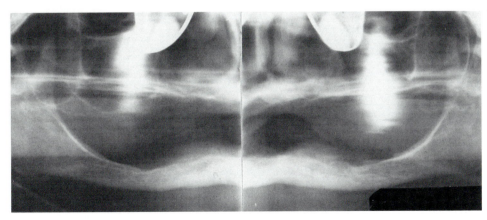

Case 10.4

CASE 10.6

1. The positioning error(s) in this case is (are):

    1. Too far forward.
    2. Too far back.

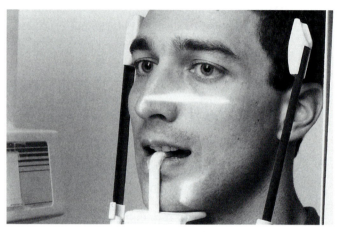

Case 10.6

3. Lips open.
4. Patient twisted.
5. Patient tilted.
A. 2 and 3.
B. 1 and 4.
C. 1 and 3.
D. 3 and 5.
E. 2 and 4.

BIBLIOGRAPHY

Christen AG, Segretto VA. Distortion artifacts encountered in Panorex radiography. J Am Dent Assoc 1968;77:1096–1101.

Farhood VW, Steed DS. Pseudocysts: two cases. Oral Surg 1979;48:491.

Langland OE, Langlais RP, McDavid WD. Panoramic radiology. 2nd ed. Philadelphia: Lea & Febiger, 1989:224–271.

McVaney TP, Kalkwarf KL. Misdiagnosis of an impacted supernumerary tooth from a panoramic radiograph. Oral Surg 1976;41:678–681.

Sämfors KA, Welander U. Distortion in the pantomogram due to object movement. Sven Tandläk Tidskr 1992;65:21–26.

Schiff T, D'Ambrosio J, Glass BJ, et al. Common positioning and technical errors in panoramic radiography. J Am Dent Assoc 1986;113:422–426.

Note to Instructors: An optional workshop, entitled "Troubleshooting Panoramic Errors," is possible if the instructor can make sets of films with panoramic errors for the students to share. Ask the students to identify the error(s) and state how to correct them.

A set of panoramic errors can be made available by the authors to instructors for duplication and student use. Multiple sets are available on a low cost-recovery basis. Please call (210) 567-3340 or fax (210) 567-3334.

Special Radiographic Techniques

11

OBJECTIVES

Upon successful completion of this unit, the student will be able to:

1. *Explain special techniques for use in children and edentulous patients as well as in endodontics, implants, and digital imaging.*

2. *Describe the minimum standard of care in implant imaging.*

3. *List specific extraoral techniques for the imaging of the skull, paranasal sinuses, and temporomandibular joint.*

4. *Test his or her knowledge by answering the Review Questions.*

KEY WORDS/PHRASES

buccal-object rule
cassette
cephalometric radiography
charge coupled device
Clark's rule
computed tomography
cross-sectional tomography
digital detectors
digital imaging
edentulous radiography
endodontic radiography

hypocycloidal tomography
image storage phosphor
implant imaging
intensifying screens
linear tomography
localization
magnetic resonance imaging
minimum standard of care for
  implants
panoramic temporomandibular
  joint projection

pediatric radiography
Richards' technique
sagittal tomography
T-Mat film
temporomandibular joint
  tomography
transcranial lateral
  temporomandibular joint
  projection
tube-shift method

INTRODUCTION

There are several special radiographic examinations that can be used in the diagnosis and prevention of diseases and abnormalities of the head and neck region. These radiographic examinations include techniques for specific circumstances and extraoral radiography.

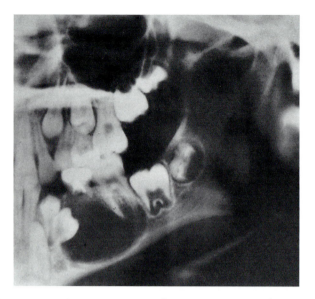

Figure 11.1. Dentigerous Cyst. Large dentigerous cyst surrounding a mandibular second premolar in a 9-year-old child.

TECHNIQUES FOR SPECIFIC CIRCUMSTANCES

PEDIATRIC RADIOGRAPHY

Radiographs of children reveal many conditions that cannot be discovered by any other method. Without radiographs, it is often impossible to identify dental disease and to plan appropriate treatment (Fig. 11.1). Congenital and pathologic disorders are often detected during childhood. Many of these disorders produce changes in the teeth. Most of the odontogenic tumors and cysts arise within the jaw bones during the period of tooth development. Additionally, some malignant disorders—such as histiocytosis X, Ewing's sarcoma, other sarcomas, Burkitt's lymphoma, and leukemia—all occur in children. The decision to take radiographs should be based on the expected benefit to the patient (Fig. 11.2).

Radiographic Surveys for Children

If it has been determined that a child requires a complete radiographic survey, the final factor to be considered

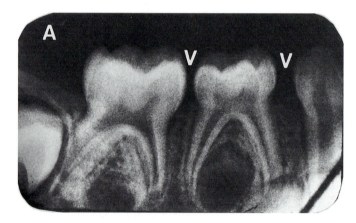

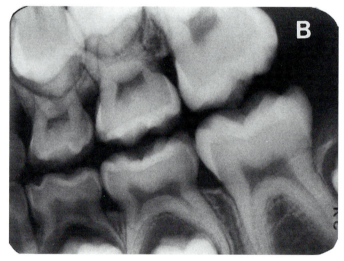

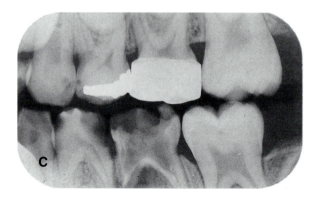

Figure 11.2 Selection Criteria (5 Years of Age and Younger). **(A)** Children 5 years and younger often have spaces (white arrows) between their posterior teeth, and one should defer taking bitewing radiographs until all posterior spacing is closed. (Note the beginning of calcification of premolars.) **(B)** Posterior bitewing radiograph of child with no dental caries and tooth contact. (Note erupting premolars underneath the primary molars.) If indicated, bitewing radiographs for caries detection are usually taken every 12 to 18 months in the absence of dental caries with primary tooth contact, as seen here, or every 24 months with permanent tooth contact. **(C)** Posterior bitewings of a child (6 years of age or younger) with a high risk for caries. A child with a **high risk** of dental caries should have bitewing radiographs made as soon as posterior primary teeth are in contact.

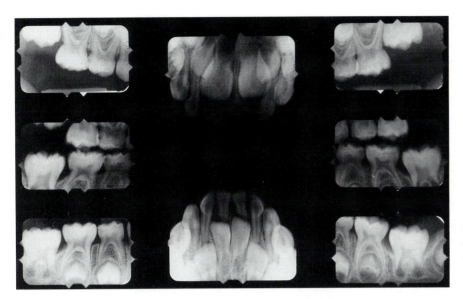

Figure 11.3. The Early Eruptive Stage (5 Years of Age and Younger). A no. 2 regular periapical film is used as an occlusal film for maxillary and mandibular anterior teeth. No. 0 pedo film is used for the posterior periapical and bitewing films.

is the number and size of films to be used in the survey. The age and behavior of the child may very well determine the type of radiographic survey to be made. However, irrespective of the size and number of films, the radiographic survey must be complete to be considered diagnostic. It must reveal all the present and developing dentition and oral conditions of the patient.

Periapical Complete-Mouth Survey in Children

If a panoramic x-ray machine is not available, the following complete periapical radiographic surveys are recommended for those children in the following three groups: (1) the early eruptive stage (5 years and younger) (Fig. 11.3), (2) mixed dentition group (6 to 9 years) (Fig. 11.4A), and (3) preadolescent group (10 to 12 years) (Fig. 11.4B). Of course, these are only guidelines; some children are large or more advanced dentally for their age. The important thing to remember is that radiography for children has to be **flexible** and **individualized,** and the type of radiographic technique, film size, and the number of films to be ordered is unique for each child. It is recommended that to minimize exposure to children, radiographs should be taken with a long beam indicating device (BID) paralleling, high-kilovoltage technique using the fastest dental film available (E+), rectangular collimation (if possible), and film-holders with beam-aiming devices. The patient should be shielded with a torso leaded apron (to protect the body and gonads) and a leaded cervical collar (to protect the thyroid) (Fig. 11.5). Children in the younger age groups may require a child's chair attached to the adult chair to take radiographs conveniently (Fig. 11.6). When these surveys are used, there will always be more radiation dose to the child than with panoramic radiography.

Panoramic Radiography in Children

If a panoramic x-ray machine is available, the panoramic radiograph with or without posterior bitewings, as required, is the baseline radiographic survey of choice (Fig. 11.7). Panoramic radiography is unequaled in evaluating growth and developmental patterns in the young child, preadolescent, and adolescent. There is no simpler, quicker technique, nor is there an alternate method of examining the teeth and jaws with less radiation dose to the child.

ENDODONTIC RADIOGRAPHY

The endodontic radiograph is much more difficult to take than the routine periapical radiograph. The major reason for this difficulty is that exposure of the film is made under adverse visual conditions, because the endodontic working radiographs are made with the rubber dam and other instruments in place. Although the basic principles of dental radiography do not change, the problem is related to visualization of the tooth for proper film positioning and cone (BID) angulation due to the presence of endodontic instruments. Because the patient cannot close on a biteblock, it becomes necessary to stabilize the film by means of various film-holders (Figs. 11.8–11.10) used in endodontic procedures. The figures should be consulted for hints in using the hemostat and the Dentsply/Rinn Snapex (Elgin, IL) endodontic film-holders to make endodontic radiography simpler and more accurate (Figs. 11.11 and 11.12). Having the patient hold the film with a finger is **not** recommended.

A single radiograph taken from one direction only may not provide sufficient diagnostic information when

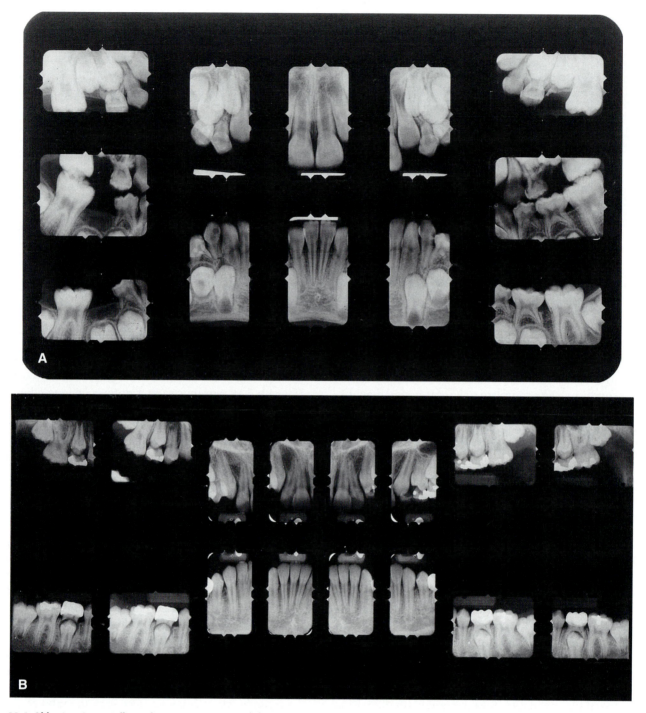

Figure 11.4. Older Age Group Full-Mouth Surveys. **(A)** Mixed dentition stage (6 to 9 years of age). This full-mouth radiographic survey is completed with no. 1 narrow films. A no. 2 regular film is used for the posterior bitewings (as seen here) if the child is large enough. **(B)** Preadolescent group (10 to 12 years of age).

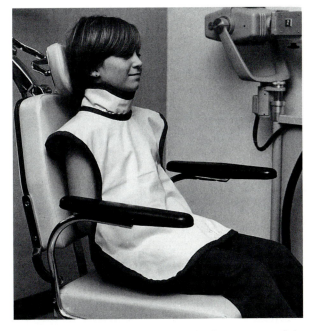

Figure 11.5. Leaded Torso Apron and Thyroid Collar. Torso and thyroid leaded shields for a child.

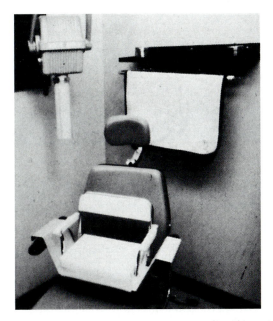

Figure 11.6. Child Chair Used In Dental Radiography. A commercial child's chair used in dental radiography.

multirooted teeth or teeth with curved roots are involved endodontically. Under these circumstances, at least two periapical radiographs should be taken to aid in gaining a three-dimensional perspective. One radiograph should be taken at a normal vertical and horizontal angulation, the other at a 20° horizontal angle either from the mesial or distal direction.

LOCALIZATION TECHNIQUES

Localization is indicated in the following instances: endodontic treatment of some teeth, foreign bodies, broken needles, broken instruments, filling materials in the alveolar process, retained roots, impacted supernumerary and unerupted teeth, calculi in a gland or duct of salivary glands, fractures of the maxilla and mandible, fracture of condyles, and expansion of the alveolar process in cyst formation. The methods of localization are as follows: tube-shift method (Clark's technique), and the buccal-object rule (Richards' technique).

Tube-Shift Method of Localization

This method was first described by Clark in 1909. It is used to determine the buccolingual relationship of foreign objects and impacted or unerupted teeth within the jaws. The method requires two periapical radiographs of the area in question, shifting the tube horizontally between exposures. The rule governing the tube-shift method of

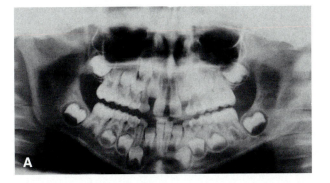
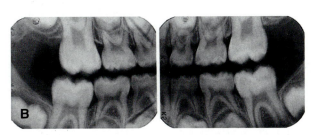

Figure 11.7. Panoramic Radiographic Survey and Posterior Bitewings. Panoramic survey with posterior bitewings of the same patient. Radiographs supplement each other and significantly reduce the radiation dose over intraoral surveys. **(A)** Panoramic radiograph. **(B)** Posterior bitewings.

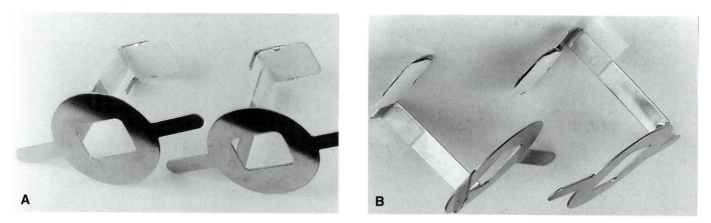

Figure 11.8. Masel Precision Endodontics Instruments. The arm is offset in these instruments so the radiograph may be taken without removing the files, reamers, or rubber dam clamp. (**A**) Anterior instruments. (**B**) Posterior instruments.

localization is as follows. If the unerupted tooth or foreign body moves in the **same direction** when the tubehead (not the cone [BID]) is shifted horizontally, the unerupted tooth or foreign body is located on the **lingual** side. If it moves in the **opposite direction** when the tubehead (not the cone [BID]) is shifted horizontally, the location of the unerupted tooth or foreign object is on the **facial or buccal/labial.** (SLOB rule: *s*ame on *l*ingual/*o*pposite on *b*uccal.) If a full-mouth survey has been taken of a patient, an unerupted tooth or foreign object could be localized as facial or lingual to the erupted teeth by the simple application of the tube-shift rule (Fig. 11.13). This would negate the necessity of taking another film to locate the unerupted tooth, foreign object, anomalies, or pathosis.

Buccal-Object Rule Method of Localization

This method of localization of pathoses, supernumerary teeth, fractures, and foreign bodies was first suggested by Richards in 1952. The rule states that when two different radiographs are made of a pair of objects, the image of the most buccal (facial) object moves, relative to the image of the lingual object, in the same direction that the x-ray beam (cone [BID]) is directed (Fig. 11.14). The horizontal (left and right) angulation of the x-ray beam (cone [BID]) should be changed when locating vertically aligned images on the radiograph, such as root canals; the vertical (up and down) angulation of the x-ray beam (cone [BID]) should be changed when locating a horizontally aligned image on the radiograph, such as the mandibular canal. The successful application of the buccal-object rule requires two different radiographs taken of the same region. These radiographs will reveal necessary clues to locate the position of the hidden object (such as an unerupted tooth) in relation to known objects (such as erupted teeth). If buccal and lingual objects are superimposed, the two may be separated and identified by applying the buccal-object rule. In making the second

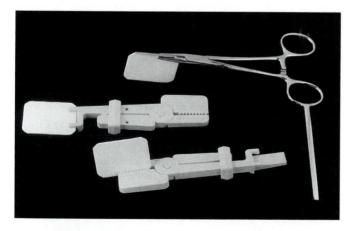

Figure 11.9. Film-Holders That Can Be Used for Endodontic Radiography. (*Lower*) Dunvale Snap-A-Ray film-holders. (*Upper*) Hemostat to hold film in patient's mouth.

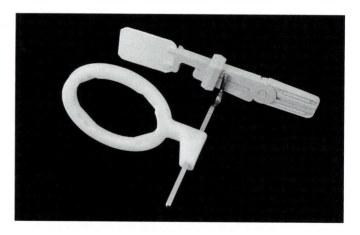

Figure 11.10. Dentsply/Rinn Snapex Film-Holders.

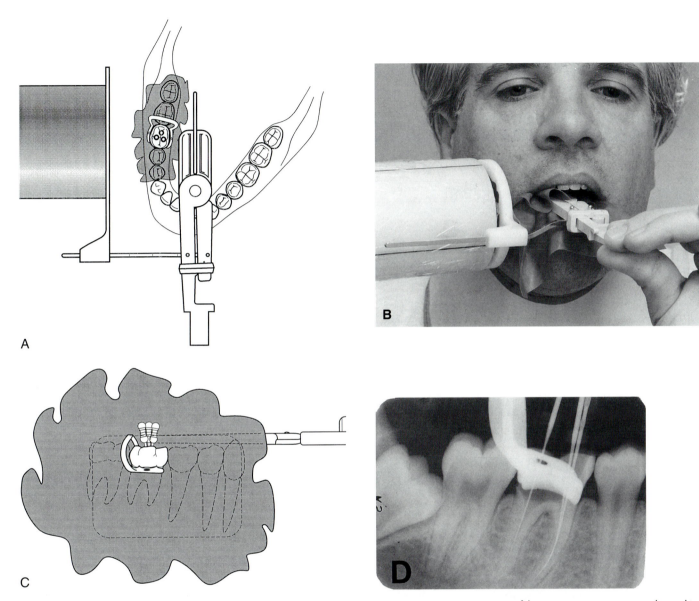

Figure 11.11. Using Dentsply/Rinn Snapex Endodontic Film-Holder in Mandibular Posterior Region. (**A**) Top view of the instrument in position to take working radiograph of mandibular first molar. (**B**) Patient with instrument in place for mandibular right first molar endodontic working radiograph. (**C**) Lateral view of instrument in position to take working radiograph of mandibular first molar. (**D**) Right first molar radiograph taken with Snapex Film-Holder.

radiograph, the horizontal or vertical angulation of the beam should be altered. When the second radiograph is compared with the first (original), the buccal object will appear to have moved in the same direction as the beam.

EDENTULOUS RADIOGRAPHY

Studies have shown that approximately one of four edentulous patients have pathologic conditions such as residual roots, unerupted and supernumerary teeth, cysts, residual areas of infection, and foreign bodies as well as other less frequently seen abnormalities. Clinical examination of the edentulous ridges alone is an insufficient basis on which to determine the health of the edentulous ridges and their surrounding tissues.

Panoramic Edentulous Survey

If a panoramic x-ray machine is available, the panoramic radiograph is the baseline radiographic survey of choice. The panoramic technique produces an image that provides exceptional coverage of both jaws on one radiograph and results in much less radiation dose than the edentulous complete mouth survey (Fig. 11.15).

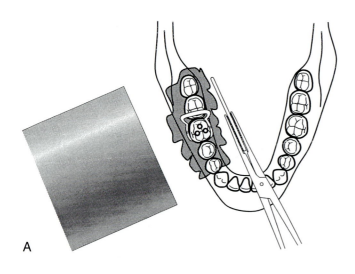

A

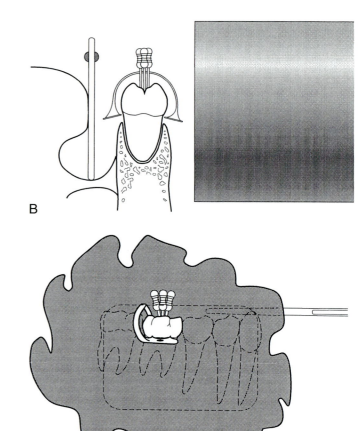

B

C

Figure 11.12. Posterior Mandibular Paralleling Technique Taking Endodontic Radiograph Using the Hemostat. In taking endodontic radiographs of the mandibular premolar and molar teeth, the paralleling technique can easily be followed without difficulty using the hemostat technique. This is because the teeth are, in most cases, parallel to the midsagittal plane. (**A**) Top view. (**B**) Front view. (**C**) Lateral view.

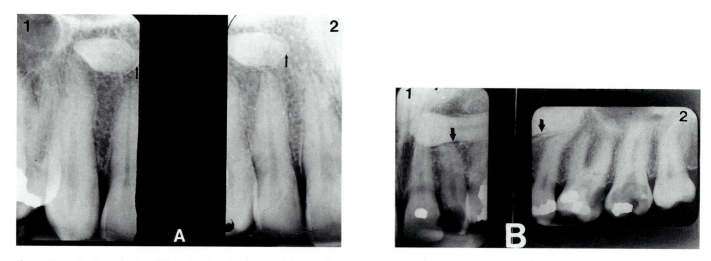

Figure 11.13. Horizontal Tube-Shift Method Localization. **A**(1) Note the position of mesiodens in lateral periapical radiography (*arrow*). (2) In central incisor periapical, the mesiodens moves in direction of tube-shift (*arrow*); therefore, mesiodens is lingual to other anterior teeth in the arch. **B**(1) Lateral incisor periapical radiograph of impacted canine. (2) Molar periapical radiograph. The impacted canine moves horizontally in the direction of the tube-shift to the posterior. The cementoenamel junction of canine (*arrows*) moves from distal of lateral incisor to mesial of second premolar. Therefore, canine is lingual to other teeth in left maxillary arch.

Edentulous Complete-Mouth Periapical Survey

If no panoramic x-ray machine is available, the edentulous survey may be taken by either the paralleling or bisecting angle technique. As much of the ridge as possible should be covered with the film, and the central ray should be directed to the center of the film. The objective is to show as much of the bone as possible on the film. A 14-film survey using no. 2 film is recommended for the edentulous complete radiographic survey (Fig. 11.16). If there is minimal resorption of the edentulous ridge, the paralleling technique using film-holders can be used. Cotton rolls, blocks of Styrofoam, or a combination can be used with the paralleling instruments. Generally, the exposure time is decreased slightly for edentulous patients.

IMPLANT IMAGING

Radiography offers the sole method of noninvasive analysis of bone required for implant therapy. It helps the clinician determine the quantity of bone present, quality of bone available, and location of critical anatomic structures. Generally, it is sound practice to obtain multiple views of the proposed site to assess it adequately.

Minimum Standard of Care in Implant Imaging

Following the clinical examination, the minimum standard of care for the radiologic assessment before initiating implant therapy consists of sagittal and cross-sectional linear tomograms of each implant site. Periapical, occlu-

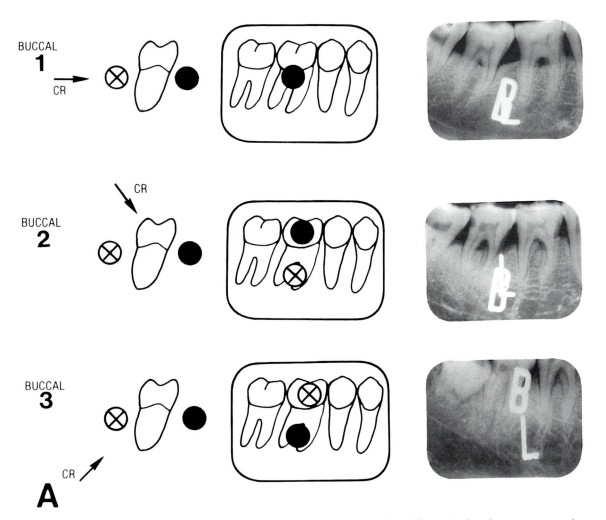

Figure 11.14. Buccal-Object Rule (Vertical and Horizontal Shift). (**A**) *Vertical shift.* Buccal and lingual foreign bodies change position with vertical shift of x-ray beam. (*1*) The original radiograph. Buccal and lingual objects are superimposed. (*2*) The beam is directed inferiorly (positive vertical angulation). The buccal object (*B*) moves inferiorly while the lingual object (*L*) moves superiorly. (*3*) The beam is directed superiorly (negative vertical angulation). The buccal object (*B*) moves superiorly while the lingual object (*L*) moves inferiorly. (*Horizontal shift continued on page 274*)

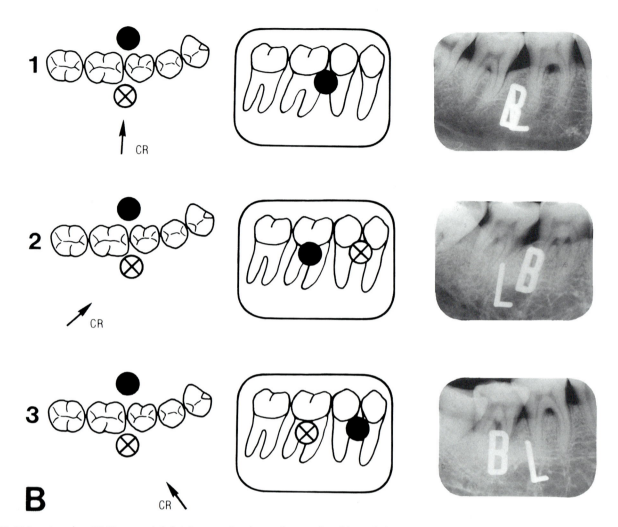

Figure 11.14 (continued). **(B)** *Horizontal shift.* (*1*) Original radiograph. Buccal and lingual objects are superimposed. (*2*) The beam is directed mesially. The buccal object (*B*) moves mesially while the lingual object (*L*) moves distally. (*3*) The beam is directed **distally**. The buccal object (*B*) moves distally while the lingual object (*L*) moves mesially.

sal, cephalometric, and sometimes panoramic radiography are used commonly instead of tomograms. Although these images may be used in conjunction with the minimum standard, such images or combination of images do **not** represent the minimum standard of care for implant imaging.

Cross-Sectional and Sagittal Tomography for Implants (Fig. 11.17)

The minimum standard of care and the most cost-effective method of radiographic assessment of one to several implant sites are both cross-sectional (coronal) and sagittal tomography, either linear or multidirectional. These tomographic radiographs are made on special tomographic equipment. Use of **both** cross-sectional and sagit-

tal tomograms is necessary to obtain a three-dimensional view of each implant site and to make accurate measurements. Vertical measurements should only be made on the sagittal tomogram.

Computed Tomography for Implants (Fig. 11.18)

Computed tomography (CT) is probably the most useful imaging modality for presurgical implant assessment when multiple implant sites in multiple arches are involved. In addition, most contemporary work stations and the software used to process the CT image data are rapid, detailed, and allow visualization of the proposed sites on a 1:1 ratio, that is, life-sized. The disadvantages of CT for use in implant imaging are (1) the cost of a CT exami-

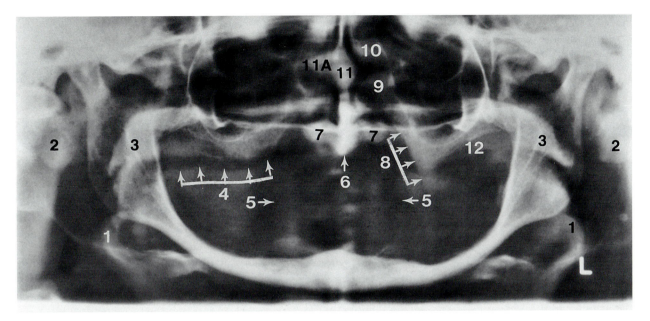

Figure 11. 15. Panoramic Edentulous Survey. Note severely resorbed edentulous ridges. Epiglottis (bilateral) (*1*), ear lobe (*2*), soft palate (bilateral) (*3*), dorsum of tongue (*4*), upper and lower lips (*5*), tip of nose (*6*), ala of nose (*7*), nasolabial fold (*8*), inferior turbinate (*9*), middle turbinate (*10*), soft tissue of nasal septum (*11*), spreading out effect of nasal septum (*11A*), and gingiva at crest of maxillary left ridge (*12*).

nation, (2) the significantly higher amounts of radiation exposure, (3) the artifacts from dental restorations that can compromise the image at the selected site, and (4) common to all tomographic techniques, the CT images may not reveal with sufficient detail the important vital structures such as the mandibular canal.

DIGITAL IMAGING (Fig. 11.19)

Digital radiography is an image acquisition process that produces **radiographic images** in digital form. Digital radiographic images may be acquired by radiographic film (**indirect digital radiography**) or by detectors (**direct digital radiography**). The direct digital systems can be grouped into two main system categories: (1) the **charged coupled device** (Trophy RVG [Trophy Radiologie, Paris, France], Regam Sens-A-Ray [Regam Medical Systems AB, Sundsvall, Sweden], Gendex Vixa [Gendex Co., Des Plaines, IL], and Villa Flash-Dent [Villa Sistemi Medicale, Srd., Buccinasco, Italy]) with small active image areas with wire connections from sensor to computer and an instantaneous image display, and (2) the image plate (storage phosphor) Sordex Digora System (Soredex Medical Systems, Soredex Orion Corp., Helsinki, Finland). The most

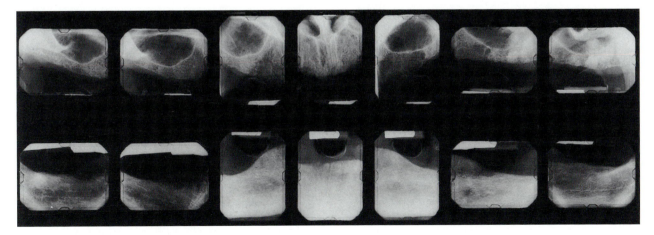

Figure 11.16. Edentulous Complete-Mouth Periapical Survey. Fourteen-film survey using no. 2 periapical film only.

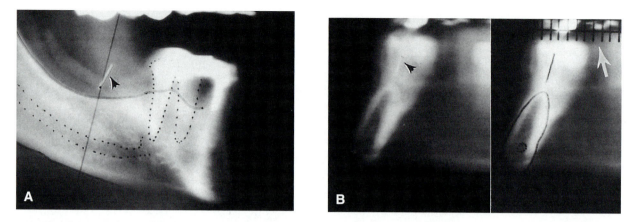

Figure 11.17. Linear Tomography for Implants. (**A**) Sagittal cut with tracings of structures of interest. (**B**) Cross-sectional cut. A magnified scale (*arrow*) is included with the tracing. (A radiopaque pin [*arrowhead*] identifies the desired placement of the implant as marked on the cast.)

common detector is the **charged coupled device** (CCD), which is a solid state electronic device. In the Digora System, a fundamentally different concept for **digital image** acquisition is used. The Digora System does not use a CCD, but uses storage phosphors instead. With either system, the digital image may be stored for future use, printed when a hard copy is required, or transmitted electronically to a remote site (teleradiography). Advantages of the digital techniques include immediate image display with no waiting for darkroom processing; the ability to manipulate the image by contrast enhancement or grayscale reversal; reduction in patient radiation dose; elimination of film, darkroom, processors, processing chemicals, film mounts, and film mounting; and significantly less cost, including supplies (such as film, film mounts, processing chemicals, processor maintenance, repairs and replacement) and the space required to accommodate a darkroom or processor with a daylight loader.

EXTRAORAL RADIOGRAPHY

An extraoral radiograph is made by placing the film in a cassette against the side of the head or face and projecting the x-rays from the other side. Extraoral radiographs are taken using screen film and appropriate intensifying screens within a cassette. Intensifying screens are used because they decrease the x-ray dose (less mAs) to the patient, yet still afford a properly exposed radiograph. The x-ray film used with intensifying screens has a photosensitive (light-sensitive) emulsion on both sides of the film and is called screen film. The film is sandwiched between two intensifying screens in a cassette, so that the emulsion on each side of the film can be exposed to the light from the intensifying screen adjacent to it (Fig. 11.20). The intensifying screen functions to absorb the energy of the x-ray beam that has penetrated the patient. The screen then converts this energy into light, which

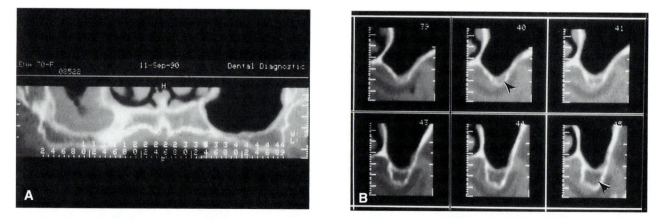

Figure 11.18. CT for Implants. (**A**) Panoramic-like reformatted image of the maxilla. Note the 1-to-1 mm and cm measuring scales on the edges of the image. Numeric references along the bottom indicate the location of the numbered cross-sectional cuts. (**B**) Numbered cross-sectional cuts from the left maxilla with the 1-to-1 measuring scale on the edges. Note the difference in the available bone for implants between cuts 40 and 45 (*arrowheads*).

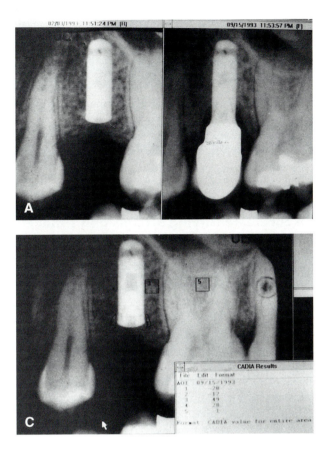

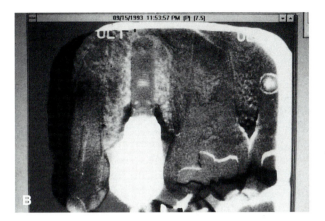

Figure 11.19. Digital Imaging of Implants. **(A)** Periapical radiographs showing the implant in February 1991 (left) versus September 1993 (right). **(B)** Subtracted image from radiographs in **A**; qualitatively, whitish areas around the implant indicate new bone formation since February 1991. **(C)** Five small area of interest (AOI) regions indicate quantitative differences in bone density. At the neck of the implant there has been bone loss (AOI *1* and *2*). At the middle of implant there has been bone gain (AOI *3* and *4*). In the control area there has been no change in the bone (AOI *5*).

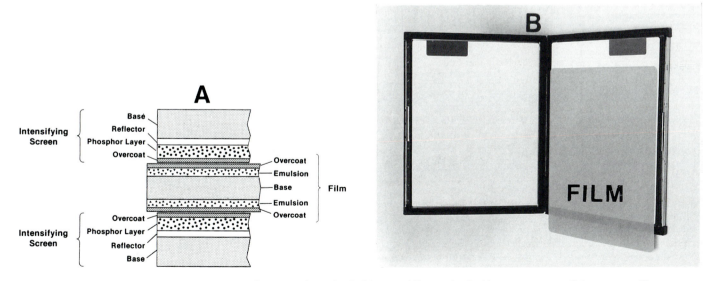

Figure 11.20. Intensifying Screens and Cassette. **(A)** Illustration shows the double-coated film sandwiched between two intensifying screens. All components of film-screen combination are shown, but not drawn to scale. For example, the thickness of the phosphor layer of the top screen may differ from that of the lower screen. **(B)** Photograph of 8- × 10-inch cassette with two white intensifying screens. The film is placed between them in the darkroom, and the cassette is closed tightly to hold the film between the two intensifying screens during exposure.

carries the same information as the original x-ray beam, to form a latent image on the x-ray film. The latent image is made visible by processing the film in chemical solutions under darkroom conditions.

FACTORS COMMON TO ALL EXTRAORAL RADIOGRAPHIC TECHNIQUES

Screen/Film Size and Screen/Film Systems

For dental use, the following screen film sizes are available: 5 × 7 inches, 5 × 12 inches (panoramic), 6 × 12 inches (panoramic), 8 × 10 inches, and 10 × 12 inches. A characteristic of x-rays is that they cause certain materials to fluoresce, that is, give off ultraviolet and/or visible light radiation. Such fluorescent materials are called phosphors. The ability of phosphors to fluoresce when excited by x-rays makes the intensifying screen possible (Fig. 11.21). Fluorescence is a form of luminescence, which refers to the emission of light by a substance caused by various kinds of stimuli such as light, chemical reactions, and ionizing radiation. The phosphor of the intensifying screen has one purpose: the conversion of the x-ray beam into visible light. This action of the phosphor can be viewed by opening a cassette in a darkened room and, while standing behind a protective barrier, exposing the intensifying screen to x-radiation. The screen will glow brightly. Depending on the phosphor selected and its treatment during manufacture, light of almost any desired color may be obtained.

Screen or photographic films are selective in their response to light of various wavelengths. When a certain type of film is exposed to light, its speed varies. It is said that certain films are more sensitive to one part of the light spectrum than to another. A film's response to various wavelengths (color) is referred to its **spectral sensitivity**. The speed of the screen/film combination is dependent on the matching of the spectral sensitivity of the film (whether it is blue, blue-green, ultraviolet, or green light) with the color emitted by the intensifying screen.

Rare Earth Intensifying Screens and T-Mat Film

Some of the newer phosphor screens are the rare earth screens. The term rare earth is used because these elements are difficult and expensive to separate from the earth and each other, not because the elements are rare. Lanthanum (La) and gadolinium (Gd) are used as rare earth phosphors. The rare earth screens emit light in approximately 60% of the green portion of the light wave spectrum. Therefore, **green-sensitive** films were developed that gave a greater sensitivity and speed to the rare earth screen-film combinations and, in turn, provided dramatic reduction in patient exposures. In 1983, T-grain film was introduced by Eastman Kodak (Rochester, NY). T-grain film contains silver halide grains that are tabular or flat, rather than pebble shaped. These flat grains have a greater cross-section, which increases their ability to absorb light from the intensifying screens. When green-sensitive T-grain film (T-Mat film) is used with rare earth green-light–emitting screens, it was found that this film-screen combination is twice as fast as calcium tungstate screen film combinations. Also, screen/film systems are designed for various applications. For instance, Kodak T-Mat L film combined with Kodak Lanex regular screens (gadolinium rare earth) provides good soft tissue visualization with a wide range of densities (long-scale contrast), whereas Kodak T-Mat G film with the same screens gives higher-contrast (short-scale contrast) radiographic images.

Cassettes

The cassette is the rigid holder that contains the screens and the film. The front surfaces or the side facing the tube should be made of material containing elements with low atomic numbers—such as in plastics, cardboard, or Bakelite—and should be as thin as practical to allow as much radiation through as possible. Attached to each cover is an intensifying screen, and the radiographic film is loaded between them. Between each screen and cover is a compression device, such as felt or rubber, which maintains close film contact with the screens when the cassette is closed and latched. The back cover is usually made of

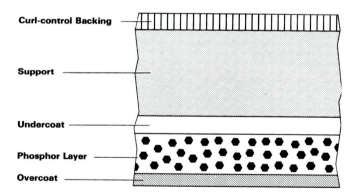

Curl-control Backing

Support

Undercoat

Phosphor Layer

Overcoat

Figure 11.21. Intensifying Screen, Physical Characteristics. Curl-control backing prevents warping or distortion of screen. The support layer is made of paper, plastic, or cardboard to impart required stiffness to the screen. Undercoat may be light-reflective, light-absorptive, or simply transparent, depending on the desired performance characteristics of the screen. Using the desired undercoat as a reflector of light will increase the speed of the screen. The phosphor layer consists of tiny phosphor crystals embedded in binder. Overcoat is a plastic protective coat. (X-rays will penetrate the overcoat layer first.)

heavy metal (aluminum, lead lined) to minimize backscatter. The hinges and hold-down clamps are usually made of stainless steel. Some of the newer cassettes feature a curved construction for more efficient expulsion of trapped air (Fig. 11.22). Some of the panoramic units use flexible plastic cassettes that wrap around a drum that rotates during the exposure cycle. A high-quality screen film radiograph depends on intimate contact maintained between the film and intensifying screen. If there is any space between the screen and the film, a loss of sharpness of the outline of the radiographic images will occur.

Identification

It is important to identify the right and left sides of the patient on the extraoral radiograph. This can be done by placing "R" and "L" lead markers on the cassette. Extraoral radiographs can be produced in the dental office using conventional dental and panoramic x-ray machines. Also, the patient can be identified by "burning-in" the information in the emulsion with the use of a simple identification photographic device before processing.

Extraoral Radiographic Units Used in Dentistry

Panoramic units are used to achieve better overall coverage of the maxillomandibular structures than conventional intraoral dental techniques can provide. Although the large medical x-ray units are specifically designed for extraoral radiography, smaller conventional dental x-ray units can be used in extraoral radiography.

SKULL RADIOGRAPHY

The skull radiographic projections used by the dentist pertain mostly to cephalometric skull radiography and temporomandibular joint (TMJ) radiography.

CEPHALOMETRIC RADIOGRAPHY

Cephalometric radiography is used by orthodontists and pediatric dentists for evaluation of the skull for prediction of growth. The technique is also used by oral surgeons for treatment planning purposes in orthognathic surgery. A head-holding device, called a cephalometer or cephalostat, is used in cephalometric radiography (Figs. 11.23 and 11.24). The cephalostat makes it possible to position and reposition the patient's head in a predetermined relationship to the x-ray beam and to the Frankfort horizontal line, which is a line connecting the superior border of the earpost of the cephalostat (porion) and the inferior border of orbit (orbitale). The most common view used in cephalometric radiography is the lateral or profile view. The lateral view is always made with the left side located nearest the cassette. In cephalometrics, the accepted distance from x-ray source to patient is 5 feet or 152.4 cm. The patient location point is measured from the midsagittal plane, which is determined as the midpoint between the earposts. The cephalostat immobilizes the patient's head by means of the nasion positioning rod and the

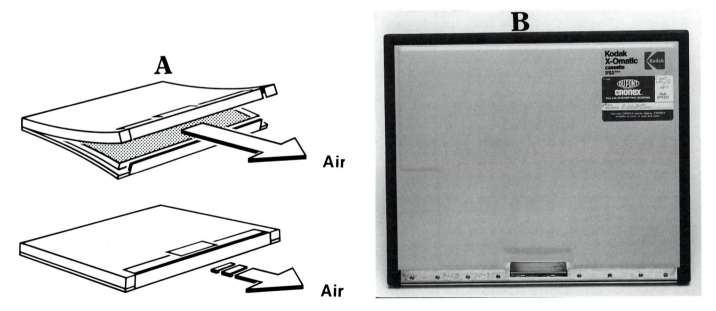

Figure 11.22. Kodak X-Omatic Cassette. **(A)** Curved construction for more efficient expulsion of trapped air and better maintenance of contact without springs. **(B)** Front of cassette in closed position.

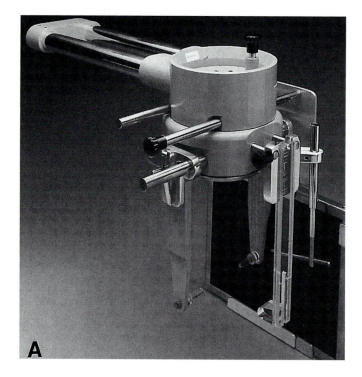

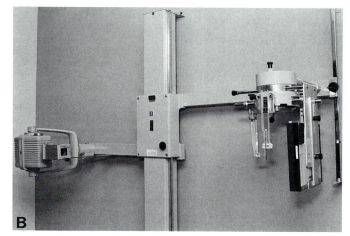

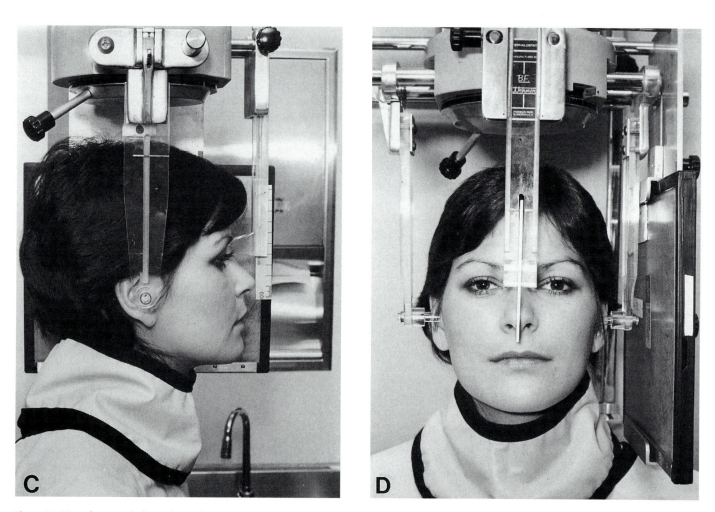

Figure 11.23. Wehmer Cephalostat for Cephalometric Radiography. (**A**) Cephalostat, close-up view. (**B**) Cephalostat and fixed dental x-ray tubehead. (**C**) Side view of lateral cephalometric projection. (**D**) Front view of lateral cephalometric projection.

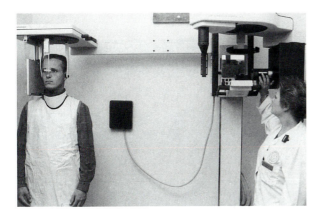

Figure 11.24. Panoramic Cephalometric Technique.

earpost plugs. The patient's head is aligned to the Frankfort plane by use of infraorbital marker. The midsagittal plane should be parallel to the horizontally placed film inside the cassette. A lateral (profile) skull cephalometric radiograph is shown in Figure 11.25. It is used to measure facial relationships and to predict or analyze growth patterns in orthodontic treatment. This is done by means of cephalometric (skull) tracings of key structures, which are then evaluated by measurements of angles and linear dimensions between the various parts.

TMJ RADIOGRAPHY

There are two TMJ radiographic techniques that can be used in the dental office: the transcranial lateral TMJ projection and the panoramic TMJ projection. There are

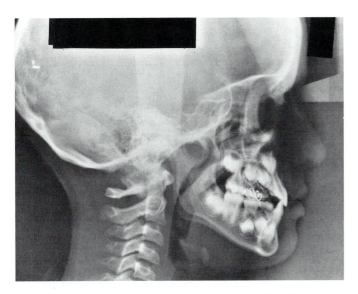

Figure 11.25. Lateral Cephalometric Radiograph. Lateral (profile) cephalometric radiograph of a child.

three TMJ radiographic techniques of such specialized character that they require equipment mostly found in hospitals, institutions, and specialty offices. These are linear or multidirectional tomography, CT, and magnetic resonance imaging (MRI).

Transcranial Lateral TMJ Projection (Fig. 11.26)

In all **transcranial** techniques, the x-ray beam is directed down across the top of the **petrous portion** of the temporal bone to the condylar head on the opposite side of the skull. This is done to avoid superimposing the petrous portion of the temporal bone over the TMJ. This oblique projection of the x-ray beam causes distortions of the three-dimensional head of the condyle and the glenoid fossa. The most that can be accomplished by transcranial projections of the TMJ is to view the lateral border of the glenoid fossa and laterosuperior border of the head of the condyle. The superior border of the condyle between the lateral and medial poles of the condyle cannot be seen on the transcranial lateral TMJ. Unfortunately, this is where most of the changes occur in TMJ disorders.

Panoramic TMJ Projection

All rotational panoramic units have special TMJ projections. The panoramic TMJ views are usually of sufficient clarity to evaluate the condyles for gross osseous changes such as erosions, masses, or displaced fractures. This view is limited because the central ray is not directed through the long axis of the condyle. The TMJ area is usually revealed as an anteroposterior oblique view. This view is not generally accepted for close examination of the TMJ. It cannot be used to evaluate the disc or the position of the condyle in the fossa (Fig. 11.27).

TMJ Tomography

Tomography is a special x-ray technique that blurs out the shadows of superimposed anatomical structures that obscure information in the radiograph. It is **not** a method of improving sharpness of the radiographic image, but is a process of controlled blurring that leaves some parts of the image less blurred than others. The tomogram is made by a special mechanism in which the x-ray tube and the film cassette are attached to a rigid connecting rod that rotates around a fixed fulcrum.

When the tube moves in one direction, the film cassette moves in the opposite direction. Tomographic techniques blur all points that lay outside the focal plane (Fig. 11.28). The fulcrum around which the system rotates is adjustable, so that any desired image layer in an anatomical structure can be selected for radiographing (Fig. 11.29).

Another factor to consider in tomography is the type of motion or movement of the x-ray tube. If the x-ray tube and the film move in a straight line, it is called a **linear tomography**. It has an advantage in that this

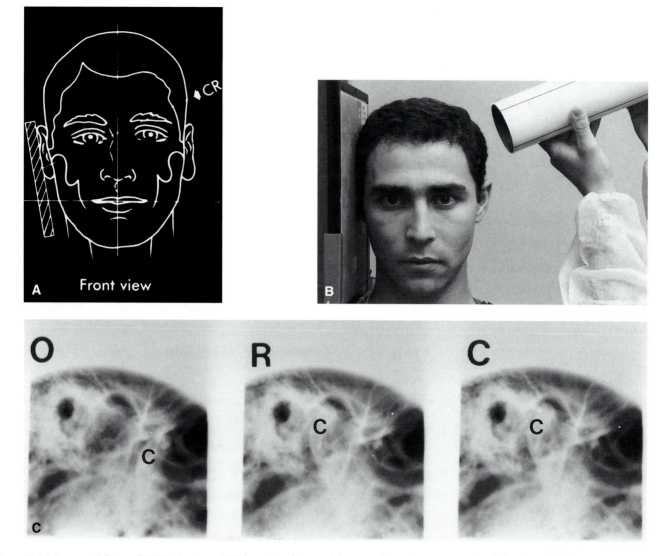

Figure 11.26. Transcranial Lateral TMJ Projection. (**A**) The point of entry of the central ray (*CR*) is 0.5 inches behind and 2 inches above the external auditory meatus on the opposite side. The CR is directed with a 25° downward vertical angulation at the condyle on the opposite side. The condylar head in the transcranial radiograph will reveal only the laterosuperior border of the condylar head because of the mandatory oblique angulation of the CR. (**B**) Position of the patient in transcranial lateral TMJ projection. (**C**) Transcranial lateral TMJ radiograph, *O*, open; *R*, rest; *C*, closed. (Smaller "*C*" indicates head of condyle in each radiograph.)

x-ray equipment is relatively inexpensive; however, it has a disadvantage in that linear structures aligned parallel to the direction of motion of the tube are not blurred as well as those lying at an angle to the tube. Therefore, tomographic equipment has been developed to produce complex types of motion that produce more effective blurring of unwanted structures (Fig. 11.30). The most complex trajectory or tube motion available is the **hypocycloidal movement**, which results in highly effective blurring; it is sometimes described as a **cloverleaf**. It has no dominant direction and is especially suitable for tomography of

small bony structures of the head (e.g., the auditory ossicles and the TMJs). Lateral tomographic slices provide a series of images that includes extensive viewing of the medial and lateral aspects of the joint (Fig. 11.31). Several tomographic units have been designed specifically for dentistry.

CT of the TMJ (Fig. 11.32)

CT scanners create digital images by measuring the transmission of an x-ray beam through tissue as the x-ray tube rotates around the patient. CT imaging offers

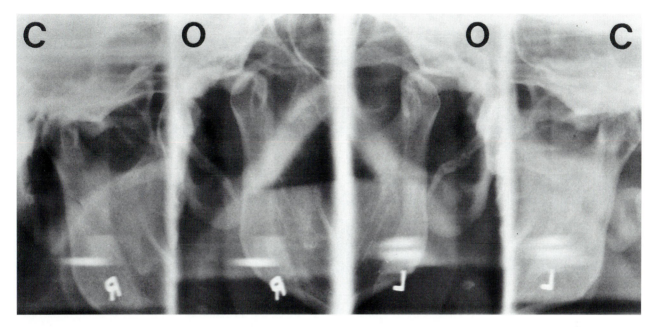

Figure 11.27. Panoramic TMJ Projection. Panoramic view of the TMJ. This is an anteroposterior oblique view of the condyles and can be used only to rule out gross pathology. *C,* closed; *O,* open.

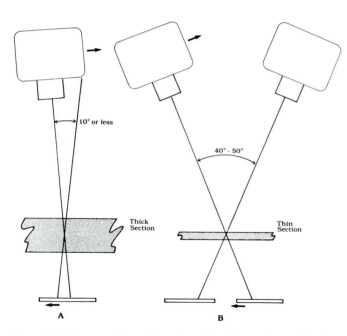

many diagnostic advantages, including the ability to produce reconstructed images in selected projections and low-contrast resolution (detail) far superior to that of all other x-ray imaging modalities. CT appears to reveal more bony detail of the TMJ than conventional tomography; how-

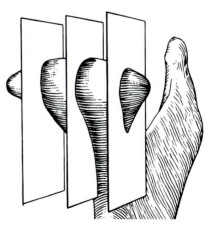

Figure 11.28. Tomography. When the tubehead moves in one direction, the film cassette moves in the opposite direction. Tomographic techniques blur all points outside the focal plane. The angles of exposure of tomography determine the thickness of the focal plane or the body section. (**A**) Zonography (narrow angle tomography). (**B**) Wide-angle tomography is best for high-contrast tissues (bone).

Figure 11.29. TMJ Tomography. The fulcrum of the TMJ tomographic system can be adjusted so that lateral condylar cuts or slices of the condylar head can be made.

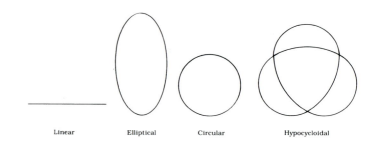

Linear   Elliptical   Circular   Hypocycloidal

Four Varieties of Tomographic Trajectory

Figure 11.30. Types of Tube Motion in Tomography. Four varieties of tomographic trajectory are shown. The hypocycloidal (cloverleaf) movement is the most complex and results in highly effective blurring of structures outside the focal plane.

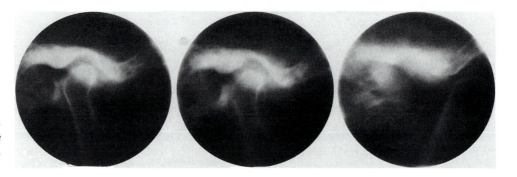

Figure 11.31. TMJ Tomographic Radiographs. Linear tomographs taken of left normal TMJ. From left to right: closed, rest, and open.

ever, in general, both imaging techniques appear to be comparable. Also, conventional tomography is less costly and delivers a smaller absorbed dose of radiation than CT.

MRI of the TMJ (Fig. 11.33)

Ionizing radiation is not used in MRI. Instead, the patient is placed in an uniform magnetic field, and electromagnetic energy temporarily changes the alignment and orientation of the hydrogen protons within the body. The area being examined is then subjected to radiofrequency waves that displace the equilibrium magnetization vector. As the magnetization vector returns to equilibrium, it gives off a signal that allows for indirect detection of the magnitude and molecular characteristics of the magnetized hydrogen protons. Using this information, a sophisticated mathematical operation, called a Fourier transformation, converts it into the final magnetic resonance image. MRI is the only imaging technique that can simultaneously image both the disc and posterior attachment as well as the condyle and mandibular fossae of both joints during

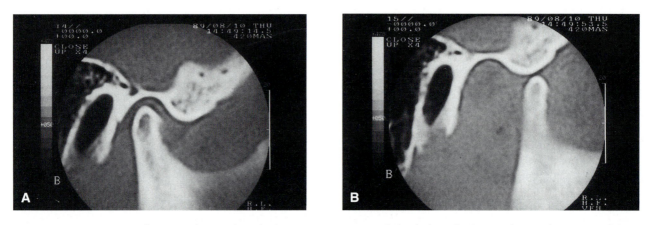

Figure 11.32. CT of TMJ. Computed tomography is indicated when a greater amount of detail about the form and internal structures of the osseous structures are required. (**A**) Closed. (**B**) Open.

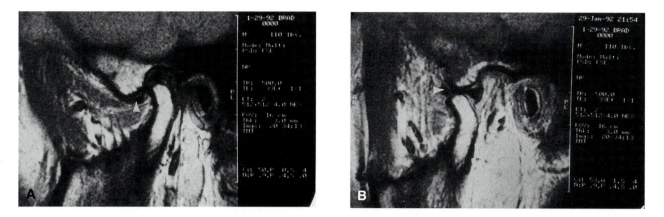

Figure 11.33. MRI of TMJ. MRI is the only imaging technique of TMJ that can simultaneously image both the disc and posterior attachment as well as the condyle and mandibular fossae of both points during a TMJ examination. (**A**) Closed anterior disc displacement (*arrowhead*). (**B**) Open. Disc has reduced to normal position (*arrowhead*). Disc and cortical bone appear black because of low water content.

a TMJ examination. Because of the high incidence of bilateral abnormalities in patients with TMJ dysfunction, this is a definite advantage. As in tomography, slices in the corrected lateral and frontal views are preferred. Both open and closed images are used to evaluate the position of the disc (Fig. 11.33).

WORKSHOP/LABORATORY EXERCISES

EXERCISE 11.1 LOCALIZATION

Materials and Equipment Needed

1. Manikin, skull, animal jaw.
2. Four no. 2 periapical films.
3. One BB (small metal ball or other metal object such as a screw).
4. X-ray machine and processing facility.

Instructions

Step 1: Obtain a manikin, skull, or animal jaw and place a radiopaque object (BB) on the buccal or lingual side. Do **not** mark the film packet. Take a standard periapical view of this object and then vary the horizontal angle by approximately 20° and expose a second film.

Step 2: Now leave the BB in the same spot on the buccal or lingual side as in Step 1. Do **not** mark the film packet. Take a standard periapical view of the object and then vary the vertical angle by approximately 20° and expose a second film.

Step 3: Process all four films and mount the films in a bitewing mount. Place the two images with the horizontal movement on one side and the two images with the vertical movement on the other side.

Step 4: Place your name on the bitewing mount and, because you know where the BB was, exchange your mount with a classmate and take your classmate's mount.

Step 5: Working in pairs, try to figure out the location of your classmate's BB.

___

CASE-BASED PROBLEM-SOLVING

In the future, you will become aware of the hassles of keeping track of inventories of x-ray supplies such as film, chemicals, bitewing tabs, biteblocks and film-positioning devices, and barrier envelopes. Also, you will begin to understand the maintenance problems associated with automatic processors, the infection control procedure problems associated with the daylight loader and the darkroom, and the time it takes to get a radiograph processed (especially with manual processing) in a tiny cubbyhole darkroom with no air circulation. So you are wondering about digital imaging. Should you trade one set of hassles for another? To help you decide, develop a comparison chart comparing the advantages and disadvantages of the two systems as you see it. What is your final decision?

REVIEW QUESTIONS

1. Which of the following statements are true concerning cephalometric radiographs?

   1. The Frankfort horizontal plane is the classic plane used in cephalometrics.
   2. It is not necessary to record the soft tissue profile in the lateral cephalometric radiograph.
   3. The posteroanterior cephalometric is the most common cephalometric radiograph produced.
   4. The accepted distance from the x-ray source to patient in cephalometric radiography is 5 feet.
   A. 1, 2, and 3.
   B. 3 and 4.
   C. 1 and 4.
   D. 2, 3, and 4.
   E. 1, 2, 3, and 4.

2. A cephalometric radiograph:

   A. Is often used to measure changes and predict growth patterns.
   B. Contains a soft tissue outline.
   C. Is commonly used by orthodontists.
   D. All of the above.

3. A radiographic image that looks like a picture of a skull taken back to front is called a:

   A. Cephalometric lateral radiograph.
   B. Posteroanterior view.
   C. Lateral.
   D. Panoramic radiograph.

4. The anatomic structures of primary importance on TMJ projections are:

   A. The condyle, joint space, and glenoid fossa.
   B. The condyle and the maxillary tuberosity.
   C. The coronoid process and the articular eminence.
   D. The articular eminence, glenoid fossa, joint space, and condyle.

5. Which of the following does not use ionizing radiation?

   A. Tomography.
   B. CT.
   C. MRI.
   D. Digital radiography.

6. Computed tomography (CT):

   A. Has the ability to distinguish minor differences between body tissues.
   B. Allows manipulation of image contrast.
   C. Uses a computer to reconstruct images.
   D. All of the above.

7. A cassette:

   A. Emits light.
   B. Is a container for film and screens.
   C. Is an instrument to align the x-ray cone.
   D. Records the patient's exposure.

8. A grid is:

   A. Used to focus a beam of electrons on the focal spot.
   B. Used to limit the size of the beam and reduce radiation exposure.
   C. Never used because it has insignificant effects.
   D. Used to reduce scatter radiation to the film.
   E. Used to reduce the patient exposure to x-rays by removing deflected photons.

9. Intensifying screens are used with extraoral films to:

   A. Increase the exposure time.
   B. Improve image quality.
   C. Decrease radiation to the patient.
   D. Increase the kVp.

10. Screen films are used with intensifying screens because these films are:

   A. More sensitive to x-rays than to light.
   B. More sensitive to light than to x-rays.
   C. Coated with silver sulfide crystals.
   D. Coated with calcium tungstate crystals.

11. A cassette was opened in the darkroom to remove and process the exposed film. A piece of black paper was discovered on the surface of the intensifying screen. The paper most likely would produce:

   A. A white or light artifact.
   B. A black artifact.
   C. No artifact.
   D. Reticulation.

BIBLIOGRAPHY

Astrand K, Reichmann S. Optimized tomography. Acta Radiol 1974;(Suppl 338).

Ballinger PW. Radiographic positions and radiologic procedures. St. Louis: CV Mosby, 1986.

Benz C, Mouyen F. Evaluation of the new Radio VisioGraphy system image quality. Oral Surg 1991;72:627–631.

Braham RL, Morris ME. Textbook of pediatric dentistry. Baltimore: Williams & Wilkins, 1980.

Broadbent, Holly B. A new technique and its application to orthodontia. Angle Orthod 1931;1:45.

Caldwell EW. Skiagraphy of the accessory sinuses of the nose. Am O Roentgenol 1906;27(2):.

Carlton RR, McKenna AA. Principles of radiographic imaging. Albany: Delmar, 1992.

Cederberg RA. Temporomandibular joint space analysis. J Craniomandib Pract 1994;12:172–177.

Clark CA. A method of ascertaining the relative position of unerupted teeth by means of film radiography. Odont Sec R Soc Med Trans 1909;3:87.

Del Rio CE, Canales ML, Preece JW. A radiographic technique for endodontics. San Antonio: University of Texas Health Science Center at San Antonio, 1982.

Downs WB. Cephalometrics in orthodontic case analysis and diagnosis. Am J Orthod 1952;38:162.

Flash Dent Product Brochure. Buccinasco, Italy: Villa Sistemi Medicali Srl, 1990.

Furkart AJ, Dove SB, McDavid WD, et al. Direct digital radiography for the detection of periodontal bone lesions. Oral Surg 1992;74:652–660.

Griffiths BM, Brown JE, Hyatt AT, et al. Comparison of three techniques for assessing working length. Int Endodont J 1992;25:279–287.

Hansson LG, Westesson PL, Katzberg RW, et al. MR imaging of the temporomandibular joint: comparison of images of autopsy specimens made at 0.3T and 1.5T with anatomic cryosections. Am J Roentgenol 1989;152:1241–1244.

Hasso AN, Christiansen EL, Alder ME. The temporomandibular joint. Radiol Clin North Am 1989;27:301–314.

Heffez L, Jordan S, Rosenberg H, et al. Accuracy of temporomandibular joint space measurements using corrected hypocycloidal tomography. J Oral Maxillofacial Surg 1987;48:137–142.

Hintze H, Wenzel A, Jones C. In-vitro comparison of D- and E-speed film radiography and RVG and Visualix digital radiography for the detection of enamel approximal and dentinal occlusal carious lesions. Caries Res 1994;28:1–9.

Hoffman DC, Berliner L Manzione J, et al. Use of direct sagittal computed tomography in diagnosis and treatment of internal derangements of the temporomandibular joint. J Am Dent Assoc 1986;113:407–411.

Horner K, Thearer AC, Walker A, et al. Radiovisiography: an initial evaluation. Br Dent J 1990;168:244–248.

Katzberg RW. Temporomandibular joint imaging. Radiology 1989;170:297–307.

Katzberg RW, Schenck J, Roberts D, et al. Magnetic resonance imaging of the temporomandibular joint meniscus. Oral Surg 1985;59:332–339.

Kodak film screen combinations. Publication M3-138. Rochester, NY: Eastman Kodak, 1983.

Larheim TA, Kolbenstvedt A. Osseous temporomandibular joint abnormalities in rheumatic disease: computed tomography versus hypocycloidal tomography. Acta Radiol 1990;31:383–387.

Molteni R. Direct digital dental x-ray imaging with Visualix/Vixa. Oral Surg 1993;76:235–243.

Mongini F. The importance of radiography in the diagnosis of TMJ dysfunctions: a comparative evaluation of transcranial radiograph and serial tomography. J Prosthet Dent 1981;45:186–198.

Musgrave MT, Westesson PL, Tallents RH, et al. Improved magnetic resonance imaging of the temporomandibular joint by oblique scanning planes. Oral Surg Oral Med Oral Pathol 1991;71:525–528.

Nelvig P, Wing K, Welander U. Sens-a-Ray: a new system for direct digital intraoral radiography. Oral Surg 1992;74:818–823.

Paquette OE, Segall RO, Del Rio C. Modified film-holder for endodontics. J Endodont 1979;5:158–160.

Richards A. Roentgenographic localization of the mandibular canal. J Oral Surg 1952;10:325.

Richards AG. The buccal object rule. Dent Radiogr Photogr 1980;53:33–56.

Rosenberg HM, Silha RE. TMJ radiography with emphasis on tomography. Dent Radiogr Photogr 1982;55:1–9.

Rosenberg HM, Greczyk R. Temporomandibular articulation tomography: a corrected anteroposterior and lateral cephalometric technique. Oral Surg Oral Med Oral Pathol 1986;62:198–204.

San Giacomo T. Topics in implantology III, radiographic treatment planning. RI Dental J 1990;12:5–11.

Sanderink GCH, Huiskens R, van der Stelt PF, et al. Image quality of direct digital intraoral x-ray sensors in assessing root canal length. Oral Surg 1994;78:125–132.

Schwaighofer BW, Tanaka TT, Klein MV, et al. MR imaging of the temporomandibular joint: a cadaver study of the value of coronal images. Am J Radiol 1990;154:1245–1249.

Shearer AC, Horner K, Wilson VHF. Radiovisionography for length estimation in root canal treatment: an in-vitro comparison with conventional radiography. Int Endodont J 1991;24:233–239.

Shelhas KP. Temporomandibular injuries. Radiology 1989;173:211–216.

Skoczylas CJ, Preece JW, Langlais RP, et al. Comparison of x-radiation doses between conventional and rare earth panoramic techniques. Oral Surg 1989;68:776–781.

Thurow RC. Atlas of orthodontic principles. St. Louis: CV Mosby, 1970.

Unger JM. Head and neck imaging. New York: Churchill Livingstone, 1987.

Van der Kuijl B, Vencen LM, de Bont LG, et al. Temporomandibular joint computed tomography development of a direct sagittal technique. J Prosthet Dent 1990;64:709–715.

Welander U, Nelvig P, Tronje G, et al. Basic technical properties of a system for direct acquisition of digital intraoral radiographs. Oral Surg 1993;75:506–516.

Winter GB. Impacted mandibular third molars. St. Louis: American Medical Book Publishers, 1926.

SECTION 4:
Radiation Health

Radiation Biology

12

John W. Preece

OBJECTIVES

Upon successful completion of this unit, the student will be able to:

1. *Relate a general knowledge of radiation biology.*

2. *Explain how tissues are affected by radiation.*

3. *Explain the various radiation factors involved in tissue damage.*

4. *Describe the host factors involving radiation injury.*

5. *State the factors affecting radiation sensitivity.*

6. *Define the various units used for radiation measurement.*

7. *Describe various concepts relating to radiation dose.*

8. *Relate a broad knowledge of specific risks to various body tissues.*

9. *List various radiation protection organizations.*

10. *Test his or her knowledge by answering the Review Questions.*

KEY WORDS/Phrases

accumulative effects
background radiation
Biological Effects of Ionizing
  Radiations Committee
Bureau of Radiological Health
deterministic effect
direct effect
dose

dose equivalent
effective dose equivalent
Environmental Protection Agency
excitation
exposure
exposure unit (X)
free radical
gray (Gy)

hydrogen radical
hydroxyl radical
indirect effect
International Commission of
  Radiological Protection
ionization
latent period
linear energy transfer

millirad (mRad)

millirem (mrem)

National Council on Radiation
    Protection and Measurements

National Evaluation of X-Ray
    Trends

nonthreshold dose

nonstochastic effect

Nuclear Regulatory Commission

Occupational Safety and Health
    Administration

quality factor

radiation-induced cancer

radiolysis of water

radioresistant tissue

radiosensitive tissue

risk

risk estimate

roentgen (R)

sievert (Sv)

stochastic effect

threshold dose

tissue doses

United Nations Scientific
    Committee on the Effects of
    Atomic Radiation

HOW TISSUES ARE AFFECTED BY RADIATION

Radiation biology is a portion of science that studies the effects of ionizing radiations on living organisms. It is virtually impossible to describe or discuss the effects of radiation without using some sort of descriptive phrase or word to describe the amount or quantity of radiation. Specific definitions will be given later, but for now the terms **exposure** and **dose** will be used to refer to the amount of radiation. Simply expressed, if individuals run through a water sprinkler they are *exposed* to a certain amount of water, but not all of it hits them and makes them wet (*dose*). The more times they run through the sprinkler, the more exposure they have and the wetter (the higher the dose) they get.

EFFECTS IN ATOMS AND MOLECULES

Everything in the world is made of atoms. Atoms can be considered to be the building blocks used to make the world. There are approximately 105 different kinds of atoms making up the world as we know it today. Different atoms can be combined (added together in specific ways) to form molecules. Molecules can be small or big and can have a variety of different shapes and functions. Life as we now understand it takes place through a complex, integrated sequence of chemical reactions that occur within the cells of an organism. The very first effect of radiation occurs when the energy of the ionizing radiation (e.g., x-rays) is deposited within the chemicals that make up the living (biologic) tissue. When this energy is deposited within an atom or molecule, two effects may take place: **excitation** and **ionization**, which can result in molecular damage.

Excitation

Excitation occurs when an x-ray photon interacts with an atom's outer electron, causing the electron to vibrate momentarily at a higher energy (Fig. 12.1). The vibration, or excitation, of the electron causes a change in the force that binds atoms into molecules. The energy of excitation may be released harmlessly through the emission of light and heat; if the energy of excitation is too large, it may produce a break in the molecular bond and disrupt the molecule. When a person drinks too much coffee, tea, or soda containing caffeine and has the "shakes," that is excitation.

Ionization

The principle means by which ionizing radiation dissipates its energy in matter is by removing orbital electrons from an electrically neutral atom/molecule. When an atom loses an electron, it is said to be ionized. An ionized atom (called ion) is no longer electrically neutral and becomes more reactive as it attempts to find an electron to replace the missing one (Fig. 12.2).

Breaking of Molecular Bonds

When an atom is ionized, its chemical-binding properties change. If the atom is a part of a larger molecule

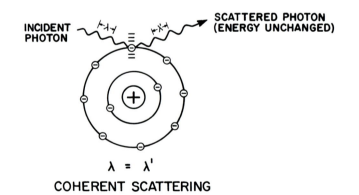

Figure 12.1. Excitation by Coherent or Unmodified Scattering. An incident x-ray photon (usually of low energy) interacts with one of the outermost electrons. They are essentially free because they are so loosely bound. The electron starts to vibrate at the frequency of the incident photon. Because the electron is a charged particle, it emits radiation with the same frequency of the incident radiation and the atom returns to its stable state again (γ = wavelength).

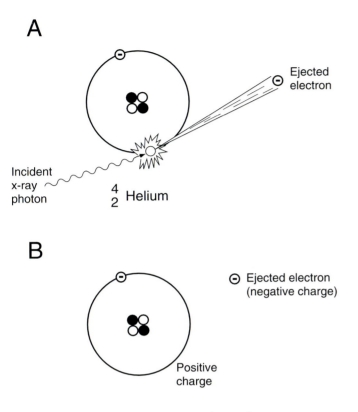

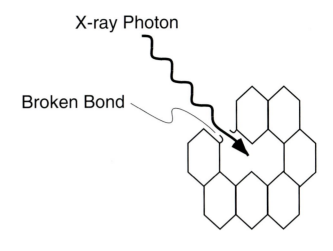

Figure 12.3. Breaking of Molecular Bonds. Breakage of a molecule's chemical bonds by direct action of radiation.

A

B

Figure 12.2. Ionization of a neutral atom by x-rays. (A) Neutral atom with x-ray photon ejecting an orbital electron. **(B)** Ion pair formed by ejected electron (− charge) and the ionized atom with more protons than electrons (+ charge).

(macromolecule), the ionized atom may cause a breakage of the molecule into two or more pieces. (A molecule is a chemical combination of two or more atoms that form a specific chemical substance.) (Fig. 12.3). The broken molecule will no longer "work" chemically; if enough molecules are damaged, then loss of function, impairment, or death of the cell may occur.

RADIOLYSIS OF WATER (INTERACTION OF RADIATION WITH H₂O)

The human body contains an abundance of water molecules (water constitutes approximately 80% of the body's total weight). Thus, x-ray photon interaction with water is a major factor in the production of early radiation damage. These interactions are referred to as the radiolysis of water. X-ray photons **remove electrons** from water molecules contained within the human body. The interaction between an x-ray photon and a water molecule creates an ion pair consisting of the ejected electron and a water molecule with an impaired outer orbital electron called a

free radical. Free radicals, molecules containing an unpaired electron, are extremely reactive. They may produce undesirable chemical combinations within the cell that may cause biologic damage. The *radiolysis of water* is extremely complex; however, water is largely converted to hydrogen (H*) and hydroxyl (OH*) free radicals.

Hydrogen and Hydroxyl Radicals

Hydrogen and hydroxyl radicals are not the only destructive elements that can be produced during the hydrolysis of water. A hydroxyl radical (OH*) can bond with another hydroxyl radical (OH*) and form hydrogen peroxide (OH* + OH* = H_2O_2), a substance poisonous to the cell. In addition, hydroperoxyl radical (HO_2*) is formed when a hydrogen free radical (H*) combines with molecular oxygen (O_2). Hydroperoxyl and hydrogen peroxide are believed to be the main toxic or poisonous substances that produce important chemical changes that can lead to the formation of biologic damage (Fig. 12.4).

BIOLOGIC EFFECTS OF RADIATION

X-rays are tiny bundles of energy that cannot be seen or felt. The injury they cause occurs to the chemicals located within the cells of the human body and cannot be seen directly. The energy deposited by the x-ray photons damages the *chemicals of life* within each cell. The more x-ray energy absorbed/deposited, the more chemicals of life are damaged.

Chemicals of life are various kinds of "biologically active" chemicals. Examples of these complex molecules are listed on the next page.

> ## EXAMPLES OF CHEMICALS OF LIFE
>
> Deoxyribonucleic acid (DNA)
> Ribonucleic acid (RNA)
> Adenosine diphosphate (ADP)
> Adenosine triphosphate (ATP)
> Nicotinamide adenine dinucleotide (NAD)
> Cytochrome oxidase
> Glucokinase
> And many more

Cells

Under normal circumstances, the various chemicals of life work together to produce what we commonly call "life." In living organisms (humans and animals), the smallest unit in which these chemical reactions of life can occur is within the cell. The cell is divided into two compartments: the nucleus and the cytoplasm. The nucleus is considered to be more radiosensitive than the cytoplasm because it contains the cell's DNA.

Tissues

Groups of the same kind of cell are called **tissues. Different kinds of tissues may be combined to form organs and systems** in the human body. Organs and organ systems serve specific purposes, such as food digestion, blood production and circulation, reproduction, and breathing.

The human body is a highly complex grouping of cells that are not visible to the human eye. These cells contain about 80% water and 20% of various kinds of biologically active chemicals (molecules with very long names) that, for simplicity, we call the chemicals of life.

TWO TYPES OF BIOLOGIC EFFECTS

Biologic effects are the result of damage to the biologically active molecules. These effects may be of two types: **direct effects** or **indirect effects.**

Direct Effect

When ionizing particles transfer their energy to biologically active molecules such as DNA, RNA, proteins, or enzymes, damage occurs as a result of what is called **direct action.** The ionization or excitation of the atoms of these molecules results in breakage of the molecules' chemical bonds, which may alter their precise three-dimensional chemical structure and provide opportunities for other chemicals in their vicinity to form inappropriate chemical bonds. DNA is an important cell molecule that carries the genetic information necessary for cell replication and regulates all cellular activity. Current experimental data strongly support the concept that DNA is the irreplaceable "master" or "key" molecule within the cell that serves as the critical biomolecular target. If the master molecule is irreparably damaged by exposure to radiation, the cell will die. When non-DNA cell molecules are destroyed by radiation exposure, the cell most likely will not show any evidence of injury following irradiation because the cell will repair itself. Direct effects of radiation are similar to a bullet through the heart or brain and result in immediate "death" of the molecule; the only difference is that the effect is occurring at the atomic/molecular level rather than at the organismal (organ) level. Cells and tissues can regenerate and recover from radiation injury. Most of the x-ray photons probably pass through, causing little or no damage. Also, the body contains so many cells that the

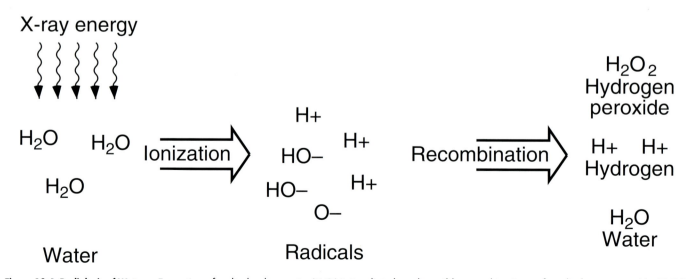

Figure 12.4. Radiolysis of Water. Formation of radicals when water (H₂O) is irradiated, and possible recombination to form hydrogen peroxide (H₂O₂).

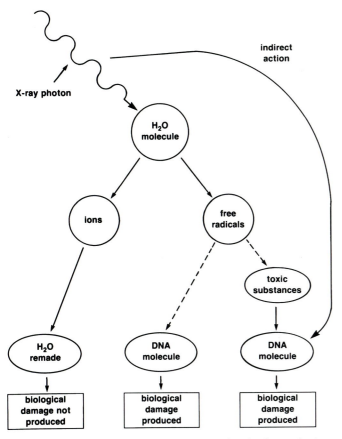

Figure 12.5. Indirect Effect. When DNA is acted on by free radicals or toxic products of free radicals, it is called an indirect action. This is because the deposition of radiation energy (x-ray photon) was not the immediate cause of damage to the biologically active molecule. Also, if ions produced by radiation energy on the H_2O molecule are remade into H_2O, again no biologic damage is produced.

destruction of a single cell or a small group of cells usually has no observable effect.

Indirect Effect

Destructive chemical changes to the chemicals of life can result from what is called indirect action of ionizing radiation. When a specific biologically active molecule such as DNA is acted on by free radicals previously produced by the interaction of radiation with water molecules, the destructive action of the ionizing radiation on the biologically active molecule is indirect in the sense that the deposition of radiation energy was not the *immediate* cause of the damage to the biologically active molecule (Fig. 12.5). The bonding of free radicals produced by the irradiation of water, oxygen, or a host of other chemical nutrients found within the cell to any of the chemicals of life results in a change in the chemical properties of the

chemicals of life; this change results in the "death" of that molecule. Under ordinary circumstances, even when these poisonous or toxic substances are formed in cells by radiolysis of H_2O, other cells in the area are not affected and the overall functions of the tissue or organ may not be affected, providing time for the irradiated cell to potentially repair the damage. However, cellular destruction is not the only biologic effect; the potential exists for the cell to become malignant.

Time-Scale of Radiation Damage

For radiation damage to become visible, hours, days, months, and even years may pass before a change is seen. The time interval between irradiation and development of the observed biologic effect is known as the **latent period.** It is important to remember that almost every cell has the ability to repair radiation damage. The lower the dose of radiation to the cell, the more capable the cell is in repairing the damage. Higher doses of radiation produce more severe damage to the cell, and it is less likely that the cell will be able to repair all the damage. Similarly, a scratch will heal quicker than a large, deep jagged cut. Radiation-induced changes are not unique to radiation and mimic other changes produced by toxic chemicals, normal aging processes, and various disease states. A squamous cell carcinoma induced by radiation exposure appears histologically similar to a squamous cell carcinoma in a patient without previous radiation exposure.

Accumulative Effects of Radiation

Whenever biologic tissue is exposed to radiation, there is some injury that is followed by repair. Radiobiologic studies indicate that repair processes exist in humans at all levels of cellular repair or replacement. Because the repair of every cell is probably never substantially complete, residual injury **may** remain within the DNA or the cytoplasm; just like a small scar may remain after a cut. Each succeeding radiation injury adds a small amount to this increment of residual damage that is known as the **accumulative effect of radiation.** The same situation exists for other agents, such as bacterial infections, viral disease, and trauma. The sum of this process is considered to be the basis for aging. At the low levels of radiation given to a patient in diagnostic radiography, permanent residual injury will be virtually impossible to detect because it will be masked by the gradual accumulation of normal aging injury within the tissues (Fig. 12.6). Thus, the effects of radiation are said to be cumulative from the standpoint that cellular repair procedures never completely repair, and unrepaired damage may lead to future health problems such as cancer, cataracts, birth defects, or premature aging. Some of the tissues and organs that are considered "critical radiologically" that could be affected are listed below.

Critical Organs in Dental Radiography	
Critical Organ	Resulting Disorder
Lens of eye	Cataracts
Gonads	Genetic abnormalities
Fetus	Congenital defects
Bone marrow	Leukemia
Thyroid gland	Cancer
Salivary gland	Cancer
Skin	Cancer
Bone	Cancer

Determinants of Radiation Injury

Like most things in life, nothing is as simple as it may first appear; so it is with radiation effects. There are many factors that determine the severity of tissue damage after exposure to radiation. The importance of only a few factors will be discussed as they relate to dental radiation exposure. Some factors that influence radiation effects are listed below.

Factors Influencing Radiation Effects

Host Factors	Radiation Effects
Species of animal	
Intrinsic resistance	Local area versus whole body exposure
Type and sensitivity of tissue	Type of radiation (linear energy transfer)
Rate of cell division	Penetrating ability of radiation
Sensitivity of tissue to radiation	Total dose
Phase of cell cycle	Acute versus chronic exposure

RADIATION FACTORS

There are many physical factors that ultimately influence the radiobiologic effect. Some of the following are major contributors.

Type of Radiation

Sparsely ionizing radiations, such as X-rays and gamma rays, deposit their energy in widely separated energy-depositing events when compared with densely ionizing radiation. Alpha particles deposit all their energy in a very short distance. The potential biologic effect of x-rays is less than that associated with alpha particles. In fact, alpha particles are approximately 20 times more effective in producing certain radiobiologic effects. The type of radiation used to make dental radiographs is a sparsely ionizing type; therefore, it has less radiobiologic effect than other types.

Linear Energy Transfer Linear energy transfer (LET) is the amount of energy transferred to tissue per distance traveled in that tissue. Large, slow-moving charged particles (such as alpha particles) have a high rate of LET, that is, they deposit most of their ionizing energy in a short distance where the distance between ionizations is very small. **High** LET radiations cause more damage than the widely separated ionizing events of x-rays (low LET radiations). A simple analogy might be how wet one gets in a cloud burst (high LET) versus a soft, fine drizzle (low LET). High LET radiations are capable of creating significantly more hydrogen peroxide radicals and inducing double strand breakage in the DNA relative to low LET radiations.

Total Dose

The larger the amount of energy deposited in a tissue (total dose of radiation), the more severe the radiobiologic effect. Most dental radiographic procedures require very small amounts of radiation to produce a radiographic image, especially compared with some medical radiographic procedures (see "Effective Dose Equivalent" in this chapter).

Penetrating Ability of Radiation (Quality of Beam)

The more penetrating (higher energy) the ionizing radiation, the more severe the radiobiologic effect will be on tissues lying within deeper parts of the body. Low energy radiations tend to be absorbed by the superficial layers of the skin and, therefore, the potential harm to deeper tissues is reduced. The dental x-ray unit contains a filter to selectively remove long wavelength x-rays and reduce skin dose.

Acute Versus Chronic Exposure

An acute exposure to an ionizing radiation occurs when all the energy is given in a very short period. Dose for dose, an acute exposure produces more severe radiobiologic effects than chronic exposures. Chronic exposure occurs when a small amount of radiation is given over a prolonged period. For chronic radiation exposures, the radiobiologic effect is less because the body/tissue has an opportunity to repair the damage between successive exposures. Dental radiographic exposures more closely resemble chronic exposure situations, because the patient is radiographed at widely separated periods.

Local Area Versus Whole Body

Exposure of the entire organism to radiation produces more severe systemic effects than exposure of a small (local) area. Dental radiographic units expose a small,

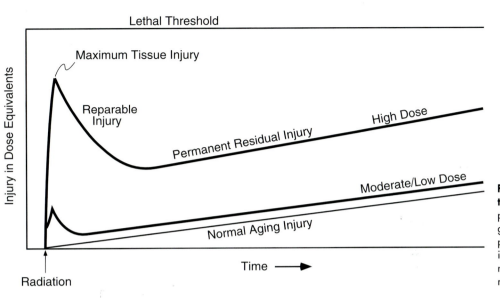

Figure 12.6. Accumulative Effects of Radiation. Radiation injury and repair after exposure to radiation. At diagnostic radiographic dose levels (moderate/low doses), permanent residual injury will be virtually impossible to detect because it will be masked by the gradual accumulation of normal aging injury within the tissues.

well-defined area of the head and neck (depending on the procedure). Thus, dental radiographic procedures are not considered to result in significant exposure to the whole body. In dentistry, the circular beam or radiation is limited to only the area of diagnostic concern, and this circular area (2.75 inches in diameter) may be further reduced by the use of rectangular collimation.

HOST FACTORS

Species of Animal

Different species of animals have differing sensitivities to lethal effects of radiation. Most mammals have approximately the same sensitivity and are relatively sensitive to radiation effects when compared to reptiles, insects, and bacteria.

Intrinsic Resistance of the Organism

Just as humans have differing "natural" sensitivities to contracting the flu during flu season, there are similar differences in "intrinsic resistance" to radiation effects. Individuals who might potentially be more or less sensitive to radiation effects cannot be identified by any physical characteristic or feature.

Type and Sensitivity of Tissue

Different tissues of the body have differing sensitivities to developing radiation effects. Some tissues are very sensitive to radiation (blood-forming tissues such as bone marrow), and others are quite resistant to the lethal effects of radiation (muscle and nerve such as the masseter muscle and inferior alveolar nerve).

Rate of Cell Division

Cells that divide rapidly during their normal "life" tend to be more sensitive to radiation damage than cells that do not divide at all. For example, malignant tumor cells divide rapidly and can be destroyed by radiation, whereas enamel does not divide and is insensitive to radiation.

Tissue and Organ Sensitivity

Relative Sensitivity	Tissue/Organ
High	Small lymphocyte
	Bone marrow
	Reproductive cells
	Intestinal mucosa
Fairly high	Skin
	Lens of the eye
	Oral mucosa
Medium	Connective tissue
	Small blood vessels
	Growing bone and cartilage
Fairly low	Mature bone and cartilage
	Salivary gland
	Thyroid gland
	Kidney
	Liver
Low	Muscle
	Nerve

Sensitivity of Tissue to Radiation

Experiments clearly demonstrate that some of the cells and tissues of the human body are more sensitive to x-radiation than others and may die following relatively low amounts of x-radiation; they are called **radiosensitive** tissues and organs. Cells that appear to be less harmed by large amounts of x-radiation are called **radioresistant**. Cells and tissues that are not particularly sensitive or resistant to radiation are **intermediate** in their sensitivity to radiation. A list of some types of tissues and their sensitivity to radiation are listed on the previous page.

Damage at the Organismal Level

Radiation biologists, scientists who study the effects of radiation on living things, divide the human body into two basic types of tissues: **somatic** and **genetic/reproductive**. **Somatic** tissues are tissues of the body that are not inherited from one generation to the next. Examples of somatic tissues are salivary glands, muscles, bones, nerves, kidneys, connective tissues, and skin. **Genetic/reproductive tissues** are those tissues responsible for producing the next generation of offspring and specifically include the oocytes (eggs) in the female ovary and spermatogonia (male sperm-forming cells). The main reason for classifying tissues as somatic or genetic is that radiation damage to somatic tissues only influences the individual who has been exposed to the radiation. Radiation damage to genetic/reproductive tissues is inherited from one generation to the next, just like eye and hair color. The only difference is that all radiation changes passed from one generation to the next are considered to be harmful. Genetic effects are, therefore, considered to be more serious and to have a long-term negative influence on the health and welfare of a population, because they involve more than the person originally exposed to radiation.

Threshold Dose

When animals are exposed to radiation, small amounts of radiation exposure to somatic tissues do not appear to produce any visible changes in the tissue until a certain **threshold dose** is reached (Fig. 12.7) This threshold dose depends on the kind of tissue exposed to radiation. When toasting marshmallows over a fire, one can see the "threshold effect." If the marshmallow is placed too high over the fire, there is not enough heat to toast the outside; if it is too close to the fire, instant cremation, flames, and charcoal on the outside result. Somewhere between these two extremes there is a distance and a length of time over the fire that will produce the first golden brown change in the surface of the marshmallow. This is a sign that it is time to begin turning the marshmallow to produce the golden brown perfection with a warm, soft center. Once the surface of the marshmallow begins to turn golden brown, then the longer it stays in that position, the darker

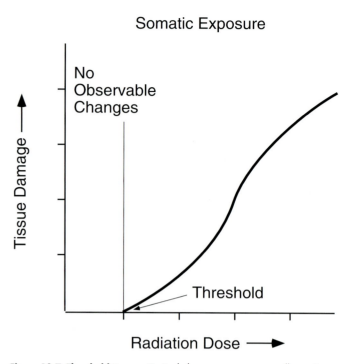

Somatic Exposure

Figure 12.7. Threshold Dose. Typical dose–response curve illustrating a threshold nonlinear (curved-line) type of biologic response.

it gets until it begins to blister, burn, and turn black. If this sounds much like sunburn, it is—the longer the exposure to sunshine, the more severe the burn once the threshold at which the skin first begins to turn pink is passed. So it is with all human somatic tissues. Small exposures produce no observable change. With increasing levels of exposure, a threshold will be reached, at which time a specific radiation effect becomes visible. Higher exposures produce progressively more severe changes. Changes such as hair loss (epilation), skin reddening (erythema), cataract formation, and sterility follow a **threshold**, nonlinear (curved-line) type of dose–response curve.

Nonthreshold Dose

Exposure of genetic tissues to radiation causes mutations. Mutations are changes in the information contained by the chromosomes within the sperm and egg cells. It is indicative of a change in the DNA of the cell. Genetic changes are always considered bad, and once incorporated into the eggs or sperm of the parent, can subsequently be passed from the affected parent(s) to their children, grandchildren, and great grandchildren. The result of mutations is the potential production of children with a wide variety of birth defects including leukemia, increased susceptibility to developing cancers, and physical deformities of various types. The formation of mutations does not appear to follow a threshold type of dose response like somatic tissues. Instead, genetic tissues follow a "non-

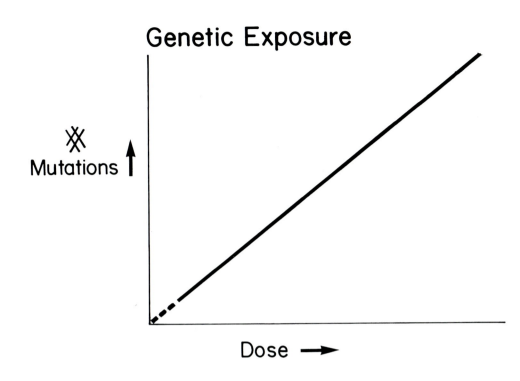

Figure 12.8. Genetic Exposure. Typical dose–response curve illustrating a nonthreshold linear (straight-line) type of biologic response.

threshold" or linear (straight-line) type of dose response (Fig. 12.8). What this means is that small amounts of radiation have the potential to produce a small number of mutations in chromosomes; with progressively increasing doses, more and more mutations are formed. When one drives a car, the car's speed follows a nonthreshold or linear pattern. When the gas pedal is depressed a little, the car goes slowly; when the pedal is pressed down more and more, the car goes faster and faster. Similarly, the number of mutations increases with increasing exposure to radiation.

Stochastic and Nonstochastic (Deterministic) Radiation Effects

Stochastic radiation effects are similar to nonthreshold radiation effects. Stochastic effects are defined as ones in which the probability of occurrence increases with increasing absorbed dose, but the severity in the affected individual does not depend on the magnitude of the absorbed dose. Stochastic effects do not have a dose threshold. Typical stochastic radiation effects include **genetic mutations** and **cancer/tumor** induction.

Nonstochastic (deterministic) radiation effects are defined as somatic effects that increase in severity with increasing absorbed dose in affected individuals and appear to have a threshold. Typical nonstochastic radiation effects include erythema, epilation, cataract formation (opacification of the lens of the eye), and impaired fertility (decreased sperm count). In general, nonstochastic effects

require larger doses to cause serious impairment of health compared with the dose to increase cancers or mutations. Nonstochastic radiation effects may also be referred to as "deterministic" radiation effects.

RADIATION UNITS AND MEASUREMENTS

UNITS OF MEASURING RADIATION

The following paragraphs mention several different units of measurement for radiation and for radiation risk. The dental health-care worker must know that there is an "old system" and a "new system" for measuring radiation units. How did this come about? In 1985, a new International System (SI) of measurement was adopted worldwide. However, before 1985, an old terminology was used in textbooks and journals. Both systems are presented here. It is frustrating to have to deal with two different sets of units, and it would be better if only one could be used. However, that is not the case.

RADIATION MEASUREMENT

To understand the potential harmful effects of radiation, it is important to know the amount of radiation associated with the harmful effects. It may seem difficult to measure something that cannot be seen, touched, felt, or smelled, but to scientists it is possible to measure the amount of x-ray energy produced by an x-ray unit and absorbed by the body. Scientists do it in the same way that others have determined a measure for a gallon of gasoline, a liter of soda, an ounce of gold, a pound of sugar, a ton of steel, or a kilowatt of electricity. The units, gallon, liter, ounce, pound, ton, and kilowatt represent certain quantities or amounts that are accepted by custom and tradition of usage for hundreds of years. The units **roentgen, rad, rem, gray,** and **sievert** are the units by which radiation is measured and refer to relatively large quantities of x-ray energy. For dental radiographic procedures, the term **milliroentgen (mR), millirad (mrad),** and **millirem (mrem)** are frequently used to refer to a unit of measurement 1000 times smaller; thus, 1 rad is equivalent to 1000 millirads, and 1 mrad = 1/1000 rad. To keep the relative size of these radiation units in perspective, one should try imaging a small glass jar containing 1000 grains of rice. This would represent the "quantity" referred to as the roentgen, rad, and rem. If someone removes one grain of rice from the jar, he or she has the equivalent of 1 mR, 1 mrad, or 1 mrem. The radiation unit called the gray (Gy) and sievert (Sv) is equal to 100 rads, or 100 rems. Therefore, 1 Gy would be equivalent to 100,000 grains of rice in the previous example. Converting rads, rems, grays, and sieverts can be a bit confusing at times. The dose conversion table below illustrates common conversions.

Dose Conversion Table for Changing Rads to Grays (Gy) and for Changing Grays (Gy) to Rads

mrad	rad (rem)	Gy (Sv)	mGy (Sv)	μGy (Sv)
1	0.001	0.00001	0.01	10
1000	1	0.01	10	10000
100000	100	1	1000	1000000
100	0.1	0.001	1	1000
0.1	0.0001	0.000001	0.001	1

m = milli or 1000th; μ = micron or 1,000,000th.

In dental radiography: 1 rad = 1 rem; 1 gray (Gy) = 1 Sievert (Sv).

EXPOSURE

How Much Radiation Comes Out of the X-Ray Machine?

Exposure is a property of the x-ray beam. Exposure is a measure of photon flow and is related to the energy transferred from the x-rays to a specified volume and mass

of **air**. The *old unit of exposure* was the **roentgen (R)**. The roentgen is still used by many persons. A roentgen is defined as the quantity of photons that will produce a defined number of ion pairs (about 2 billion) in a cubic centimeter of air at standard temperature and pressure. Physicists convert the number of ion pairs released into an electrical charge that they measure in a unit called coulombs (C). One dental bitewing or periapical radiograph exposes the patient to approximately 0.3 R (300 mR). The *new unit of exposure* is simply called the "exposure unit" (**X**). The X unit is the quantity of photons that will produce in air, ions carrying 1 C of charge per kilogram of air (1 X unit = 1 C/kg air). Actually, the SI definition of a roentgen is meaningless to most radiologists; the coulomb is not a part of the daily vocabulary. When a state inspection is performed on the x-ray machine in a dental office, the physicist or technician will measure the exposure in roentgens of C/kg produced by the machine at certain mA, time, and kVp settings. Exposure is independent of area or field size. **Exposure is like rainfall, in that rainfall is measured in inches without regard to area.** A 1-inch rainfall produces a 1-inch deep layer of water in a drinking glass, a washtub, or a swimming pool, provided each has a flat bottom and perpendicular sides. Therefore, an exposure measurement does not describe the size of the x-ray beam. When a patient asks the question, "How dangerous are dental x-rays?" one can respond, "The exposure from one bitewing film is 300 milliroentgens." However, this answer would be of no value to anyone but a physicist or a radiation biologist. Rather than answering the question with a dry, technical, accurate, but unhelpful statement of exposure, the dental health-care worker should consider how much radiation is being absorbed by the patient, which leads to the topic of **dose**.

Dose

Dose is the amount of x-**ray energy absorbed by a unit mass of tissue.** Tissue absorbs x-ray energy differently than air, depending on the density (compactness) and atomic composition of the tissue. Because some x-rays pass through the patient and others are partially or completely absorbed by the patient, dose does not equal exposure. The old unit expressing absorbed dose is the rad, defined as 100 ergs of energy absorbed per gram of tissue (1 rad = 100 erg/gm). The new unit is the gray (Gy) and is defined as 1 joule of energy absorbed per kilogram tissue (1 Gy = 1 J/kg). Some authorities use gray, whereas others use rad. These units can be simply converted by using the following formula: 1 Gy = 100 rad or 1 rad = 0.01 Gy = 1 cGy (cGy is the abbreviation for centigray, which people who were accustomed to rad like to use because 1 rad = 1 cGy). Dose is of more interest to biologists and health-care workers than exposure, because dose describes how much energy is deposited in the tissues, which in turn indicates how much biologic damage may occur from the radiation. Dose is independent of the volume of tissue irradiated. Exposure and dose are two different concepts. They should not be confused. Radiation **exposure** refers to the amount of radiation that comes out of the x-ray unit and reaches the person. Because radiation has the capability of passing through the body, not all the energy that a person is exposed to is actually absorbed by the body. The amount of x-ray energy actually absorbed or deposited within the tissues of the body is called the **dose** or **absorbed dose**. The absorbed dose is typically used as an indication of potential harm. In most cases, the effect of radiation increases with absorbed dose. That is, the higher the absorbed dose, the greater is the biologic effect (or the greater is the probability of the biologic effect, depending on the endpoint under consideration).

Perhaps a patient has a laboratory job in which he works with radioactive materials. This patient could say, "How does my dose from x-rays in your dental chair compare to the dose I get at work from alpha particles?" To answer this question, the dental health-care worker needs to know something about the concept of "dose equivalent."

Dose Equivalent

X-rays and alpha particles give different bangs for the buck. Dose equivalent is a concept that allows the comparison of the biologic effect of different types of ionizing radiation. Alpha particles, beta particles, gamma rays, protons, and neutrons are other types of ionizing radiation. **Equal doses** of **different types of radiation** produce **different amounts of biologic damage**. For example, 50 cGy (rad) of neutrons would cause much more biologic damage than 50 cGy (rad) of x-rays. The dose equivalent takes differences in biologic damage into consideration by using a **quality factor (QF)** to adjust the dose. The **QF** is **1 for x-rays, beta particles, and gamma rays; 5 for low-energy neutrons; and 20 for alpha particles, protons, and higher-energy neutrons.** For some strange reason, dose equivalent is abbreviated **H**. Therefore, to calculate dose equivalent, the following formula is used:

$$H \text{ (dose equivalent)} = D \text{ (dose)} \times QF \text{ (quality factor)}$$

The old unit for dose equivalent is the **rem**. The new unit for dose equivalent is the **sievert (Sv)**. A rem can be converted to a sievert by the following formula:

$$1 \text{ Sv} = 100 \text{ rem}.$$

X-rays are the standard against which all other radiations are measured, so the QF for x-rays is 1. Therefore,

for x-rays, if a patient received 10 Gy, the dose would be 10 Gy and the dose equivalent would be:

$$10 \text{ Gy} \times 1 = 10 \text{ Sv}.$$

In contrast, if the patient received 10 Gy of low-energy neutrons, the dose equivalent would be:

$$10 \text{ Gy} \times 5 = 50 \text{ Sv}.$$

This simply reminds us that low-energy neutrons are approximately 5 times as damaging to the cell as an equal dose of x-rays. Dose equivalent is of little concern in dentistry, because only x-rays that have a QF of 1 are dealt with. Therefore, **dose** is as useful as **dose equivalent** in dentistry. Whenever someone uses **dose** (in Gy or rad) when referring to x-rays, they could just as well use **dose equivalent** (in Sv or rem), because for x-rays 1 Gy = 1 Sv and 1 rad = 1 rem. Why does anyone bother to distinguish between **dose** and **dose equivalent**? Radiation therapists and nuclear reactor operators have to be concerned about dose equivalent because they use several different types of radiation with different QFs. With regard to dental x-ray exposure, it is acceptable to consider the roentgen, rad, and rem **roughly** equivalent, although each term has a specific definition and use. Therefore, we may assume that 1 R = 1 rad = 1 rem, or 1 Gy = 1 Sv.

Effective Dose Equivalent

It has already been noted that both exposure and dose are independent of the size of the x-ray beam, or the volume of tissue irradiated. However, common sense would (correctly) suggest that 1 Sv of x-rays to the right hand would be less dangerous than 1 Sv of x-rays to the whole body. The right hand has relatively few cancer-susceptible tissues (bone marrow and skin) and is a relatively small body part. In contrast, the whole body has many cancer-susceptible tissue types and has a much greater volume. **The doses in each situation are the same, yet the risk is obviously much greater in the whole-body situation.** Another example: 1 Sv of x-rays to the right hand would be much less hazardous than 1 Sv of x-rays to the right breast. Although both tissue volumes involved are about the same, breast tissue is much more susceptible to radiation-induced cancer than are any of the tissues of the hand. It is important to understand that when a complete-mouth set of dental radiographs are taken, the cone (beam indicating device [BID]) does not stay in the same place for each radiograph. The cone (BID) is moved around the patient's face so that total amount of x-ray energy is **not** concentrated over one area; in this way, the tissues of the face receive relatively small amounts of radiation.

To help **compare the biologic consequences** of radiation to various parts of the body, the **effective dose equivalent** has been introduced. We will ignore the mathematics, and simply summarize by stating that **effective dose equivalent** is the dose equivalent with an adjustment for (1) the **volume** of tissue irradiated, and (2) the **radiosensitivity** of the tissue irradiated. Effective dose equivalent is abbreviated H(E), with units of Sv (usually stated in μSv or millionths of a sievert). The risks taken into account with H(E) are cancer induction and the induction of genetic mutations. **Therefore, if one wants to compare the risk from two different x-ray exposures (e.g., comparing the risk of four bitewings versus one panoramic radiograph), effective dose equivalent rather than dose equivalent should be used.** Because both dose equivalent and effective dose equivalent are stated in units of Sv, one must carefully look at each table's caption to determine which concept is under consideration. See below for **effective dose equivalents** from diagnostic x-ray examinations in microsieverts (μSv):

Effective Dose Equivalents from Diagnostic X-Ray Examinations (microsieverts [μSv])

Examination	Effective Dose Equivalent (μSv)
Panoramic radiograph	7
Full-mouth intraoral radiographs (20 films)	
D-speed film, round collimation	84
E+ speed film, rectangular collimation	33
Bitewing radiographs (4 films)	
D-speed film, round collimation	17
E+ speed film, rectangular collimation	7
Chest	80
Upper gastrointestinal tract	2400
Barium enema	4060
Abdomen	560
Effective dose equivalent to average U.S. resident from background radiation per year	3000
1000 μSv = 1 mSv = 100 mrad.	

Because the effective dose equivalent takes into account risk estimates (with a wide margin of error) and actual dose equivalent (little margin of error), the **effective dose equivalent** for a given radiographic procedure will change whenever the **risk estimates** change. For example, the esti-mated risk of cancer from a given dose of x-rays increased by approximately 4 times between 1980 and 1990. In the next 10 years, the risk estimates will possibly change again as radiation research progresses. That means that the effective dose equivalents will also change.

There is no doubt that x-rays are potentially dangerous. Therefore, the dental health-care worker is ill advised to take a casual attitude or approach to the use of x-rays. Telling a patient, "Trust me, they are not dangerous. I would not use them if they were harmful," is a paternalistic response to the patient's question, "Are dental x-rays dangerous?" and will alienate rather than reassure the patient. When a patient asks this question, he or she may simply want to know whether the operator is using x-rays carefully and has respect for their hazards. A simple "No" response to the question may seem to contradict what the patient has read in magazines or seen on television about x-rays. A discussion of chemical or cellular effects, or even irrelevant organismal effects, would probably waste both the operator and the patient's time. However, the operator might want to help the patient consider the real but very small risk from dental radiography, which is carcinogenesis.

ASSESSING RISKS FROM DENTAL RADIOGRAPHY

Many of the biologic effects described previously are not a risk in dental radiography. Some of these effects (cataracts, osteoradionecrosis, xerostomia, erythema, epilation) have a **threshold** dose much higher than that used in dentistry. Some effects require not only high doses, but also whole-body exposure (bone marrow destruction, gastrointestinal necrosis, cerebrovascular syndrome). Other effects may occur at lower doses but are not a risk in dental radiography, because that particular area of the body is not irradiated (fetal abnormalities, genetic mutations).

Risk Estimates to the Eye

The threshold for induction of cataracts is about 2000 mSv. Dental single exposures to the lens and cornea of the eye are primarily from scattered radiation and are reported to be less than 0.5 mSv when open, round cones (BID) are used and 0.16 mSv when rectangular collimation is used. Panoramic radiographic exposures to the lens and cornea of the eye are extremely small (approximately 0.09 mSv per radiograph). The risk of dental radiographic procedures contributing significantly to occurrence of eye problems appears to be extremely remote (Gibbs et al.; Weissman and Sobkowski).

Gonadal Dose

Heritable (genetic) effects are those seen in the progeny of irradiated persons. There is little information about genetic effects of radiation exposure in humans; to date, no such effects have been clearly demonstrated. There is no statistically significant increase in genetically related disease in the children of atomic bomb survivors. Current knowledge of heritable defects from radiation exposure is derived mainly from research on mice. One method to measure the risk from genetic exposure is by determining the doubling dose. This is the amount of radiation a population requires to produce in the next generation as many additional mutations as arise spontaneously. In humans, the genetic doubling dose for mutations resulting in death is approximately 1 Sv (1000 mSv) [HEW publication (FDA) 76-8034, 1976]. The gonadal dose to patients from a full-mouth survey (FMX) is approximately of 2 μSv (0.002 mSv) (NCRP report 54, 1977) (note: 1 μSv is 1 millionth of 1 Sv). The gonadal dose is so small from dental radiography that the risk of heritable defects is negligible.

Risk Estimates for Pregnancy

Exposure of a fetus during gestation would be similar in magnitude to that of genetic tissues. Previous studies suggest that the production of congenital defects from doses below 100 mSv is very small when compared with the normal risk of 4.6% for congenital defects and is negligible at 50 mSv or less (NCRP report 54, 1977). Studies of groups such as the survivors of Hiroshima have shown that damage to the newborn is not expected for doses below 200 mSv (ICRP pub. 16, 1970). It is estimated that there is a 4% chance of mental retardation per 100 mSv at 8 to 15 weeks gestational age, with less risk from exposure at other gestational ages. Again, the exposure to the embryo from dental radiography is in the range of 0.002 mSv with rectangular collimation. If the patient wears a leaded apron, the exposure drops to virtually zero in the 0.001 to 0.003 mSv range. However, it is prudent to routinely use leaded torso aprons on all girls and women during the first trimester of pregnancy, and radiation exposure should be held to a minimum. Actually, a leaded torso apron should be used on all patients.

Cancer Is the Principal Biologic Risk in Dental Radiography

The principal biologic risk from dental radiography is radiation-induced cancer. As mentioned above, cancer induction probably has no threshold dose. Even a small radiation dose may increase the patient's statistical probability of cancer development, similar to the statistical probability that as a vehicle's speed increases, the probability of getting a ticket or being involved in a fatal accident increases. There are no cancers that are uniquely caused by x-rays. X-rays simply **increase the probability** that a patient may die of cancer (approximately 20% of us will die of cancer), and dental radiography increases this probability by a very tiny amount (one extra fatal cancer per

million dental radiographic examinations is a reasonable estimate of this increased risk). The estimated number of deaths attributable to low-level radiation exposure is a small fraction of the total number that occur spontaneously.

The estimation of the number of cancers induced by diagnostic use of radiation is very difficult to determine. Most of the exposed individuals studied by UNSCEAR, BEIR , and ICRP (see Radiation Protection Organizations) have received radiation exposure well above the diagnostic range. By far, the largest group of individuals studied are the Japanese atomic bomb survivors. Thus, the probability that cancer will result from a small dose of diagnostic radiation can be estimated only by extrapolation from the rates observed following exposure to larger doses. Some patient questions may require the health-care worker to explain which tissues are at risk for radiation carcinogenesis. The worker's demonstration of this knowledge plus the explanation of how the dose to these tissues is minimized will indicate a concern for patients that should enhance their trust. Because of the slight risk of cancer associated with dental radiography, the following statements should be considered.

---

1. Any dose of radiation may be potentially harmful.
2. The probability of occurrence of radiation-induced cancer increases with dose.
3. Radiation carcinogenesis may be an additive effect.
4. Children are approximately twice as radiosensitive for cancer induction as adults.

Which Tissues Have the Highest Risk for Cancer from Dental Radiation?

The risk of cancers resulting from a dental radiographic exposure is the sum of the risks of individual radiosensitive organs. The highest estimate of risks in dental radiography are for **leukemia** (cancer of the **bone marrow**) and cancer of the **thyroid**.

Leukemia Risk The region of the mandible and maxilla involved in dental radiography contains a very small percentage of active bone (blood-producing) marrow. The skull contains approximately 10% of the available bone marrow in the body, with the mandible accounting for less than 1% of the total marrow. An increased incidence of leukemia (other than chronic lymphocytic leukemia) arises following x-ray exposure to the red bone marrow and is directly related to the total amount, or percentage, of bone marrow irradiated. The mean active bone marrow dose is that dose of radiation averaged over the entire bone marrow (Bushong, 1993). The mean active marrow dose resulting from an intraoral FMX of 20 films exposed with round collimation has been reported to be 0.142 mSv, and one exposed with rectangular collimation only 0.06 mSv (White, 1992). Panoramic radiography was found to contribute a mean active bone marrow dose of approximately 0.01 mSv per film. For comparison, the mean active bone marrow dose from one chest film is 0.03 mSv [DHHS publication (FDA), 1984]. Studies have found no relationship between the level of background radiation (3 mSv or 3000 μSv/year effective dose) and the incidence of leukemia (Court-Brown et al., 1960; Craig and Seidman, 1961), congenital malformations (Schuman, 1970), and neonatal deaths (Grahn et al., 1963).

Thyroid Cancer Risk   Under most circumstances, the thyroid gland is not irradiated by the primary beam of radiation during intraoral radiography; however, the scatter radiation to the gland from an FMX (open-ended rectangular BID and E+ speed film) is reported to be less than 0.3 mSv. The dose to the thyroid from intraoral radiography can be reduced by half by use of a thyroid collar. The thyroid dose from panoramic radiography has been reported to be about 0.74 mSv, or 1% of the cervical spine (5.5 mSv) examination. The thyroid gland is fairly resistant to radiation in an adult. Nevertheless, thyroid cancer has been reported in children exposed to an estimated dose as low as 500 mSv to the thyroid following exposure to high levels of radiation for thymus gland enlargement and ringworm of the scalp. There is only a remote chance that dental radiation could cause thyroid cancer when every means to reduce radiation exposure to the patient has been used.

Comparison of Risks of Dental X-Rays with Other Risks in a Patient's Life

A patient may say, "You have told me that the cancer risk from dental x-rays is very small, but I do not have anything to compare it with. How dangerous are dental x-rays compared to something else in my life?" Comparing risks of x-rays to other activities with higher risk to demonstrate the relative safety of x-rays may or may not be helpful to patients. See below for "One In One Million Risk of Fatal Outcome."

For example, one may say, "Your risk from dental x-rays is much less than your risk of cancer from those cigarettes in your pocket." This is an apples-and-oranges comparison, and many patients will not call this a fair comparison. Most persons find it helpful to compare radiation risk from dental radiography to radiation risk from the general environment, such as **background radiation** that they receive daily.

Background Radiation

Every day, humans are exposed to radiation from within the environment. This environmental radiation is called **background radiation**. It is important because we

One in One Million Risk of Fatal Outcome

	Risk	Nature
20 minutes	As 60-year-old man	Death (CVD, cancer)
2 months	In Denver, CO	Cancer
10 miles	By bicycle	Accident
300 miles	By automobile	Accident
10 days	Typical factory work	Accident
One	Cigarette	CVD, cancer
500 ml	Wine	Alcohol-related death
125 ml	Whiskey	Alcohol-related death
1500 ml	Beer	Alcohol-related death
30 cans	Diet soda	Cancer

cannot do anything about it. **The average annual background effective exposure to the U.S. population resulting from external and internal natural sources is about 3000 μSv (3.0 mSv).** External exposure background radiation is due to cosmic and terrestrial radiation, or that radiation originating from the environment. These sources contribute to approximately 16% of the radiation exposure to the population. At sea level, the exposure from cosmic radiation is about 240 μSv per year; at Denver, Colorado, 1 mile high in elevation, the cosmic radiation exposure is about 500 μSv per year. The average cosmic radiation exposure in the United States is calculated to be 270 μSv per year. Therefore, the effective background exposure of cosmic radiation in Denver is 230 μSv higher than the U.S. average. Therefore, if a person living in the United States in an average location had an FMX (33 μS effective dose equivalent) and a panoramic radiograph (7 μS effective dose equivalent) taken by the very best techniques (rectangular collimation, E+ speed film, and rare earth screens), each year it would be only one sixth of the risk (40 μS) of a person living in Denver (230 μS per year of cosmic radiation higher than average) who was not exposed to dental radiation. The effective dose equivalent also allows for comparison of radiation doses resulting from dental diagnostic radiography and those doses received everyday from natural or background radiation. This type of data may be used by the dentist to discuss radiation risk with patients in terms that are more easily understood by them (see the following table).

Natural or background radiation is by far the largest contributor (82%) to the radiation exposure of persons living in the United States today (NCRP report 93, 1987;

NCRP report 94, 1987; NCRP report 95, 1987). Diagnostic radiation (medical and dental) accounts for approximately 11% of all exposure from major sources of radiation to U.S. populations (see following table). Only about 1% of this 11%, or about 0.1% of the total exposure, results from dental radiography (United Nations, 1988). This can be compared with radon, which is estimated to contribute to more than half (55%) of human exposure.

Summary of Radiation Risks

Available evidence indicates that all radiation, no matter how small the dose, has the potential for producing undesirable effects on both somatic and genetic tissues. Although repair processes occur within the cell, complete recovery from the effects of radiation may not occur, and the residual damage persists and is cumulative. As a patient's dose increases, the risk of developing some adverse sequelae such as the induction of cancer, leukemia, cataracts, or mutated reproductive tissues increases. The severity of the consequences can be minimized by using every means to reduce patient exposure no matter how small, insignificant, or unimportant one may consider the exposure modifications. The current estimate of the average effective dose from natural or background sources (based on fatal cancers) is 3000 μSv per year. This figure becomes 4400 μSv per year (12 μSv per day) when nonfatal cancer and severe hereditary effects (the probability of stochastic affects) are included. With the figure of 4400 μSv per year, we can estimate that an FMX taken with E+ speed film and rectangular collimation (33 μSv) is equivalent to 3 days of background exposure.

The risks from dental radiography are numerically very small but cannot be ignored. Therefore, it appears reasonable to accept the notion that the information gained from a properly justifiable radiographic examination outweighs the potential risk of harm. However, sooner or later, a patient will ask this (or a very similar) question, "How dangerous are dental x-rays?" This chapter was designed to help the dental health-care worker answer patient questions about dental radiation safety and hazards. This chapter does not provide a canned answer or a one-size-fits-all response. Each patient who asks such a question may ask it in a different way, for a different reason, or from a different educational background. The dental health-care worker must tailor the answer to the patient's need. Because there is no single best answer to radiation questions, the worker must listen carefully to determine what the patient wants to know and frame the answer in terms that he or she can understand. Although there may not be a final answer to every patient's question, there may be a "bottom line" basic understanding of the biologic effects of diagnostic radiation that may be gained from all the technical/scientific detail covered in this chapter.

Science is increasingly discovering that there are mechanisms within the cell nucleus that continually monitor and repair damage to the DNA strand. Such damage occurs as a result of "spontaneous" or "endogenous" damage, which is produced by the continuous interaction of various atoms and molecules together through the dynamics of cellular metabolism. Every hour, human and other mammalian cells undergo **at least 50 to 100 times more** spontaneous or "natural" DNA damaging events than would result from the absorption of 1 cGy (rad) of ionizing radiation. The miracle is that this spontaneous or natural damage appears to be successfully repaired minute by minute, hour by hour, year after year. If the process did not work effectively, there would be no humans left alive.

Average Annual Effective Dose of Ionizing Radiations (μSv) to a Person in the United States (1000 μSv = 1mSv)

Source	μSv	Percentage of Annual Average Effective Dose
Natural		
(environmental)		
External		
Cosmic	270	8.00%
Terrestrial	280	8.00%
Internal		
Radon	2000	55.00%
Other	400	11.00%
Rounded total	3000	82.00%
(natural)	(3.0 mSv)	
Artificial		
Medical		
X-ray diagnosis	386	10.90%
Nuclear medicine	140	4.00%
Dental		
X-ray diagnosis	4	0.10%
Consumer products	100	3.00%
Other		
Occupational	<10	0.03%
Nuclear fuel cycle	<10	0.03%
Fallout	<10	0.03%
Miscellaneous	<10	0.03%
Rounded total	600	18.00%
(artificial)	(0.6 mSv)	
Natural plus artificial	3600	100.00%
	(3.6 mSv)	

From National Council on Radiation Protection and Measurements. NCRP reports 93, 94, 95, 100. Bethesda, MD: NCRP, 1987, 1987, 1987, 1989.

Billen (1990) estimates that there are about 8000 to 10,000 DNA-damaging events of various kinds occurring in *each* cell every hour. The absorption of 1 cGy of radiation would produce *an additional* 80 DNA damage sites. The question to the reader is this, "If the nucleus can effectively handle the repair of 8000 to 10,000 natural DNA damaging events per hour, shouldn't it be able to handle an additional 80 (1%) without overloading or short circuiting?"

As a way of maintaining perspective on this issue, think of dinner guests who would presumably leave a few more dirty dishes for the dishwasher to "deal with." In the majority of instances, the dishwasher would simply wash the extra dishes without complaining or breaking down. Although there were more dishes to wash, there was the benefit of the pleasurable social interaction with friends that makes the added work and inconvenience of doing the extra dishes well worth the effort. It is the author's opinion that this is the way the nuclear repair process treats the extra damage produced by low levels of diagnostic radiation—no big deal, simply a "few more dishes to wash." Similarly, significant health benefits can be derived because of the diagnostic information obtained through the judicious, prudent use of ionizing radiation.

RADIATION PROTECTION ORGANIZATIONS

Radiation protection organizations and the interrelation of the various committees whose reports have been quoted in this chapter deserve a brief explanation. First, there are the committees who summarize and analyze data and suggest risk estimates for radiation-induced cancer and genetic effects. At the international level, the **United Nations Scientific Committee on the Effects of Atomic Radiation (UNSCEAR)** was established. This committee has widespread international representation. Reports appeared in 1958, 1966, 1972, 1977, and 1982, with the latest report in 1988. The United States committee is appointed by the **National Academy of Sciences (NAS)** and is known as the **Biological Effects of Ionizing Radiations (BEIR) Committee.** The first report appeared in 1956 when the group was known as the Biological Effects of Atomic Radiation (BEAR) Committee. Subsequent reports appeared in 1972 (BEIR II), 1988 (BEIR III), and 1990 (BEIR V). These committees are scholarly committees in the sense that when information is not available on a particular topic, they do not feel compelled to make a recommendation.

Second, there are the committees that formulate the concepts for use in radiation protection and recommend maximum permissible levels. At the international level, the **International Commission of Radiological Protection (ICRP)** was established in 1928 after a decision by the

Second International Congress of Radiology. In 1950, this commission was restructured and given its present name. The ICRP often takes the lead in formulating concepts in radiation protection and in recommending dose limits. As an international body, it has no jurisdiction over anyone and can do no more than recommend. It has established considerable credibility, however, and its views carry great weight. Its most recent report is ICRP publication 90, published in 1991. In the United States, the **National Council on Radiological Protection and Measurement (NCRP)** was chartered by Congress to be an impartial watchdog. The NCRP consists of 70 experts from the radiation sciences. The NCRP often but not always follows the lead of the ICRP. Their most recent report on dose limits (NCRP report 116, published in 1992) differs from ICRP in several important respects. The ICRP and NCRP suggest dose limits and safe practices, but in fact neither body has any jurisdiction to enforce their recommendations. **Each state also has its own bureau of radiation safety, which governs practices within that state. These state bureaus are responsible for upholding the state practice acts governing radiation practices.** Up to the present time, the various regulating bodies in the United States have accepted, endorsed, and used the reports issued by the NCRP, but they are not obligated to do so.

The **International Commission on Radiation Units and Measurements (ICRU)** is an agency that makes recommendations on radiologic units of measurement. The organization that establishes radiation protection regulations is the **Nuclear Regulatory Commission (NRC)**, formally known as the Atomic Energy Commission. Its regulations apply to nuclear reactors, reactor fuel, and radioactive materials produced by reactor operation. The **Environmental Protection Agency (EPA)** has the responsibility in the United States for providing guidance to federal agencies. For example, the EPA sets the action level for radon. The **Occupational Safety and Health Administration (OSHA)** is responsible for all occupational radiation protection regulations that are not regulated by the NRC. OSHA can choose to transfer its responsibility to the states. The **Bureau of Radiological Health (BRH)**, now called the **National Center for Devices and Radiological Health**, regulates the manufacture of radiation-producing equipment such as x-ray machines, microwave ovens, video display terminals, and medical ultrasound equipment. The **Center for Devices and Radiological Health** is an organization within the United States Food and Drug Administration. The **U.S. Food and Drug Administration (FDA)** is a part of the **Department of Health, Education and Welfare (DHEW)** of the U.S. government.

In addition to these agencies and bureaus, an important program has provided the dental community with valuable information concerning radiation exposure practices. It is called the **National Evaluation of X-Ray Trends (NEXT)** and is carried out jointly by the state and federal governments to compile nationwide data on radiation exposure in dental offices. These data are collected yearly and analyzed to provide the most recent dose comparisons, depending on technique and examination type.

REVIEW QUESTIONS

1. Cell sensitivity to radiation is more pronounced:

   1. During mitosis.
   2. During periods of increased metabolism.
   3. During embryonic development.
   4. In muscle cells.
   5. In nerve cells.
   A. 1, 2, and 3.
   B. 1, 2, and 5.
   C. 1, 3, and 5.
   D. 2, 3, and 4.
   E. 2, 3, and 5.

2. Which of the following tissues is most susceptible to radiation?

   A. Nerve tissue.
   B. Muscle tissue.
   C. Brain tissue.
   D. Blood-forming tissue.

3. Theoretically, the biologic response to a given dose of radiation would be greater (more severe) with:

   A. An anoxia of the tissue being irradiated.
   B. A higher dose rate.
   C. A smaller area of tissue exposure.
   D. Lower linear energy transfer (LET).

4. Which of the following latent effects can be associated with low-dose, whole-body radiation?

   A. Shock.
   B. Epistaxis.
   C. Epilation.
   D. Leukemia.

5. To a person in the United States, the average effective dose of ionizing radiation from natural background radiation is about:

   A. 10 mSv/year.
   B. 3 mSv/year.
   C. 6 mSv/year.
   D. 50 mSv/year.

6. A certain amount of radiation is needed before the clinical signs of damage to somatic cells appear. The amount of radiation after which visible damage can be produced is called the:

   A. Latent dose.
   B. Threshold dose.
   C. Hazard dose.
   D. Scattered radiation dose.
   E. Background radiation dose.

7. The acute radiation syndrome:

   A. Invariably results in the death of the individual exposed.
   B. Could be induced in a sensitive individual with a radiation dose of 5 rem.
   C. Occurs when the head and neck area is exposed to a radiation dose of 400 to 500 rem.
   D. None of the above.

8. Which of the following is a unit of radiation absorbed dose expressed in joules per kilogram of irradiated tissue?

   A. Roentgen (R).
   B. Curie.
   C. rem.
   D. Gray (Gy).

9. The unit of exposure of air is called:

   A. Coulomb per kilogram.
   B. Gray.
   C. Rad.
   D. Relative biologic effectiveness (RBE).

10. A radiation-damaged cell can pass along damage to offspring cells. This is an example of:

    A. Somatic effect.
    B. Genetic effect.
    C. Latent effect.
    D. Indirect effect.

11. X-radiation affects the incidence of cancer, leukemia, and other abnormalities by:

    A. Increasing their incidence among the general population.

B. Increasing the patient's incidence of each disease.

C. Producing specific types of cancer or other abnormalities more often.

D. Storing the radiation within the tissue, creating continual damage after exposure has ceased.

12. Which of the following is **not** considered a critical organ?

A. The brain and spinal cord.
B. The bone marrow.
C. The gonads.
D. The thyroid gland.

BIBLIOGRAPHY

Accident Facts. Chicago: National Safety Council, 1979.

Alcox RW. A dosimetry study of dental exposures from intraoral radiography. HEW publication (FDA) 73-8029. Rockville, MD: US Department of Health, Education and Welfare. 1972.

Alcox RW, Jameson WR. Patient exposures from intraoral radiographic examinations. J Am Dent Assoc 1974;88:568–575.

Antoku S. Doses to critical organs from dental radiography. Oral Surg 1976;42:251–257.

Antoku S, Hoshi M, Russell WJ, et al. Dental radiography exposure of the Hiroshima and Nagasaki populations. Oral Surg Oral Med Oral Pathol 1989;67:354–360.

Bengtsson G. Maxillofacial aspects of radiation protection: focus on recent research regarding critical organs. Dentomaxillofac Radiol 1978;7:5–14.

Bennett J. Oral care of cancer patients undergoing head and neck irradiation. Dent Hyg 1979;53:209–212.

Billen D. Spontaneous DNA damage and its significance for the "negligible dose" controversy in radiation protection. Radiat Res 1990;124:242–245.

Bomberger A, Dannenfelser BA. Radiation and health principles and practice in therapy and disaster preparedness. Rockville, MD: Aspen, 1984.

Bushong SC. Radiologic science for technologists: physics, biology, and protection. 5th ed. St. Louis: CV Mosby, 1993:654.

Court-Brown WJ, Doll R, Spiers FW, et al. Geographical variation in leukemia mortality in relation to background radiation and other factors. Br Med J 1960;88:1753–1759.

Craig L, Seidman H. Leukemia and lymphoma mortality in relation to cosmic radiation. Blood 1961;17:319–327.

Curry III TS, Dowdy JE, Murry RC Jr. Christensen's physics of diagnostic radiology. 4th ed. Philadelphia: Lea & Febiger, 1990.

Danforth RA, Gibbs SJ. Diagnostic dental radiation: what's the risk? J Calif Dent Assoc 1980;28:12–19.

Duncan W, Nias AHW. Clinical radiobiology. Edinburgh: Churchill Livingstone, 1977.

Edwards C, et al. Radiation protection for dental radiographers. St. Louis: CV Mosby, 1984.

Fletcher GH. Textbook of radiotherapy. 3rd ed. Philadelphia: Lea & Febiger, 1980.

Gibbs SJ, Pujol A, Chen T-S, et al. Radiation doses to sensitive organs from intraoral dental radiography. Dentomaxillofac Radiol 1987;16:67–77.

Gibbs SJ, Pujol A, Chen T-S, et al. Patient risk from intraoral dental radiography. Dentomaxillofac Radiol 1988;17:15–23.

Gibbs SJ, Pujol A, McDavid WD, et al. Patient risk from rotational panoramic radiography. Dentomaxillofac Radiol 1988;17:25–32.

Goaz PW, White SC. Oral radiology principles and interpretation. 3rd ed. St. Louis: CV Mosby, 1994.

Gonad doses and genetically significant dose from diagnostic radiology: U.S. 1964 and 1970. HEW publication (FDA) 76-8034. Rockville, MD: US Department of Health, Education and Welfare, 1976.

Grahn D, Kratchman J. Variation in neonatal death rate and birth weight in the United States and possible relations to environmental radiation, geology, and attitude. Am J Hum Genet 1963;15:29–35.

Granier R, Gambini DJ. Applied radiation biology and protection. New York: Ellis Horwood, 1990.

Gregg EC. Radiation risks with diagnostic x-rays. Radiology 1977;123:447–452.

Hall EJ. Radiobiology for the radiologist. 4th ed. Philadelphia: JB Lippincott, 1994.

Hendee WR. Health effects of low-level radiation. Norwalk, CT: Appleton-Century-Crofts, 1984.

Horiot JC, Bone MC, Ibrahim E, et al. Systematic dental management in head and neck irradiation. Radiat Oncol Biol Phys 1981;7:1025–1029.

International Commission on Radiation Protection. Radiation protection. ICRP pub. 16, 1970.

International Commission on Radiological Protection. Radiation protection. ICRP pub. 90, 1991.

Keifer J. Biological radiation effects. New York: Springer-Verlag, 1990.

Khan, FM. The physics of radiation therapy. 2nd ed. Baltimore: Williams & Wilkins, 1994.

Langland OE, Sippy FH, Langlais RP. Textbook of dental radiology. 2nd ed. Springfield: Charles C. Thomas, 1984.

Langland OE, et al. Panoramic radiology. 2nd ed. Philadelphia: Lea & Febiger, 1989.

Linus, A, et al. Low dose radiation and leukemia. N Engl J Med 1980;302:1101–1105.

Manson-Hing LR, Greer DF. Radiation and distribution measurements for three panoramic machines. Oral Surg 1977;44:313–318.

Matteson SR, Whaley C, Secrist VC. Dental radiology. 4th ed. Chapel Hill: University of North Carolina Press, 1988.

Mettler FA, Upton AC. Medical effects of ionizing radiation. 2nd. ed. Philadelphia: WB Saunders, 1995.

Miles DA, VanDis ML, Jensen CW, et al. Radiographic imaging for dental auxiliaries. Philadelphia: WB Saunders, 1989.

National Council on Radiation Protection and Measurements. Basic radiation protection criteria. NCRP report 39. Washington, DC: NCRP, 1971.

National Council on Radiation Protection and Measurements. Medical radiation exposure of pregnant and potentially pregnant women. NCRP report 54. Washington, DC: NCRP, 1977.

National Council on Radiation Protection and Measurements. Ionizing radiation exposure of the population of the United States. NCRP report 93. Washington, DC: NCRP, 1987.

National Council on Radiation Protection and Measurements. Exposure of the population in the United States and Canada from natural background radiation. NCRP report 94. Washington, DC: NCRP, 1987.

National Council on Radiation Protection and Measurements. Radiation exposure of the U.S. population from consumer products and miscellaneous sources. NCRP report 95. Washington, DC: NCRP, 1987.

National Council on Radiation Protection and Measurements. Exposure of the U.S. population from diagnostic medical radiation. NCRP report 100. Bethesda, MD: NCRP, 1989.

National Council on Radiation Protection and Measurements. Exposure of the U.S. population from occupational radiation. NCRP report 101. Bethesda, MD: National Academy Press, 1990.

Nationwide evaluation of x-ray trends: representative sample data. January 1, 1983 to December 31, 1983. Department of Health and Human Services publication (FDA). Washington, DC: DHHS, 1984.

North Carolina Department of Environment, Health and Natural Resources, Division of Radiation Protection. North Carolina regulations for protection against radiation. Raleigh, NC: NCDEHNR, 1991.

Nygaard O, Sinclair WK, Lett JT. Advances in radiation biology. San Diego: Academic Press, 1992.

Pizzarello DL, Witcofsky RL. Medical radiation biology. 2nd ed. Philadelphia: Lea & Febiger, 1982.

Pochin EE. Why be quantitative about radiation risk estimates? LS Taylor Lecture Series, no. 2. Washington, DC: NCRP, 1978.

Schuman LM. Background radiation and Down's syndrome. Ann NY Acad Sci 1970;171:441–453.

Silverman C, Hoffman DA. Thyroid tumor risk from radiations during childhood. Prev Med 1975;4:100.

Smith QW, Preece JW, Hefley DC, et al. Radiation exposure in the dental setting: an update. Radiol Technol 1983;55:546.

Stenstrom B, Henrikson CO, Holm B, et al. Absorbed doses from intraoral radiography with special emphasis on collimator dimensions. Swed Dent J 1986;10:59–71.

Sullivan DM, Fleming TJ. Oral care for the radiotherapy-treated head and neck cancer patient. Dent Hyg 1986;60:112–114.

Taylor LS. Let's keep our sense of humor in dealing with radiation hazards. Perspect Biol Med 1980;12:325–334.

Underhill TE, Chilvarquer I, Kimura K, et al. Radiobiologic risk estimation from dental radiology: part I. absorbed doses to critical organs. Oral Surg Oral Med Oral Pathol 1988;66:111–120.

United Nations Scientific Committee on the Effects of Atomic Radiation. Source, effects and risks of ionizing radiation. New York: United Nations, 1988.

Velders XL, Van Aken J, Vander Selt PF. Absorbed dose to organs in head and neck from bitewing radiography. Dentomaxillofac Radiol 1991;20:161–165.

Wall BF, et al. Doses for patients from pantomographic and conventional dental radiography. Br J Radiol 1979;52:727.

Wall BF, Kendall GW. Collective doses and risks from dental radiology in Great Britain. Br J Radiol 1983;56:5-11.

Weissman D, Sobkowski F. Comparative thermoluminescent dosimetry of intraoral periapical radiography. Oral Surg Oral Med Oral Pathol 1970;20:376–386.

Whitcher BL, Gratt BM, Sickles EA. Leaded shields for thyroid dose reduction in intraoral dental radiography. Oral Surg 1979;48:564–570.

Whitcher BL, Gratt BM, Sickles EA. A leaded apron for use in panoramic dental radiography. Oral Surg 1980;49:467.

White SC, Rose TC. Absorbed bone marrow dose in certain radiographic techniques. J Am Dent Assoc 1979;98:553.

White SC. 1992 Assessment of radiation risks from dental radiography. Dentomaxillofac Radiol 1992;21:118–126.

Wilson R. Risks caused by low levels of pollution. Yale J Biol Med 1978;51:37.

Radiologic Health and Protection

13

OBJECTIVES

Upon successful completion of this unit, the student will be able to:

1. *State the basic factors affecting radiologic health.*

2. *Explain how to minimize patient radiation doses.*

3. *Describe all concepts associated with operator protection.*

4. *Test his or her knowledge by answering the Review Questions.*

KEY WORDS/PHRASES

As Low As Reasonably
  Achievable Concept
collimation
constant potential
distance
dosimetry monitoring
E+ speed film
electronic timers

film-holders
filtration
kilovoltage
long beam indicating device
  (round and rectangular)
maximum permissible dose
milliamperage
nonoccupational exposure

occupational exposure
position
protective aprons (torso and
  poncho)
rare earth screens
selection of radiographs
shielding
thyroid collar

RADIOLOGIC HEALTH

INTRODUCTION

Because the effects of x-rays at low-level radiation doses cannot currently be measured, the basic assumption is made that every dose of radiation produces some potential biologic damage. It is a goal to keep radiation exposures to the minimum that are necessary to meet diagnostic requirements. Therefore, efforts have been made to determine the most appropriate balance between the potential risk to the patient and the obvious benefits of radiation in terms of improved diagnosis and treatment. Efforts to identify this acceptable balance point have resulted in the establishment of radiation protection standards by various national committees on radiation protection.

NATIONAL COUNCIL ON RADIATION PROTECTION AND MEASUREMENTS

The National Council on Radiation Protection and Measurements (NCRP) is a private organization of scientists who are experts in various aspects of radiation and operate under a congressional charter, but **do not have legal status.** They make **maximum permissible dose (MPD)** recommendations that are published periodically in handbooks. The **NCRP** is purely advisory, but most state and federal laws are based on NCRP recommendations.

MPD

By definition, **the MPD is the amount of radiation that an individual is allowed to receive from artificial sources of radiation,** such as x-ray machines, except when the individual is a medical or dental patient. This is a level of radiation dose that represents an acceptably low risk of harmful effects. Since the first recommendation of by the NCRP in 1931 of 50 Roentgens per year (0.2 R per workday), the MPD has been lowered on three occasions. The MPD is now only one tenth of its initial level. Recommended exposures have been lowered because of growing concern over the increasing use of diagnostic radiation and apprehension about the mounting evidence that small doses can cause leukemia and carcinoma.

MPD for Two Groups

The MPD is defined for two groups of persons: **occupationally exposed,** i.e., those persons who are normally expected to use or work around radiation as a normal part of their job (dentists, assistants, hygienists), and **nonoccupationally exposed,** i.e., those persons who do not work with radiation (front office staff, general public, family in waiting rooms). Also, in the event of **pregnancy,** an occupationally exposed woman would be permitted to receive the same dose as a nonoccupationally exposed person. In addition, there are dose limits recommended for different organs or parts of the body because of their different sensitivities to radiation. The permissible levels for each of these three groups are listed below:

Maximum Permissible Doses

Class of Exposed Individual	Maximum Permissible Dose (mSv)
Radiation workers (dentists, assistants, hygienists) (annual)	
Effective dose equivalent limit (whole body)	50
Partial body dose equivalent limits	
Skin	150
Forearms	300
Hands	750
Other organs and organ systems (e.g., red bone marrow, breast, lung, and gonads)	500
Lifetime cumulative exposure	10 (times age in years)
Public exposures (annual)	
Effective dose equivalent limit, continuous or frequent exposure	1
Effective dose equivalent limit, infrequent exposure	5
Dose equivalent limits for lens of eye, skin, and extremities	50
Trainees younger than 18 years of age (annual)	
Effective dose equivalent limit	1
Dose equivalent limit for lens of eye, skin, and extremities	50
Pregnant women (with respect to fetus)	
Total dose equivalent limit	5 (during gestation period)
Dose equivalent limit in 1 month	0.5

Summary of National Council on Radiation Protection and Measurements. Exposure of the U.S. population from diagnostic and medical radiation. NCRP report 116. Washington, DC: NCRP, 1993. Recommendations for radiation dose limits, excluding background and medical exposures but including both internal and external exposures.

With a properly designed office, properly functioning x-ray machines, and proper dental radiography procedures, x-ray machines should not cause any occupational or nonoccupational person to receive anywhere near the MPD. In fact, if a dental office's dosimetry service indicates that the office is receiving even one tenth of the MPD, office procedures should be carefully evaluated because routine dental radiography should result in almost no increase above background levels to any member of the dental staff or public. When calculating the MPD or dose limits for occupationally or nonoccupationally exposed persons, radiation received from environmental background and diagnostic medical and dental exposures (for the individual's personal health care) are specifically **excluded** from calculations, primarily because medical and dental exposures and environmental background radiation cannot be effectively controlled or limited. Therefore, **the concept of MPD does not apply to doses that someone receives as a dental or medical patient.** The government does not limit the radiation dose that patients receive because it recognizes that to set such a limit might prevent physicians and dentists from prescribing radiographs that would greatly benefit the patient. However, radiation operators are required to use the minimum amount of radiation possible to obtain the information required to diagnose and treat each patient. Therefore, one of the many responsibilities of a licensed or certified dental health-care worker is to use x-rays carefully and only for each patient's benefit, as described in the following paragraphs.

ALARA Concept

An important radiation protection concept is the **As Low As Reasonably Achievable (ALARA)** concept. In principle, this concept does not specify a specific level of radiation dose for exposed persons as the MPD concept does. Simply stated, ALARA means that every reasonable measure will be taken to assure that occupationally and nonoccupationally exposed persons will receive the smallest amount of radiation possible. The implications of this concept will be discussed more fully in the section on operator and patient protection. Currently, **ALARA** is considered the most appropriate, relevant radiation concept for the 1990s and should be considered the radiation protection concept of choice for our modern society.

PATIENT RADIATION PROTECTION

Patients may want to know how careful a dental health-care worker is with x-rays and may ask a question such as, "I have heard that x-rays are dangerous. What do you do to protect me against them?"

RADIATION PROTECTION

The following recommendations are designed to minimize the somatic and genetic exposures to patients from dental diagnostic radiographic procedures. Many of the factors have been discussed elsewhere in this book and are included in this section as a means of integrating information on radiation protection. It should be noted that all suggestions will secondarily minimize the exposure. The radiation operator and consequently the results may be considered of potential double benefit to the patient and the dental health-care worker.

Decisions for Selection of Radiographs

First, the operator should expose no one to x-rays without a good reason. This means that "routine radiographs," which are radiographs taken without considering the patient's clinical findings and history, should **not** be taken. An example of routine radiographs would be to make a full-mouth series or a panoramic radiograph on every new patient without a prior examination. Another example would be bitewing radiographs on every patient every 6 months. A further example would be to take a full-mouth survey when a panoramic radiograph would serve equally well. Instead of this approach, the dental health-care worker should examine and question the patient **before** deciding whether to make radiographs and, if radiographs are needed, which radiographs should be made. A Food and Drug Administration (FDA) panel has published a set of radiographic selection criteria—which include patient signs, symptoms, developmental stage, and historical features—that help in the decision about which radiographs to take and when to take them (U.S. Department of Health and Human Services, 1989). If a radiograph would not change the diagnosis or treatment or if a radiograph is highly unlikely to provide any additional helpful information, it should probably not be taken. Postoperative radiographs should be taken only when there is a clinical indication and not as verification for third-party payment plans. It is always prudent to use only the minimum number of films required to adequately treat a patient, i.e., a panoramic radiograph rather than the full-mouth survey. This applies to all patients, whether pregnant, young, old, new, or recall. Pregnancy is not a contraindication for dental radiography.

Decisions Made at the X-Ray Machine

Kilovoltage (kVp) The x-ray machine should be operated at the highest kilovoltage (kVp) consistent with a good image, usually 70 to 90 kVp. An x-ray machine that is incapable of being operated at least at 60 kVp should **not** be used. High-kilovoltage operation produces more "useful" x-rays and fewer low-energy rays that are absorbed by the patient without contributing to the quality of the image. Dental x-ray techniques using higher kilovoltages reduce the effective dose delivered per intraoral examination. It has been reported by Gibbs et al. (1988) that the effective dose to the patient was reduced up to 23% in one study by increasing kilovoltages from 70 to 90 kVp.

Constant Potential X-Ray Machines This generator design converts the alternating current (AC) to direct current (DC) to produce a homogeneous beam of consistent wavelengths during the whole exposure. This type of dental x-ray machine can reduce the patient exposure by 20% over conventional machines. Because this is an integral design feature, older machines cannot be converted to constant potential. Because lower exposures are necessary, it is important to follow the manufacturer's instructions.

Filtration The x-ray beam should be properly filtered. Filtration preferentially removes soft, low-energy, long-wavelength x-rays from the beam (Fig. 13.1). These rays are undesirable because they are absorbed by the patient (increasing the patient's dose) without contributing to the formation of the radiographic image (no increased benefit). Filtration is stated in millimeters of aluminum (mm Al), which is the material most commonly used. A dental x-ray machine operating at 50 to 69 kVp should have at least 1.5 mm Al equivalent filtration, whereas a machine operating at 70 kVp or more should have at least 2.5 mm Al equivalent filtration.

Minimum Total Filtration	
Operating Voltage (kVp)	**Aluminum Filtration (mm)**
50 to 69	1.5
70 and above	2.5

From National Council on Radiation Protection and Measurements. Dental x-ray protection. NCRP report 35. Washington, DC: NCRP, 1970.

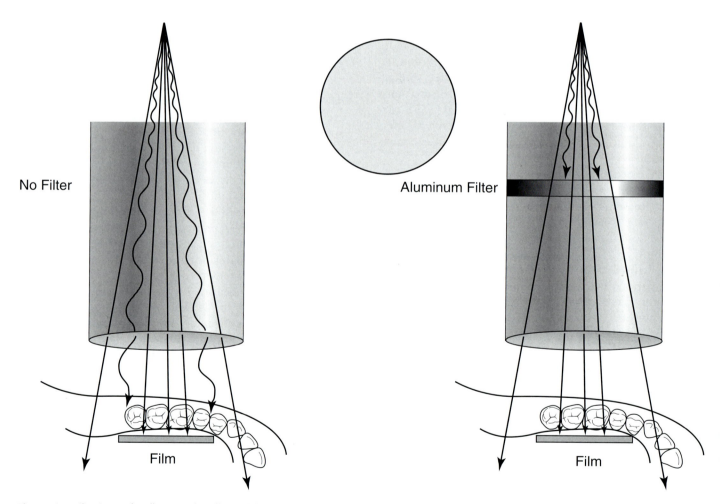

Figure 13.1. Filtration. This illustrates the effects of filtration on skin exposure of patient. (*Left*) No filter. (*Right*) With filter, long low-energy x-rays are filtered out.

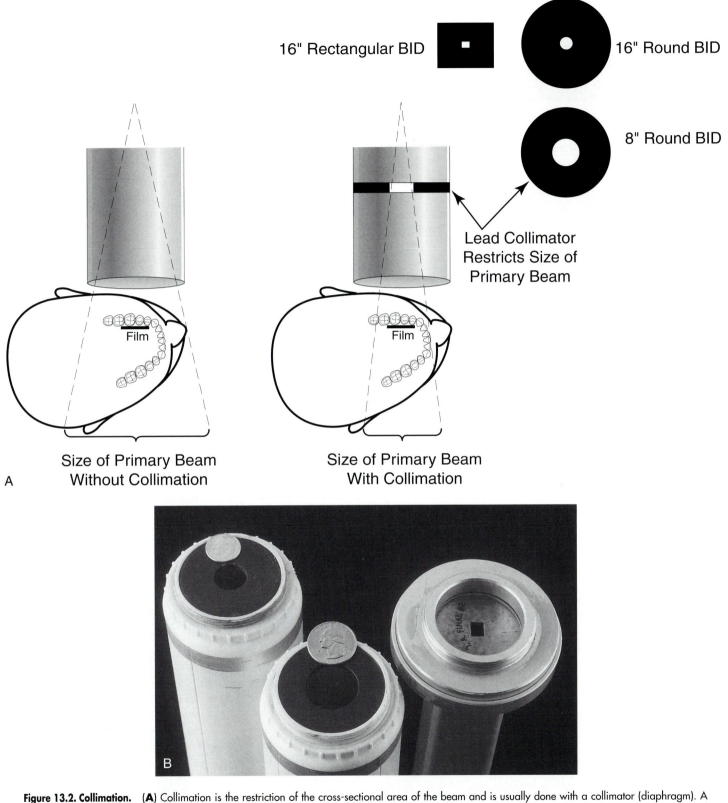

16" Rectangular BID

16" Round BID

8" Round BID

Lead Collimator
Restricts Size of
Primary Beam

Film

Film

Size of Primary Beam
Without Collimation

Size of Primary Beam
With Collimation

A

B

Figure 13.2. Collimation. (**A**) Collimation is the restriction of the cross-sectional area of the beam and is usually done with a collimator (diaphragm). A collimator can be a flat piece of lead with a round hole in it to restrict the useful beam to an area no larger than 2.75 inches in diameter when measured at the end of the beam indicating device (BID). The size and shape of the hole in the center depends on whether the BID is short/long or rectangular/round. The collimators on the right are for long round cones (*upper*) and short round cones (*lower*). (**B**) Collimator aperture sizes: (*left*) long round BID—dime size; (*middle*) short round BID—quarter size; (*right*) rectangular long BID—smallest.

A. Round Collimator

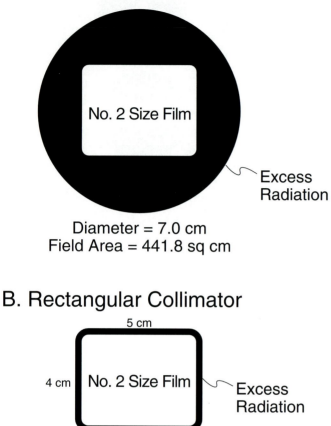

No. 2 Size Film

Excess Radiation

Diameter = 7.0 cm
Field Area = 441.8 sq cm

B. Rectangular Collimator

5 cm

4 cm | No. 2 Size Film

Excess Radiation

Field Area = 200 sq cm

Figure 13.3. Rectangular Collimation. By using a rectangular collimator (**B**) rather than a round cylinder beam restrictor (**A**), the area irradiated has been decreased by more than 55%.

In panoramic and cephalometric x-ray machines, selective filtration of both low- and high-energy photons with rare earth materials, in combination with aluminum filtration, has reduced patient exposure by 20 to 80% compared with conventional aluminum filtration alone. Adequate filtration should be confirmed by expert (such as a factory representative or state inspector) periodic inspection of the x-ray machine.

Collimation of the Beam It is required by federal law to collimate (limit) the field of radiation at the patient's skin surface to a circle having a diameter of no more than 7 cm (2.75 inches). Collimation means restriction of the cross-sectional area of the beam, and this is usually done with a lead diaphragm (collimator) within the tubehead or at the end of a lead-lined cylinder (incorrectly referred to as a cone) (Fig. 13.2). Because the dimensions of a no. 2 intraoral regular film is 3.2 × 4.1 cm, the patient exposure using the circular collimation as required by law (7-cm diameter) is actually almost 3 times the area necessary to expose the film. Therefore, the patient exposure can be significantly reduced by limiting the beam even more. It is highly recommended that instead of using round collimation, rectangular collimation (which restricts the beam to approximately the size of the film) be used. Use of rectangular collimation reduces the patient dose approximately 55% compared with round collimation (Fig. 13.3). Rectangular collimation also improves image quality by reducing fog from scatter, resulting in a radiograph with better resolution and better contrast. Rectangular collimation of the x-ray beam can be accomplished by one or a combination of methods. Dentsply/Rinn XCP film-holders (Elgin, IL) used in conjunction with a rectangular BID or with a round BID with a Dentsply/Rinn Universal rectangular collimator attached to it can be used to reduce

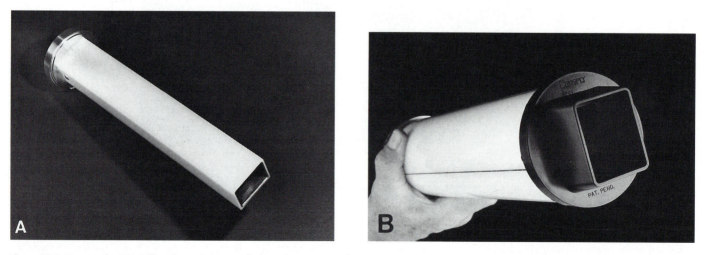

Figure 13.4. Rectangular BID Collimation. (**A**) Dentsply/Rinn long rectangular BID. (**B**) Dentsply/Rinn Universal Rectangular Collimator attached to long round BID.

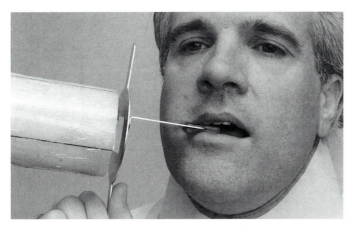

Figure 13.5. Masel Precision Instruments. The Masel Precision Instruments collimate the circular x-ray beam to a rectangular-shaped beam at the patient's face, reducing unnecessary radiation exposure to the patient.

patient exposure (Fig. 13.4). Also, the Precision Instrument (Masel, Philadelphia, PA) can be expected to produce similar results (Fig. 13.5).

Use of Long BID (Cone) The lead-lined cylinder or rectangular collimator protruding from the x-ray machine functions as a beam indicating device (BID). The BID serves to show the radiographer where the beam will strike the patient. There are three lengths of BIDs: 8 inches, 12 inches, and 16 inches (Fig. 13.6). A lead-lined long BID is preferred because they result in less beam divergence.

Therefore, there is less volume of patient's tissue irradiated per exposure (Fig. 13.7). Pointed plastic cones **are not recommended** because they increase scattered radiation to all areas of the patient's head, neck, and reproductive organs (Fig. 13.8). In addition, a much greater volume of tissue is irradiated due to scattered radiation from the plastic pointed cone (Fig. 13.9). Also, by use of the lead-lined, long open-ended BID rather than the shorter BID, the diagnostic quality of the radiographic image is improved because less scatter radiation is produced.

Use of Electronic Timers The timer on the x-ray machine should be electronic. Mechanical timers are imprecise when used for the short exposures needed in modern dental radiography. Mechanical timers are also not accurate for exposures **less** than 1 second and are not recommended (Fig. 13.10). The timer on the x-ray machine should have a "dead man" control, which shuts the machine off immediately, regardless of timer setting, unless finger or foot pressure is held continuously on the timer switch throughout the desired exposure. The electronic timer is calibrated in sixtieths of a second, corresponding to the 60 cycles per second of alternating current that powers the machine. Each one sixtieth of a second exposure results in one pulse of x-rays produced.

Decisions Made at the Chair

E+ Speed Film The fastest and most appropriate film should be used. Speeds of dental x-ray film are described with letters: A, B, C, D, and E, with A being the slowest

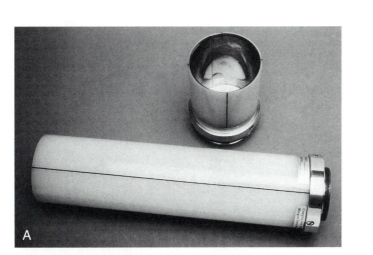

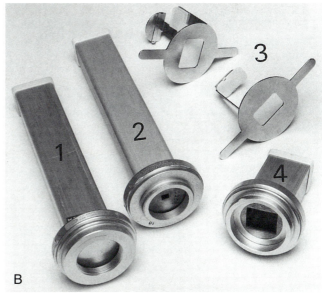

Figure 13.6. Long and Short BIDs. (**A**) Short (*above*) and long (*below*) round open-ended, lead-lined cylinders or BIDs. (**B**) Types of rectangular collimators (*1*) and (*2*) long Dentsply/Rinn rectangular BIDs for different x-ray machines. (*3*) Masel Precision Instruments (anterior and posterior instruments). (*4*) Short Dentsply/Rinn rectangular BID for recessed anode tubeheads.

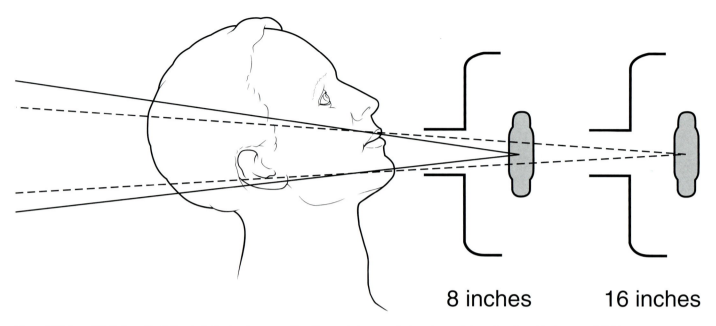

8 inches   **16 inches**

Figure 13.7. Long BID Reduces Radiation to Patient. As source-film distance is increased, the volume of tissue irradiated is decreased. White areas represent the extra volume of tissue exposed when an 8-inch distance is used rather than the 16-inch distance.

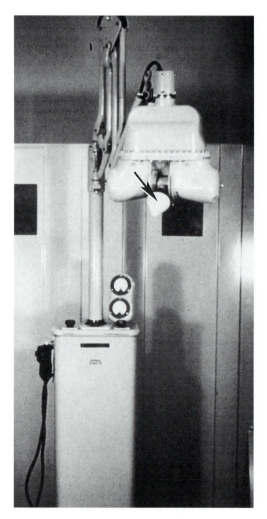

Figure 13.8. Plastic Pointed Short Cone. Plastic pointed short cone (*arrow*) on older vintage x-ray machine.

POINTED BID

OPEN ENDED BID

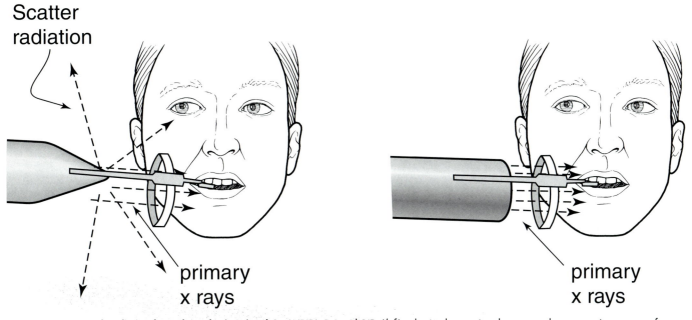

Figure 13.9. Scattered Radiation from Short Plastic Pointed Cone (BID). Pointed BID (*left*): plastic short pointed cone produces a major source of scatter radiation when irradiated by the primary x-ray beam. Open-ended BID (*right*): the source of scatter radiation is eliminated when the open-ended cylinder is used.

and E being the fastest. A, B, and C film are no longer commercially available. E-speed film requires half the exposure that D-speed film requires to produce the same amount of film density. E-speed film is technically more difficult to process (develop and fix) satisfactorily, and tighter quality control is needed. In 1994, Eastman Kodak (Rochester, NY) developed a Kodak Ekta speed Plus (E+) dental film that gives diagnostic detail that rivals D-speed film.

Rare Earth Intensifying Screens Patient x-ray exposure during panoramic and other extraoral projections can be further reduced by using rare earth intensifying screens and high-speed film. The higher speed of the rare earth/T-Mat grain film (flattened silver halide grains) combinations have been found to be twice as fast as conventional calcium tungstate screen/film combinations (Miles et al., 1989; Ponce et al., 1986).

Film-Holding Devices A film-holding device should be used. The purposes of this device are to **avoid** using the patient's fingers to hold the film in place, thus avoiding an unnecessary dose to the fingers; to more accurately align the film with the teeth, and the BID with the film;

and to avoid retaking radiographs caused by improper alignment. Film-holding devices are essential if rectangular collimation is used, because the smaller, narrow beam leaves almost no room for error in aiming the BID at the film.

Leaded Protective Aprons and Thyroid Collars or Shields The patient should be provided with a leaded torso apron and a leaded thyroid shield (Fig. 13.11). Although exposure to the gonads is negligible, a leaded apron provides shielding and thus further reduces genetic and carcinogenic risk to pelvic, abdominal, and thoracic tissues. Breast and bone marrow are the somatic tissues of greatest concern here. Leaded torso (body) aprons will reduce genetic exposure by 98% for panoramic radiography, and the apron should cover both the front of the patient's chest as well as the shoulders and back because the tubehead exposes the film from this position (Fig. 13.12). Additionally, for intraoral radiography, a **thyroid shield** will reduce the dose to the thyroid gland by approximately 50%. An added benefit of both leaded apron and thyroid shield is that patients appreciate this precaution.

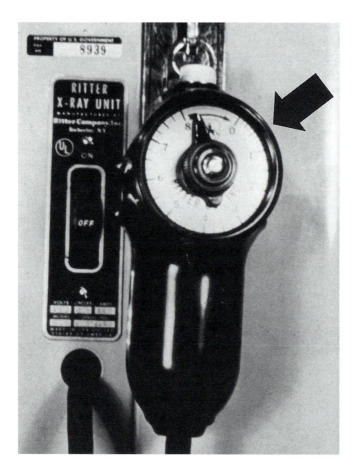

Figure 13.10. Mechanical Timers. A mechanical timer (*arrow*) on an older dental x-ray machine. When the button is pushed, it closes the circuit and allows the current to flow without interruption. These timers are inaccurate for exposure times shorter than 1 second.

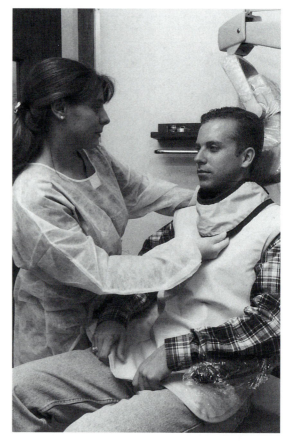

Figure 13.11. Leaded Torso Apron and Thyroid Collar. Example of a protective leaded torso apron and thyroid collar.

Decisions Made in the Darkroom

Correct film processing procedures necessarily include a wide variety of subcategories, because each factor will significantly improve the quality of the radiograph. If neglected, these same factors will severely degrade the quality of the radiograph.

Darkroom Lighting Decisions The darkroom must be kept free from light leaks. White light should not be allowed to leak in around doors, plumbing, air conditioning ducts, windows, and so on because it will produce film fog. An appropriate safelight filter should be used in the darkroom to permit the operator to work in the dark without producing film fog during various stages in film processing. The Kodak GBX-2 (red) safelight filter is a universal safelight filter that can be used in darkrooms where both intraoral and extraoral, such as panoramic and cephalometric films, are handled. This includes films that are used with the rare earth screens. A standard 15-W bulb should be used with most films, and the safe-

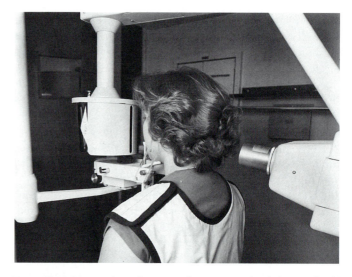

Figure 13.12. Panoramic Lead Apron. The panoramic leaded apron should cover both the front and the back of the patient because both sides of the patient are exposed in panoramic x-ray projections. The leaded thyroid shield cannot be used because it interferes with the panoramic image.

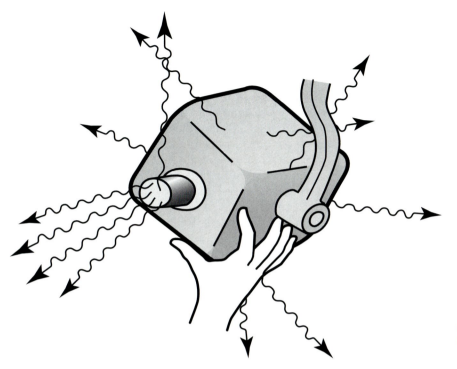

Figure 13.13. Tubehead Leakage Radiation. Never hold the cone (BID) or tubehead during exposure because of leakage radiation from tubehead.

light lamps should be placed at a minimum of 4 feet from the working area. The ML-2 (light orange) filter should **not** be used with panoramic or other extraoral films. The ML-2 is designed to be used with the intraoral D speed dental film only. It will fog panoramic and E+ intraoral films.

Full Development Processing Decisions When radiographs are to be processed by the manual (hand-dip) method, time/temperature processing is absolutely essential because it is the only way to ensure maximum development of the radiographic image. In all instances, full development should be used (e.g., 5 minutes at 70°F). The exposure time can be reduced when the film is given full development. For example, the radiation exposure may be decreased by 25% without interfering with the quality of the film image. It has been estimated that to shorten developing time by 1 minute, it would be necessary to increase the patient's exposure by at least 30%—an extremely unwise thing to do. Sight or visual development techniques are prohibited because they encourage overexposure of the patient and underdevelopment of the radiographic image.

Decisions about Processing Solutions Processing solutions should be changed regularly, stirred thoroughly twice each day, kept covered to prevent oxidation when not in use, and not subjected to excessively high temperatures. Weekly quality control checks should be performed to ensure optimal processing and quality radiographs. (It

should be done daily with automatic processors.) Chemicals should also be replenished according to the manufacturer's instructions. Depleted or contaminated chemicals can result in a nondiagnostic radiograph that necessitates a retake, thus doubling the patient's dose for that image. Manual processing tanks or automatic processor tanks and rollers should be cleaned and checked regularly and frequently. The darkroom should be immaculate, and the counter tops devoid of wet or dried chemicals, which could adversely affect the quality of the films before or after processing.

Decisions about a Quality Assurance Program Every dental office should have a written quality control program. There should be one staff member who is responsible for implementing the plan daily and for monitoring all exposure, processing, and equipment maintenance steps. In this way, the cause of any substandard radiographs can be quickly detected and corrected, thus preventing future retakes (see Chapter 8).

Decisions about the Viewbox

Radiographs should be properly mounted in opaque mounts and viewed in a dimly lit room with a properly functioning illuminator (viewbox). An illuminator with variable intensity is helpful when viewing radiographs that have been overexposed (too dark) or underexposed (too pale). Many retakes can be avoided by adjusting the light source on the viewbox. If all other steps have been followed but the radiographs are not viewed under ideal conditions, the radiographic image could be misinterpreted.

OPERATOR RADIATION PROTECTION

General Concepts

The operator should be ready to answer clearly and completely when asked about the precautions taken on behalf of the patient when radiographs are made. In addition, new members of the office staff will surely have their own welfare in mind. They have already learned that humans may develop cancer from an overexposure to radiation. What should they be told when they ask, "What is done in this office to protect me from occupational radiation exposure?" There are several procedures operators can use to minimize their occupational exposure in the dental office. Most of them are based on certain fundamental concepts concerning x-rays, which are that (1) x-rays travel in a straight line from their source, (2) x-radiation intensity of the beam decreases as the distance from the source increases (inverse square law), and (3) x-rays can be scattered in their path of travel.

The operator of dental x-ray equipment may be potentially exposed to primary radiation from the useful beam, leakage radiation from the tube housing, and scattered radiation usually from the patient's skull. Leakage radiation is radiation other than the useful beam that escapes through the protective shielding of an x-ray tube housing. Because x-rays radiate in straight lines from the source, there is need for a metal housing for the tube. Despite the metal tube housing, there is a small amount of radiation that will leak. The operator should never hold the cone or tube housing to steady it during exposure (Fig. 13.13).

Three Basic Methods to Reduce Occupational Exposure

There are three basic methods to reduce the occupational dose from x-rays: position, distance, and shielding. These methods can be used to the operator's advantage, as summarized in the following paragraphs.

Position and Distance The most effective way of reducing operator exposure to primary radiation is to enforce strict application of the **position and distance rule** (i.e., the operator should stand at least 6 feet away from the patient and in a safe quadrant at an angle between 90 and 135° to the primary beam) (Fig. 13.14).

If the operator cannot stand at least 6 feet from the patient during the exposure, he or she should stand behind an appropriate protective barrier or outside the operatory behind a wall (Fig. 13.15). Dental personnel should **not** hold films in the patient's mouth. Squamous cell carcinoma of the fingers can be caused by this practice (Fig. 13.16). The tubehead or cone should **never** be held or stabilized during exposure, and the operator should **never** stand directly in line with the primary beam of radiation (Fig. 13.17). Dentists, dental hygienists, dental assistants, and dental radiology technicians should **never** stand in the primary beam to restrain a patient during x-ray exposure. When a patient has to be restrained during exposure, a relative or friend of the patient should do so. The relative or friend should be provided with a leaded apron and gloves so they have maximum protection during exposure.

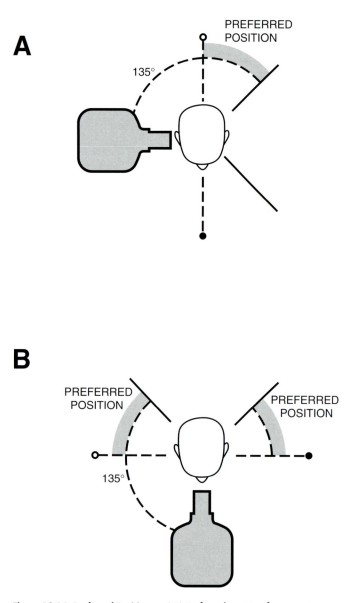

Figure 13.14. Preferred Positions. (**A**) Preferred position for posterior radiographs. (**B**) Positions of greatest safety for operator during x-ray exposure to patient for anterior radiographs. The circles represent 90° positions; the operator should stand in the area designated "preferred position," at least 6 feet away from the cone (BID) tip.

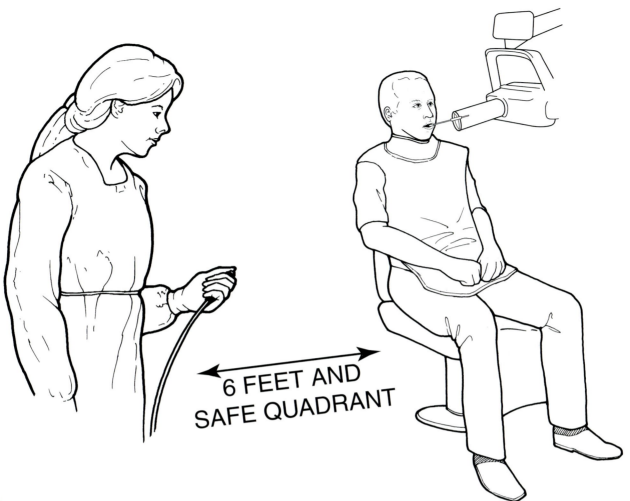

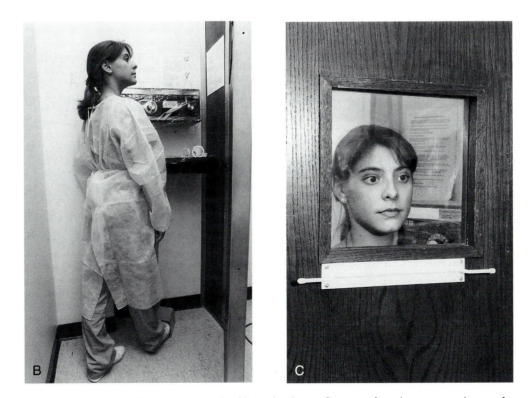

Figure 13.15. Distance and Protective Barrier. (**A**) The operator should stand at least 6 feet away from the patient and in a safe quadrant at an angle between 90° and 135° to the primary beam. (**B**) If the radiographer cannot stand at least 6 feet away from the patient, he or she should stand behind a leaded protective barrier or behind a gypsum wallboard (drywall). (**C**) Operator viewing patient through leaded window of leaded protective barrier.

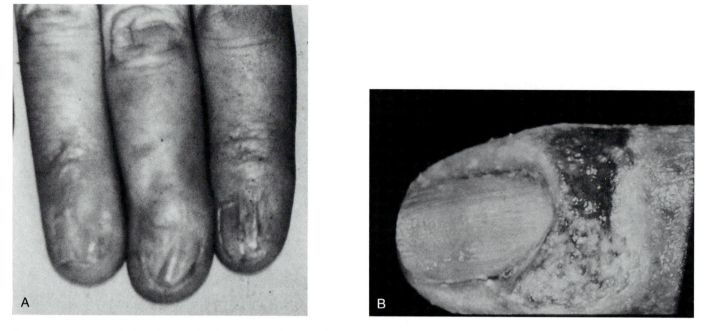

Figure 13.16. Squamous Cell Carcinoma. **(A)** Dystrophic nail changes from radiation. **(B)** Squamous cell carcinoma of dentist's finger caused by holding films in patient's mouth.

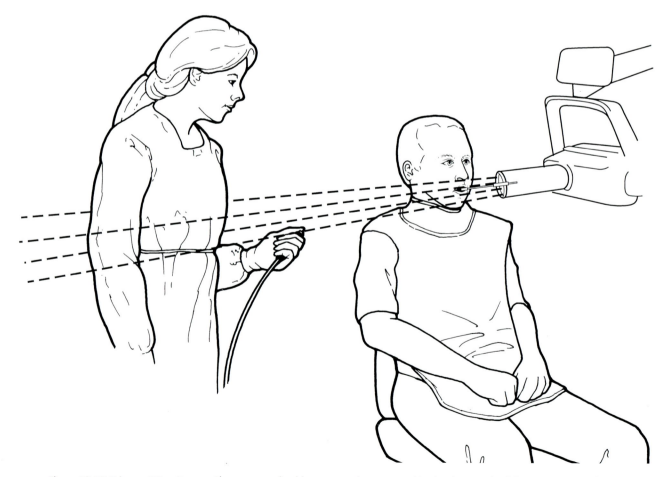

Figure 13.17. Primary X-Ray Beam. The operator should never stand unprotected in the direct path of the primary x-ray beam.

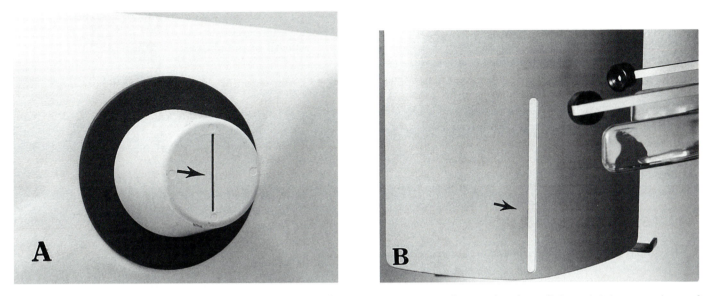

Figure 13.18. Panoramic X-Ray Collimation. The scattered radiation from panoramic x-ray machine is relatively small due to (**A**) the narrow beam of radiation from the tubehead and (**B**) the narrow shielding collimation at the cassette carrier.

Scattered radiation from panoramic x-ray units is relatively small, owing to the narrow beam of radiation and the narrow shielding collimation at the cassette carrier (Fig. 13.18). Using the MPD guidelines for occupationally exposed persons of 1 mSv per week, an operator could conceivably expose 4000 panoramic radiographs per week with safety if he or she stood 2 meters from the unit (2 meters is approximately 6 feet). However, to be prudent, the operator should stand behind a barrier if he or she cannot stand 6 feet from the panoramic x-ray machine.

Shielding If the operator must stand closer than 6 feet from the patient and machine, he or she should leave the room or take a position behind a suitable wall during exposure of the film. Minimal shielding requirements for dental operatories are provided the NCRP (NCRP report 35, 1970). A physicist or radiography inspector can determine how much shielding is needed for a given situation. The walls of the dental x-ray operatory must be of sufficient density or thickness to limit the exposure of nonoccupationally exposed persons (for instance, persons working in an adjacent office) to legally acceptable levels. Usually, it is not necessary to line the walls with lead to meet this requirement. A wall constructed of gypsum wallboard (drywall) has been determined to be sufficient for the average dental office (MacDonald et al., 1983).

Radiation Dosimetry Monitoring Service Subscribing to one of the many film badge services provides an excellent tangible way to express concern for reducing and monitoring radiation exposure to office staff (Fig. 13.19). Quarterly reports (monthly or semiannually are also avail-

able) from a film badge service provide appropriate legal documentation that staff members have or have not received excessive radiation exposure during their employment in the office. These reports also serve as a direct way of monitoring the staff's willingness to abide by office

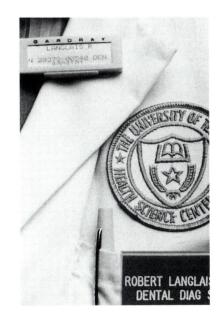

Figure 13.19. Radiation Dosimetry Monitoring Service. Personal monitoring badge. The film badge contains a lithium fluoride crystal. When returned to the company, the badge is processed and compared optically with known amounts of radiation. The resulting exposure is reported to the dental office. The dosimetry badge is usually worn on the clothing over the front of the hip or chest, as shown here.

safety rules regarding radiation exposure procedures. An additional advantage to monitoring office personnel is that a series of radiation reports indicating little or no exposure serves to allay any apprehension the office staff may have about receiving potentially damaging exposure to x-radiation. If the doses are high, it alerts the staff to look for improper procedures followed in the office or for problems in barrier design. It also provides a written record of staff exposures in the unlikely but possible event that one of the staff members develops cancer and blames it on the office x-ray procedures.

CASE-BASED PROBLEM-SOLVING

1. You have a pregnant patient who is concerned about getting dental x-rays. Outline the available protective measures for this patient. What is your final recommendation?

2. You have an employee who takes dental radiographs and is fearful that small daily doses of exposure could lead to cancer or a deformed fetus. Outline the protective measures available to allay this employee's fears.

REVIEW QUESTIONS

1. Greater beam limitation is achieved when the BID is _____ and the diameter of the opening is _____.

   A. Shorter, smaller.
   B. Longer, bigger.
   C. Shorter, bigger.
   D. Longer, smaller.

2. Which type of radiation is produced when the primary beam of x-ray photons interact with the pointed plastic cone?

   A. Primary radiation.
   B. Scattered radiation.
   C. Characteristic radiation.
   D. Remnant radiation.

3. Which of the following procedures will reduce your x-ray exposure as an x-ray operator?

   A. Standing at least 6 feet away from the tubehead when making an exposure.
   B. Standing behind an appropriate barrier or outside the x-ray room.

   C. Never holding or stabilizing the tubehead during exposures.
   D. All of the above.

4. Collimation of a beam refers to what?

   A. The selective removal of soft radiation from the beam.
   B. The selective removal of hard radiation from the beam.
   C. The reduction of the beam diameter.
   D. The process of reducing the beam intensity by 50%.

5. Filtration is used in dental x-ray machines to remove:

   A. Scatter radiation.
   B. High-energy photons.
   C. Long-wavelength photons.
   D. Low-energy electrons.

6. All of the following are good ways to reduce exposure **except:**

   A. Using fast film; E-speed is the fastest.
   B. Using an 8-inch BID.
   C. Using the paralleling technique.
   D. Using higher kilovoltage settings.

7. Depending on the circumstances, when films are to be held in the mouth of a child, the dental radiographer should:

   1. Hold them him/herself.
   2. Ask the assistant to hold the film.
   3. Ask a parent or guardian to hold the film.
   4. Use film-holders.
   A. 1 and 4.
   B. 2 and 3.
   C. 2 and 4.
   D. 3 and 4.

8. A dental health-care worker is using a film badge service to measure his or her radiation exposure. The service reports that the badge was exposed to 5 mSv in the previous month. The worker should:

   A. Stop taking x-ray films immediately.
   B. Report to a physician for a blood count.
   C. Ignore the report because the reading is insignificant.

D. Evaluate x-ray procedures and take steps to reduce unnecessary radiation.

9. During pregnancy, a patient:

   A. Should be advised of her legal rights before being irradiated.
   B. Should be warned about possible miscarriage.
   C. Should never be irradiated for dental radiographs.
   D. May be irradiated for dental radiographs by taking the necessary precautions.

10. As a radiation worker, you should not be exposed to more than an effective dose of 50 mSv a year. But in x-raying yourself for dental treatment, you are exposed to about 50 mSv. Which of the following reconciles these contradictory statements?

   A. Because you need dental radiographs, you can be given an unlimited amount of radiation.
   B. As a patient you can be given any amount of radiation, regardless of damage.
   C. Exceptions can be made.
   D. Whole-body radiation is different from specific-region radiation.

11. The dental health-care worker should not hold the:

   A. Film during exposure.
   B. Tube during exposure.
   C. Patient during exposure.
   D. All of the above.

12. Some of the most effective means of controlling secondary radiation are:

   1. Shielding.
   2. Increasing kVp.
   3. Using filters.
   4. Decreasing film speed.
   A. 1 and 3.
   B. 2 and 3.
   C. 1, 2, and 3.
   D. 2, 3, and 4.

13. X-ray filters are usually made of:

   A. Copper.
   B. Lead.
   C. Aluminum.
   D. Stainless steel.

14. Collimators are usually made of:

   A. Copper.
   B. Lead.
   C. Aluminum.
   D. Stainless steel.

15. A film badge:

   1. Is affected by ionizing radiation.
   2. Is affected by other forms of radiant energy such as heat.
   3. Should be worn by all occupationally exposed persons.
   4. Is used to identify x-ray films.
   A. 2 and 4.
   B. 1 and 3.
   C. 1, 2, and 3.
   D. 1, 3, and 4.

BIBLIOGRAPHY

ADA State Legislative Clearing House. Dental radiography survey results. Chicago: American Dental Association, 1983.

Bengtsson G. Maxillofacial aspects of radiation protection: focus on recent research regarding critical organs. Dentomaxillofac Radiol 1978;7:5–11.

Brown RF, Shaver JW, Lamel DA. The selection of patients for x-ray examinations. HEW publication (FDA) 80-8104. Rockville, MD: US Department of Health, Education and Welfare, 1980.

Bushong SC. Radiologic science for technologists: physics, biology, and protection. 4th ed. St. Louis: CV Mosby, 1990.

Council on Dental Materials, Instruments and Equipment. Recommendations in radiographic practices: an update, 1988. J Am Dent Assoc 1989;118:115–117.

Court-Brown WM, Doll R, Spiers FW, et al. Geographical variation in leukemia mortality in relation to background radiation and other factors. Br Med J 1980;88:1753–1759.

D'Ambrosio JA, Schiff TG, McDavid WD, et al. Diagnostic quality versus patient exposure with five panoramic screen-film combinations. Oral Surg 1986;61:409–411.

Domon M, Yoshino N. Factors involved in the high radiographic sensitivity of E-speed films. Oral Surg 1990;69:113–119.

Frommer HH, Jain RK. A comparative clinical study of group D and E dental film. Oral Surg 1987;63:738–742.

Gelskey DE, Baker CG. Energy-selective filtration of dental x-ray beams. Oral Surg 1981;52:565–567.

Gibbs SJ, Pujol A, Chen TS, et al. Patient risk from intraoral dental radiography. Dentomaxillofac Radiol 1988;17:15–23.

Gonad doses and genetically significant dose from diagnostic radiology: U.S. 1964 and 1970. HEW publication (FDA) 76-8034. Rockville, MD: US Department of Health, Education and Welfare, 1976.

Horton PS, Sippy FH, Kohout FJ, et al. A clinical comparison of speed groups D and E dental x-ray films. Oral Surg 1984;58:104–105.

Kaffe I, Littner MM, Kuspet ME. Densitometric evaluation of intraoral x-ray films: Ekta speed versus Ultraspeed. Oral Surg 1984;57:338–342.

Kaffe I, Littner MM, Shlezinger T, et al. Efficiency of the cervical lead shield during intraoral radiography. Oral Surg 1986;62:732–736.

Kapa SF, Tyndall DA. A clinical comparison of image quality and patient exposure reduction in panoramic radiography with heavy metal filtration. Oral Surg 1989;67:750–759.

Kapa SF, Tyndall DA, Quellette TE. The application of added beam filtration to intraoral radiography. Dentomaxillofac Radiol 1990;19:67–74.

Kircos LT, Vandre RH, Lorton L. Exposure reduction of 96% in intraoral radiography. J Am Dent Assoc 1986;113:746–750.

Kircos LT, Staninec M, Chou L. Rare earth filters for intraoral radiography: exposure reduction as a function of kV(p) with comparisons of image quality. J Am Dent Assoc 1989;118:605–609.

MacDonald JCF, Reid JA, Berthoty D. Drywall construction as a dental radiation barrier. Oral Surg 1983;55:319–326.

Miles DA, Van Dis ML, Peterson MG. Information yield: a comparison of Kodak T-Mat G, Ortho L, and RPX-Omat films. Dentomaxillofac Radiol 1989;18:15–18.

National Council on Radiation Protection and Measurements. Dental x-ray protection. NCRP report 35. Washington, DC: NCRP, 1970.

National Council on Radiation Protection and Measurements. Medical x-ray and gamma-ray protection for energies up to 10 MeV structural shielding design and evaluation. NCRP report 49. Washington, DC: NCRP, 1976.

National Council on Radiation Protection and Measurements. Recommendations on limits for exposure to ionizing radiation. NCRP report 91. Bethesda, MD: NCRP, 1987.

National Council on Radiation Protection and Measurements. Ionizing radiation exposure of the population of the United States. NCRP report 93. Bethesda, MD: NCRP, 1987.

National Council on Radiation Protection and Measurements. Exposure of the population in the United States and Canada from natural background radiation. NCRP report 94. Washington, DC: NCRP, 1987.

National Council on Radiation Protection and Measurements. Exposure of the U.S. population from diagnostic medical radiation. NCRP report 100. Washington, DC: NCRP, 1989.

National Council on Radiation Protection and Measurements. Exposure of the U.S. population from diagnostic medical radiation. NCRP report 116. Washington, DC: NCRP, 1993.

New Mexico Health and Environment Department, Environmental Improvement Division. Radiation protection regulations. Santa Fe: NMHED, 1989.

Ponce AZ, McDavid WD, Underhill TE, et al. Use of E-speed film with added filtration. Oral Surg 1986;61:297–299.

Preece JW, Morris CR. The efficient and effective use of x-radiation in the dental office: III. office assessment. GP Texas Acad Gen Dent Pub 1980;6:1–5.

Reid JA, MacDonald JDF. Use and workload factors in dental radiation: protection design. Oral Surg 1984;57:219–224.

Richards AG, Colquitt WN. Reduction in dental x-ray exposures during the past 60 years. J Am Dent Assoc 1981;103:713–718.

Sikorski PA, Taylor KW. The effectiveness of the thyroid shield in dental radiology. Oral Surg 1984;58:225–236.

Texas Department of Health, Division of Occupational Health and Radiation Control. Texas regulations for control of radiation. Austin: TDH, 1991.

U.S. Department of Health and Human Services. The selection of patients for x-ray examinations: dental radiographic examinations. HEW publication (FDA) 88-827. Rockville, MD: Public Health Service, Food and Drug Administration, Center for DRH, 1989.

Wall BF, Kendall GM. Collective doses and risks from dental radiology in Great Britain. Br J Radiol 1983;56:511–516.

Weissman DD, Longhurst GE. Clinical evaluation of a rectangular field collimating device for periapical radiography. J Am Dent Assoc 1971;82:580–682.

Whitcher BL, Gratt BM, Sickles EA. Leaded shields for thyroid dose reduction in intraoral dental radiography. Oral Surg 1979;48:564–570.

Whitcher BL, Gratt BM, Sickles EA. A leaded apron for use in panoramic dental radiography. Oral Surg 1980;49:467.

White SC, Rose TC. Absorbed bone marrow dose in certain radiographic techniques. J Am Dent Assoc 1979;98:553.

White SC. 1992 Assessment of radiation risks from dental radiography. Dentomaxillofac Radiol 1992;21:118–126.

Winkler KG. Influence of rectangular collimation on intraoral shielding on radiation dose in dental radiography. J Am Dent Assoc 1968;77:95–101.

SECTION 5:
Radiographic Image Interpretation

Normal Intraoral Radiographic Anatomy

14

OBJECTIVES

Upon successful completion of this unit, the student will be able to:

1. *Recognize the anatomical features of the teeth and periodontium.*

2. *Recognize the anatomical features of the maxilla in radiographs.*

3. *Recognize the anatomical features of the mandible in radiographs.*

4. *Test his or her knowledge by answering the Review Questions.*

KEY WORDS/PHRASES

alveolar bone	inferior alveolar canal	median maxillary suture
antrum	inverted-Y	mental foramen
coronoid process	lamina dura	mental ridge
dentin	lateral fossa	mylohyoid line
enamel	lingual foramen	nasal fossa
external oblique line	malar bone	periodontal ligament space
genial tubercles	mandibular canal	pulp
hamular process	mandibular foramen	zygomatic arch
incisive canal	maxillary sinus	zygomatic bone
incisive foramen	maxillary tuberosity	zygomaticomaxillary suture

TEETH AND SUPPORTING STRUCTURES

INTRODUCTION

Radiologically, the thicker, more mineralized or denser a tissue, the more radiopaque it will appear in the image; less dense, thinner or demineralized tissue appears less dense or radiolucent in the image. Strictly speaking, the terms radiolucent (dark/black) and radiopaque (light/white) are used in plain or ordinary radiographic images, such as intraoral, panoramic, and extraoral radiographs. In plain film radiography, the images are usually referred to as radiographs. When x-ray images are obtained by computed tomography (CT), they are referred to as images or scans. Structures and diseases, as viewed in CT images, are referred to as areas of increased density (radiopaque) or decreased density (radiolucent). The exact density can be measured by the computer in Hounsfield units, and this measurement is referred to as the CT number. Today, CT and advanced imaging terminology has trickled down into our everyday usage in dental imaging.

ENAMEL (RADIOPAQUE)

Enamel is the most radiopaque (white) of any tissue seen radiologically and covers the coronal portion of the tooth. When a radiograph has been correctly exposed and processed, there is a difference in density between the enamel and the underlying dentin (Fig. 14.1). The line of demarcation between enamel and dentin is referred to as the dentinoenamel junction (DEJ). The most common disease affecting enamel is caries.

DENTIN (RADIOPAQUE)

Dentin may be seen immediately beneath the enamel in the coronal portion of the tooth and also makes up most of the root structure. In a correctly exposed and processed radiograph, dentin appears less dense or lighter than the underlying pulp but darker than the overlying enamel (Fig. 14.1). The most common disease affecting dentin is caries, which has extended through the enamel of the crown or cementum of the root to the dentin.

PULP SPACE (RADIOLUCENT)

The pulp is contained within the pulp chamber and root canal portions of the tooth. The pulp tissue is not visible radiographically. The spaces that contain the pulp are visible and are the most radiolucent (dark) portions of the tooth (Fig. 14.1). In younger individuals, the pulp spaces tend to be large; they decrease in size with advancing age. The root canal space is also radiolucent and is centered within the root. In normal instances, the root canal space tapers gently toward the apex. The apical foramen is the terminal portion of the root canal space at the apex of the tooth through which the vital elements of the tooth pass (Fig. 14.1). The most common disease affecting the pulp is inflammation due to bacterial infection as a sequela of deep caries, trauma, or advanced periodontal disease.

LAMINA DURA (RADIOPAQUE)

The lamina dura is the thin layer of compact alveolar bone that lines the tooth socket. The lamina dura forms a continuous white (radiopaque) line around the tooth root (Fig. 14.2). In reality, it is perforated by many small openings (cribriform plate) that carry branches of the intraalveolar nerves and vessels to the periodontal ligament and the cementum of the tooth. A thickened lamina dura at the apical region of a developing tooth is a sign of tooth eruption. Thinning or absence of the lamina dura is seen in pulpal and periodontal disease and in diseases such as

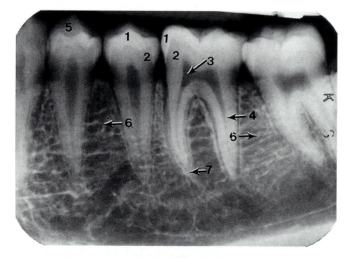

Figure 14.1. Normal Anatomy of Tooth and Supporting Structures. The enamel and dentin line of demarcation is very sharp. The enamel is whiter than dentin, because enamel is much denser. Enamel (1), dentin (2), pulp chamber (3), pulp canal (4), buccal cusp (5), alveolar bone (6), and root apex (7).

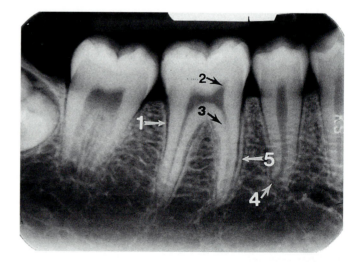

Figure 14.2. Periodontal Ligament Space and Lamina Dura. The periodontal ligament space is a distinct radiolucent line just outside the root portion of the tooth and inside the lamina dura. Periodontal ligament space (1), pulp horn (2), two root canals in mesial root (3), apex of root (4), and lamina dura (5).

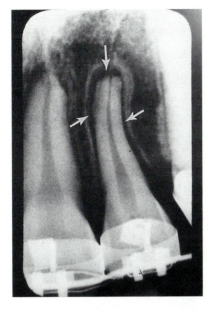

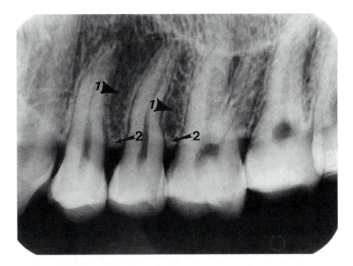

Figure 14.5. Alveolar Bone. Radiograph of maxillary premolar region alveolar bone, trabeculae, and narrow spaces (*1*) as well as alveolar bone crest with thin, white (radiopaque) cortical bone (*2*).

Figure 14.3. Tooth Mobility from Periodontal Ligament Thickening. Note thickening of PDL and lamina dura (*arrows*) of maxillary incisor being moved posteriorly by orthodontic appliances.

fibrous dysplasia, hyperparathyroidism, and Paget's disease.

PERIODONTAL LIGAMENT SPACE (RADIOLUCENT)

The periodontal ligament is not visible radiographically but is contained within the periodontal ligament space (PDLS). In the radiograph, it is seen as a distinct radiolu-

cent line just outside the root portion of the tooth and inside the lamina dura (Fig. 14.2). The PDLS is wider in younger individuals and narrows with advancing age. The PDLS may become widened due to tooth mobility (Fig. 14.3) or the presence of disease, such as scleroderma, metastatic disease, osteosarcoma, and chondrosarcoma (Fig. 14.4). The PDLS disappears in ankylosis.

ALVEOLAR BONE (RADIOPAQUE)

The alveolar bone is made up of the inner and outer cortical plates, the cancellous or spongy alveolar bone

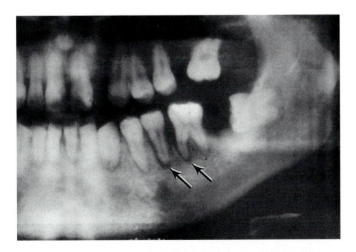

Figure 14.4. Periodontal Ligament Space Thickening in Chondrosarcoma. Panoramic radiograph of patient with chondrosarcoma of mandibular left mandible. Widening of the periodontal ligament space of the mandibular second premolar and the first molar (*arrows*) are signs of possible osteosarcoma or chondrosarcoma of the jaws, in addition to periodontal disease.

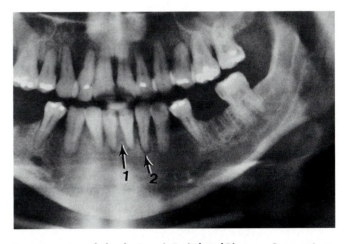

Figure 14.6. Loss of Alveolar Bone in Periodontal Disease. Panoramic radiograph of a young adult with rapidly progressive periodontitis. (*1*) Severe alveolar bone loss. (*2*) Periodontal ligament thickening noting possibility of tooth mobility. (Patient has generalized advanced horizontal bone loss.)

proper, and the lamina dura (Fig. 14.5). The cortical bone at the alveolar crest should be intact and may be seen as a thin, white (radiopaque) line. A loss of alveolar bone is commonly seen in periodontal disease (Fig. 14.6). Cortical bone thinning is seen in osteoporosis.

ANATOMICAL STRUCTURES OF THE MAXILLA

MEDIAN MAXILLARY SUTURE (MEDIAN PALATAL SUTURE) (RADIOLUCENT)

This suture lies between the two palatal (palatine) processes of the maxilla. It appears as a dark (radiolucent) line extending in the midline between the maxillary central incisors back to the posterior aspect of the palate (Fig. 14.7). There is sometimes a funnel-shaped widening at the anterior aspect, known as the **anterior median maxillary cleft**. This is sometimes associated with a diastema (space) between the central incisors and represents a variation of normal anatomical structure (Fig. 14.8).

NASOPALATINE (INCISIVE) FORAMEN (RADIOLUCENT)

The nasopalatine (incisive) foramen is located just posterior to the maxillary central incisors and is formed by the union of the two palatal processes of the maxilla. It may be a symmetrically oval, round, or heart-shaped radiolucency and may be small or large (Fig. 14.9). It rarely has a cortical (white) outline (border). Yet, if a cortical border is present, it usually indicates transformation into a nasopalatine (incisive) cyst. The nasopalatine (incisive) foramen transmits the nasopalatine nerves and vessels. The **nasopalatine nerve** is a branch of the spheno-palatine ganglion, supplies the nasal roof and septum, and extends downward and forward in a groove in the vomer bone and the cartilaginous septum. On reaching the anterior portion of the floor of the nose, the nasopalatine nerve enters and traverses the canal of Stensen and finally emerges on the hard palate through the nasopalatine (incisive) foramen. There is one canal of Stensen on each side of the nasal septum, and both lateral canals of Stensen terminate at the nasopalatine (incisive) foramen. Sometimes, the two canals of Stensen further subdivide into the four canals of Stensen and Scarpa. When the additional two smaller canals of Scarpa are found, they are

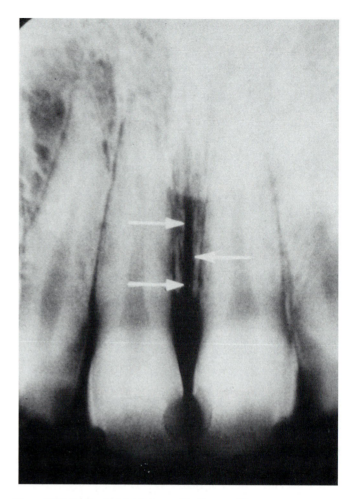

Figure 14.7. Median Palatal Suture. Median maxillary suture appears as a dark (radiolucent) line in the midline between the central incisors extending back to posterior aspect of the palate (arrows).

seen in the midline—one in front of the other—and serve as passageways for the nasopalatine nerves (Fig. 14.10).

NASAL FOSSAE (RADIOLUCENT)

In some cases, particularly when excessive vertical angulation is used, the nasal fossae may be seen in the intraoral radiograph. They are divided by the nasal septum (white) in the midline (Fig. 14.11). The nasal fossae, being cavities in bone, appear in radiographs as dark images. They are radiolucent or dark because they contain air, at least in some part. Hazy gray images may be seen arising from the lateral walls of both fossae and may extend almost to the septum; these represent the anterior portions of the inferior turbinate, the soft tissue of which covers the thin leaf-like conchae bones.

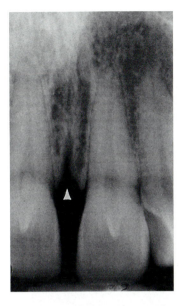

Figure 14.8. Anterior Median Maxillary Cleft. Note funnel-shaped widening of anterior median maxillary cleft (*arrowhead*). This is sometimes associated with diastema between maxillary central incisors, as shown here.

MAXILLARY AND MANDIBULAR (INCISIVE) LATERAL FOSSAE (RADIOLUCENT)

Incisive fossae represent depressions in the outer surface of the alveolar bone between the maxillary lateral incisor and canine teeth and between the mandibular ca-

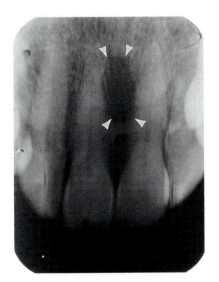

Figure 14.9. Radiograph of Nasopalatine (Incisive) Foramen. Nasopalatine (incisive) foramen is the oval radiolucency between the maxillary centrals (arrowheads).

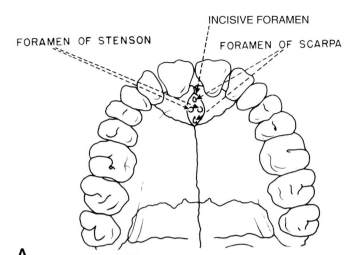

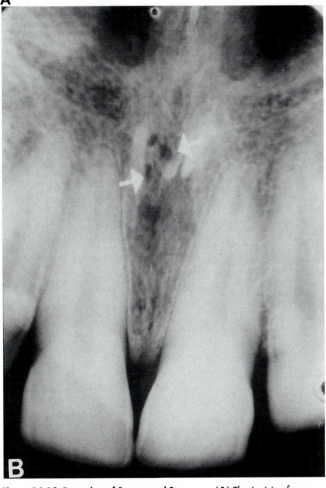

Figure 14.10 Foramina of Scarpa and Stensen. (**A**) The incisive foramen, just behind the upper central incisors, is formed by the union of halves of the maxilla. Lateral canals within this fossa, on each side of the midline (foramina of Stensen), transmit the nasopalatine nerves and the terminal branch of the descending palatine artery. In some individuals, additional canals within the fossa (canals of Scarpa) are found in the midline. When present, these also serve as passages for the nasopalatine nerves. (**B**) Radiograph revealing four small radiolucent holes (*arrows*) representing the foramina of Stensen and Scarpa.

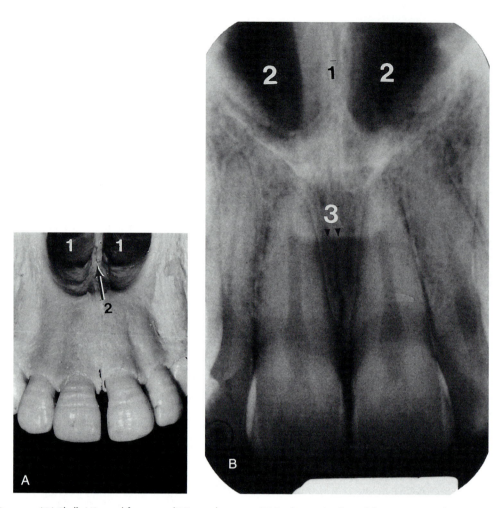

Figure 14.11. Nasal Fossae. **(A)** Skull: (*1*) nasal fossae and (*2*) nasal septum. **(B)** Radiograph of nasal fossae: (*1*) nasal septum, (*2*) nasal fossa, and (*3*) tip of nose.

nines. The lateral fossa (incisive) produces a relatively more radiolucent (dark) area in the alveolar bone (Fig. 14.12). This radiolucency or darkness in the bone may sometimes give the impression that there is disease in the bone. When a cyst occurs here, it is referred to as the globulomaxillary cyst.

LATERAL-CANINE AREA (RADIOPAQUE)

The **inverted-Y** is an important anatomical landmark. It is especially useful in locating the maxillary canine area in edentulous surveys. It is formed by the cortical lining of the anterior wall of the maxillary sinus and the floor of the nasal fossa (Fig. 14.13). The Y-shaped landmark is valuable in identifying and differentiating cysts in this region, because this anatomical landmark tends to be altered or obliterated by adjacent pathology. The most com-

mon cyst found in this region is the globulomaxillary cyst.

MAXILLARY SINUS (MAXILLARY ANTRUM) (RADIOLUCENT)

The maxillary sinus is one of the paranasal sinuses, and only the maxillary sinus is referred to as the antrum. The antrum is an air-filled cavity that communicates with the nasal fossa via the maxillary sinus ostium, an opening (orifice) that is not visible in the periapical radiograph. The lower half of the maxillary sinus is revealed on the radiograph as a dark shadow. The margin of the cavity is a thin layer of dense bone (the cortex) that appears as a white line (Fig. 14.14). This line tends to be irregular, much like a pencil-line on an artist's sketch that has a rough surface texture. Although it may not always look

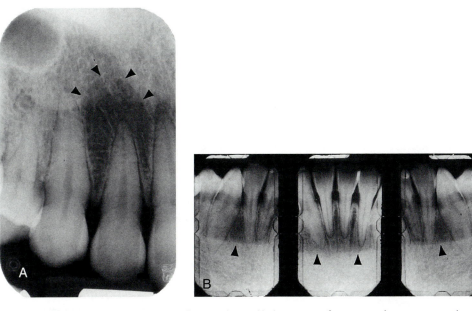

Figure 14.12. Maxillary and Mandibular Incisive Fossae. Maxillary and mandibular incisive fossae are depressions in alveolar bone. The following anatomical structures are identified: the canine eminence, mental foramen, and mental ridges. **(A)** Note radiolucent maxillary incisive (lateral) fossa (arrowheads). **(B)** Note radiolucent mandibular lateral fossa (arrowheads).

like it on the radiograph, there is usually a lamina dura surrounding root apices immediately adjacent to the antral (sinus) floor except in disease. The antrum proper (cavity or sinus) sometimes extends down between the roots of the maxillary posterior teeth, especially the lingual (palatal) and buccal roots of the maxillary first molars, which may give the appearance that one or more roots protrude into the antrum (sinus) (Fig. 14.15). This downward extension of the maxillary sinus is known as **pneumatization**. Pneumatization occurs with advancing age, especially when the maxillary first molar is extracted prematurely (Fig. 14.16). Pneumatization can be accelerated by chronic sinus disorders such as infection and allergy.

MAXILLARY TUBEROSITY (RADIOPAQUE)

The alveolar process of the maxilla is arranged in the form of a curve (dental arch curve) that extends to the maxillary tuberosity, a rounded elevation on the posterior region of both sides. Tuberosities are important in the retention of dentures (Fig. 14.17).

The tuberosities may be completely occupied by the maxillary sinus. When extracting a third molar, such an affected area of the whole body of the tuberosity may be removed with the tooth. The tuberosity may contain pathology, such as odontogenic tumors and cysts.

ZYGOMATIC (MALAR) BONE AND ZYGOMATIC ARCH (RADIOPAQUE)

The zygomatic bone is the small quadrangular (cheek) bone sometimes called the malar bone or zygoma (Fig. 14.18). The general shape of the inferior border of the malar bone on the radiograph roughly resembles the letter "U." The limbs of the "U" represent the lateral walls of the maxillary sinus where the anterolateral and posterolateral walls meet. The dark area between them represents a recess or extension of the maxillary sinus into the malar (cheek) bone. When this recess or air space is deep into the malar bone, the image is dark; when there is no recess, the area is gray or white. The zygomatic arch is formed by the temporal process of zygomatic bone and the zygomatic process of the temporal bone, with the zygomatico maxillary suture in between.

HAMULAR PROCESS (RADIOPAQUE)

This landmark consists of a hook-like process arising from the inferior tip of medial pterygoid plate of the sphenoid bone. It is the posterior boundary of pterygomaxillary notch or fissure, which is an important prosthodontic landmark in the construction of maxillary complete dentures. This process is seen just posterior to the maxillary tuberosity (Fig. 14.19).

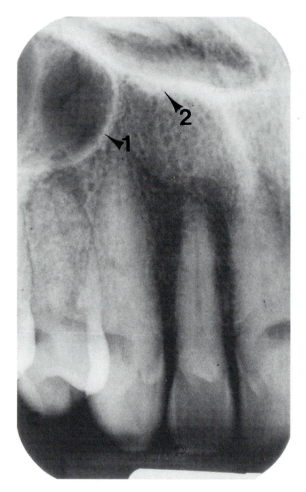

Figure 14.13. Maxillary Lateral Canine Region. Radiograph of the maxillary lateral canine region that illustrates the inverted-Y formed by the floor of the nasal fossa (2) and the anterior wall of the maxillary sinus (1).

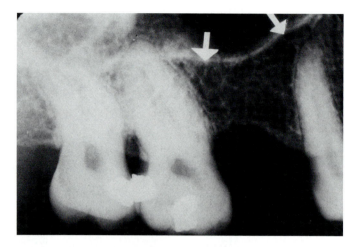

Figure 14.14. Maxillary Sinus (Antrium). The floor of the maxillary sinus is revealed as a thin, white line (*arrows*).

MENTAL RIDGES OR TUBERCLES (RADIOPAQUE)

The mental protuberance is a triangular eminence of denser bone on the inferior, anterior aspect of the mandible. The raised portions of this bone on either side of the midline form the mental ridges or tubercles (Fig. 14.21).

MENTAL FORAMEN (RADIOLUCENT)

The mental foramen conducts the mental vessels and nerves; a circular radiolucent area is seen below the premolar teeth on either side, midway between the upper and lower border of the body of the mandible (Figs. 14.21A and 14.22). The location varies from the distal of the canine to the second premolar area. It may be located at

ANATOMICAL STRUCTURES OF THE MANDIBLE

CORONOID PROCESS OF MANDIBLE (RADIOPAQUE)

This structure is a thin, triangular eminence of the mandible that is flattened lateromedially. It lies medial to the zygomatic arch, and on its medial surface is the insertion of the temporalis muscle. It is the anterior slope of the sigmoid notch of the mandible. The coronoid process is sometimes seen on the maxillary posterior molar periapical radiograph (Fig. 14.20). The coronoid process may become enlarged due to hypertrophy (bilateral) or tumor such as osteochondroma (unilateral); in either case, this causes limited jaw opening.

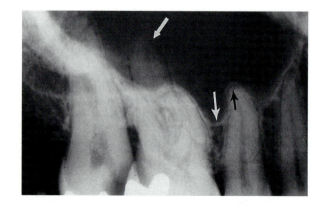

Figure 14.15. Radiographic Appearance of Maxillary Sinus Molar Roots. The maxillary sinus sometimes extends down between the roots of the posterior teeth and may give the appearance that one or more roots are protruding into the sinus (antrum).

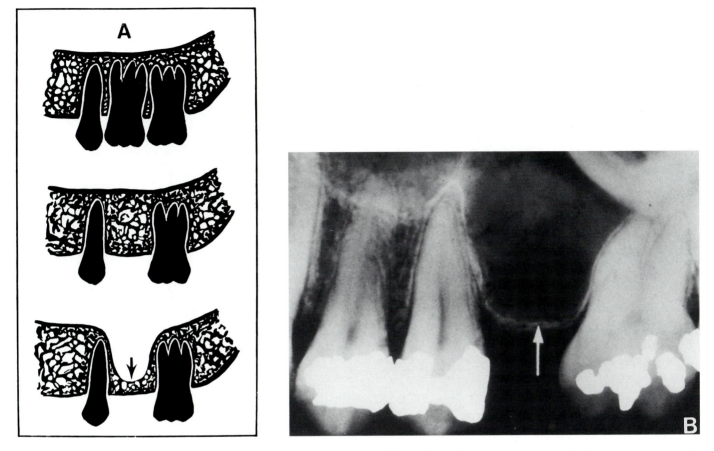

Figure 14.16. Pneumatization of Maxillary Sinus. (**A**) After the premature removal of maxillary molars, it is not uncommon for the antrum to pneumatize down to the alveolar crest in the premolar/molar areas. (**B**) Radiograph showing pneumatization of the maxillary first molar area by the antrum into the alveolar bone after removal of the maxillary first molar. The *arrow* identifies the floor of the maxillary sinus.

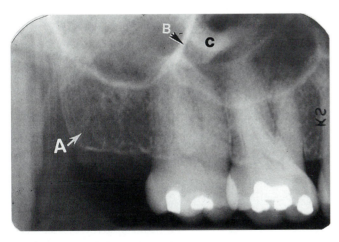

Figure 14.17. Maxillary Tuberosity. The maxillary tuberosity (*A*) is a rounded elevation on the posterior region or both sides. Maxillary sinus septum (*B*). Zygomatic or malar bone (*C*).

the apex of either premolar and may resemble periapical pathology of pulpal origin or cementoma.

EXTERNAL OBLIQUE LINE OR RIDGE (RADIOPAQUE)

This ridge is located on the buccal side of the mandible and may be followed in an obliquely upward direction from the mental tubercle to the anterior border of the ramus. It is seen as a radiopaque (white) line of varied width and density that passes across the molar region. The triangularis and inferior labial quadratus muscles are attached to anterior portion of the line (ridge). It serves as a mark of division between the reticular (net-like) alveolar bone above and the denser mandibular bone below (Fig. 14.23).

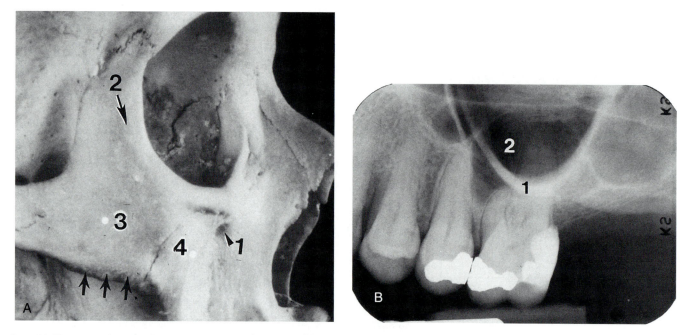

Figure 14.18. Zygomatic (Malar) Bone. **(A)** Anatomical structure of lateral facial side of skull. Infraorbital foramen (*1*), frontal process of zygomatic bone (*2*), zygomatic or malar bone (arrows indicate lower border of zygomatic bone) (*3*), and zygomatic process of maxilla (*4*). **(B)** Radiograph of U-shaped zygomatic bone (lower cortical border) (*1*) with dark radiolucent maxillary sinus above (*2*).

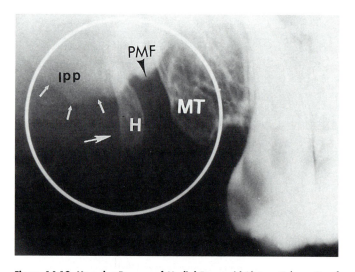

Figure 14.19. Hamular Process of Medial Pterygoid Plate. Tuberosity of maxilla, and the pterygomaxillary notch or fissure (prosthodontic landmark). Radiograph of hamular process (*H*), pterygomaxillary fissure (*PMF*), maxillary tuberosity (*MT*), and lateral pterygoid plate (*lpp*).

MYLOHYOID LINE OR RIDGE (RADIOPAQUE)

The mylohyoid ridge is located on the lingual aspect of the mandible and is sometimes referred to as the **internal oblique ridge**. It serves as the point of attachment for the mylohyoid muscle of the floor of the mouth and extends from the molar region to the premolar area. Radiographically, the mylohyoid ridge is a radiopaque (white) line, often seen below the apices of the molar teeth and the external oblique ridge (Fig. 14.23).

GENIAL TUBERCLES OR MENTAL SPINES AND LINGUAL FORAMEN (RADIOPAQUE/RADIOLUCENT)

The genial tubercles are located on the inner surface of the body of the mandible in the midline. These tubercles are the points of insertion of the genioglossus and geniohyoid muscles bilaterally to the upper and lower genial tubercles, respectively. On the periapical radiograph, the genial tubercles appear as roundish, localized areas of increased density (radiopaque) with a small, dark (radiolucent) round spot in the middle representing the small radiolucent *lingual foramen* for the passage of a small lingual nutrient vessels (Fig. 14.24).

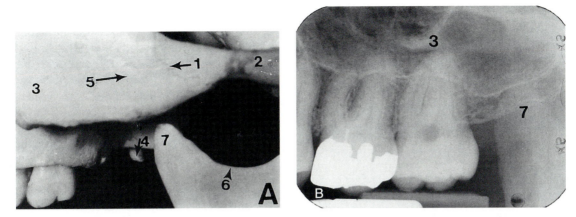

Figure 14.20. Coronoid Process of Mandible. (**A**) Anatomical structures of the skull in the posterior maxillary region. Zygomaticotemporal suture (*1*), zygomatic process of temporal bone (*2*), zygomatic bone (malar) bone (*3*), hamular process of medial pterygoid plate of sphenoid (*4*), temporal process of zygomatic bone (*5*), sigmoid or mandibular notch of mandible (*6*), and coronoid process of mandible (*7*). Note: *5* and *2* form zygomatic arch. (**B**) Radiograph of coronoid process of mandible. Coronoid process (*7*) of mandible seen in maxillary molar radiograph, and zygomatic bone (*3*).

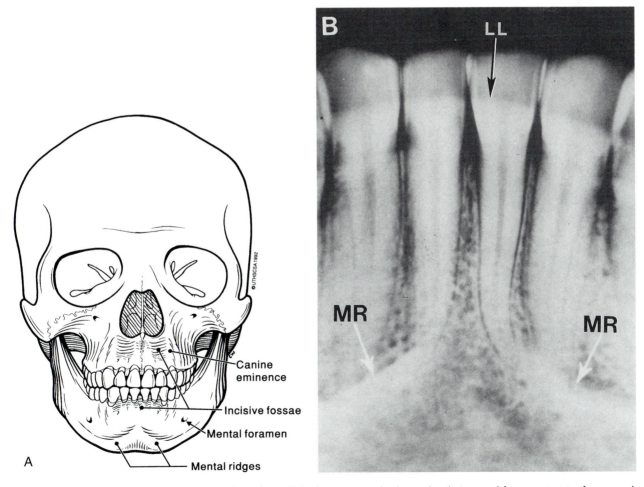

Figure 14.21. Mental Ridges (Tubercles). (**A**) Outer surface of mandible showing mental ridges (tubercles), mental foramen, incisive fossae, and canine eminence. (**B**) Radiograph showing mental ridges (*MR*) and lip line (*LL*).

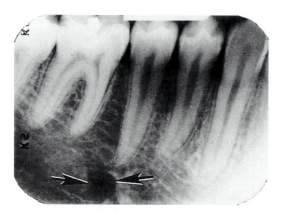

Figure 14.22. Mental Foramen. Radiograph of mental foramen (*arrows*).

MANDIBULAR CANAL OR INFERIOR ALVEOLAR CANAL (RADIOLUCENT)

The mandibular canal starts at the mandibular foramen on the inner aspect of the ramus and passes in a downward and forward direction through the mandible. As it passes forward, it also moves from the lingual side of the body of the mandible in the third molar area to the buccal

side in the premolar region. It appears as a narrow, dark (radiolucent) ribbon between two white (radiopaque) lines representing the canal walls (Fig. 14.25). In the region of the mental foramen, the mandibular nerve bifurcates into its terminal branches known as the incisive and mental nerves. The smaller incisive canal can sometimes be seen on some radiographs and runs anteriorly from the mental foramen area. The exact location of the mandibular canal is important in the placement of implants, the removal of third molars, and the implementation of planned surgical procedures. Interruptions in the wall(s) of the canal or displacement of the canal indicate a close relationship to pathology. The canal may also be widened due to the presence of vascular or neural pathology within.

FOREIGN MATERIALS OVERVIEW

The recognition of foreign materials in dental radiographs is usually self-evident. The foreign material may be within an air space, soft tissue, bone, or tooth. Foreign materials usually represent a permanent record of something that has been done to the patient therapeutically, iatrogenically (introduced by treatment), or as a result of accident or voluntary procedure.

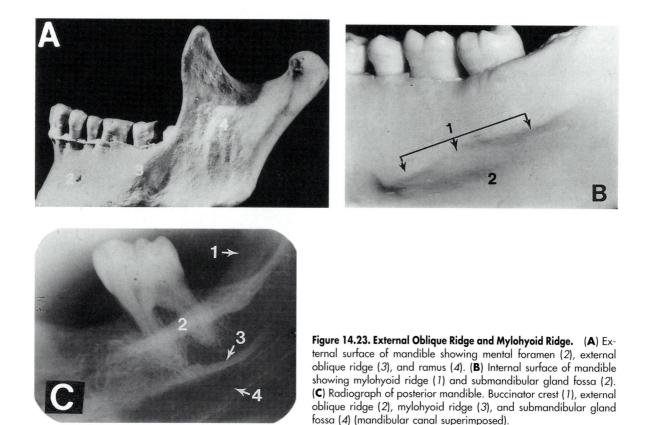

Figure 14.23. External Oblique Ridge and Mylohyoid Ridge. (**A**) External surface of mandible showing mental foramen (*2*), external oblique ridge (*3*), and ramus (*4*). (**B**) Internal surface of mandible showing mylohyoid ridge (*1*) and submandibular gland fossa (*2*). (**C**) Radiograph of posterior mandible. Buccinator crest (*1*), external oblique ridge (*2*), mylohyoid ridge (*3*), and submandibular gland fossa (*4*) (mandibular canal superimposed).

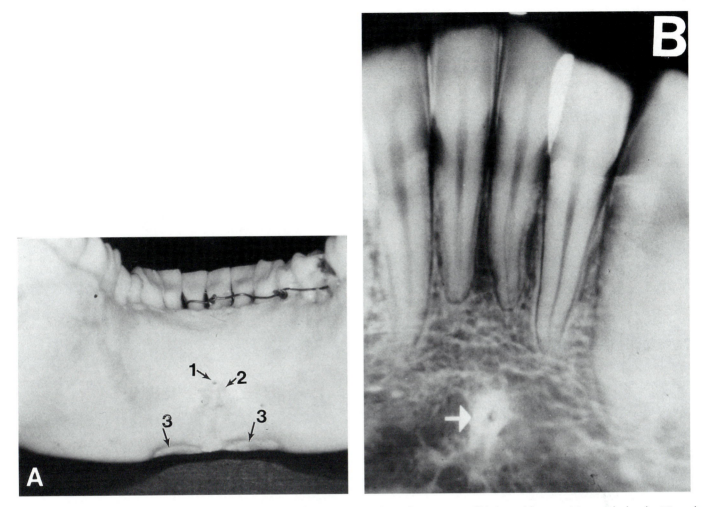

Figure 14.24. Genial Tubercles (Mental Spines) and Lingual Foramen. (**A**) Inner surface of anterior mandible lingual foramen (*1*), genial tubercles (*2*), and digastric fossae (*3*). (**B**) The doughnut-shaped radiopacity (*arrow*) is the genial tubercles, and the radiolucent center is the lingual foramen that transmits a small lingual nutrient artery.

Probably the most important reason for the recognition of a foreign material is to observe signs of the patient's reaction or nonreaction to the foreign substance. Occasionally, older radiolucent dental materials no longer in current use may be seen in older patients, and their appearances must also be recognized.

Endodontic Materials (Fig. 14.26)

During the endodontic procedure, the temporary presence of broaches, files, rubber dam clamp, and frame as well as film-holding devices are noted. Endodontic restorative materials include gutta percha, gutta percha alloy, silver points, and root canal sealer material. Each of these is progressively more radiopaque than the other. Several types of post materials may be seen to fill the cervical portion of the root canal. These posts may be preformed scored metal types, screw types, and cast gold types. The posts are cemented in place with a radiopaque crown and bridge type cement. Retrograde amalgam may be seen at the apex of an endodontically treated tooth that had previously undergone an apicoectomy. Broken endodontic instruments, such as files, may sometimes remain within the root canal space as part of the permanent filling material of that space.

Restorative Materials (Fig. 14.27)

The most important outcome after the evaluation of a restorative material is to identify any defects radiographically that may cause the material to fail. Defective restorations may actually contribute to the recurrence of disease, such as caries along deficient margins of restorations, and alveolar bone loss beneath an overhang or an open con-

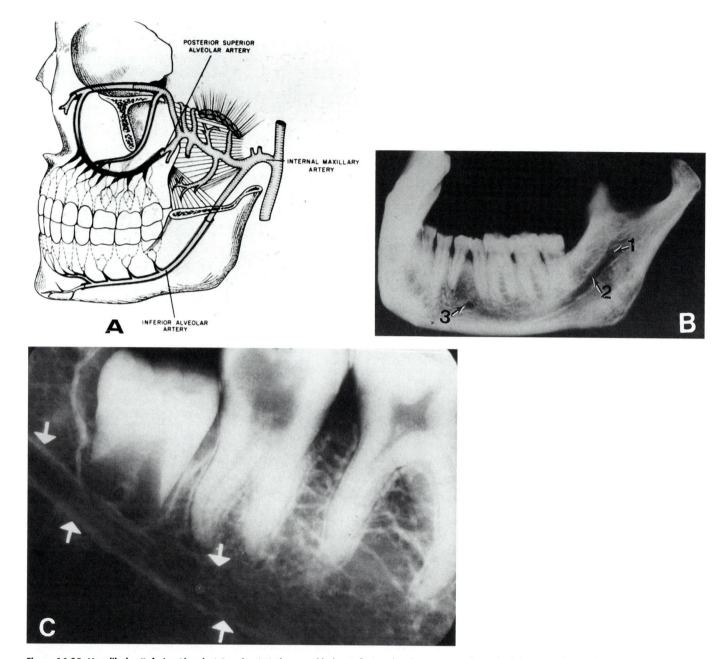

Figure 14.25. Mandibular (Inferior Alveolar) Canal. (**A**) The mandibular (inferior alveolar) artery, a branch of the internal maxillary artery, descends with the mandibular (inferior alveolar) to the mandibular foramen on the medial side of the ramus of the mandible. It runs along the mandibular canal and is accompanied by nerve and veins. It gives off a few branches to the cancellous bone and roots of the teeth. Opposite the second premolar teeth, the nerve and vessels divide into the incisive and mental branches. (**B**) Radiograph of a dry mandible revealing the mandibular foramen (*1*), mandibular canal (*2*), and mental foramen (*3*). (**C**) Intraoral radiograph of mandibular molar region revealing mandibular canal (arrows).

tact. Some older restorative materials and cements no longer in current use may be present in older patients. For example, a 50-year-old patient could have a 30-year-old tooth-colored restoration in a central incisor that may mimic a carious lesion on the radiograph. These older tooth-colored materials are radiolucent on the radiograph, whereas newer tooth-colored materials are radiopaque.

Principal among these esthetic restorative materials are older resins, porcelain veneer gold crowns, porcelain crowns, and silicates. Cements include those used as subbases or for crown cementation. Radiolucent materials in current use (such as temporary crowns and bridges, denture bases, and denture teeth) are invariably made of acrylic. Radiopaque materials include tooth-colored com-

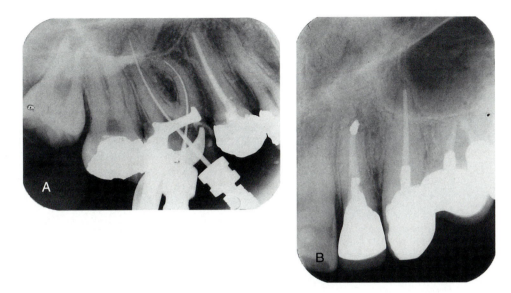

Figure 14.26. Endodontic Materials. **(A)** Rubber dam clamp, endodontic files, and gutta percha root canal filling. **(B)** Retrograde amalgam, gutta percha, post and core, and crown restorations (from apex toward crown).

posite restorations, sealants, pins, cements, bases, amalgam, gold foil, cast gold, nonprecious alloys, and porcelain fused to metal crowns. Aluminum temporary crowns and stainless-steel full-faced and open-faced crowns are also seen in children.

Orthodontic/Pediatric Materials (Fig. 14.28)

Some of the main advantages of direct bonded orthodontic brackets include more pleasing esthetics than bands, easier and faster placement than bands, and no need for separating wires to open contacts. However, many orthodontists still prefer to use bands, especially in combination with direct bonded brackets. A principal disadvantage of bands is that caries, such as interproximal caries, cannot be detected beneath them. Other orthodontic materials include wires, springs, space maintainers, fixed retainers, inclined planes, habit-breaking appliances, and similar materials including radiopaque cement for bands. Pediatric materials include most other materials in addition to sealants, stainless-steel crowns, and space maintainers.

Trauma/Oral Surgery Materials (Figs. 14.29–14.31)

One of the most commonly encountered foreign materials are those associated with implants. These include the implant itself or the fixture, the healing caps (used for 3–6 months after placement), the post that screws into the implant after removal of the healing cap, and the final restoration that is usually some type of casting either as a single unit or as a part of a fixed bridge. In the evaluation of implants, the persistence of bone right to the edge of

the implant and minimal vertical loss of bone at the neck or cervical portion of the implant are important. Other materials include wires, plates, and screws used after trauma or orthognathic survey and transplanted bones such as ribs to fill surgical defects. Patients with a retrognathic profile may sometimes have an acrylic button implanted to fill out the chin. Other foreign materials often seen in American patients include broken surgical burs and instrument tips, radiopaque automobile glass fragments, pellets, birdshot, bullets, and explosive fragments. These may provide information about the patient's history. Amalgam fragments may sometimes cause an amalgam tattoo (presence of amalgam fragments in oral tissue). The diagnosis is confirmed by the presence of very minute to large-sized amalgam fragments around the cervical portion of a full crown, within the crestal portion of the alveolar bone, or within the soft tissues including the tongue or cheek.

Prosthodontic Materials (Fig. 14.32)

Any removable prosthodontic device, such as a complete or partial denture, should usually be removed before taking radiographs. This is because any metallic or porcelain part of these prostheses may obscure the image of other structures, such as abutment teeth or alveolar bone. Sometimes "flippers" or temporary partial dentures are left in; because they are often all-plastic, only the wrought wire clasp may be visible. Fixed bridges may involve only one missing tooth or an entire arch. These fixed bridges involve materials mentioned previously in the restorative section.

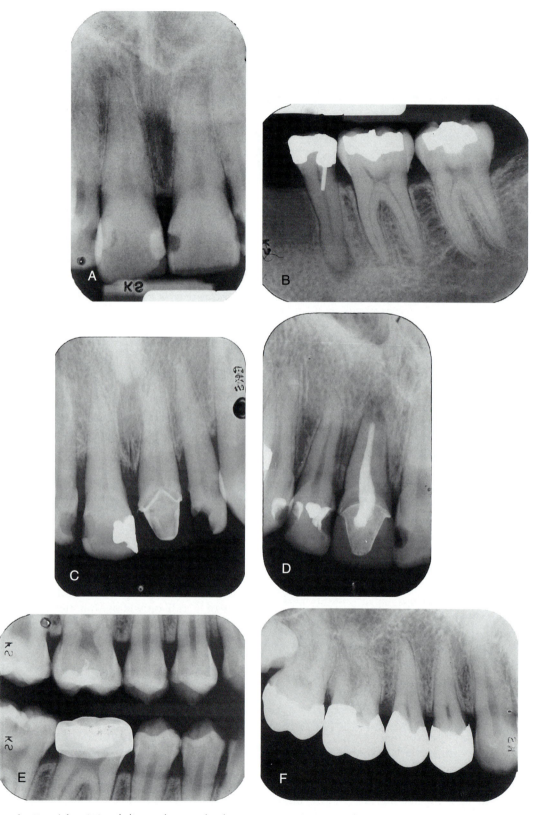

Figure 14.27. Restorative Materials. (**A**) Radiolucent silicate and radiopaque composite. (**B**) Amalgam restorations, pin in pulp, resulting periapical lesion. (**C**) Radiopaque cement and temporary acrylic crown, and cast gold anterior restoration. (**D**) Porcelain crown, radiopaque cement, and gutta percha root canal filling. (**E**) Temporary aluminum crown. (**F**) Cast gold crowns.

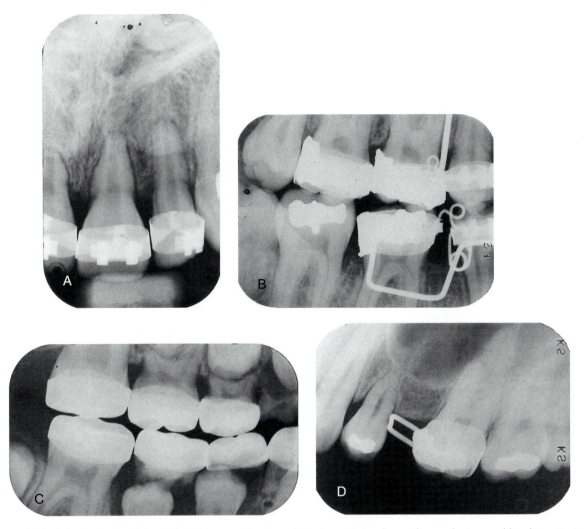

Figure 14.28. Orthodontic/Pediatric Materials. (**A**) Stainless-steel bands and brackets. (**B**) Bands, stainless-steel wires, and brackets. (**C**) Stainless-steel crowns. (**D**) Space maintainer and stainless-steel band.

Periodontal/Hygiene Materials (Fig. 14.33)

Materials relating to periodontal/hygiene procedures are seen infrequently. These materials may include stainless-steel wires used for tooth splinting, broken scalers, curette tips, or prophy paste containing radiopaque materials such as zirconium. Films contaminated with stannous fluoride causes black fingerprints on the processed film. Metallic measuring devices are sometimes placed within periodontal pockets or bony defects to more accurately assess the periodontal problem.

Radiographic Materials (Fig. 14.34)

Most radiology equipment is now made of heat-sterilizable plastic materials and disposable materials made of paper, plastic, or Styrofoam that are primarily radiolucent. Occasionally, metallic biteblocks, attachments of metallic positioning rods, and film-holding devices (such as hemostat forceps) may be seen on the radiograph. Additionally, various radiographic artifacts mentioned elsewhere may be radiolucent or radiopaque.

OTHER MATERIALS (Fig. 14.35)

The above discussion includes the most commonly seen materials. However, others may be encountered, including retained injected radiopaque materials for sialogram (radiogram of salivary glands and ducts) or the opacification (making opaque) of lesions such as cysts in soft tissues or the maxillary sinuses. Also, jewelry in the ears, nose, tongue, and lips may be seen in radiographs, as well as eyeglass frames and some types of wigs. Unusual foreign objects, such as a thumb tack in the nose, straight pin in a salivary duct, or broken syringe needle, have all been reported.

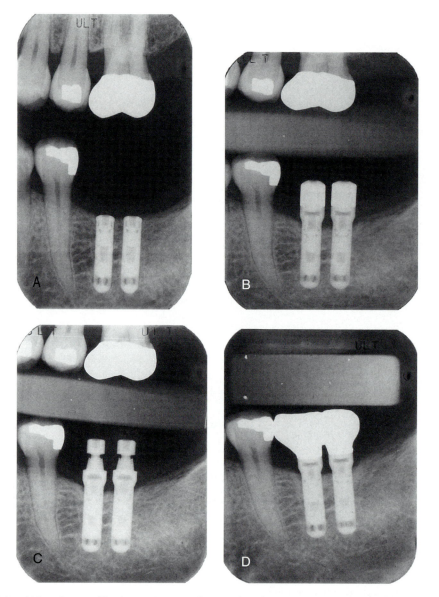

Figure 14.29. Implant Materials. (**A**) Implants and healing caps. (**B**) Implants and appliance. (**C**) Prepared with screw tips. (**D**) Crowns screwed in place.

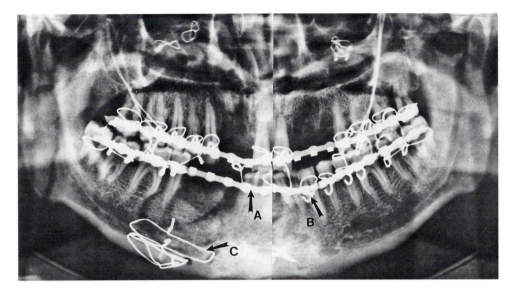

Figure 14.30. Trauma/Oral Surgery Materials. Winter arch bars (**A**), stainless-steel wires holding arch bars in place (**B**), and surgical wires stabilizing fractures (**C**).

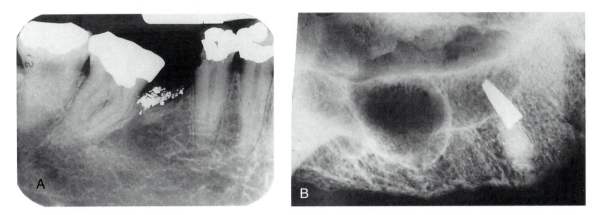

Figure 14.31. Trauma-Related Materials. (**A**) Amalgam fragments of amalgam tattoo. (**B**) Elevator tip in maxillary sinus. (Note the retained root tip.)

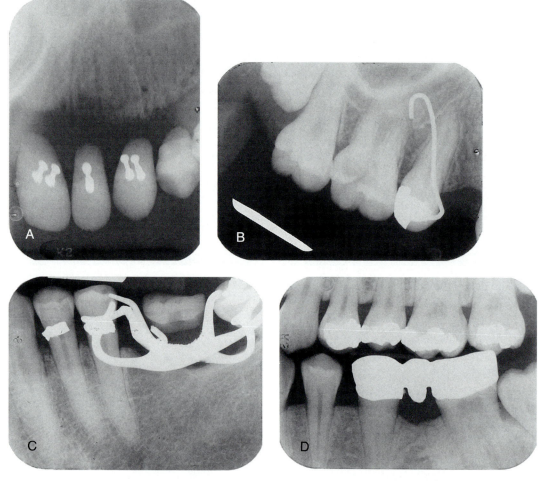

Figure 14.32. Prosthodontic Materials. **(A)** Anterior porcelain denture teeth with metal pins and radiotransparent acrylic denture base. **(B)** Acrylic temporary partial denture with radiotransparent plastic tooth and wrought wire clasp. **(C)** Cast chrome-cobalt partial denture framework, porcelain posterior denture tooth, and radiotransparent acrylic. **(D)** Posterior cast gold three-unit fixed bridge.

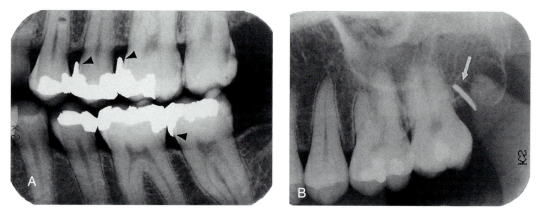

Figure 14.33. Periodontal/Hygiene Materials. **(A)** Overhangs. **(B)** Broken scaler tip.

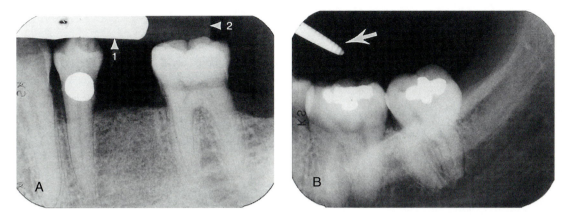

Figure 14.34. Radiographic Materials. (**A**) Metal (*arrow 1*) and plastic biteblock (*arrow 2*). (**B**) Hemostat tip (*arrow*) used to hold film.

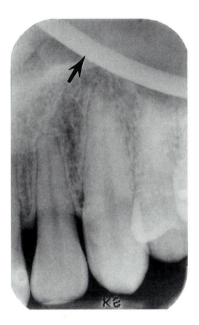

Figure 14.35. Other Materials. Glass eyeglass lens and metal frame (*arrow*).

WORKSHOP/LABORATORY EXERCISES

EXERCISE 14.1 NORMAL INTRAORAL ANATOMY AND MATERIALS

Materials and Equipment Needed

1. The mounted half- or full-mouth survey from the previous workshop on the paralleling technique or a duplicated set of full-mouth radiographs on a patient from the instructor.
2. Plastic orthodontic tracing sheets.
3. Sharp pencil and paper.

Instructions

Step 1:   Using transparent tape, attach the orthodontic tracing sheet on top of the full-mouth survey.

Step 2:   Use the viewbox and magnifying lens.

Step 3:   Using neat tracings and numbered arrows, identify as many anatomical landmarks and materials as you can.

Step 4:   On a separate sheet of paper, name the landmarks that correspond to the numbered arrows.

Note to Instructors: This workshop can be simplified if several **different** full-mouth surveys are each duplicated on a single panoramic-sized duplicating film. Label each original set with numbered arrows using a fine sharp pen. Ask the students to identify the numbered arrows on a separate sheet of paper and include structures and materials. This will eliminate the tracing and simplify correction.

CASE-BASED QUESTION

You are trying to sort out which structures in the **mandible** are within the bone, which ones are on the buccal surface, and which ones are on the lingual surface. Create a table that locates these structures by region, including anterior, premolar, and molar/retromolar areas. Indicate which are radiolucent and which are radiopaque.

Note to Instructors: Half of the class (group) can be asked to do the mandible as a bone and half can be asked to do the maxilla; then trade with a classmate who has done a different jaw (upper or lower) and critique the table.

REVIEW QUESTIONS

1. Which of the following structures appear radiopaque on the radiograph?

   1. Nasal fossa.
   2. Mylohyoid ridge.
   3. Maxillary sinus.
   4. External oblique ridge.
   5. Coronoid process.
   A. 2, 4, and 5.
   B. 1, 3, and 4.
   C. 1, 4, and 5.
   D. 1, 2, and 5.
   E. 1, 2, and 3.

2. What is the hamular process?

   A. A hooked bony projection of palatine bone.
   B. A bony projection of the medial pterygoid plate.
   C. A bony projection of the lateral pterygoid plate.
   D. A hooked bony projection of maxillary tuberosity.
   E. A bony projection of the coronoid process of the mandible.

3. Which of the following can mimic a periapical radiolucent lesion on dental radiograph?

   1. Apical foramen of tooth not closed in an immature tooth.
   2. Mental foramen.
   3. Nasopalatine foramen.
   4. Greater palatine foramen.
   A. All of the above.
   B. 1, 2, and 4.
   C. 1, 2, and 3.
   D. 3 and 4.
   E. 1 and 2.

4. Which of the following is usually a sign of active eruption of a tooth?

   A. The lamina dura forms a continuous line around the tooth root.
   B. The lamina dura is perforated by many small openings.
   C. There is widening of the periodontal ligament space.
   D. There is a thickening of the lamina dura at the root apex region.

5. Match the following terms with the proper definitions:

Column A

1. Fossa _____
2. Canal _____
3. Foramen _____
4. Sinus _____
5. Septum _____
6. Suture _____
7. Cortical _____
8. Cancellous _____

Column B

A. Hole or opening in bone
B. Broad shallow depression in bone
C. Cavity, recess, or hollow space in bone
D. Passageway through bone
E. Sponge-like bone
F. Bony partition that separates two spaces
G. Immovable joint found between bones
H. Hard or compact bone

6. Which of the following affects the form of the alveolar crest?

A. Tooth inclination.
B. State of eruption.
C. The shape of the interproximal tooth surfaces.
D. All of the above.

CASE-BASED QUESTIONS

CASE 14.1

1. Identify the anatomical structures by matching the columns.

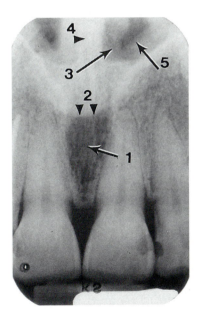

Column A

Arrow 1 _____
Arrow 2 _____
Arrow 3 _____
Arrow 4 _____
Arrow 5 _____

Column B

A. Nasal fossa
B. Nasal septum
C. Tip of nose
D. Incisive foramen
E. Nasal mucosa

CASE 14.2

1. Identify the radiopaque line indicated by the arrow.

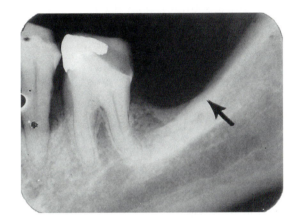

A. Mylohyoid ridge.
B. External oblique ridge.
C. Mental ridge.
D. Retromolar triangle.
E. Buccinator ridge.

CASE 14.3

1. Most likely, what is the dark area identified by the arrowhead in this radiograph?

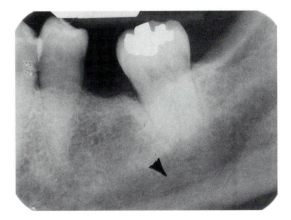

A. Periapical cyst.
B. Tumor of some kind.
C. Mylohyoid fossa.
D. Submandibular gland fossa.
E. Sublingual gland fossa.

CASE 14.4

1. The landmark known as the inverted-Y is well demonstrated. It is composed of which structures?
   A
   1. Inferior border of nasal cavity
   2. Anterior border of maxillary sinus.
   B
   1. Floor of orbit.
   2. Inferior border of nasal cavity.
   C
   1. Inferior border of left nasal cavity.
   2. Anterior border of right nasal cavity.
   D
   1. Floor of maxillary sinus.
   2. Floor of orbit.
   E
   1. Palatal extension of maxillary sinus.
   2. Anterior border of maxillary sinus.

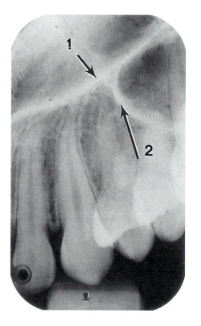

CASE 14.5

1. In all probability, what is the dome-like structure (arrow) above the roots of the molars on this radiograph?

   A. Mucocele.
   B. Sinusitis.
   C. Mucous retention cyst (phenomenon).
   D. Radicular cyst.
   E. Osteoma.

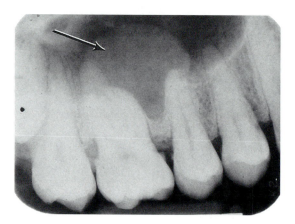

CASE 14.6

1. Identify the radiolucent circle identified by the arrow in this radiograph. The premolars are vital.

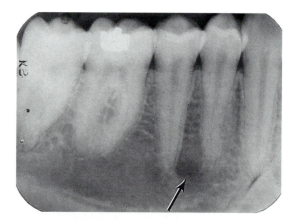

   A. Medullary space.
   B. Lingual foramen.
   C. Apical granuloma.
   D. Mental foramen.
   E. Nasopalatine foramen.

CASE 14.7

1. In all probability, what are the white radiopacities in this radiograph (arrows)?

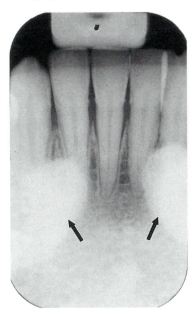

A. Cementomas.
B. Osteomas.
C. Tori.
D. Exostoses.
E. Foreign bodies.

CASE 14.8

1. What are the several dark lines within the edentulous alveolar bone? The patient has no signs or symptoms.

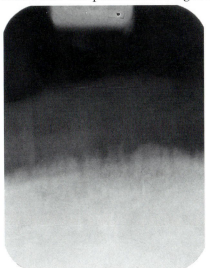

A. Fracture lines.
B. Medullary spaces.
C. Nutrient canals.
D. Trabecular spaces.
E. Osteomyelitis.

BIBLIOGRAPHY

Brand RW, Isselhard DE. Osteology of the skull. In: Anatomy of orofacial structures. 4th ed. St. Louis: CV Mosby, 1990:227–233.

Dental Auxiliary Education Project. Normal radiographic landmarks. New York: Teachers College Press, 1982.

Frommer HH. Radiology for dental auxiliaries. St. Louis: CV Mosby, 1987:232-252.

Goaz PW, White SC. Oral radiology principles and interpretation. 3rd ed. St. Louis: CV Mosby, 1994:126–150.

Kasle MJ. An Atlas of dental radiographic anatomy. Philadelphia: WB Saunders, 1977.

Langlais RP, Kasle MJ. Intraoral radiographic interpretation. Philadelphia: WB Saunders, 1978.

Langlais RP, Bentley KC. Advanced oral radiographic interpretation. Philadelphia: WB Saunders, 1979.

Langland OE, et al. A textbook of dental radiology. 2nd ed. Springfield: Charles C. Thomas, 1984:380–411.

Miles DA, Van Dis ML, Jensen CW. Radiographic imaging for dental auxiliaries. Philadelphia: WB Saunders, 1989:165–217.

Radiologic Diagnosis of Periodontal Disease

15

OBJECTIVES

Upon successful completion of this unit, the student will be able to:

1. *Understand the limitations of the radiograph in the evaluation of periodontal disease.*

2. *Understand the benefits of the radiograph in the evaluation of periodontal disease.*

3. *Recognize the presence of etiologic factors in radiographs.*

4. *Test his or her knowledge by answering the Review Questions.*

KEY WORDS/PHRASES

alveolar bone height	faulty restorations	occlusal trauma
bone defects	food packing	pocket formation
bone loss	furcation involvement	pocket wall(s)
bruxism	generalized bone loss	ramping
calculus	hemiseptum	root morphology
clenching	horizontal bone loss	thick periodontal ligament space
crater	infrabony pocket	tooth mobility
crestal changes	juvenile periodontitis	triangulation
crown-root ratio	localized bone loss	vertical bone loss

Introduction

The term periodontal disease represents a group of diseases that affect the surrounding and supporting tissues of the teeth. The most common periodontal diseases are caused by microbiological infections associated with local accumulation of bacterial plaque, pathogens, periodontal flora, restorations, and calculus. Periodontitis is characterized by gingival inflammation, periodontal pocket formation, destruction of the periodontal ligament and alveolar bone, and gradual loosening of the teeth. It is associated with apical migration of the junctional epithelium on the root surface. Hoag and Pawlak (1990) report that the incidence of periodontitis is approximately one in four for adults. The incidence of periodontal disease with pocket formation is about 4 in 10 adults at 50 years of age.

ROLE OF THE RADIOGRAPH IN PERIODONTAL DISEASE

There are limitations to the use of the radiograph in the diagnosis of periodontal disease. Radiographs give a two-dimensional representation of three-dimensional anatomical structures. The radiographic image lacks the third dimension of depth, which results in bone and tooth structures being superimposed over each other. However, if the limitations of the radiograph are recognized, the radiograph can still be considered an important diagnostic aid in the initial examination and diagnosis of patients with periodontal disease. To minimize the limitations of radiography, the intraoral radiograph must be taken with the long-cone (beam indicating device [BID]) paralleling technique. This provides a radiograph that is the most anatomically accurate. Also, it is important that a high-kilovoltage (80–90 kVp) technique be used, because radiographs with long-scale contrast are produced. Such images are superior to lower-kVp images in the interpretation of bony lesions because of the varying degrees of opacities and lucencies.

Although the radiograph provides crucial information regarding the presence of periodontal disease, it does not provide data concerning the activity or rate of periodontal destruction at the time of the examination. Sequential radiographic examinations performed after bone destruction has occurred can demonstrate disease activity retrospectively, because succeeding radiographic examinations of a patient can be compared both visually and more accurately by digital subtraction techniques. Early et al. (1979) estimated that a 30–50% change in bone mineral content is needed before bone loss can be detected in the radiograph. Small amounts of alveolar bone loss are difficult to see when dental radiographs are compared visually. Webber et al. (1982), Jeffcoat (1984), Jeffcoat et al. (1987), and McHenry et al. (1987) reported that small osseous changes can be detected by subtracting all unchanged bony structures from a set of dental radiographs, leaving only the area of change in the resultant subtraction radiograph. Lesions with less than 5% bone loss can be detected by digital subtraction radiography. Digital subtraction can also be used to detect bone regeneration as a result of periodontal therapy.

The digital subtraction radiograph may be used routinely in the dental office in the future. In digital subtraction, one image of an anatomical region from, for example, the previous year can be superimposed on a second image of the same anatomical region from the current year. The superimposition of the two images is done in the computer using special software. When one image is subtracted from the other, only the **differences** between the two images are seen. Thus, **even minute** changes in alveolar bone density can be detected and quantified.

LIMITATIONS OF THE RADIOGRAPH

With respect to periodontal disease, the role of the radiograph is misunderstood, and the limitations of radiographs must be understood. Some of the important limitations are listed below.

Presence or Absence of Periodontal Pockets

Because the periodontal pocket is a pathologically deepened gingival sulcus, the only reliable method of locating a periodontal pocket and evaluating its extent is by careful periodontal probing. The periodontal pocket is composed of soft tissue, so it will not be visible on the radiograph (Fig. 15.1); however, if a radiopaque material

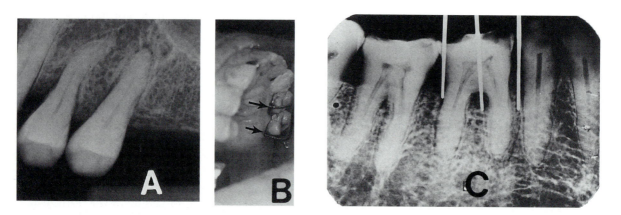

Figure 15.1. Absence of Periodontal Pockets on Radiograph. (**A**) Radiograph of a patient with 10-mm pockets on the palatal surface of maxillary premolars. (**B**) Photograph of patient in **A** showing 10-mm pockets on lingual surfaces of premolars by periodontal probes (*arrows*). (**C**) Silver points were used on mandibular first molar to assess base of periodontal pockets.

such as gutta percha root canal points or Hirschfeld calibrated silver points are inserted into the pocket, the base of the pocket can usually be recorded on the radiograph (Fig. 15.1).

Early Bone Loss

In a study by Pauls and Trott (1966), interseptal bony defects smaller than 3 mm could not be seen on radiographs by the use of visual methods. The sensitivity of radiographs in quantifying early bone destruction is only fair. The status of bone on facial and lingual aspects of the teeth is difficult to evaluate because the dense tooth structures are superimposed over the bone. Ramadan and Mitchell (1962) reported that by the time periodontal bone destruction becomes detectable on the radiograph, it has usually progressed beyond the earliest stage. Therefore, the very earliest signs of periodontal disease must be detected clinically.

Early Furcation Involvement

Furcation involvement is detected by clinical examination, which includes careful examination with a specialized probe such as the Nabors probe. Radiographs are helpful but usually show less bone loss than is actually present (Fig. 15.2). The furcation area of a tooth should be examined clinically, even if the radiograph shows a very small radiolucency or an area of diminished radiodensity at the furcation. Variations in the alignment of the x-ray beam may obliterate the presence or extent of furcation involvement. The facial and lingual aspects of the alveolar bone will often be superimposed over the furcation.

Dental Calculus

Radiographs may be useful in detecting subgingival calculus, which appears as a radiopaque line that increases in density with increased mineralization. The detection of calculus radiographically will depend on its degree of mineralization and on the angulation of the x-ray beam.

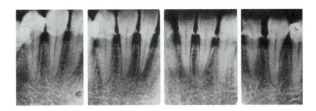

Figure 15.3. Dental Calculus. Interproximal spur-like calculus in lower anteriors.

The radiograph may show heavy calculus deposits and calculus spurs or spicules interproximally (Fig. 15.3), sometimes even on the facial and lingual surfaces; however, it cannot be relied on for the thorough detection of calculus. Here the radiograph is an adjunct to the clinical examination.

Tooth Mobility

Radiographs do not record tooth mobility. However, in most cases, a widening of the periodontal ligament space (PDLS) on the radiograph does indicate an increase in mobility (Fig. 15.4). In such instances, the PDLSs are wider around the mobile tooth or teeth than the remainder of the teeth. Traumatic defects manifest themselves more readily in the faciolingual aspects of the supporting structures, because in the mesiodistal aspects the contact areas of the adjacent teeth provide added stability. Because the tooth is superimposed over the faciolingual structures, a widened PDLS on these surfaces cannot be seen on the radiograph. Such changes will require a thorough clinical assessment of mobility for the final diagnosis.

Morphologic Characteristics of Bone Deformities

The presence of osseous defects or bone deformities may be suggested on the radiograph, but careful periodontal probing and surgical exposure are necessary to deter-

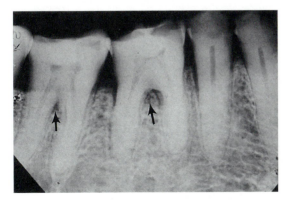

Figure 15.2. Furcation Involvement. Radiograph showing furcation involvement (*arrows*) of lower first and second molars.

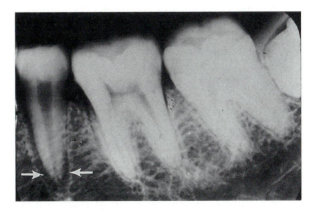

Figure 15.4. Periodontal Ligament Space (PDLS) Widening. The lower second premolar PDLS is widened (*arrows*), and the tooth is mobile.

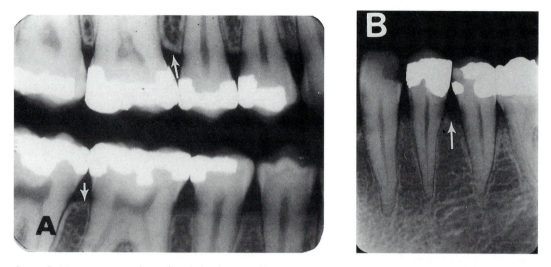

Figure 15.5. Crestal Irregularities. (**A**) Normal interdental alveolar crestal bone (*arrows*). The coronal border of the alveolar bone (alveolar crest) extends normally to approximately 1.5 mm from the cementoenamel junction (CEJ) of the teeth. (**B**) Note fuzziness and break of continuity of lamina dura at crest of alveolar bone between first and second premolars (*arrow*).

mine the shape and dimensions of bone deformity. Because the radiograph lacks depth, it will not accurately record the true picture of a bone deformity (e.g., showing the number of remaining walls of an infrabony bony pocket).

BENEFITS OF THE RADIOGRAPH

Despite its limitations, the periodontal examination is incomplete without accurate radiographs, which can show most bony changes in association with periodontal disease when viewed under good lighting conditions. The remainder of this chapter will be devoted to the benefits of the radiograph in the diagnosis of periodontal disease.

Early Radiographic Changes in Periodontitis

Although the radiograph is not sensitive enough to detect the earliest signs of periodontal disease, it is still an essential part of the clinical examination. Glickman (1972) listed the following sequence of early radiographic changes that occur in periodontitis:

1. Crestal irregularities,
2. Triangulation (funneling),
3. Interseptal bone changes.

Crestal Irregularities One of the first radiographic signs of periodontitis is the indistinctness and interruption in the continuity of the lamina dura (radiopaque) seen along the mesial or distal aspect of the interdental alveolar crest (Fig. 15.5). This bone resorption results from extension of the inflammation into the interdental bone, with

an associated widening of the vessel channels within the bone, and a reduction in calcified tissue per unit of bone at the septal margin.

Triangulation (Funneling) Triangulation is the widening of the PDLS by the resorption of bone along either the mesial or distal aspect of the interdental (interseptal) crestal bone. The sides of the triangle are formed by the alveolar bone and root surfaces, the base is toward the tooth crown, and the apex of the triangle is pointed toward the root (Fig. 15.6). This is an early sign of bone degeneration and necessitates a search for possible etiologic factors, such as plaque, calculus, gingivitis, or food impaction.

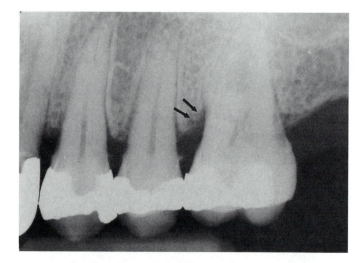

Figure 15.6. Triangulation (Funneling). Note the wedge-shaped radiolucencies on the mesial aspects of the first molar (*arrows*). Spur calculus can be seen on distal of second premolar.

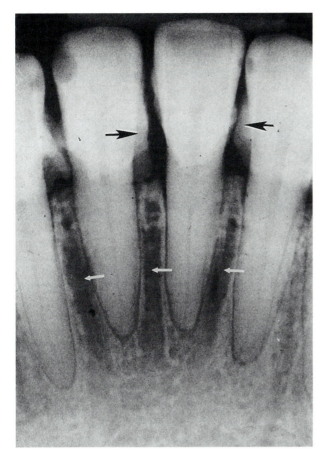

Figure 15.7. Interseptal Bone Changes. Note the increased bone resorption along endosteal margins of medullary spaces, which results in increased radiolucency of interseptal bone (*white arrows*). Also note the gross amounts of interproximal deposits of calculus (*black arrows*).

Interseptal Bone Changes One of the earliest radiographic signs of periodontitis is the finger-like radiolucent projections extending from the crestal bone into the interdental alveolar bone. These projections are a result of a deeper extension of the inflammation from the connective tissue of the gingiva. They represent widened blood vessel channels within the alveolar bone that allow for the passage of inflammatory fluid and cells into the bone. It results in a reduction of mineralized tissue per unit area (Fig. 15.7). When all the alveolar bone support is lost and the tooth seems to "float in air" on the radiograph, it is called the "terminal stage" of chronic destructive periodontitis (Fig. 15.8). Reactive sclerosis (radiopaque) can sometimes be seen at the margin of the remaining bone of terminal, chronic destructive periodontitis. Reactive sclerosis is a defense mechanism by the host bone whereby more bone is laid down at the margins of benign bone diseases, causing the area to appear more radiopaque in the radiographic image.

Evaluation of Bone Loss

The radiograph is used indirectly to determine the amount of bone loss attributed to periodontal disease. Actually, the radiograph indicates the amount of bone remaining and not the amount of bone loss. The amount of bone loss is the difference between the remaining coronal (pertaining to crown of tooth) height and the assumed normal coronal bone level for the patient. In a normal individual, the alveolar bone height is located 1–1.5 mm apical (toward apex of tooth) to the cementoenamel junction (CEJ). The evaluation of bone loss is made primarily by examining the interproximal septal bone on the radiograph. Of course, bone loss occurs on all surfaces, but the thickness of the tooth tends to obscure facial and lingual bone loss on the radiograph. If the bone loss occurs in isolated areas, it is described as **localized bone** loss (Fig. 15.9). When the bone loss is evenly distributed throughout the dental arches, it is called **generalized bone loss** (Fig. 15.10). The inflammation of periodontitis may spread from the gingiva into the alveolar bone and periodontal ligament, and reach the pulp through the root apices or accessory pulp canals near the apex or the furcation of a tooth. In these cases, retention of the tooth will depend on a combined periodontal/endodontic treatment plan (Fig. 15.11). If the alveolar bone loss from periodontitis is severe in the posterior maxillary molar region, the radio-

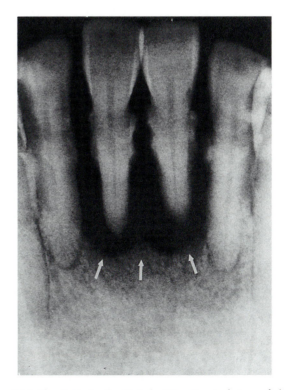

Figure 15.8. Chronic Destructive Periodontitis. Terminal stage of chronic destructive periodontitis (*arrows*). The teeth seem to be hanging in the air.

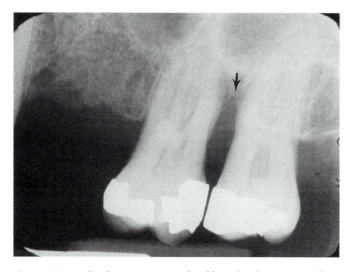

Figure 15.9. Localized Bone Loss. Localized bone loss between maxillary molars. Note the deficient contact between the molars providing an excellent food packing area.

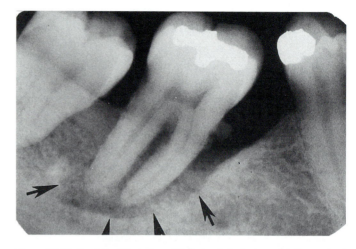

Figure 15.11. Combined Periodontal-Endodontic Pathoses. Radiograph of nonvital second molar which is periodontally involved.

graph is useful in determining the approximation of the crestal bone level to the floor of the maxillary sinus. This is especially important if bone surgery is being planned in this region.

Direction of Bone Loss The direction of bone loss or bone destruction, whereby areas previously occupied by healthy bone become radiolucent due to pathologic dissolution of the bone, is determined using the CEJ as the plane of reference.

Horizontal Bone Loss When the bone loss occurs on a plane that is parallel to a line drawn from the CEJ of a tooth to that of an adjacent tooth, it is called horizontal bone loss (Fig. 15.12).

Vertical Bone Loss When there is a greater degree of bone destruction on the interproximal aspect of one tooth than on the adjacent tooth, the bone level is angular or not parallel to a line joining the CEJs. This type of bone loss is called *angular or vertical bone loss* (Fig. 15.13). Vertical bone loss usually consists of one or many infrabony pockets, because the base of the pocket is usually located apical to the crest of the surrounding bone. Traditionally, horizontal bone loss was thought to be a result of a uniform resorptive response when inflammation from local irritating factors was the sole cause; vertical bone loss resulted from a more complex etiology, such as systemic disease, with a combination of occlusal trauma and local irritation. Proof of these theories have not been demonstrated conclusively. Thus, patterns of bone loss are now less important in the clinical diagnosis of periodontal disease than they were once thought to be.

Localized Juvenile Periodontitis Vertical bone loss

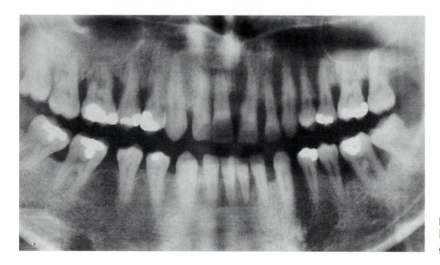

Figure 15.10. Generalized Bone Loss. Generalized bone loss in maxilla and mandible revealed in a panoramic radiograph.

around the first molars and incisors in an otherwise healthy adolescent with little or no accumulation of plaque and little or no clinical inflammation represents the classic diagnostic features of *localized juvenile periodontitis* (LJP). The classic radiographic finding in LJP is an arch-shaped loss of alveolar bone extending from the distal surface of the second premolar to the mesial surface of the second molar. Also, there is almost always a distolabial migration of the maxillary incisors with diastema formation (Fig. 15.14). The rate of bone loss is three to four times faster than in typical adult periodontitis. The definitive etiologic factors of LJP are not known, but most authorities believe that the principal cause is bacterial, with the possibility of an altered host response.

Evaluation of Bone Height

Because the density of the tooth obscures the coronal bone level of the alveolar bone on the facial and lingual surfaces, it is difficult to assess bone loss on the facial and lingual surfaces of teeth.

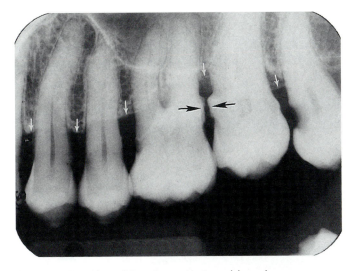

Figure 15.12. Horizontal Bone Loss. Horizontal bone loss occurs on a plane parallel with a line drawn from the CEJ of one tooth to that of an adjacent tooth (*white arrows*). Note trifurcation involvement of maxillary first molar and gross amounts of interproximal calculus between first and second molars (*black arrows*).

At times it is possible to estimate facial and lingual bone levels by using two procedures in combination:

1. Tracing the lamina dura line coronally until it loses its maximal opacity. This provides a rough estimate of the true height of the interseptal bone. The bone coronal to this level is the facial bone that has been cast coronally by excessive vertical angulation. This is especially true if the bisecting angle technique has been used. (The relationship of the buccal and lingual cusps of the teeth to each other should be checked.)

2. Starting at the apex of the tooth, the trabecular pattern of the bone on the root of the tooth should be traced coronally until it terminates at some level on the tooth root. A line running across the tooth will be noted. This line separates the denuded portion of the root from the root portion covered by bone (Fig. 15.15). The line usually represents the lingual height of the alveolar crest because of its greater detail. This line will join the terminal portion of the maximal coronal lamina dura opacity, as described in the first procedure.

Evaluation of Bone Defects

There are different types of bone deformities produced by periodontal disease. The accurate radiograph will usually show a bony defect in the interseptal bone, but its exact form or shape can be determined only by careful periodontal probing and/or by direct vision during surgical exposure. In most instances, the bony defect in periodontal disease is angular or vertical with an accompa-

nying infrabony pocket. As suggested by Goldman and Cohen (1958), infrabony pockets can be classified according to the number of bony walls associated with the infrabony pocket. Infrabony pockets may be classified as one-walled, two-walled, three-walled, or four-walled bony defects (Fig. 15.16).

Osseous Crater The *osseous crater* is a radiolucent defect and is thought to be the most common bony defect occurring in periodontal disease. Manson and Nicholson

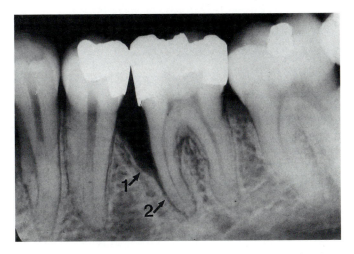

Figure 15.13. Vertical Bone Loss. (*1*) Vertical bone loss occurs when there is greater bone loss on the proximal of one tooth than the adjacent tooth. (*2*) Thickened PDL space.

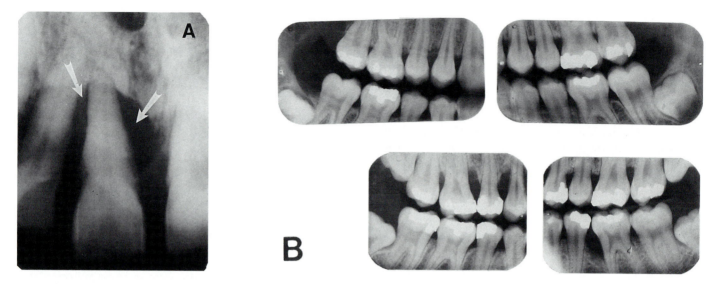

Figure 15.14. Localized Juvenile Periodontitis (LJP). (**A**) Classic arch-shaped anterior alveolar bone destruction found in LJP. (**B**) A 17-year-old girl with LJP. Clinically, there were few signs and symptoms of inflammation. Upper radiographs: patient at age 13. Lower radiographs: patient at age 17. (Note the severe bone loss between premolars and molars.)

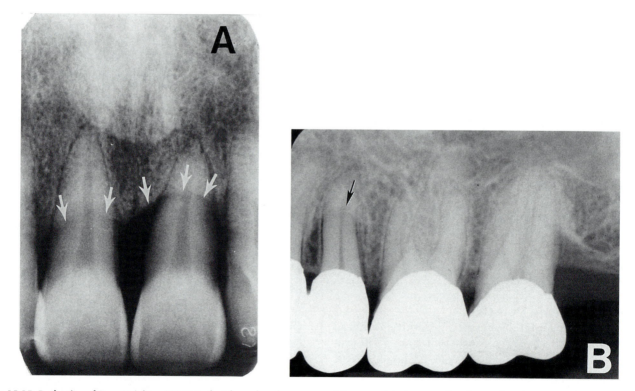

Figure 15.15. Evaluation of Bone Height. (**A**) Note that the trabecular pattern of the central incisors can be observed as the eye scans apically from the arrows. Below the arrows, the root appears denuded of bone. This is the true line of the bone height. (**B**) Note the severe bone loss on lingual surface of the maxillary second premolar. This is most likely bone level on the lingual surfaces because of its clarity (*black arrow*).

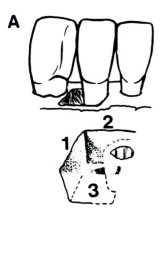

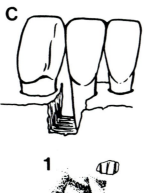

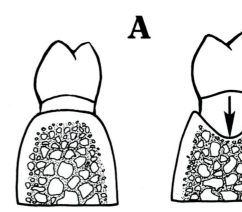

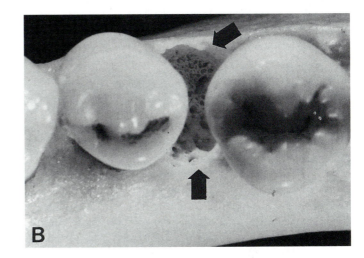

Figure 15.16. Bony Defect. (**A**) Three-wall bony defect. (**B**) Two-wall bony defect. Another type of two-wall bony defect is the osseous crater where the facial and lingual walls are intact but the interdental alveolar crest has been resorbed, forming a crater in the bone. (**C**) One-wall bony defect. This is also called the hemiseptum defect in which one wall of the interdental septum remains after the facial and lingual walls have been destroyed. Ramping is another form of one-wall defect when a facial wall is left standing and the interdental septal wall slopes toward the destroyed wall, forming a ramp-like appearance. (**D**) Four-wall bony defect completely surrounds the tooth.

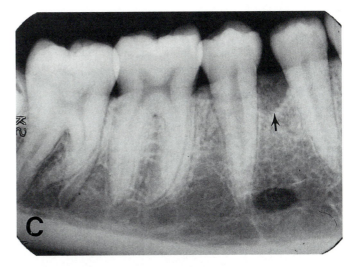

Figure 15.17. Osseous Crater (Two-Wall Bony Defect). (**A**) Diagram of an osseous crater between two mandibular premolars. (*Left*) Normal bone contour. (*Right*) Osseous crater within interdental septal bone (*arrow*). (**B**) Osseous crater between two premolars in dry specimen. (**C**) Radiographic appearance of osseous crater between first and second premolars.

(1974) found that craters constitute approximately one third (35.2%) of all bony defects and two thirds (62.0%) of all mandibular bony defects; they were also twice as common in the posterior segments compared with anterior segments. An osseous crater is a concavity in the crest of the interdental bone confined within the facial and lingual walls (Fig. 15.17). It is a **two-wall infrabony** crater deformity. A less-common, two-wall (crater) defect occurs when the facial or lingual cortical plate of bone is missing (Fig. 15.18). When the remaining facial or lingual wall is very thin or if a high-contrast/low-kilovolt technique is

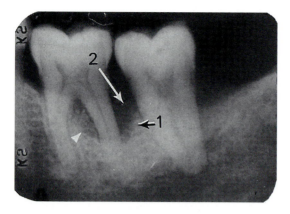

Figure 15.18. Less Common Two-Wall Bony Defect. Radiograph of less frequently seen two-wall infrabony defect found here on the distal of the first molar. Distal wall (*1*) and lingual wall (*2*) were intact, with furcation involvement (*white arrowhead*) confirmed by probing.

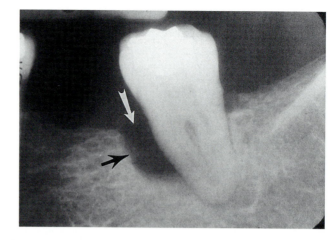

Figure 15.19. Radiograph of Two-Wall Bony Defect With Burnt-Out Lingual Wall. Radiograph of two-wall infrabony defect on mesial of molar with mesial wall (*black arrow*) and lingual wall (*white arrow*). The lingual remaining wall in this case is irregular and thin as well as "burnt out" and erased from the radiograph. This lingual wall was confirmed by probing.

used, this defect may not be seen on the radiograph. This is because the thin bony wall will be **burnt out** and erased from the radiograph (Fig. 15.19).

Hemiseptum and Ramping Defects In the one-wall angular defect, one bony wall of the interseptal bone remains after the mesial or the distal portion of the interseptal bone has been destroyed. It is called a *hemiseptum defect* and is identical to vertical or angular bony deformities (Figs. 15.20 and 15.21). The one-wall defect will sometimes take the *form of a ramp* or slanted area when the facial or lingual cortical bone is destroyed. This defect is called ramping.

Furcation Involvement

Extension of the periodontal pocket between the roots of multirooted teeth is called furcation involvement. The mandibular first molars are the most common sites of furcation involvement, and the maxillary first premolars are the least common locations. The number of furcation involvements increases with age. Examination of the extent of the furcation involvement is made by exploration with a Nabors periodontal probe or dental explorer inserted into the roof of the furcation. Visualization can be

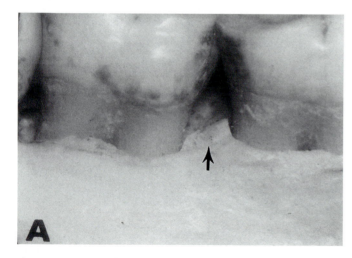

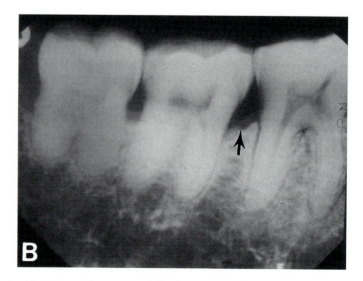

Figure 15.20. One-Wall Vertical Angular Bony Defect (Hemiseptum Appearance). (**A**) One-wall hemiseptum defect between mandibular first and second molars of dry specimen. (**B**) Radiograph of **A** showing one-wall hemiseptum defect between first and second molars.

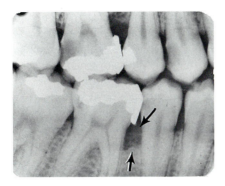

Figure 15.21. One-Wall Bony Defect (Ramp-Like Appearance). The defect has formed a ramp-like appearance (*arrows*), because the interdental septal bone slopes down from the facial/lingual wall crest of bone toward the crest of the destroyed facial/lingual bone. In this case, probing confirmed that the lingual wall was destroyed, and the ramping sloped down from intact facial wall toward the lingual crest of bone.

In using the radiograph to aid in the detection of furcation involvement, the following rules should be kept in mind:

1. If there is a slight thickening of the PDLS in the furcation area, the area should be investigated clinically. It is a general rule that furcation involvement is often greater than the radiograph shows.
2. If there is severe bone loss on the mesial or distal surface of a multirooted tooth, furcation involvement should be suspected.

facilitated by use of warm compressed air. Radiographs can be helpful in locating furcation involvement; however, the furcation involvement will not be seen unless the bone resorption extends apically beyond the furca. Mandibular molar furca is much more sharply defined than the maxillary molar furca, mainly because the palatal root is not superimposed over the furca as with the maxillary molar (Fig. 15.22).

RECOGNITION OF ETIOLOGIC FACTORS

The primary cause of inflammatory periodontal diseases is the accumulation and growth of bacterial plaque on the teeth near the gingival margin or in the sulcus or pocket. However, the periodontal tissue response to the bacteria is influenced by local, immune, and systemic factors.

Local factors are found in the immediate environment of the periodontal tissues and can be divided into **local**

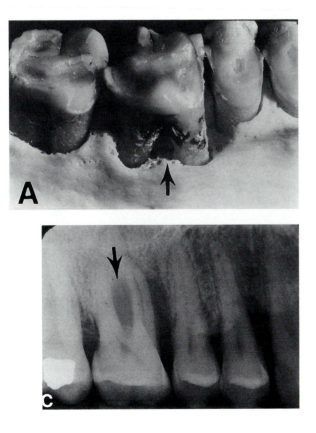

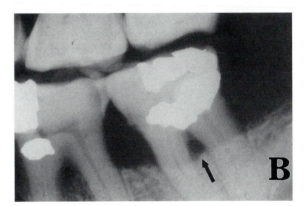

Figure 15.22. Furcation Involvement. (**A**) Furcation involvement of lower first molar of a dry specimen. (**B**) Radiograph of "through-and-through" bifurcation involvement of second molar (*arrow*). (**C**) Through-and-through trifurcation involvement of maxillary first molar. The radiolucency is not as dark as the radiolucency of a bifurcation involvement of a lower molar because of superimposition of palatal root of maxillary molars over the furca.

irritating and **functional factors**. Local irritating factors are separated **into local initiating** and **local predisposing factors**. Bacterial plaque is the **local initiating factor** because it causes gingival inflammation when it accumulates on the teeth adjacent to the gingiva.

Local predisposing factors, such as overhanging restorations, calculus, and food retention areas, create a dentogingival environment that favors the accumulation of bacterial plaque. **Local functional factors**, such as bruxism and occlusal trauma, create occlusal forces that are associated with destruction of the periodontal ligament and alveolar bone but do not affect the inflammatory process directly.

Detection of Local Predisposing Factors

Several local predisposing factors may be detected on the radiograph: calculus deposits, faulty restorations, and food packing areas. The radiograph plays no role in determining the cause of the predisposing factors in periodontal disease, it only detects them.

Dental Calculus Deposits Calculus is bacterial plaque that has been mineralized. It can form on all tooth surfaces and on dental prostheses. Calculus is classified into two groups, according to its location and source: supragingival (salivary) and subgingival (serumal).

The primary etiologic role of calculus in periodontal tissues is that it acts as a holding mechanism for nonmineralized bacterial plaque and keeps the bacterial plaque in direct contact with the tissue.

Dental Calculus Detection The radiograph shows heavy radiopaque calculus deposits interproximally and sometimes even on the facial and lingual surfaces. The ability to diagnose and detect calculus radiographically depends on its degree of mineralization and the angulation factors of the x-ray beam. Sometimes the detection of calculus spicules is useful in diagnosing and monitoring periodontal disease (Figs. 15.23 and 15.24).

Faulty Restorations Inadequate dental restorations and prostheses are common causes of gingival inflammation, periodontitis, and alveolar bone resorption.

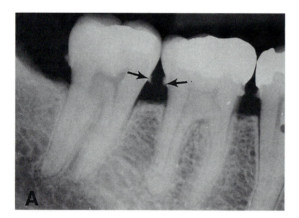

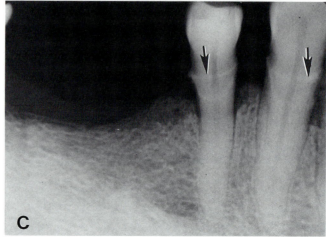

Figure 15.23. Dental Calculus. (**A**) Spur-like calculus of interproximal surfaces of lower molars and second premolars (*arrows*). (**B**) Ledge-like smooth veneer type of calculus (*arrows*). (**C**) Ring-like (line) calculus (*arrows*) on lower canine and premolars (*arrows*).

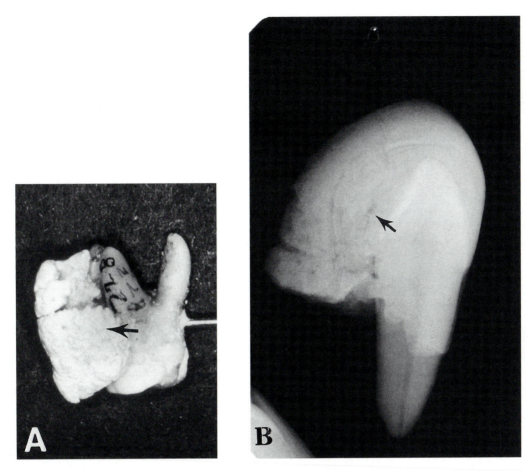

Figure 15.24. Gross Amounts of Dental Calculus. **(A)** Gross amounts of calculus deposits on buccal crown and roots of extracted maxillary first molar (*arrow*). **(B)** Radiograph of extracted lower canine with gross amounts of supragingival calculus (*arrow*).

Some problems with restorations and prostheses include the following:

1. Overhanging margins of dental restorations (Fig. 15.25).
2. Open interproximal contacts of dental restorations (Fig. 15.26).
3. Deficient margins of crowns and aesthetic porcelain restorations.
4. Fixed and removable prostheses that are improperly adapted.
5. Overcontoured restorations and pontics that create excessive buccolingual contours and inadequate interproximal embrasure spaces.
6. Clasps of partial dentures that retain plaque adjacent to the gingiva or exert excessive occlusal forces.

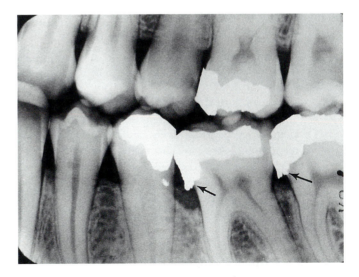

Figure 15.25. Overhanging Restorations. Overhanging restorations on mesial surfaces of first and second molars (*arrows*).

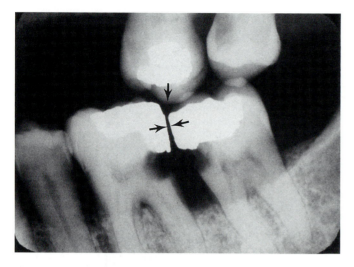

Figure 15.26. Open Interproximal Contact. Plunger maxillary molar cusp causes food wedging between lower first and second molar, followed by caries and periodontal bone destruction.

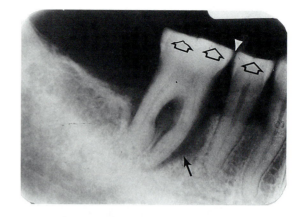

Figure 15.27. Attrition and Open Contact. Severe attrition has caused a loose contact and food packing area between second premolar and first molar, with resultant periodontal destruction of alveolar bone.

Food Packing Areas Food impaction is the forceful wedging of food through occlusal pressure into the interproximal spaces. The absence of tooth contact or presence of an unsatisfactory interproximal relationship is conducive to food impaction. As the teeth wear down and the flattened surfaces replace normal convexities, the wedging effect of the opposing cusp into the interproximal space is exaggerated and food impaction results. Cusps that tend to forcibly wedge food interproximally are known as "plunger cusps."

when occlusal forces exceed the adaptive capacity of the supporting periodontal tissues. Clinically, it is characterized by breakdown of the periodontal ligament fibers, resorption of bone, widening of the PDLS, and loosening of the teeth. The diagnosis of periodontal or occlusal traumatism is made from clinical mobility tests, tooth percussion, probing, palpation, observation of wear patterns, observation of masticating movements, and the history of the patient's oral habits (bruxism, clenching). The radiograph is used only as a supplemental aid in determining periodontal or occlusal traumatism.

Some factors leading to food impaction include the following:

1. Wear from attrition, opening contact points (Fig. 15.27).
2. Loss of occlusal support by extraction of adjacent teeth, which will open contacts by shifting the teeth.
3. Opening of the contact areas by caries (Fig. 15.28).
4. Supraeruption of teeth, opening contact points when opposing teeth are not replaced.
5. Partially impacted teeth, producing food-lodging areas around the impaction.
6. Improperly constructed restorations.

Local Functional Factors

Periodontal Occlusal Traumatism Periodontal occlusal trauma gives rise to a degenerative lesion that develops

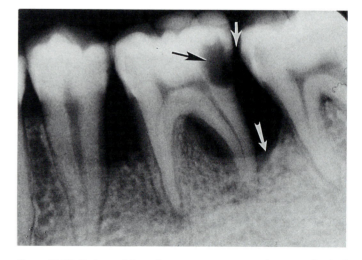

Figure 15.28. Caries and Open Contact. Large carious lesion on distal of first molar has created a food packing area, which has contributed to the severe amount of destruction of alveolar bone supporting the first molar.

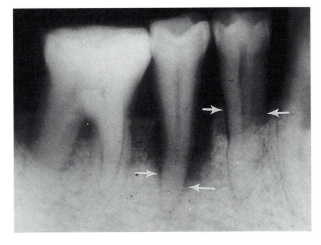

Figure 15.29. Clinical Crown-to-Root Ratio. Note poor clinical crown-to-root ratio of lower first and second premolars (*arrows*).

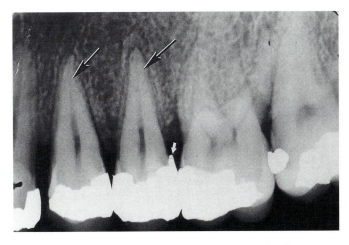

Figure 15.30. Spiked Roots. Note short, spiked roots of maxillary premolars with thickened PDLS and overhanging restoration on distal of second premolar.

The radiographic signs of trauma from occlusion include the following:

1. The increased width of the PDLSs of the mesiodistal surfaces due to resorption of the lamina dura, and
2. Vertical or angular bone destruction.

Crown-Root Ratio and Root Morphology Tooth stability is influenced by the amount of leverage placed on the periodontium. The type of leverage is dependent on the amount of tooth that is within bone (clinical root) in relation to the amount of tooth not within bone (clinical crown). An increase in length of the clinical crown produces unfavorable leverage on the periodontium (Fig. 15.29). In any patient the clinical root may be short or

spike-like because of a morphologic variation in the normal anatomy of the root. Some Hispanic Americans have significantly shortened roots as a result of the shovel-shaped incisor syndrome; any patient may have shortened roots from excessive orthodontic forces. If there is a loss of alveolar bone surrounding these short or spike-shaped teeth, the leverage exerted on the periodontium becomes exceedingly great (Fig. 15.30).

Activity of the Destructive Process

The approximate activity of the destructive process of periodontal disease can be evaluated by comparing standardized radiographs taken over regular intervals. When the interdental septal bone crest is rough and irregular and the alveolar bone below the crest is devoid of any suggestion of bone opacity, it is most likely that the resorptive process is **active** (Fig. 15.31A). Nutrient canals indi-

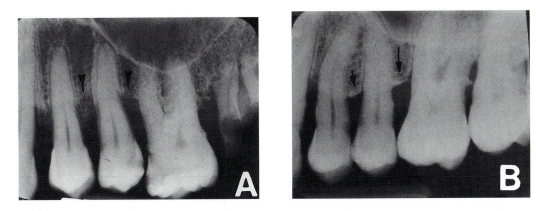

Figure 15.31. Activity of Destructive Process. **(A)** Radiograph of patient with appearance of an actively destructive process. **(B)** Radiograph of a patient with a static destructive periodontal disease. The crests of the interseptal alveolar bone between first and second premolars are smooth and radiopaque.

cate active and even rapid bone resorption. If a smooth surface of the alveolar bone with condensation of remaining alveolar bone is seen in the presence of bone loss, a static destructive process or slowly destructive process is indicated (Fig. 15.31B).

Prognosis

The prognosis cannot be estimated until all available information has been secured. Radiographic information is part of the diagnostic data that are used in determining the prognosis. The prognosis is reasonably good if the destructive process is not generalized, the past bone response to local irritants has been good, only a limited amount of bone has been lost, the destructive activity is minimal, correctable etiologic factors can be identified (radiographs can only identify certain local predisposing irritants and cannot determine etiology), occlusal deformities can be corrected, the location of the periodontal pocket is favorable (a patient with deep pockets and little bone loss has a better prognosis than a patient with shallow pockets and severe bone loss), the number and distribution of remaining teeth is favorable for the adequate support of a prosthesis (the crown-root ratio of abutment teeth is favorable), the patient's general health is good, the patient's teeth are normal in size and shape (not short and spike-shaped), and the patient is motivated to save the remaining teeth and is capable of performing all routine and specialized home care procedures as dictated by the extent and distribution of the periodontal disease.

REVIEW QUESTIONS

1. Identify information that cannot be obtained from radiographs concerning the diagnosis of periodontal disease.

    1. Root length and shape.
    2. Existence or absence of periodontal pockets.
    3. Morphology (shape) of bone deformities.
    4. Clinical crown to clinical root ratio.
    5. Approximate gross amount of bone destruction.
    6. Position of maxillary sinus in relation to periodontal deformity.
    7. Position or condition of structures on the facial and lingual aspects of the tooth.
    A. 1, 3, 4, 5, and 6.
    B. 2, 3, and 7.
    C. 1, 2, 3, 6, and 7.
    D. 3, 4, 5, 6, and 7.
    E. 1, 2, 3, 5, and 7.

2. Which of the following are benefits of the dental radiograph in periodontal diagnosis?

    1. The position of the septal bone between the teeth is usually recorded in one plane.
    2. The clinical crown to clinical root ratio is documented.
    3. Root length and root morphology are recorded.
    A. 1 and 2.
    B. 1, 2, and 3.
    C. 2.
    D. 1 and 3.
    E. 2 and 3.

3. Which of the following statements are true concerning periodontitis?

    1. Juvenile periodontitis is a localized periodontitis occurring in teen-agers and young adults.
    2. A normal crown-to-root ratio is 1:2.
    3. Calculus plays a primary inflammatory role in initiating periodontal disease.
    4. The crater bone deformity is the most common osseous deformity in periodontitis.
    5. The infrabony osseous deformity is a three-wall infrabony pocket.
    A. 1 and 3.
    B. 2 and 4.
    C. 1, 2, 3, and 5.
    D. 1, 3, 4, and 5.
    E. 1, 2, 4, and 5.

CASE-BASED QUESTIONS

CASE 15.1

This patient is an older man with calculus.

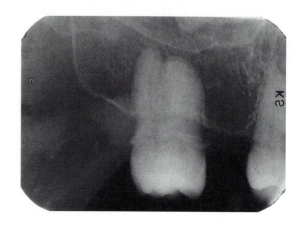

1. In the maxillary molar, the distribution and location of the calculus is:

   A. Circumferential.
   B. Subgingival.
   C. Supragingival.
   D. Generalized.
   E. A and B.

CASE 15.2

This 45-year-old woman has moderately severe horizontal bone loss and calculus.

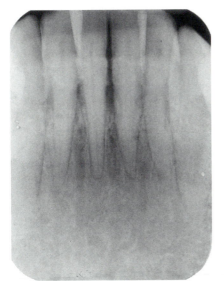

1. The presence of prominent nutrient canals indicates:

   A. Hyperemic and bleeding gingiva.
   B. A good host response.
   C. The patient is prone to posttreatment infection.
   D. Rapidly destructive periodontitis.

CASE 15.3

This patient is a 58-year-old man who has long denied he has any problems; he states that he "doesn't get cavities."

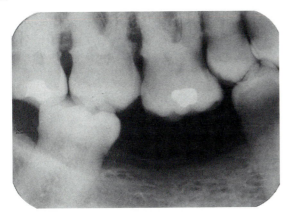

1. There is a problem with the maxillary first molar. What term best describes its **position**?

   A. Supraerupted.
   B. Elongated.
   C. Ectopic.
   D. Infraerupted.

CASE 15.4

This patient is a 35-year-old woman who has regularly seen her hygienist and dentist for many years but had to come to a dental school due to financial problems.

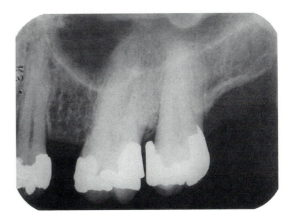

1. The periodontal problem between the maxillary molars is due to:

   A. Not replacing the second premolar.
   B. Open contact.
   C. An overhang.
   D. Poorly contoured restorations.
   E. All of the above.

CASE 15.5

This patient is a 50-year-old man who is without any major dental complaint.

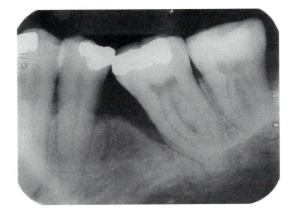

1. What is the **primary** cause of the bone destruction at the mesial of the second molar?

    A. Nonreplacement of the first molar.
    B. Poor home dental care.
    C. Juvenile periodontitis.
    D. Toothpick misuse.

CASE 15.6

This 42-year-old woman is not prone to accept regular recalls and feels she has had little need for dental care. Her teeth have always been described by others as "beautiful."

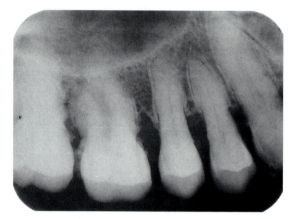

1. Which problems listed below do you think she has?

    A. Moderate to severe calculus formation.
    B. Horizontal bone loss.
    C. Vertical bone defect(s).
    D. Multiple open contacts of teeth.
    E. All of the above.

BIBLIOGRAPHY

Animo J, Tammisalo EH. Comparison of radiographic and clinical signs of early periodontal disease. Scand J Dent 1973;81:548–554.

Brekhus PS. Dental disease and its relation to the loss of human teeth. J Am Dent Assoc 1929;16:2237–2247.

Brown LJ. Periodontal disease in the U.S. in 1981: prevalence, severity, extent and role in tooth mortality. J Periodontol 1989;60:363–669.

Early PJ, et al. Textbook of nuclear medicine technology. 3rd ed. St. Louis: CV Mosby, 1979:379.

Glickman I. Bifurcation involvement in periodontal disease. J Am Dent Assoc 1950;40:528–531.

Glickman I. Clinical periodontology. 4th ed. Philadelphia: WB Saunders, 1972:499–505.

Goldman HM, Cohen DW. The infrabony pocket: classification and treatment. J Periodontol 1958;29:272–276.

Hausmann E. Progression of untreated periodontitis as assessed by subtraction radiography. J Periodont Res 1986;6:716–724.

Hausmann E. Radiographic examination. In: Genco RJ, Goldman HM, Cohen DW, eds. Contemporary periodontics. St. Louis: CV Mosby, 1990:334–344.

Hirschfeld I. Food impaction. J Am Dent Assoc 1930;17:1504–1511.

Hirschfeld I. A calibrated silver point for periodontal diagnosis and recording. J Periodontol 1953;24:94–97.

Hoag PM, Pawlak EA. Essentials of periodontics. 4th ed. St. Louis: CV Mosby, 1990:69–88.

Hormand J, Frandsen A. Juvenile periodontitis localization of bone loss in relation to age, sex and teeth. J Clin Periodontol 1979;6:407–415.

Jeffcoat MK. A new method for comparison of bone loss measurement on nonstandardized radiographs. J Periodontal Res 1984;19:434–441.

Jeffcoat MK, et al. Extraoral control of geometry for digital substraction radiology. J Periodontal Res 1987;22:398–406.

Kay S, Forseher BK, Sackett LM. Tooth root length-volume relationships: an aid to periodontal prognosis. I: anterior teeth. Oral Surg 1954;7:735–739.

Krill DB, Fry HR. Treatment of localized juvenile periodontitis (periodontosis). J Periodontol 1987;58:1–11.

Larato DC. Furcation involvements: incidence and distribution. J Periodontol 1970;41:491–497.

Larato DC. Infrabony defects in the dry human skull. J Periodontol 1970;41:496–501.

Larato DC. Some anatomical factors related to furcation involvements. J Periodontol 1975;46:608–613.

Manson JD. Bone morphology and bone loss in periodontal disease. J Clin Periodontol 1976;3:14–320.

Manson JD, Lehner T. Clinical features of juvenile periodontitis (periodontosis). J Periodontol 1974;45:636–641.

Manson JD, Nicholson K. The distribution of bone defects in chronic periodontitis. J Periodontol 1974;45:88–92.

Manson JD. Bone morphology and bone loss in periodontal disease. J Clin Periodontol 1976;3:14–19.

McHenry K, et al. Methodical aspects and quantitative adjuncts to computerized substraction radiology. J Periodontal Res 1987;22:125–133.

Nielsen JJ, Glavina L, Karring T. Interproximal periodontal infrabony defects: prevalence, localization and etiological factors. J Clin Periodontol 1980;7:187–196.

Orban B, Weinmann JP. Diffuse atrophy of the alveolar bone (periodontosis). J Periodontol 1952;13:31–41.

Patur B, Glickman I. Roentgenographic evaluation of alveolar bone changes in periodontal disease. Dent Clin North Am 1960;48:47–58.

Pauls V, Trott JR. A radiological study of experimentally produced lesions of bone. Dent Pract 1966;16:254–261.

Ramadan A-BE, Mitchell DF. A roentgenographic study of experimental bone destruction. Oral Surg 1962;15:934–941.

Updegrave WJ. Accurate radiography for diagnosis of periodontal disease. In: Ward H, ed. A periodontal point of view. Springfield: Charles C. Thomas, 1973:389–419.

Webber RL, et al. X-ray image subtraction as the basis for assessment of periodontal changes. J Periodontal Res 1982;17:509–517.

Abnormalities of Teeth

16

OBJECTIVES

Upon successful completion of this unit, the student will be able to:

1. *Recognize alterations in numbers of teeth on radiographs.*

2. *Identify alterations in tooth size, shape, and structure on radiographs.*

3. *Identify acquired defects of teeth on radiographs.*

4. *Identify alterations in tooth eruption on radiographs.*

5. *Test his or her knowledge by answering the Review Questions.*

KEY WORDS/Phrases

abrasion	embedded tooth	malformation
amelogenesis imperfecta	enamel hypoplasia	microdontia
anodontia	enamel pearl	migration
anomaly	enameloma	oligodontia
attrition	erosion	peg lateral
concrescence	familial	regional odontodysplasia
dens evaginatus	fusion	schizodontism
dens in dente	gemination	supernumerary roots
dens invaginatus	ghost teeth	supernumerary teeth
dentinal dysplasia	hyperdontia	synodontism
dentinogenesis imperfecta	hypodontia	taurodontism
dilaceration	impacted tooth	translocation
drift	Leong's premolar	transposition
ectopic eruption	macrodontia	variation

INTRODUCTION

A **developmental abnormality** is a departure or divergence from what is considered the normal process of growth and differentiation. A developmental disturbance or abnormality may be classified according to severity. A **variation** is a minor deviation from normal (e.g., enlarged medullary bone space), and **anomalies** are more severe deviations that do not interfere with function (e.g., peg laterals). **Malformations** are more severe deviations that do interfere with function (e.g., cleft palates). The most common anomalies are those that affect the teeth; those that result from faulty development of the supporting structures of the teeth are more rare. Anomalies discussed in this chapter may be caused by local conditions, inherited dental disorders, or manifestations of systemic disturbances. The anomalies of teeth are classified conventionally in this chapter to include **defects or alterations in number, size, shape, structure,** and **eruption.** In addition, **acquired defects** of teeth such as abrasion, attrition, and erosion are discussed.

ALTERATIONS IN NUMBER OF TEETH

ANODONTIA AND HYPODONTIA (OLIGODONTIA)

Anodontia means the absence of all teeth. In true anodontia, all teeth fail to develop; this is an extremely rare occurrence. Acquired anodontia is very common and results from the premature extraction of all teeth. Hypodontia (oligodontia) or partial anodontia means that one or several, but not all, teeth are missing. Hypodontia may

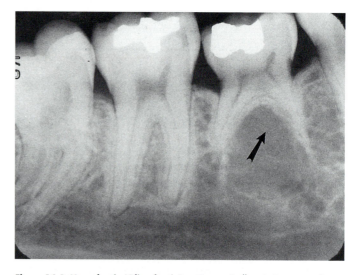

Figure 16.1. Hypodontia (Oligodontia). Congenitally missing second premolar with a retained primary second molar (*arrow*).

be congenital or acquired. The most common congenitally missing permanent teeth are the third molars, followed by the premolars and maxillary lateral incisors. When the second premolar is congenitally missing, a submerged, sometimes ankylosed (fused) second primary molar is present (Fig 16.1).

HYPERDONTIA (SUPERNUMERARY TEETH)

Hyperdontia refers to one or more extra teeth, and the problem is congenital only. Approximately 90% of all supernumerary teeth occur in the maxilla. The most common extra tooth is the maxillary **mesiodens** (extra tooth

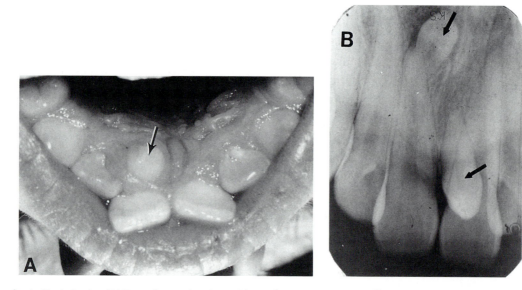

Figure 16.2. Hyperdontia (Mesiodens). (**A**) Erupted mesiodens (*arrow*) located just posterior to maxillary central incisor. (**B**) Bilateral mesiodens (*arrows*).

in maxillary midline) (Fig. 16.2). Others include upper fourth molars and mandibular premolars (Fig. 16.3). Upper fourth molars may resemble other maxillary molars or they may be small and conical. These microdontic (small) fourth molars are referred to as **distomolars** when they are distal to the third molar in location and as **paramolars** when they are seen buccal or palatal to the maxillary molars.

ALTERATIONS IN TOOTH SIZE

MACRODONTIA

Macrodontia refers to teeth that are larger than normal (Fig. 16.4). This condition may affect all teeth, as may be seen in the pituitary giant, or may be localized and involve one or several teeth. The term macrodontia should not be applied to teeth that are enlarged due to magnification, gemination, or fusion. Relative macrodontia occurs when the teeth appear to be overly large due to micrognathia, in which the jaws are too small to accommodate the teeth.

MICRODONTIA

Microdontia means teeth that are smaller than normal. This condition is much more common than macrodontia. Generalized microdontia affects all teeth, as may be seen in the pituitary dwarf. Relative generalized microdontia occurs when the teeth appear to be too small to fill all the space provided by the jaws. Microdontia of one or several teeth is more common than the generalized form. The most commonly affected teeth are the maxillary permanent lateral incisors, sometimes known as "peg laterals," and the third molars (Fig. 16.5). Peg laterals are usually cone shaped, and the condition is often bilateral and familial in occurrence. Familial means, occurring in

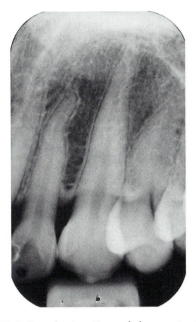

Figure 16.4. Macrodontia. Extremely long canine tooth.

or affecting more members of a family than would be expected by chance.

ALTERATIONS IN TOOTH SHAPE

SHAPE GEMINATION (SCHIZODONTISM)

Gemination consists of an aborted attempt by a single tooth bud to divide. It most frequently affects anterior teeth, particularly in the primary dentition. In gemination, the total number of teeth in the arch is normal. Radiographically, the crown is usually enlarged and the incisal edge may be notched. The pulp chamber is often Y-shaped with two coronal portions and a single root canal space (Fig. 16.6).

FUSION (SYNODONTISM)

Fusion occurs as a result of the union of two adjacent tooth buds by dentin and/or enamel. If fusion occurs between two normal teeth, a reduced number of teeth will be present in the arch. If the union is between a normal tooth and a supernumerary tooth, the distinction between fusion and gemination may be impossible. Fusion occurs mainly in the anterior region, particularly in the primary dentition. The most reliable radiographic sign of this condition is seen when two separate root canal spaces and pulp chambers are seen (Fig. 16.7).

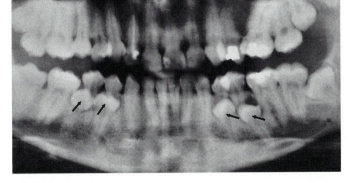

Figure 16.3. Hyperdontia (Supernumerary Teeth). Bilateral unerupted supernumerary premolars (*arrows*).

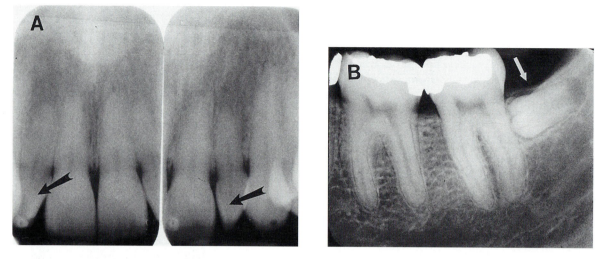

Figure 16.5. Microdontia. (**A**) Bilateral peg laterals (*arrows*). (**B**) Microdontic horizontally impacted third molar (*arrow*).

CONCRESCENCE

Concrescence occurs when there is a union between the roots of two or more teeth by cementum only. In true concrescence, the union occurs during root development and/or eruption. In acquired concrescence, the cemental union occurs after the completion of root formation, often as a result of hypercementosis (Fig. 16.8). It is usually seen in maxillary molar region. Concrescence can cause difficulty with extraction and orthodontic tooth movement.

DILACERATION

Dilaceration is a bent tooth. The root is most frequently involved, and it usually develops as a result of mechanical trauma during root formation and/or eruption. Some common causes include mechanical blockage of the path of eruption by the presence of neoplasms, cysts, supernumerary teeth, or orthodontic treatment. Dilaceration may occur at any location along the root and in any tooth. Dilaceration can result in malpositioning of teeth and can interfere with orthodontic realignment (Fig. 16.9).

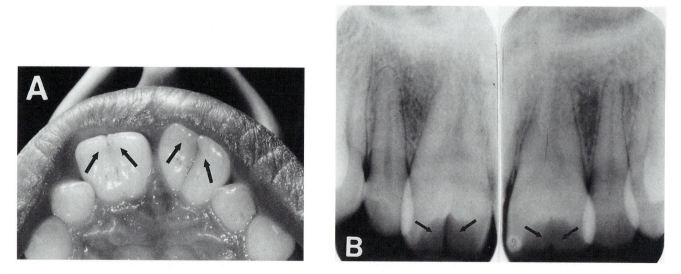

Figure 16.6. Gemination. (**A**) Photograph of a patient with bilateral gemination of maxillary central incisors (*arrows*). (**B**) Radiograph of bilateral gemination of maxillary central incisors of the patient in A.

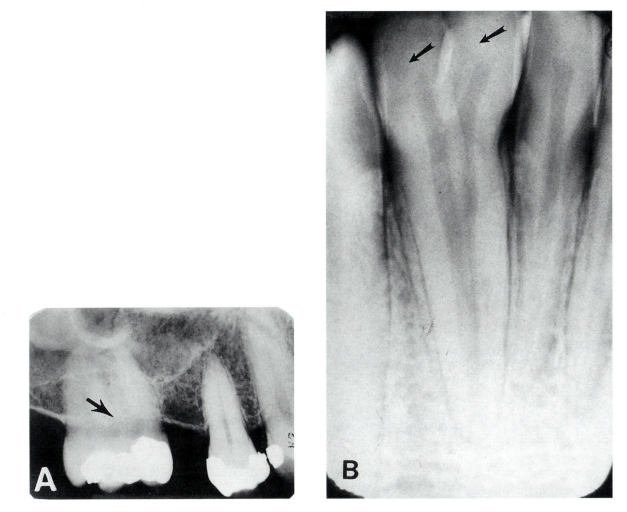

Figure 16.7. Fusion. (**A**) Fusion between two maxillary molars. (**B**) Fusion between lateral and central incisors. There is one less tooth in the mandibular incisor region. (Usually fused teeth look like two teeth stuck together; often the dentin is confluently joined together as one, as shown here. Note there are two separate pulp chambers and root canals in this radiograph. This makes the diagnosis of fusion much easier.)

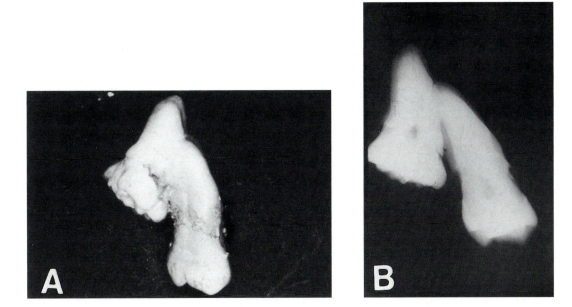

Figure 16.8. Concrescence. (**A**) Gross specimen (second and third molars) of concrescence. (**B**) Radiograph of the gross specimen in (**A**).

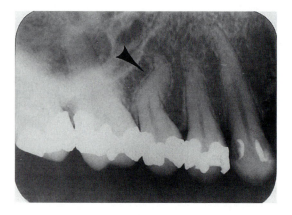

Figure 16.9. Dilaceration. Dilaceration of upper right second premolar (*arrow*).

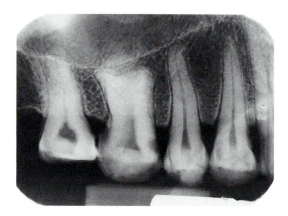

Figure 16.10. Taurodontism. Taurodontism of upper right first molar.

TAURODONTISM

Taurodontism ("tauros" meaning bull, and "odont" meaning tooth) refers to teeth that have an abnormally large pulp chamber and shortened roots, giving them the appearance of a bull. The condition often affects molar teeth, and clinically the teeth appear normal. The pulp chamber appears rectangular and lacks the usual constriction at the cervix. The roots are usually very short, although the overall length of the tooth is invariably normal (Fig. 16.10). Taurodontism may affect either the primary or permanent dentition, although permanent involvement is more common.

SUPERNUMERARY ROOTS

Extra or supernumerary roots may occur on any tooth but are more frequently seen in mandibular permanent

premolars and canines. Radiographic signs of supernumerary roots include double periodontal ligament spaces on one side of the root, the periodontal ligament space crossing roots, and an abrupt diminution in size of the root canal space with branching, producing an inverted-Y shape of the apical portion of the root canal space. The root canal will sometimes branch into two root canals within a single rooted tooth (Fig. 16.11).

ENAMEL PEARLS (ENAMELOMAS)

Enamel pearls consist of small round or ovoid radiopacities seen in the cervical portion of teeth, often molars. They are usually well defined and show the same degree of radiopacity as enamel. They may be superimposed on the pulp chamber of affected teeth and may be mistaken for pulpal calcifications. Because the enamel pearl is on the outside of the tooth, it will move away from the pulp chamber when off-angle views are taken, whereas pulp

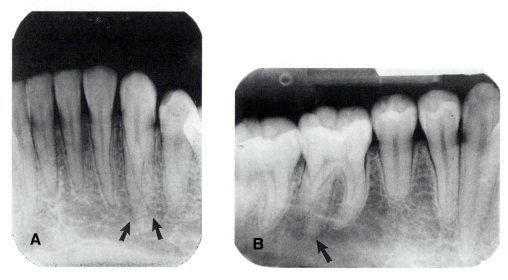

Figure 16.11. Supernumerary Roots. (**A**) Two-rooted canine (*arrows*). (**B**) Three-rooted lower molar (*arrow*).

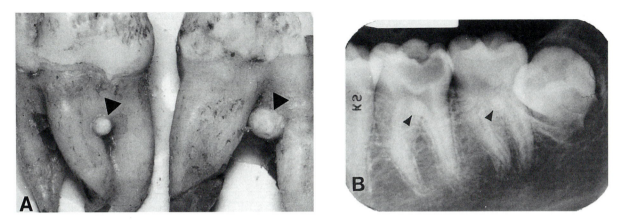

Figure 16.12. Enamel Pearls (Enamelomas). **(A)** Enamel pearls in two extracted molars (*arrowheads*). **(B)** Enamel pearls (*arrowheads*) at bifurcation of mandibular molars.

stones always remain within the confines of the pulp chamber or root canal space when supplemental views are taken (Fig. 16.12). If the enamel pearl happens to be located at the bifurcation of a molar tooth at the cementoenamel junction, it could lead to a periodontal pocket formation. If the enamel pearl is a predisposing cause of periodontal disease, it may be removed. "Pseudo" enamel pearls are seen at the bifurcation of mandibular first, second, and third molars and are caused by the superimposition of parts of the mesial root on the distal root. The cause is improper horizontal angulation of the beam.

DENS INVAGINATUS (DENS IN DENTE)

Dens invaginatus is a variation that arises as a result of an invagination or infolding of the tooth's surface before calcification. This condition most frequently affects the coronal portion of the permanent lateral incisors and may occur bilaterally. Dens invaginatus is seen in 1–5% of the population. The invagination produces a deep lingual pit, and the underlying pulp is more susceptible to exposure by caries or by mechanical pulpal exposure in the preparation of the tooth. Radiographically, a characteristic teardrop-shaped or hourglass-shaped invagination may be seen, with or without a thin layer of dentin beneath. There is often evidence of carious penetration of the base of the invaginated enamel and varying degrees of periapical disease of pulpal origin at the apex of the tooth (Fig. 16.13). Sealing of the pits at the earliest age will prevent the development of pulpal problems in many cases.

DENS EVAGINATUS (LEONG'S PREMOLAR)

The reverse of dens invaginatus is a condition called "dens evaginatus," which is an outfolding of the enamel organ on the occlusal surfaces of premolar teeth. It forms

an enamel-covered, slender supernumerary tubercle (elevation) between the buccal and lingual cusps (Fig. 16.14). The most common complications of this anomaly are pulpal inflammation and necrosis due to caries, attrition, or mechanical exposure during tooth preparation. There may be a pulp horn within the tubercle, especially in younger persons.

ALTERATIONS IN TOOTH STRUCTURE

ENAMEL HYPOPLASIA

Enamel hypoplasia is an incomplete or defective formation of the organic enamel matrix of the teeth. This causes

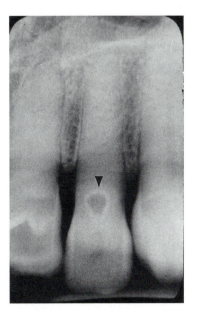

Figure 16.13. Dens Invaginatus (Dens in Dente). Dens invaginatus (*arrowhead*) of upper left lateral, demonstrating a teardrop shape.

381

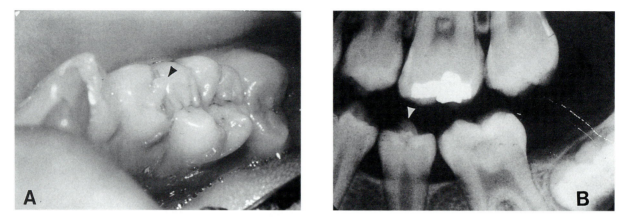

Figure 16.14. Dens Evaginatus (Leong's Premolar). (**A**) Photograph of dens evaginatus (*arrowhead*) of the occlusal surface of a mandibular second premolar. (**B**) Radiograph of dens evaginatus (*arrowhead*).

defects on the surface of the enamel that may range from a white spot to a more severe and generalized mottling, pitting, or grooving (Fig. 16.15). Some unique forms of enamel hypoplasia are due to various specific causes, such

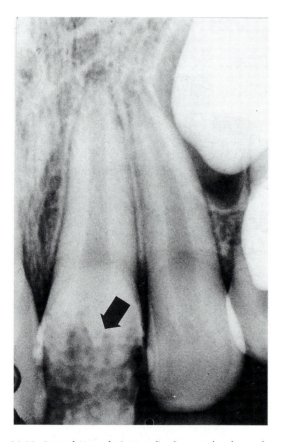

Figure 16.15. Enamel Hypoplasia (Localized). Localized pitted type of enamel hypoplasia of permanent maxillary central incisor, probably due to infection or trauma when tooth was developing.

as **notched screwdriver-shaped incisors** and **mulberry molars** associated with congenital syphilis, **mottled enamel** due to fluorosis, and **Turner's hypoplasia** (Turner's tooth) (Fig. 16.16) due to trauma or local inflammation associated with a primary tooth (especially the molars and maxillary incisors). Enamel hypoplasia may be due to various other causes, including nutritional deficiencies and high fevers associated with childhood diseases (Fig. 16.17). In many cases, the condition remains unexplained and is referred to as idiopathic.

AMELOGENESIS IMPERFECTA

Amelogenesis imperfecta is the hereditary form of enamel hypoplasia. There are three types of amelogenesis imperfecta. The **hypoplastic type** is characterized by the presence of a thin layer of normal enamel around the crowns of all the teeth (Fig. 16.18). The **hypomineralized type** consists of a normal amount of enamel that is poorly mineralized (Fig. 16.19). In the hypomineralized type, the enamel may be pitted or chalky and tends to fracture. The **hypomaturation type** is associated with snow-capped cusp tips. For some reason, all these teeth usually have a greater resistance to caries than normal teeth.

DENTINOGENESIS IMPERFECTA

Dentinogenesis imperfecta is a hereditary disorder of dentin that is transmitted as an autosomal dominant trait. (The autosome is any 1 of 22 paired chromosomes in humans, as distinguished from a sex chromosome.) The dentin and the dentinoenamel junction are affected. The teeth have a yellowish-gray opalescent (milky iridescence, like an opal) sheen, and the enamel has a tendency to chip away. In **Type 1**, the condition is associated with

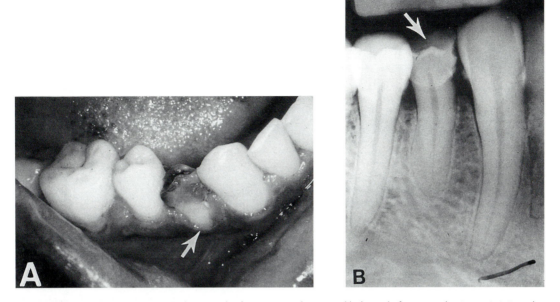

Figure 16.16. Turner's Tooth (Enamel Hypoplasia). **(A)** Photograph of Turner's tooth, a mandibular right first premolar (*arrow*). **(B)** Radiograph of Turner's tooth in **A**, *arrow*. Hypercementosis is present in the tooth.

osteogenesis imperfecta (a generalized disease of bone), in which case there will be a history of susceptibility to fracture of the long bones, possible deformities due to multiple fractures, and blue sclera ("white") of the eyes. In **Type 2**, there is no association with osteogenesis imperfecta. In **Type 3**, the Brandywine type, the teeth only are affected but more generally so. Type 3 occurs only in an inbred population of white, black, and Native American ancestry from Maryland. The radiographic features of dentinogenesis imperfecta include enamel fractures, root fractures, bulbous crowns, short tapered roots, early obliteration of the root canal and pulp spaces, and normal susceptibility to caries. Dentinogenesis imperfecta is a generalized condition affecting all the teeth, including the primary and permanent dentitions (Fig. 16.20). There is a normal susceptibility to caries, and restorations other than crowns tend to fail due to the chipping away of the enamel.

DENTINAL DYSPLASIA (ROOTLESS TEETH)

Dentinal dysplasia is a rare disturbance of dentin formation characterized by apparently normal enamel formation with an underlying, bizarre, whorl-like spherical dentinal pattern; partial or complete pulpal obliteration; pulp stones; defectively formed roots; and a predisposition for abscess and cyst formation without an obvious inciting factor, such as pulpal inflammation by caries. Dentinal

dysplasia has been subdivided into two types. **Type 1** has three subtypes (O'Carroll et al., 1991) and is more common. **Type 2**, a Shields-type (Shields et al., 1973), is characterized by a large pulp chamber and narrowed root canal space (Fig. 16.21).

REGIONAL ODONTODYSPLASIA (GHOST TEETH)

This is a rare developmental anomaly characterized by defective dentin and enamel formation and by calcification within the pulp and dental follicle. The etiology has not been determined. The pulp chambers are large, and demarcation between enamel and dentin is absent, giving the so-called ghost-like appearance to the teeth (Fig. 16.22). The affected teeth are most often localized in the jaws (regional). Eruption may be delayed, partially erupted, or not erupted at all. Ghost teeth may occur as a solitary finding or as a feature of the Goltz-Gorlin syndrome.

ACQUIRED DEFECTS OF TEETH

ATTRITION

Attrition is the physiologic wearing away of tooth structure as a result of normal function. Attrition is usually generalized and most commonly affects the incisal or occlusal surfaces. It is also seen on the interproximal surfaces at the contact points. Attrition that is confined to a single

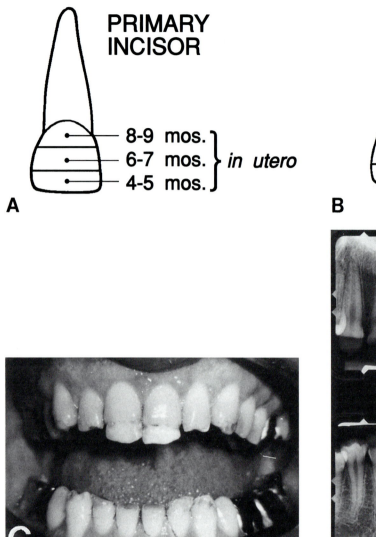

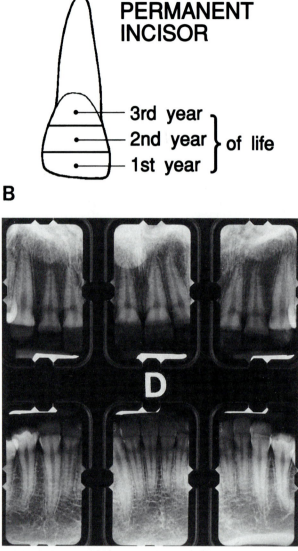

Figure 16.17. Enamel Hypoplasia Due to Serious Nutritional Deficiency or Systemic States. (**A**) Time frame and area on tooth enamel for **primary** incisors. (**B**) Time frame and area on tooth enamel for **permanent** incisors. (**C**) Photograph of anterior teeth with pit type of enamel hypoplasia on all incisors, except the maxillary lateral incisors. If the disturbance takes place in the first year, all incisors except the maxillary lateral incisors will be affected. (**D**) Anterior radiographs of the grooved type of enamel hypoplasia of upper and lower incisor teeth, including the maxillary lateral incisors. The disturbance must have taken place during second year of the patient's life (see **B**).

tooth or groups of teeth is caused by an abnormal function—such as a grinding, clenching, or bruxism habit—and is referred to as a severe or pathologic attrition. Radiographically, attrition is characterized by a flattening of the involved surfaces causing the teeth to appear worn down (Fig. 16.23).

ABRASION

Abrasion is the pathologic wearing away of tooth structure by a mechanical process or by the abrasive action of substances other than food. Some types of abrasion include **occupational abrasion**, which is seen in seamstresses and tailors who hold needles and pins between their anterior teeth, hairdressers who use their teeth to open hairpins or bobby pins, shoemakers and carpenters who hold nails between their teeth, and others including glassblowers, musicians, sandblasters, and farmers (in these cases, the abrasion is caused by dust). **Habitual abrasion** is seen between the incisal edges of anterior teeth in pipe smokers and from toothbrush and toothpick misuse. **Clasp abrasion** is caused by poorly designed removable partial-den-

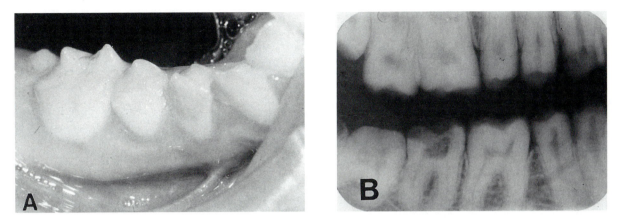

Figure 16.18. Amelogenesis Imperfecta (Hypoplastic Type). **(A)** Photograph of hypoplastic type. **(B)** Hypoplastic smooth type, right bitewings.

ture clasps. **Ritual abrasions** are mostly seen in Third World rural population groups, most often involving filing down the anterior teeth to create spaces between them. **Cocaine abrasion** occurs as a result of rubbing cocaine powder into the gingiva as an alternate method of cocaine absorption during bouts of severe nasal mucosal irritation from "line snorting."

Radiographically, the appearance varies greatly with the cause. Hairpins, nails, needles, and similar implements produce notched areas on the incisal edges. Pipe smoking, glassblowing, and similar activities produce an uneven wear pattern conforming to the shape of the object being held. Sandblasters and farmers may show an inordinate degree of interocclusal wear for their chronologic age due

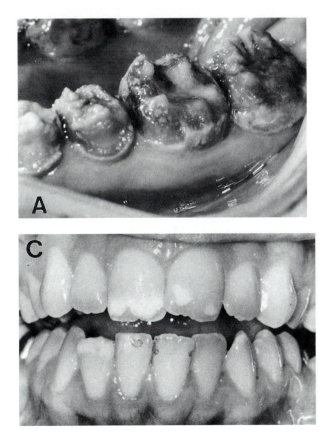

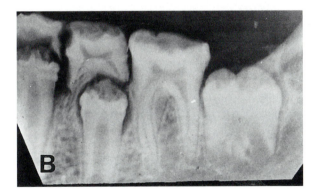

Figure 16.19. Amelogenesis Imperfecta (Hypomineralized and Hypomaturation Types). **(A)** Hypomineralized type. **(B)** Radiograph of hypomineralized type—permanent and primary teeth. **(C)** Note snow-capped hypomaturation type of amelogenesis imperfecta of upper and lower incisors. Teeth do not show radiographic findings.

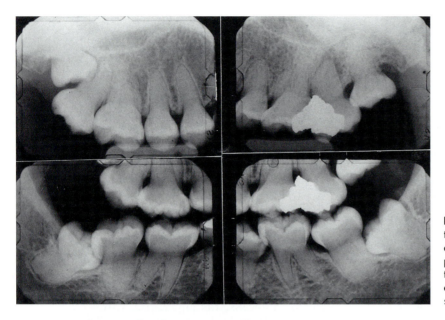

Figure 16.20. Dentinogenesis Imperfecta (Type 2). This type of dentinogenesis imperfecta does not occur in association with osteogenesis imperfecta. Bitewing and maxillary posterior radiographs of a 21-year-old woman with dentinogenesis imperfecta (Type 2) are shown. Note total obliteration of the pulps, the bulbous crowns, the short and slender roots, and the evidence of early attrition.

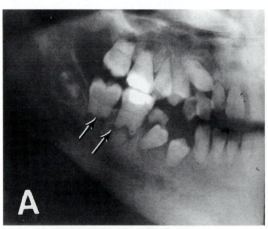

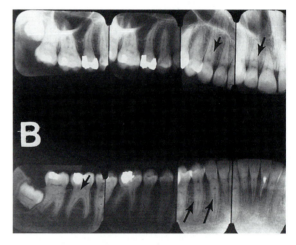

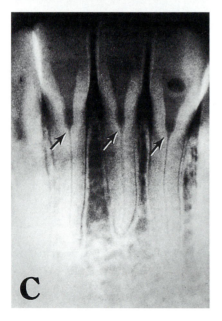

Figure 16.21. Dentinal Dysplasia (Types 1 and 2), Generalized Conditions. (**A**) Dentinal dysplasia (Type 1). Panoramic survey of a young patient with the most severe form of dentinal dysplasia. One can see complete obliteration of the pulps and minimal root development (*arrows*). (**B**) Dentinal dysplasia (Type 1). Radiographs of a patient with several teeth with two crescent-shaped horizontal lines, each concave to the other. (Note pulp stones.) (**C**) Dentinal dysplasia (Type 2) with thistle-shaped pulp chambers of lower anterior teeth (*arrows*).

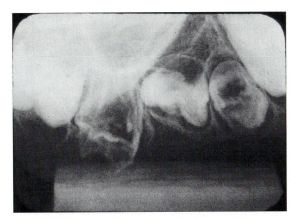

Figure 16.22. Regional Odontodysplasia (Ghost Teeth). The radiodensity of teeth in the upper right quadrant is greatly reduced. The demarcation between enamel and dentin is absent. The pulp chambers are widened. These features contribute to the ghost-like appearance of the teeth.

to the constant presence of gritty material in the mouth. In toothpick abrasion, the abnormal wear usually occurs beneath the contact points. Toothbrush abrasion produces a characteristic pattern in which there is a well-demarcated

horizontal radiolucent line crossing the cervical area in the cervical root area and is sometimes V-shaped in certain radiographic views (Fig. 16.24). Toothbrush abrasion may resemble cervical caries.

EROSION

Erosion is the loss of tooth substance by a nonbacterial chemical process. Clinically, the teeth appear smooth and glistening, and the underlying yellowish dentin may be exposed and sensitive, particularly to temperature changes. There may be a history of difficulty in retaining restorations. Known causes include chronic vomiting as in bulimia (Fig. 16.25A), chronic regurgitation (vomiting) as in hiatal hernia, excessive intake of acidic carbonated soft drinks, habitual sucking of lemons and acidic candy, use of acidic medications such as a dilute hypochloric acid and some iron preparations, and occupation in industries using acid. The radiographic findings are essentially nonspecific in most instances, although the crowns of the teeth may appear slightly more radiolucent than normal (Fig. 16.25B).

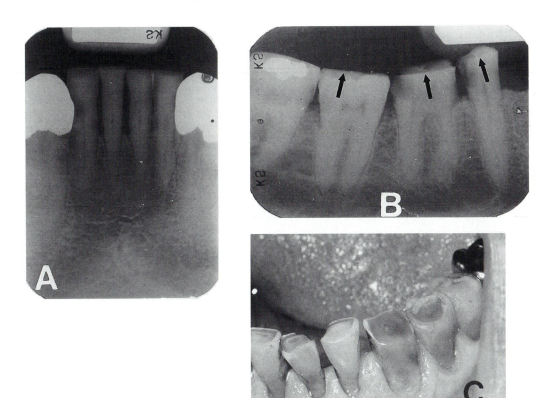

Figure 16.23. Attrition. (**A**) Severe incisal attrition, lower anterior teeth. (**B**) Attrition of occlusal surfaces (*arrows*) of an elderly man. (**C**) Photograph of severe incisal and occlusal attrition of a 70-year-old man.

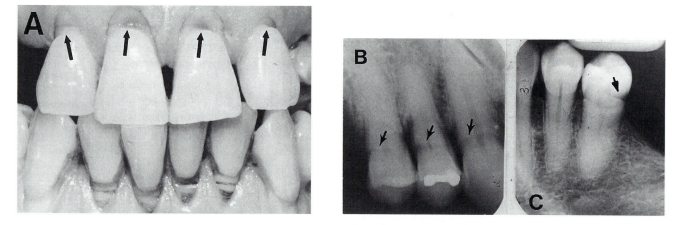

Figure 16.24. Toothbrush Abrasion. This condition is caused by brushing back and forth horizontally on the cervical neck of the teeth, rather than using the preferred up-and-down motion. **(A)** Toothbrush abrasion of maxillary (*arrows*) and mandibular anterior teeth. **(B)** Radiograph of toothbrush abrasion of cervical surfaces, right canine and premolars. **(C)** Note V-shaped toothbrush abrasion on distal of premolar. Sometimes this resembles cervical caries.

ALTERATIONS IN TOOTH ERUPTION

DRIFT AND MIGRATION

Drift refers to the movement of an erupted tooth when either mesial or distal contact is lost. **Distal drift** is the most common and is frequently seen in mandibular second premolars (Fig. 16.26). *Migration* refers to an abnormal movement of an unerupted tooth. It usually occurs in a mesial direction and is seen more frequently in the mandible. Migrated teeth usually remain embedded within the jaw (Fig. 16.27).

TRANSLOCATION (TRANSPOSITION) AND ECTOPIC ERUPTION

Translocation or transposition of teeth occurs when a tooth erupts into the normal position of another or when there is an interchange of position between two teeth. Because the translocated teeth occupy normal positions within the arch, crowding is usually absent and the curvature of the arch remains normal (Fig. 16.28). *Ectopic eruption* refers to the eruption of a tooth into an abnormal position in the arch. In this instance there may be crowding, and the wayward tooth may be located in a buccal

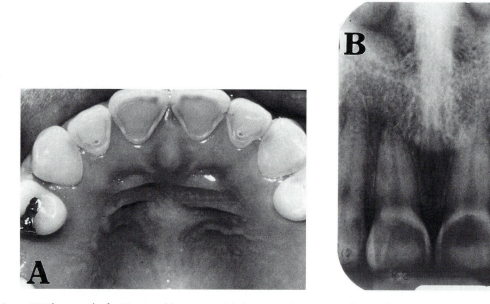

Figure 16.25. Erosion. **(A)** Photograph of a 31-year-old woman with bulimia, which causes an abnormal increase in the sensation of hunger. Note erosion on lingual surfaces of the teeth in this patient from excessive vomiting. **(B)** Radiograph of maxillary central incisor erosion of lingual surfaces of central incisors of a patient with bulimia.

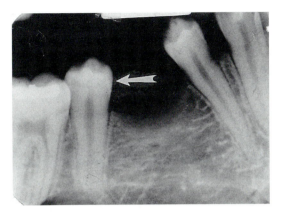

Figure 16.26. Distal Drift. Radiograph showing distal drift (*arrow*) of the erupted second premolar.

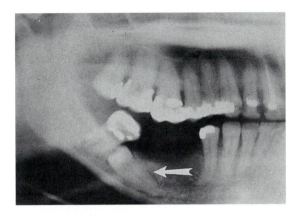

Figure 16.27. Migration of Unerupted Tooth. Panoramic view of distal migration (*arrow*) of an unerupted second premolar to mesial root region of erupted second molar.

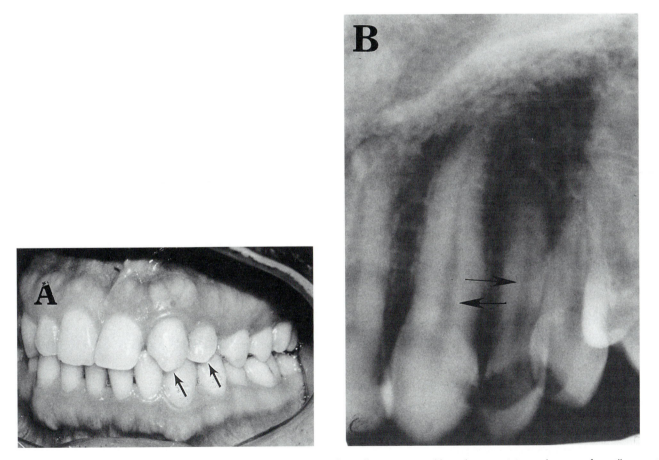

Figure 16.28. Translocation (Transposition). (**A**) Photograph of translocation of maxillary canine and lateral incisor. (**B**) Translocation of maxillary canine and lateral.

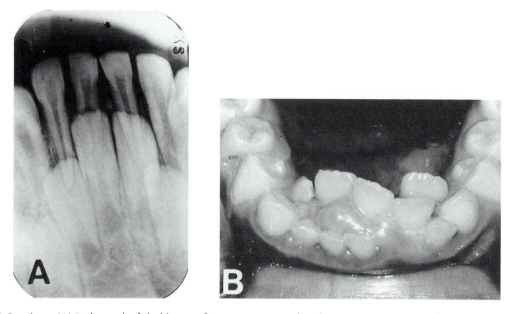

Figure 16.29. Ectopic Eruption. (**A**) Radiograph of double row of anterior incisor teeth with erupting permanent teeth. (**B**) Double row of lower anterior teeth (permanent and primary teeth) because of prolonged retention of primary incisor teeth and crowding. Permanent teeth have ectopically erupted lingually to primary incisor teeth. In a note there is no resorption of the roots of the primary teeth.

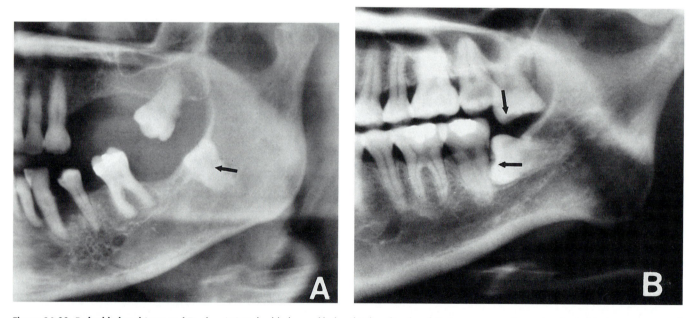

Figure 16.30. Embedded and Impacted Teeth. (**A**) Embedded mandibular third molar that failed to erupt and remains buried in bone. Note tooth is ankylosed to bone, as no periodontal ligament space can be seen. (**B**) Horizontally impacted lower third molar (*arrow*) and a supraerupted maxillary third molar (*arrow*) because there is no antagonist below.

or lingual position, producing a disruption of the even curvature of the arch (Fig. 16.29).

EMBEDDED AND IMPACTED TEETH

An *embedded tooth* is one that has failed to erupt and remains buried in the bone (Fig. 16.29). An *impacted tooth* is one in which some physical entity has prevented eruption (Fig. 16.30). The third molars and the maxillary canine are the most frequently impacted or embedded, followed by the premolars and supernumerary teeth.

REVIEW QUESTIONS

1. What is the prominent feature in taurodontism?

   A. Enamel hypoplasia.
   B. Abnormal dentin.
   C. Extension of the pulp chamber deep into the root portion of the tooth.
   D. Pulp cavity has been obliterated and the entire tooth is more opaque.

2. Radiographically, the teeth in amelogenesis imperfecta show what?

   A. Dentin with significant disturbances; enamel is normal.
   B. Dentin and enamel with significant disturbances.
   C. Pulp and dentin are abnormal.
   D. Very thin or defective enamel; dentin is normal.
   E. None of the above.

3. Radiographically, the teeth in dentinogenesis imperfecta show what?

   A. Pulp is abnormal; dentin is normal.
   B. Dentin only shows disturbances.
   C. Enamel is missing; dentin formation is normal.
   D. Shortened roots, obliterated root canal, and pulp spaces.
   E. None of the above.

4. When two teeth appear to be joined by cementum alone, the condition is termed:

   A. Fusion.
   B. Gemination.
   C. Concrescence.
   D. Dilaceration.

5. An enamel pearl is usually seen:

   A. At the cervical region of a tooth.
   B. Within the pulp chamber.
   C. As a tubercle on the occlusal surface of the tooth.
   D. On the lingual of the anterior teeth.
   E. On the cusp tips of newly erupted incisors.

6. When one tooth takes the place of another in the arch, the condition is termed:

   A. Migration.
   B. Distal drift.
   C. Translocation.
   D. Ectopic eruption.

7. When teeth are **larger** than normal, they are termed:

   A. Microdontia.
   B. Macrodontia.
   C. Distomolars.
   D. Paramolars.

8. The pathologic wearing away of tooth structure by a mechanical process is termed:

   A. Attrition.
   B. Erosion.
   C. Abrasion.
   D. None of the above.

9. What is Turner's tooth?

   A. Hereditary hypoplasia of enamel of dominant character.
   B. Hypoplasia of enamel of local origin.
   C. Hereditary hypoplasia of enamel of recessive character.
   D. Hypoplasia of enamel from congenital syphilis.
   E. A tooth characterized by significant hypoplasia and hypocalcification of enamel and dentin.

CASE-BASED QUESTIONS

CASE 16.1
This patient is a 20-year-old dental hygiene student and a daughter of an orthodontist.

Questions

1. Which anomaly(ies) is (are) present in the lateral incisor?

A. Dens in dente.
B. Dens evaginatus.
C. Orthodontic root resorption.
D. A, B and C.
E. A and C.

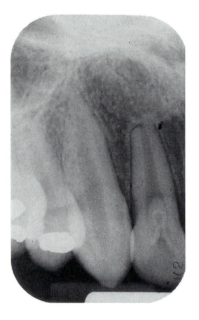

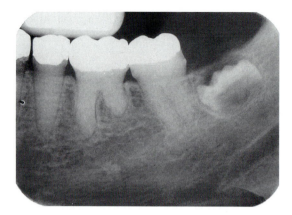

2. What, if any, procedure for the maxillary lateral incisor should this patient seek from a classmate?

A. A better radiograph.
B. A thorough prophylaxis.
C. A sealant for a lingual pit.
D. No procedure is needed.

CASE 16.3

A third-year dental student brought his grandfather in for dental treatment.

Questions

1. The condition affecting the four incisor teeth is:

A. Attrition.
B. Abrasion.
C. Erosion.
D. Dentinogenesis imperfecta.

CASE 16.2

1. This patient is a 14-year-old girl whose teeth have been crowned because the enamel was chipping away and ordinary fillings failed. This patient has:

A. Amelogenesis imperfecta.
B. Dentinogenesis imperfecta.
C. Dentin dysplasia.
D. Enamel hypoplasia.
E. None of the above.

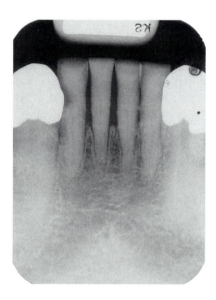

2. The problem affecting the right lateral incisor is:

A. Caries.
B. Cervical burnout.
C. Internal resorption.
D. Not a problem, it is an older radiolucent silicate restoration.

CASE 16.4

1. This patient is 9 years old, and the permanent central incisors have not erupted. The lateral incisors have erupted. What is (are) the reason(s) for the noneruption of the central incisors?

   A. Insufficient arch space.
   B. Failure to initiate orthodontic treatment.
   C. Extraction of the primary incisors at an early age.
   D. Bilateral mesiodens.
   E. A, B and C.

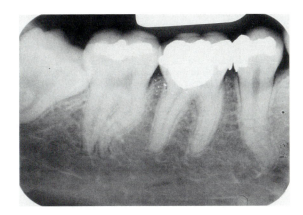

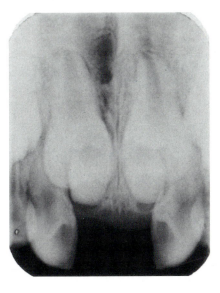

CASE 16.5

This patient is a 24-year-old dental student who needs to have his third molars removed.

Questions

1. The term that best describes the shape of the mesial root of the second molar is:

   A. Tapered.
   B. Dilacerated.
   C. Supernumerary.
   D. Hypoplastic.

2. The distal-buccal attached gingiva adjacent to the first molar appeared bluish. The problem is:

   A. An intraoral nevus.
   B. Localized gingivitis and periodontitis due to the poor restoration.
   C. Chemical (fixer) stains.
   D. Amalgam tattoo.

CASE 16.6

1. What is the anomaly in this radiograph?

   A. Microdontia
   B. Taurodontism.
   C. Congenitally missing tooth.
   D. Hypercementosis.
   E. Supernumerary molar.

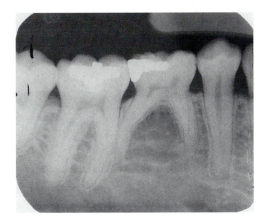

BIBLIOGRAPHY

Bernick SM. Taurodontia. Oral Surg 1970;29:549–555.

Brook AH, Winter GB. Double teeth: retrospective study of geminated and fused teeth in children. Br Dent J 1970;129:125–132.

Brook AH. Dental anomalies on number, form and size: their prevalence in British school children. J Int Assoc Dent Child 1974;5:37–42.

Brook AH, Ekanayake NO. The etiology of oligodontia: a familial history. J Dent Child 1980;48:32–38.

Buenviaje TM, Rapp R. Dental anomalies in children: a clinical and radiographic survey. J Dent Child 1984;51:42–47.

Cavanha AO. Enamel pearls. Oral Surg 1965;19:373–377.

Clayton JM. Congenital dental anomalies occurring in 3,557 children. J Dent Child 1956;23:206–212.

Dachi SF, Howell FV. A survey of 3,874 routine full-mouth radiographs: II. a study of impacted teeth. Oral Surg 1961;14:1165–1172.

Dixter C, Langlais RP, Lichty GC. Exercises in dental radiology. Pediatric radiographic interpretation. Philadelphia: WB Saunders, 1980;3:63–70, 216–221, 260–261.

Egermack-Eriksson I, Lind V. Congenital numerical variation in the permanent dentition: D. sex distribution of hypodontia and hyperdontia. Odontol Rev 1971;22:309–317.

Gardiner JH. Supernumerary teeth. Dent Pract Dent Rec 1961;12:65–70.

Gardner DG, Sapp JP. Regional odonto-dysplasia. Oral Surg 1973;34:351–356.

Gotoh T, Kawahara K, Imai K, et al. Clinical and radiographic study of dens invaginatus. Oral Surg 1979;48:88–92.

Grahnen H, Granath LE. Numerical variations in primary dentition and their correlation with the permanent dentition. Odontol Rev 1961;12:348–355.

Jorgenson RJ. Clinician's view of hypodontia. J Am Dent Assoc 1980;101:285–290.

Jorgenson RJ, Salinas CF, Shapiro SD. The prevalence of taurdontism in a select population. J Craniofac Genet Div Biol 1982;2:125–133.

Jorgenson RL, Yost C. Etiology of enamel dysplasia. Pedodontics 1982;4:325–332.

Kisling E, Hoffding J. Premature loss of primary teeth: part III. drifting patterns for different types of teeth after loss of adjoining teeth. J Dent Child 1979;46:35–41.

Langland OE, et al. Textbook of dental radiology. 2nd ed. Springfield: Charles C. Thomas, 1984:412–431.

Menczer LF. Anomalies of the primary dentition. J Dent Child 1955;22:57–67.

Miles AEW. Malformation of teeth. Proc R Soc Med (Sect Odontol) 1954;47:817–828.

Morris CR, Jerman AC. Panoramic radiographic survey: a study of embedded third molars. Oral Surg 1971;29:122–126.

O'Carroll MK, Duncan WK, Perkins TM. Dentin dysplasia: review of literature and a proposed subclassification based on radiographic findings. Oral Surg Oral Med Oral Pathol 1991;72:119–129.

Pindborg JJ. Pathology of the dental hard tissues. Philadelphia: WB Saunders, 1970:51–54, 65, 77–94.

Rose JS. A survey of congenitally missing teeth, excluding third molars in 6,000 orthodontic patients. Dent Pract (Bristol) 1967;17:107.

Sarnat BG, Schour I. Enamel hypoplasia. J Am Dent Assoc 1941;28:1989–1999.

Sarnat BG, Schour I. Enamel hypoplasia. J Am Dent Assoc 1942;29:67–78.

Sarnat BG, Shaw NG. Dental development in congenital syphilis. Am J Dis Child 1942;64:771–781.

Shields ED, Bixler P, El-Kafrawy AM. A proposed classification for heritable human dentin defects with a description of a new entity. Arch Oral Biol 1973;18:545–556.

Stafne EC, Gibilisco JA. Oral radiographic diagnosis. 5th ed. Philadelphia: WB Saunders, 1985:18–45.

Tannenbaum KA, Alling EE. Anomalous tooth development: case reports of gemination and twinning. Oral Surg 1963;18:885–890.

Turner JG. Two cases of hypoplasia of enamel. Br J Dent Sci 1912;55:227–230.

Villa VG, Bunag CA, Ramos AB. A developmental anomaly in the form of an occlusal tubercle with central canal which serves as the pathway of infection to the pulp and periapical region. Oral Surg 1959;12:345–350.

Woolf CM. Missing maxillary lateral incisors: a genetic study. Am J Hum Genet 1971;23:289–299.

Worth HM. Principles and practice of oral radiologic interpretation. Chicago: Year Book, 1963:206–207.

Radiologic Diagnosis of Caries

17

OBJECTIVES

Upon successful completion of this unit, the student will be able to:

1. *Identify and interpret caries by type and location.*

2. *Discuss and describe factors influencing caries interpretation.*

3. *Test his or her knowledge by answering the Review Questions.*

KEY WORDS/PHRASES

acute caries	dentinal caries	pulpal caries
arrested caries	facial caries	rampant caries
caries progression	incipient caries	recurrent caries
caries size	interproximal caries	restorative materials
cemental caries	lamellar caries	root caries
cervical burnout	lingual caries	root defects
chronic caries	occlusal caries	secondary caries

INTRODUCTION

A great percentage of the radiologic interpretation done in the dental office is devoted to acquiring information regarding dental caries, periodontal disease and periapical disease. Because the earliest studies conducted to determine the causes of tooth extraction (Allen, 1944; Brekhus, 1929) reached similar conclusions that caries, periodontal disease and periapical disease accounted for approximately 93% of tooth loss, it is imperative that the dental health-care worker become competent in the radiologic interpretation of these diseases.

Dental caries, or tooth decay, is a pathologic process consisting of localized destruction of dental hard tissues by organic acids produced by the microbial deposits adhering to the teeth. The carious lesions, or the localized destructions of tooth hard tissues, are the signs of the disease. Dental caries is a multifactorial disease with an interplay of three principal factors: the host (primarily the teeth and saliva), the microflora, and the substrate or diet. In addition, there is a fourth factor: time. When the three essential parameters of dental caries—a susceptible host, cariogenic oral flora, and a suitable local substrate—are present in an individual for a considerable time, dental caries may develop. Carious lesions do not develop without plaque (bacterial mucous mass). When plaque contains appreciable portions of highly acidogenic bacteria, such as *Streptococcus mutans*, and is exposed to readily fermentable dietary sugars, it produces sufficient concentrations of acids to demineralize the enamel. Therefore, the pathogenicity of plaque depends on its microbial composition and on the availability of dietary sugars. Characteristically, dental plaque resists removal by the physiologic oral cleaning forces such as saliva and tongue movement; however, plaque is removable by tooth-brushing, if the bristles can reach it. Unlike the sharp decline in caries currently being experienced in Western Europe and North America, caries is increasing rapidly in children in developing countries.

INTERPRETATION OF CARIES BY TYPE AND LOCATION

Because dental caries is essentially a process of decalcification, a certain percentage (50%) of the calcium and phosphorus must be destroyed before the decreased density can be seen on the radiograph. The classification of the radiographic appearance of caries is discussed according to the location of caries on the tooth (interproximal, occlusal, facial/lingual, pulpal, root, or cemental), recurrent or secondary caries (immediate vicinity of preexisting restoration), and arrested caries (occlusal and interproximal surfaces).

INTERPROXIMAL ENAMEL CARIES

Interproximal is defined as "between two adjacent surfaces." The use of confusing and inappropriate terms such as "approximal" and "proximal" should be discouraged. The interproximal carious lesion is the most easily recognized on the radiograph; between the posterior teeth, it is the most difficult to detect by use of clinical methods only. In an investigation by Hansen (1980), four times as many posterior interproximal carious lesions were found when posterior bitewings were used compared with clinical observations alone. Interproximal enamel caries usually begins just below the contact point and appears clinically as a chalky, white spot that becomes slightly roughened due to early demineralization (Fig. 17.1). As the carious lesion progresses, it often forms a classic V-shaped radiolucent appearance, with the base of the radiolucent triangle at the surface of the tooth and usually a rounded apex pointed toward the dentinoenamel junction. No reason can be given for this V-shaped configuration, except that the carious process tends to follow the course of the enamel rods, which are usually aligned at

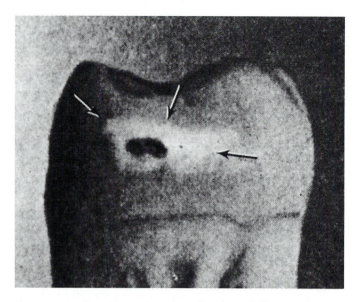

Figure 17.1. Early Carious Lesion. Note the white, chalky appearance of the interproximal area with a stained cavitation between the contact point and the cementoenamel junction of the extracted tooth. (Reprinted with permission from Black AD. Pathology of hard tissues of the teeth. 7th ed. Chicago: Medico-Dental Publishers, 1936:346.)

right angles to the dentinoenamel junction; because the interproximal enamel surfaces are usually convex, the enamel rods tend to converge at the dentinoenamel junction, producing the classic triangular V-shaped radiolucent appearance of interproximal caries (Fig. 17.2). Nevertheless, there are exceptions to this rule, and various shapes and sizes of interproximal enamel carious lesions may be seen radiographically (e.g., line-shaped, W-shaped, flame-shaped, half-moon–shaped). According to

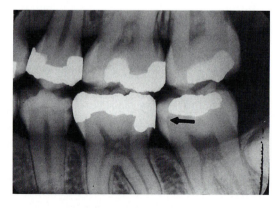

Figure 17.2. Interproximal Enamel Caries. Note classic V-shaped caries on mesial surface of the mandibular second molar (*arrow*). The enamel carious lesion on the distal surface of the mandibular second premolar has a rounded triangular-shaped appearance.

Newbrun (1989), the determinants of the shape of the carious lesions are still unknown.

Lamellar Caries

At one time, the onset of caries was thought to be related to the presence of lamellae in the enamel (proteolytic theory), which were considered pathways of primary invasion. Because lamellae are in all teeth, inevitably some of them may be involved in carious lesions; hence, they are called lamellar caries. Scott and Wyckoff (1949), however, believe that the association between lamellae and carious lesions is random and not a cause-and-effect relationship. Regardless of etiology, lamellar caries appears radiographically as a dark, thin line running completely through the interproximal enamel into the dentin, where the caries then spreads along the dentinoenamel junction (Fig. 17.3).

Incipient Caries

Incipient interproximal caries can be seen on a radiograph as a small, cone-shaped radiolucent area in the outer enamel (Fig. 17.4). At this stage, the incipient lesion may be arrested or even reversed by remineralization, if an effective preventive program is enacted. Restoration of an incipient lesion is an elective procedure that is generally not recommended, except in cases of high caries susceptibility.

Dentinal Caries

As the carious lesion reaches the dentinoenamel junction, it usually first spreads laterally, undermining normal enamel. In the dentin, it spreads much more rapidly toward the pulp, in a form much like a mushroom, with its base on the dentinoenamel junction (Fig. 17.5). Each of the dentinal tubules enlarge and act as a tract for microor-

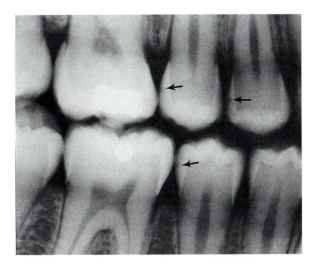

Figure 17.4. Interproximal Incipient Enamel Carious Lesion. Bitewing radiograph revealing incipient enamel carious lesions on distal interproximal surfaces of the premolars (*arrows*).

ganisms to travel. This leads to eventual destruction of dentinal tubules and the spread of the lesion.

Interproximal Caries Progression

There is a need in private practice and teaching clinics for a caries scoring code to classify interproximal carious lesions according to their radiographic depth of penetration into a tooth. Not all early or incipient interproximal carious lesions detected radiographically should be restored. Recent data have provided evidence that caries progression in many industrialized countries has slowed down, leaving adequate time for nonsurgical treatment of interproximal lesions. However, the progression rate of lesions varies among individuals and among lesions within an individual. On the basis of these observations, it is essential that decisions to treat or not to treat incipient lesions by restorative procedures should be based on combined radiographic and clinical assessments. Therefore, it is important for the dentist and his or her staff to record in the patient's chart as objectively as possible the radiographic findings related to interproximal caries penetration. An example of a caries penetration scoring code is shown in Figure 17.6. Each of the four classes of interproximal caries penetration is illustrated in Figure 17.7.

Rampant Caries Rampant caries is a sudden, rapid, and almost uncontrollable destruction of teeth. Rampant caries involves surfaces of teeth that are ordinarily relatively free of caries. Interproximal and cervical surfaces of anterior teeth, including mandibular incisors that are usually relatively caries free, may be attacked. Rampant caries is most often observed in the primary teeth of young children, in the permanent teeth of teen-agers (11–19 years), and in adult patients with xerostomia (Fig. 17.8).

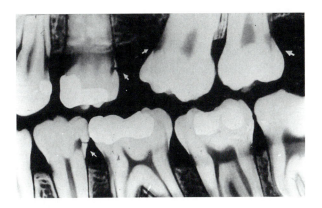

Figure 17.3. Lamellar Caries. Bitewing radiograph. Note "line-shaped" enamel caries with dentinal spread at dentinoenamel junction of distal surface of maxillary mandibular second premolar (*arrows*). The radiolucencies at mesial of the maxillary second molar and distal of the third molar are areas of cervical burnout.

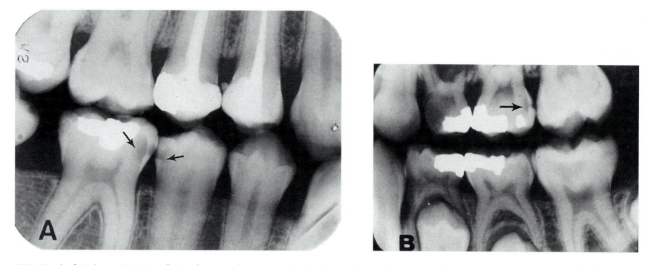

Figure 17.5. Dentinal Caries. (**A**) Note dentinal carious lesions in distal surface of mandibular second premolar (*arrow*) and mesial of mandibular first molar (*arrow*). (**B**) Note dentinal spreading of carious lesion at dentinoenamel junction of distal surface of the upper second primary molar (*arrow*).

Classification of Radiographic Caries

C-1. Enamel caries *less* than 1/2 way through enamel (sometimes called incipient caries). Do not record these lesions if doubtful of their existence.

C-2. Enamel caries penetrating at least 1/2 way through enamel, but *NOT* involving dentino-enamel junction.

C-3. Caries of enamel and dentine definitely at or through the dentino-enamel junction extending less than 1/2 way to pulp cavity.

C-4. Caries of enamel and dentine penetrating more than 1/2 way dentine toward pulp cavity.

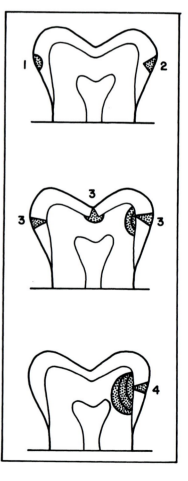

Figure 17.6. Classification of Radiographic Caries. An example of a caries penetration scoring code illustrating four classes of interproximal caries penetration.

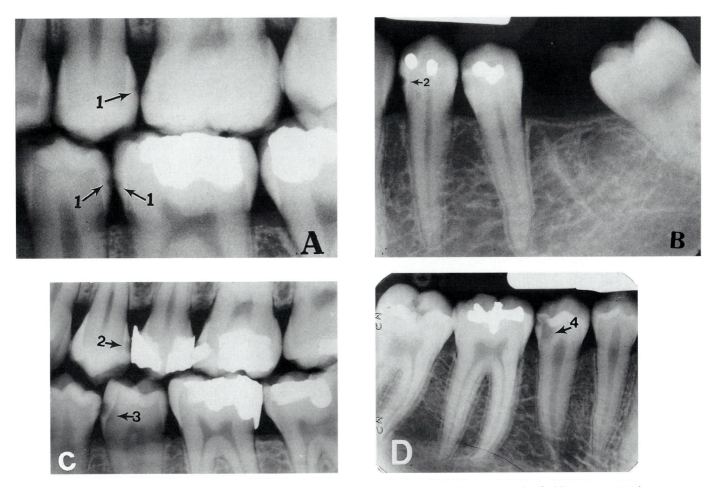

Figure 17.7. Four Classes of Interproximal Caries Penetration. (**A**) Distinct Class 1 (incipient) carious lesions identified by arrows. (**B**) Class 2 carious lesions on mesial of lower first premolar (*arrow*). (**C**) Class 3 carious lesion on mesial surfaces of rotated lower second premolar. Class 2 carious lesion on distal surface of upper first premolar. (**D**) Class 4 carious lesion on mesial surface of lower second premolar (*arrow*).

Acute and Chronic Caries In most cases of acute caries (a condition commonly seen in young adults between the ages of 15 and 25 years), there is a rapid penetration through the enamel, and the initial entrance of the carious process remains small (Fig. 17.9). In chronic caries (commonly seen in adults older than 25 years of age), there is a slower progression of the lesion, and it has a larger entrance at the surface of the enamel (Fig. 17.10).

OCCLUSAL CARIES

Occlusal caries is the most prevalent location of caries in the oral cavity. It usually occurs early in life, before smooth surface lesions appear. The irregular pit and fissure surfaces of the premolar and molar teeth are inherently more prone to occlusal caries because of their physical characteristics, which result in poor self-cleaning

fissures. Enamel caries that begins in the pits and fissures of the occlusal surfaces of teeth appears opposite to that of interproximal enamel caries, in that the apex of the triangle is toward the outer surface of the tooth and the base of the triangle is at the dentinoenamel junction (Fig. 17.11). Occlusal caries is usually not seen radiographically until it has reached the dentinoenamel junction and has spread in all directions. This is because of the great mass of enamel tissue superimposed over the occlusal enamel lesion. Caries of the occlusal surface is usually initially seen as a radiolucent dark line or area just under the occlusal enamel surface (Fig. 17.12). The radiograph is not always a reliable diagnostic aid for the detection of occlusal caries. It can only alert the clinician to occlusal surfaces that should be examined more thoroughly. A mirror and the sharp explorer (currently controversial) are the traditional diagnostic aids in the detection of occlusal caries. According to some, probing with a sharp explorer

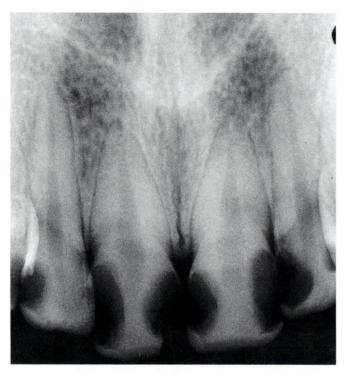

Figure 17.8. Rampant Caries. Teen-age girl with rampant caries in all her teeth. Maxillary incisors have large carious lesions.

exacerbates the spread of caries—most specifically, pit and fissure lesions.

FACIAL/LINGUAL CARIES

Smooth surface caries on the facial and lingual surfaces of the teeth begins in the pits, fissures, or cervical region of the tooth. Caries developing in pits on the facial and

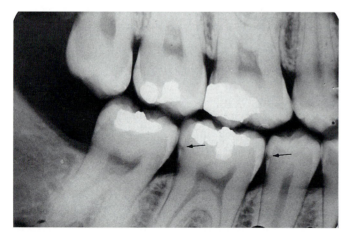

Figure 17.9. Acute Caries. Note the small entrance of the carious lesions as shown by *arrows*.

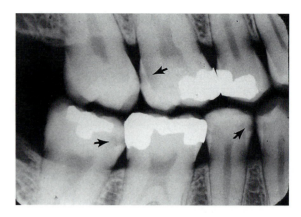

Figure 17.10. Chronic Caries. Note the large entrance of carious lesion as shown by *arrows*.

lingual surfaces appears on the radiograph as round radiolucent dots on the tooth surface. Many times, it is like looking into a small "black hole." The periphery of the black hole is especially well demonstrated if the pit or fissure is on the lingual surface, because this surface is very close to the film (Fig. 17.13). Cervical caries on the facial or lingual surfaces extend laterally toward the interproximal surfaces, forming a typical crescent-shaped, semilunar cavity, although the cavity may also be round or oval (Fig. 17.14). Facial and lingual caries almost always seems to produce a wide-open cavity unlike that found in interproximal and occlusal caries, which has a narrow area of penetration.

PULPAL CARIES

The extent and/or proximity of the caries to the pulp chamber can be evaluated with only a limited degree of

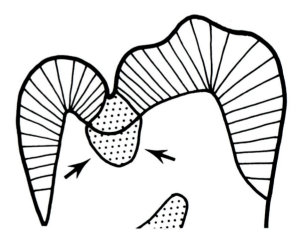

Figure 17.11. Occlusal Caries. Diagram showing the features of occlusal caries in posterior teeth (*arrows*).

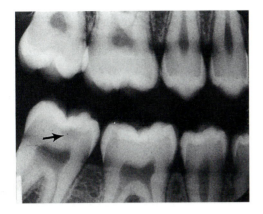

Figure 17.12. Occlusal Caries. Note occlusal caries in mandibular second molar (*arrow*).

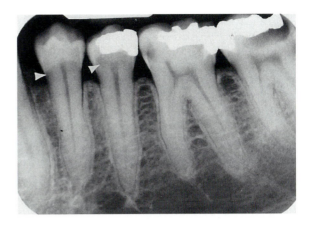

Figure 17.14. Cervical Caries. Note cervical facial caries on first and second premolars.

reliability from radiographs. This limitation stems in large part from the fact that the dental radiograph is a two-dimensional image of a three-dimensional tooth. The radiograph has length and width but lacks the dimension of depth. However, the radiograph does provide some information, and as long as it is applied with some reservation, it has a place in the evaluation of pulpal caries. If on the radiograph a carious lesion appears to have progressed right to the edge of the pulp chamber and not in the pulp, the dentist should be forewarned of a possible pulp exposure during caries excavation (Fig. 17.15). Over-angulation of the x-ray beam can create an appearance of pulpal exposure or abnormal apical periodontal ligament space widening, which is seen in advanced pulpitis. In addition, overexposure of the film causes "burnout" of dentin between the pulp and carious lesion by enlarging the carious lesion. Moreover, the radiograph does not have depth, so a large carious lesion can be superimposed over the pulp, when in reality the caries has not penetrated the pulp.

ROOT OR CEMENTAL CARIES

Root caries is known by a variety of terms including cemental caries, radicular caries, and senile caries. Sumney et al. (1973) reported that root caries is usually seen as a shallow (less than 2-mm deep), ill-defined, softened area that is often discolored and characterized by destruction of cementum with penetration of underlying dentin. As it progresses, the lesion extends more circumferentially (circular in area) than in depth. Root caries starts at or near the cementoenamel junction and appears only after the cementum is exposed.

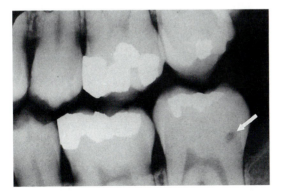

Figure 17.13. Facial/Lingual Caries. Note the round, black hole appearance of lingual caries on lower second molar.

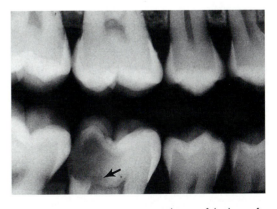

Figure 17.15. Pulpal Caries. Large carious lesion of the lower first molar that has probably reached the pulp; however, the carious lesion could be superimposed over the pulp chamber and give an impression of a pulpal penetration.

Root caries frequently occurs in the elderly for three reasons:

1. Cementum seems to be less resistant to caries than enamel and may be exposed in the elderly because of gingival recession.
2. The elderly have many more loose contacts between adjacent teeth because of attrition, periodontal disease, or poor restorations; this causes food packing areas.
3. Older persons often have xerostomia (dry mouth) for various reasons (salivary gland atrophy, drugs).

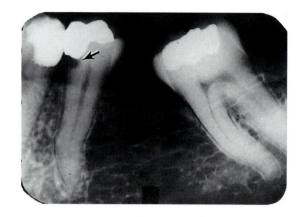

Figure 17.17. Recurrent or Secondary Caries. There is recurrent caries on the mesial surface of the lower second premolar (*arrow*).

When root surfaces are exposed to the oral environment as a result of gingival recession, plaque retention areas increase, particularly along the cementoenamel junction. Cemental or root caries start as small lesions along the cementoenamel junction and eventually coalesce and spread over the entire tooth surface. The surface becomes soft on probing, with a leathery consistency. Cementum has a laminated appearance microscopically. When the microbial deposits reach the cemental layers, they produce caries, which tends to progress laterally between the layers undermining the cementum. The radiographic appearance of root caries is described as saucer-shaped or having a cupped-out appearance. Root caries is usually located in the region of the interproximal cementoenamel junction (Fig. 17.16). Although it does not usually involve the enamel, it may undermine the enamel by spreading underneath it. Root caries may at times be misinterpreted as cervical burnout, which is normally seen in the cervical region of the teeth as a radiolucent triangular area on the interproximal surfaces of the posterior teeth and as a radiolucent band on the anterior teeth.

RECURRENT OR SECONDARY CARIES

Recurrent or secondary caries develops at the margins or in the vicinity of a restoration and may indicate an unusual susceptibility to caries, poor oral hygiene, a deficient cavity preparation, a defective restoration, or a combination of these factors. It is usually due to a "leaky margin," produced by one of the above factors. Mjor (1981) reported that clinical studies based on dentists' reports show that 60% of all replacements of amalgam restorations are due to recurrent (secondary) caries. Recurrent caries is seen under the restoration as a dark, radiolucent area (Fig. 17.17). Incomplete removal of dentinal caries before placing the restoration is also seen on the radiograph as a radiolucent area under the restoration. A radiopaque layer of dentin will sometimes be seen under the radiolucent carious lesion under the restoration (Fig. 17.18). At times, a flame-shaped, radiopaque area can be

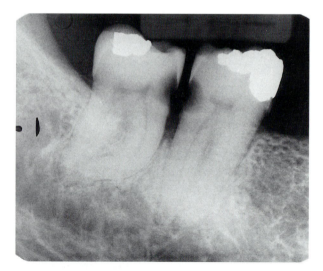

Figure 17.16. Root or Cemental Caries. Root or cemental caries with characteristic cupped-out appearance, as seen between two molars. Note the loose contact and food packing area between the teeth.

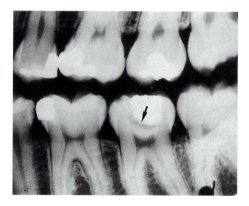

Figure 17.18. Recurrent or Secondary Caries. Note the radiolucent caries lesion under the radiopaque restoration. This is most likely from incomplete removal of dentinal caries before placement of the restoration.

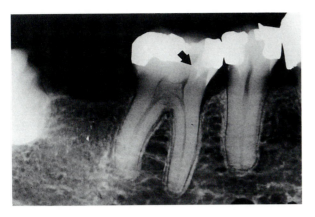

Figure 17.19. Radiopaque Dentin. Note flame-shaped radiopacity underneath margins amalgam restorations of molar and premolars. This is thought to represent tin or zinc ions from the amalgam that have been released into partially demineralized dentin.

seen in the dentin immediately adjacent to a restoration (Fig. 17.19). It was previously thought that these radiopaque areas in dentin under carious lesions and restorations represented defensive reactions. It is now thought that they represent partially demineralized dentin containing tin or zinc that has leaked out from amalgam or cement restorations due to changes in pH.

ARRESTED CARIES

Incipient and even more advanced carious lesions may become arrested if there is a significant shift in the oral environment from factors that cause caries to those that tend to slow down the caries process. According to Backer (1966), clinical longitudinal studies suggest that incipient

enamel caries can remain dormant for long periods and that some carious lesions may be reversed by remineralization. Most typically, the arrested incipient carious interproximal lesion is seen on teeth where the adjacent tooth has been extracted, so the local environmental conditions have changed completely. Clinical exploration of the lesion reveals that it is the same hardness as normal enamel. Therefore, these lesions are defined as remineralized carious lesions. Radiologically, these areas may appear as small radiolucent areas. Another form of arrested caries is seen in large occlusal carious lesions that become static or stop progressing for some reason. The appearance of arrested occlusal caries is an open cavity revealing yellow, brown, or black exposed dentin that has a polished, eburnated (hard) surface. The carious lesion most likely becomes arrested because microorganisms cannot be retained on the polished surfaces of the lesion. The radiographic appearance of arrested caries is one in which the crown of the tooth is absent, with a dark, radiolucent area on a roughened top surface of a destroyed tooth. A white sclerotic line under the radiolucent area may be present as a defensive measure of the pulp to wall-off the carious lesion (Fig. 17.20).

FACTORS INFLUENCING INTERPRETATION OF CARIES

RADIOGRAPHIC UNDERESTIMATION OF CARIES SIZE

Radiographic Appearance of Caries and Demineralization

A sufficient amount of calcium and phosphorus must be removed from the tooth for the carious lesion to be

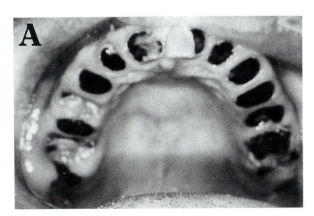

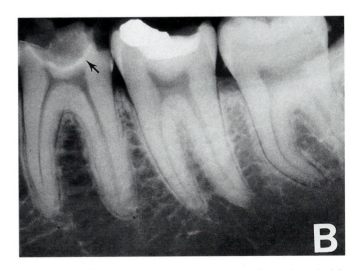

Figure 17.20. Arrested Caries. **(A)** Photograph of a patient with multiple teeth with arrested caries. **(B)** Arrested caries in lower first molar, which has a black-brown polished occlusal surface.

seen on the radiograph. Early et al. (1979) estimated that it takes approximately 50% of the calcium and phosphorus in a localized area of a tooth or bone to be absorbed before a radiolucency will be revealed on the radiograph. Therefore, the actual depth of penetration of the carious lesion is further advanced clinically and microscopically than the radiograph indicates.

Histopathologic Studies

Silverstone (1982) reported that when a lesion is first detected on a radiograph and appears to be limited to the outer enamel, the lesion has already penetrated the dentin (Fig. 17.21). This finding implies that carious lesions that may appear on radiographs to involve part of the enamel only may, at the histologic level, have reached the dentinoenamel junction, with a significant response from the pulpodentinal organ. However, this may also indicate that a slowly progressing enamel carious lesion may be attenuated by an effective defensive response in the dentin and pulp.

CARIES PROGRESSION STUDIES

The rapid decline in the rate of caries progression recognized since 1963 underlines the importance of reviewing the newer studies on caries progression. Pitts (1983) and Schwartz et al. (1984) reported that progression of interproximal carious lesions is usually a slow process and that many lesions remain unchanged for long periods. Today, more conservative criteria are being used in selecting surfaces for operative treatment than were used in the past.

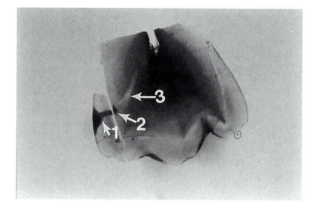

Figure 17.21. Histopathology of Carious Lesion. Thin ground section of carious lesion on distal surface of an upper first premolar. The radiograph of this lesion before extraction revealed penetration of the carious lesion to half the width of the enamel at 1. This thin ground section shows that the carious lesion has actually reached the dentinoenamel junction at 2. Note the "transparent" or sclerotic dentin at 3. This is considered a defensive mechanism of the pulpodentinal complex because its formation alters the permeability of the dentinal tubules, blocking access of irritants to the pulp.

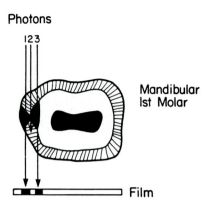

Figure 17.22. Normal Tooth-to-Caries Ratio. The film records a radiopaque area for photon 2, because the normal tooth-to-carious-tooth-structure ratio is greater in this area of the tooth compared with areas of the tooth that photons 1 and 3 are penetrating.

Thus, it may be more appropriate to institute preventive and remineralization procedures for a carious lesion than to initiate restorative treatment.

Caries to Normal Tooth Ratio

The radiograph underestimates the size of the carious lesion for another reason. It can be explained by the caries to normal tooth thickness ratio. The classic shape of the enamel caries lesion is the V shape, with the point of the V located closest to the dentinoenamel junction. Therefore, the ratio of the thickness of the enamel to the size of the carious lesion becomes greater at the "V-point" of the carious lesion. At this point, the x-ray energy becomes reduced enough to block out the registration of the radiolucent carious lesion in this region of the enamel. The carious lesion will then appear smaller on the radiograph than the actual demineralization of the enamel from dental caries. When the carious lesion reaches the dentinoenamel junction, it spreads along the junction and progresses rapidly through the dentin to the pulp. In the dentin, this creates a smaller tooth structure to caries ratio, and the radiolucency of the dentinal carious lesion is seen again on the radiograph (Fig. 17.22). This creates a radiographic appearance of interproximal caries with a small opening on the enamel periphery, a band of normal enamel, and finally carious dentin. This radiographic appearance could be misinterpreted as enamel caries only; if the dentist decided to delay restorative treatment, it could result in unnecessary carious pulpal involvement of the tooth (Fig. 17.23).

CERVICAL BURNOUT

The constricted cervical neck of the tooth, the area between the crown and the root, absorbs less x-ray energy

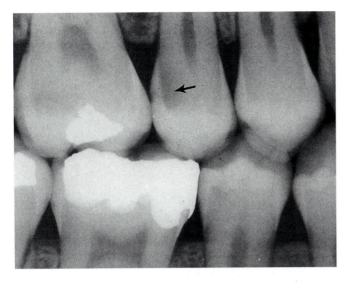

Figure 17.23. Normal Tooth-to-Caries Ratio Radiograph. Note the apparent enamel carious lesion on the mesial and distal surfaces of the upper second premolar (*arrow*). However, with a closer look, this lesion has penetrated the dentin.

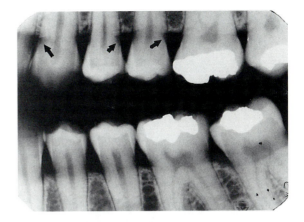

Figure 17.25. Posterior Cervical Burnout. Note radiolucent areas (*arrows*) that are cervical burnout areas and **not** caries.

than the areas above and below it. This is because of the presence of enamel above and the alveolar bone covering the root of this tooth below the cervical neck. It results in a radiolucent band running across the cervical neck of anterior teeth (Fig. 17.24) and a triangular, wedge-shaped radiolucency at the interproximal cervical neck of the posterior teeth (Fig. 17.25). This is called cervical burnout because of the great density difference between the cervical neck of the tooth and the tissues above and below it.

Other reasons for cervical burnout in addition to density tissue differences are anatomical differences such as the shape of the cementoenamel contour, various root configurations, and poor horizontal angulation of the beam. Thus, cervical burnout will often disappear if the radiograph is retaken with an improved horizontal angulation.

RESTORATIVE MATERIALS

Materials of relatively high atomic weights (such as amalgams and gold) appear radiopaque on the radiograph and are not confused with caries, although older silicate and plastic restorations tend to be radiolucent and simulate dental caries (Fig. 17.26). Older silicate materials

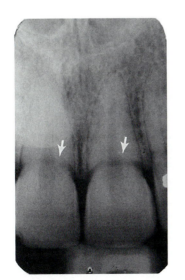

Figure 17.24. Anterior Cervical Burnout. Cervical burnout in upper centrals. Note the dark radiolucent collar at the cervical neck of the incisors (*arrows*).

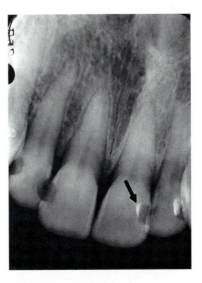

Figure 17.26. Restorative Materials that Mimic Caries. Silicates and resins are radiolucent and could mimic caries (*arrow*). Cement bases (*arrow*) under silicates are radiopaque because they contain metallic elements such as zinc in these materials.

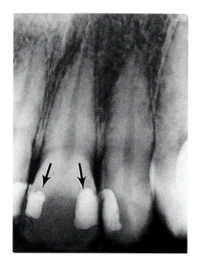

Figure 17.27. Anterior Composite Restorations. Composite restorations (*arrows*) are radiopaque because they contain metallic materials. Sometimes a radiolucent line can be seen under the composite restorations. These are sealing or bonding materials and not leaky margins or recurrent caries.

often require the use of suitable radiopaque base materials, and this assists the practitioner in differentiating silicates from caries. Anterior composite restorations are radiopaque (Fig. 17.27). Both zinc oxide-eugenol and zinc phosphate cements appear radiopaque because of the zinc used in these materials. The older calcium hydroxide materials were radiolucent; the newer ones contain additives to render them radiopaque. Calcium hydroxide is ordinarily used as a subbase between a pulpal exposure or a near exposure and conventional base materials, such as zinc phosphate cements. If the restoration is very old (before

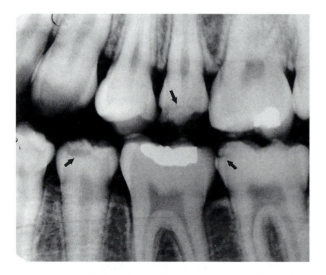

Figure 17.28. Enamel Hypoplasia Mimics Caries. Enamel hypoplasia of lower and upper second premolars and the mesial surface of the mandibular second molar (*arrows*).

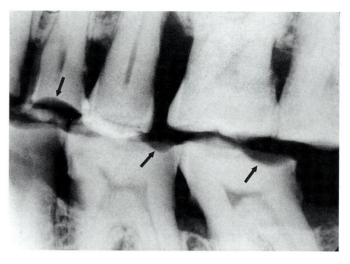

Figure 17.29. Attrition Mimics Caries. Note the severe attrition of occlusal surfaces (*arrows*) mimicking caries.

1970), the subbase area may be radiolucent on the radiograph and would be difficult to differentiate from caries.

DEVELOPMENTAL/ACQUIRED DEFECTS IN ENAMEL

Developmental defects, particularly **enamel hypoplasia,** can simulate caries radiographically (Fig. 17.28). Pits and fissures on the facial and lingual surfaces simulate caries but are readily identified by clinical examination. Because these pits tend to stain, caries is often suspected. Caries is detected clinically if the explorer point sticks on removal from the defect. The lesion is termed an enamel developmental defect without caries involvement if the explorer does not stick.

Attrition is defined as the physiologic wearing away of teeth. Clinically, the earliest change occurs as a small facet on a cusp tip or a slight flattening of the incisal edge.

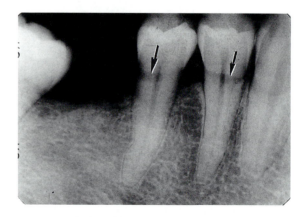

Figure 17.30. Cervical Toothbrush Abrasion Mimics Caries. Toothbrush abrasion of lower premolars mimics caries.

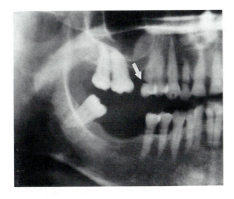

Figure 17.31. V-Shaped Toothbrush Abrasion Mimics Caries. The V-shaped depression shown here (*arrow*) in a panoramic radiograph mimics a carious lesion. Note other areas of toothbrush abrasion.

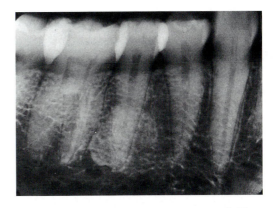

Figure 17.33. Improper Horizontal Angulation. Periapical of lower premolars showing severe overlapping that makes it impossible to interpret interproximal caries.

When the enamel has been completely worn away and the dentin has been exposed, a cavity in the tooth will appear. The attrition cavity on the occlusal or incisal surfaces of teeth may appear as dental caries on the radiograph (Fig. 17.29).

Abrasion is the abnormal wearing away of tooth substance by a mechanical process. This usually occurs on exposed root surfaces as a result of improper tooth-brushing (Fig. 17.30). A V-shaped depression is created on the root side of the cementoenamel junction where there is some gingival recession. This V-shaped depression mimics carious lesions on the radiograph (Fig. 17.31). The improper use of dental floss and toothpicks may also contribute to abrasive wearing away of the teeth, which can mimic interproximal or root caries.

TECHNIQUE ERRORS THAT WILL AFFECT CARIES DETECTION

For the dentist to interpret a radiograph properly, it is essential that the radiograph has diagnostic quality. As discussed previously, diagnostic quality can only be achieved by following the principles of good radiographic technique covered in previous chapters. The important common errors that affect caries interpretation are projection errors.

Common Errors in Projection

If the film is not placed properly in the mouth and the x-ray beam directed accurately to the teeth and film, then shape distortion and overlapping of tooth contacts of the teeth will occur.

Improper Vertical and Horizontal Angulation

Improper vertical angulation causes foreshortening of the tooth images and projects the enamel cap of the crown of the tooth over the interproximal surfaces of the tooth. This obliterates the carious lesion from view on the radiograph (Fig. 17.32). *Improper horizontal angulation* causes overlapping of the contact areas of the crowns of the teeth, which in turn makes it impossible to interpret the interproximal surfaces of the teeth for caries (Fig. 17.33).

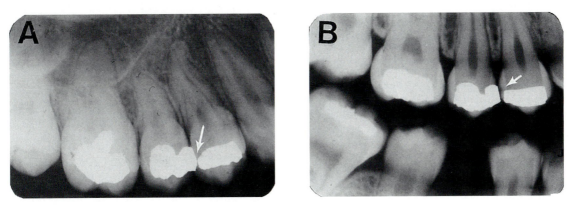

Figure 17.32. Improper Vertical Angulation. (A) Periapical radiograph taken with improper vertical angulation. Note how interproximal spaces are distorted. (B) Bitewing radiograph of same patient as in A. Note caries on distal of upper first premolar, which could not be seen on the periapical radiograph with improper vertical angulation.

WORKSHOP/LABORATORY EXERCISES

EXERCISE 17.1 ASSESSMENT OF CARIES

Set up several viewboxes with radiographs. Request students rotate at various times to answer questions or to identify carious lesions present on radiographs.

REVIEW QUESTIONS

1. In discussing radiologic caries interpretation, how is the phenomenon of cervical burnout explained?

    A. Tissue density and thickness in the cervical area of the tooth is less than the adjacent tooth and bony tissues.
    B. Tissue density in the cervical region of the tooth is greater than the adjacent tooth and bony tissues.
    C. The cervical region of the tooth is more receptive to dental caries.
    D. The cervical region of the tooth attenuates the x-ray beam more than the rest of the tooth.
    E. The exposure time used is too low.

2. In most cases, which pattern of caries development describes the smooth surface caries?

    A. Saucer-shaped with the base of the saucer toward the dentinoenamel junction.
    B. Triangular with the base toward the periphery of tooth enamel.
    C. Triangular with the base toward the dentinoenamel junction.
    D. Hair-like line penetrating enamel toward dentinoenamel junction.
    E. Flame-like configuration with the base at periphery of enamel of tooth.

3. Which of the following statements are true concerning acute caries?

    1. Initial lesion is small at the surface.
    2. Large initial lesion at the surface in its incipiency.
    3. More common in children.
    4. More common in adults.
    5. Slow progress.
    6. Rapid progress.
    A. 2, 4, and 5.
    B. 2, 3, and 6.
    C. 1, 4, and 5.
    D. 2, 3, and 5.
    E. 1, 3, and 6.

4. Recurrent or secondary caries in most cases occurs because of which of the following?

    A. Inadequate extension of the cavity preparation.
    B. Improper adaptation of the restorative material to margins of the cavity preparation.
    C. Incomplete removal of the caries from the tooth before placing the restoration.
    D. All of the above.

5. How is root (cemental) caries usually revealed on the radiograph?

    A. A radiolucent area just beneath a restoration.
    B. An ill-defined, radiolucent, saucer-shaped area located in the interproximal region just below the cementoenamel junction.
    C. A V-shaped radiolucent area in the enamel just below contact point.
    D. A black circle on either of the facial/lingual surfaces.

CASE-BASED QUESTIONS

CASE 17.1

This patient is a 35-year-old man who has been experiencing sensitivity to hot, cold, and sweets.

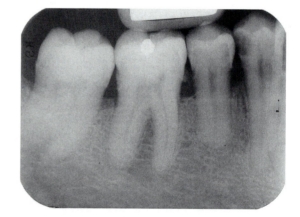

Questions

1. What term best describes the morphology of the caries on the distal of the second premolar?

    A. Interproximal.
    B. Approximal.

C. Cone-shaped.
D. Flame-shaped.
E. Linear.

2. What do you think is (are) this patient's main problem(s)?

A. Multiple caries.
B. Periodontal disease.
C. Halitosis.
D. A and B.

3. What **significant** past treatment do you think he had?

A. Operative dentistry.
B. Scaling and root planing.
C. Orthodontic treatment.
D. Oral surgery.

CASE 17.2

This is a routine bitewing of a 43-year-old man.

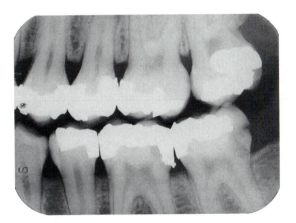

1. Which of the following carious mandibular teeth may also have significant periodontal problems?

A. Distal of first premolar.
B. Mesial of second premolar.
C. Distal of first molar.
D. Distal of second molar.

CASE 17.3

This patient is a 45-year-old woman who complains that her teeth are sensitive to hot and cold. The cervical areas are sensitive on probing.

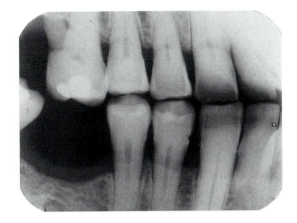

1. This patient's problems are due to:

A. Exposed cementum due to vertical bone loss.
B. Cervical caries.
C. Cocaine abrasion.
D. Toothbrush abrasion.

CASE 17.4

This patient has a slight toothache, and deep caries is discovered on the distal of the maxillary second premolar.

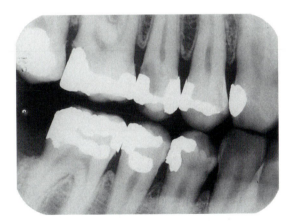

1. The term that best describes this type of caries is:

A. Interproximal.
B. Approximal.
C. Recurrent (secondary).
D. Root.

CASE 17.5

This is a 26-year-old graduate student with a toothache. You note the problem seems to be occlusal caries.

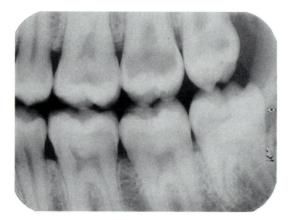

Questions

1. Which molars have occlusal caries?

   A. The uppers.
   B. The lowers.
   C. The uppers and lowers.
   D. Only the upper second.

2. At a young age, what procedure could have **prevented** his current problem?

   A. Diet counseling.
   B. Sealants.
   C. Home care.
   D. Fluoride treatments.
   E. All of the above.

CASE 17.6

This patient is a 14-year-old girl. Almost all the lower anterior teeth are carious.

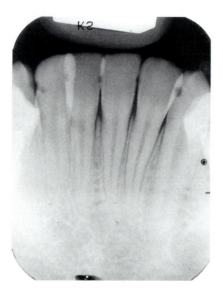

1. The most significant reason for recognizing this pattern of caries is:

   A. A strong susceptibility to caries.
   B. A response to pubertal hormonal change.
   C. A lack of proper home care.
   D. The patient did not floss properly.

CASE 17.7

This patient is a 40-year-old man. He reports periodic discomfort in his teeth, which is hard to describe and localize and is very intermittent.

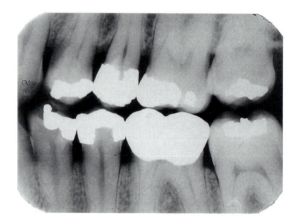

1. These radiographs indicate there is a leaky margin at:

   A. The lower first molar.
   B. The mesial of the upper second premolar.
   C. The distal of the lower first premolar.
   D. B and C.
   E. None of the above.

CASE 17.8

This 35-year-old man has made an appointment for a dental examination in your office. Bitewing radiographs were taken.

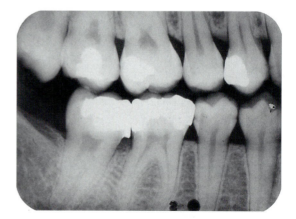

Questions

1. Which of the surfaces named (identified) have definite radiographic evidence of caries?

    1. Distal of maxillary second premolar.
    2. Distal of mandibular first premolar.
    3. Mesial of mandibular second premolar.
    4. Distal of mandibular second premolar.
    A. 2 and 3.
    B. 2, 3, and 4.
    C. 1, 2, 3, and 4.
    D. 3 and 4.
    E. 1 and 2.

2. Which area(s) on the radiograph reveal definite radiographic evidence of periodontal disease between which of the following teeth?

    A. Maxillary first molar and second premolar.
    B. Maxillary second premolar and first premolar.
    C. Mandibular premolars.
    D. Mandibular molars.
    E. All areas look normal.

BIBLIOGRAPHY

Allen EF. Statistical study of the primary causes of extraction. J Dent Res 1944;23:453–459.

Backer DO. Posteruptive changes in dental enamel. J Dent Res 1966;45(Suppl 3):503–507.

Berry HM. Cervical burnout and Mach band: two shadows in doubt in radiologic interpretation of carious lesions. J Am Dent Assoc 1983;106:622–627.

Brekhus PS. Dental disease and its relation to the loss of human teeth. J Am Dent Assoc 1929;16:2237–2245.

Early PJ, Razzak MA, Dodee DB. Textbook of nuclear medicine technology. 3rd ed. St. Louis: CV Mosby, 1979:379–385.

Grondahl HG. Radiographic caries diagnosis and treatment decisions. Swed Dent J 1979;3:109–113.

Hansen BF. Clinical and roentgenologic caries detection. Dentomaxillofac Radiol 1980;9:34–40.

Haugejorden O. A study of the methods of radiologic diagnosis of dental caries in epidemiological investigations. Acta Odontol Scand 1974;65(Suppl):.

Haugejorden O, Slack GL. A study of intra-examiner caries at different diagnostic levels. Acta Odontol Scand 1975;33:169–176.

Haugejorden O, Slack GL. The construction and use of diagnostic standards for radiographic caries incidence scores. Acta Odontol Scand 1977;35:95–102.

Lane EJ. Mach bands and density perception. Radiology 1976;121:9–17.

Mjor IA. Placement and replacement of restorations. Operative Dent 1981;6:49–54.

Newbrun E. Comparison of two screening tests for streptococcus mutants and evaluation of their suitability for mass screening and private practice. Commun Dent Oral Epidemiol 1984;12:289–296.

Newbrun E. Cardiology. 3rd ed. Chicago: Quintessence, 1989:66, 248–256.

Pitts NB. Monitoring of caries progression in permanent and primary posterior approximal enamel by bitewing radiography. Commun Dent Oral Epidemiol 1983;11:228–235.

Schwartz M, Grondahl HG, Pliskin JS, et al. A longitudinal analysis from bitewing radiographs of the rate of progression of approximal carious lesions through human dental enamel. Arch Oral Biol 1984;29:529–536.

Scott DB, Wyckoff RW. Studies of tooth surface structure by optical and electron microscopy. J Am Dent Assoc 1949;39:276–284.

Silverstone LM. The relationship between the microscopic, histological and radiographic appearance of interproximal lesions in human teeth: an in-vitro study using an artificial caries technique. In: Radiation exposure in pediatric dentistry. Pediatr Dent 1982;3(Special issue 2):414–434.

Sumney DL, Jordan HV, Englander HR. The prevalence of root surface caries in selected populations. J Periodontol 1973;44:500–508.

Thylstrup A, Fejershov O. Textbook of cardiology. Copenhagen: Munksgaard, 1986:1211–1220.

Wagg BJ. ECSI: A new index for evaluating caries progression. Commun Dent Oral Epidemiol 1974;2:219–227.

Zamir T, Fischer D, Fishel D, et al. A longitudinal radiographic study of the rate and spread of human approximal dental caries. Arch Oral Biol 1976;21:523–531.

Radiologic Diagnosis of Periapical Disease

18

OBJECTIVES

Upon successful completion of this unit, the student will be able to:

1. *Explain the role of the lamina dura and apical periodontal membrane space in the diagnosis of periapical disease.*

2. *Know how to interpret acute periapical pathogens of pulpal origin.*

3. *Know how to interpret chronic apical periodontitis and its variants.*

4. *Test his or her knowledge by answering the Review Questions.*

KEY WORDS/PHRASES

acute apical abscess

acute apical periodontitis

apical cyst

apical granuloma

chronic apical abscess

chronic apical periodontitis

condensing osteitis

dental granuloma

fistula

hypercementosis

lamina dura

periapical cemental dysplasia

pulpoperiapical disease

RADIOLOGIC DIAGNOSIS OF PERIAPICAL DISEASE

LAMINA DURA IN PERIAPICAL DISEASE

In almost every normal tooth, the lamina dura can be traced from the alveolar crest, around the root (Fig. 18.1), and into the bifurcation and trifurcation areas. In periapical disease, resorption of the lamina dura occurs at the apex of the tooth. Radiographically, it appears to have lost its continuity, its thickness, and its degree of radiopac-

ity. This usually indicates, with few exceptions, that **periapical disease** is present (Fig. 18.2).

PULPOPERIAPICAL DISEASE: INTRODUCTION

Because there is little correlation between clinical and histopathologic findings of periapical (apical) lesions of pulpal origin, diagnostic differentiation of periapical disease is usually based on the patient's clinical findings rather than on histopathologic findings. Therefore, periapical (apical) lesions are classified into six main clinical

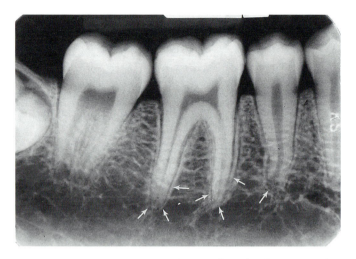

Figure 18.1. Lamina Dura. Lamina dura is a thin, white line (*arrows*) that can be traced around the apical ends of all normal teeth.

groups: (1) acute apical periodontitis (AAP), (2) acute apical abscess (AAA), (3) apical granuloma, (4) apical cyst, (5) chronic apical abscess, and (6) apical condensing osteitis (ACO). Lesions with significant symptoms, such as pain or swelling, are designated as acute and those with mild or no symptoms are classified as chronic.

ACUTE APICAL CONDITIONS

ACUTE APICAL PERIODONTITIS (ACUTE PERIAPICAL PERIODONTITIS)

AAP is an inflammatory response of the apical periodontal ligament to pulpal irritants via the root canal or from trauma. In most cases, the pulp is irreversibly inflamed or necrotic; however, AAP may be associated with a vital tooth, such as in occlusal trauma, from irregular wear of teeth, a large carious lesion, a recently inserted high restoration, or a foreign object wedged between the teeth. The clinical features of AAP are slight to severe spontaneous pain and pain from percussion. Pulp testing will result in abnormal responses. If the AAP is caused by an irreversible pulpitis, the treatment will require a complete pulpectomy followed by appropriate root canal therapy. Most cases of AAP are associated with normal apical periodontal ligament spaces and intact lumina dura. A slight widening of the apical periodontal ligament space usually indicates irreversible pulpitis or pupal necrosis (Fig. 18.3).

ACUTE APICAL ABSCESS (ACUTE ALVEOLAR ABSCESS)

AAA is a painful, localized collection of pus in the alveolar bone at the root apex of the tooth after the death of the pulp, with extension of the infection through the periapical foramen into the periapical tissue. The cause of AAA is a previously existing AAP with a necrotic pulp that has advanced to an extensive acute suppurative in-

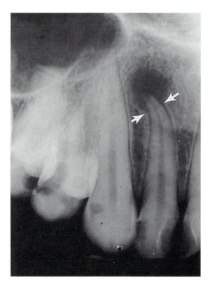

Figure 18.2. Periapical Disease. When there is an interruption in the continuity of the lamina dura (as shown here by arrows on the root of the upper lateral incisor), apical pathoses should be suspected. (Note loss of lamina dura at root apex.)

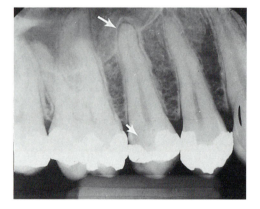

Figure 18.3. Acute Apical Periodontitis. Upper second premolar has large, recurrent (secondary) caries on distal surface. Note thickened periodontal ligament space at apical end of root. The tooth gave abnormal responses to pulp testing, elicited spontaneous pain, and was painful to percussion. The pulp was severely inflamed, and anesthesia was difficult to obtain during the pulpectomy procedure.

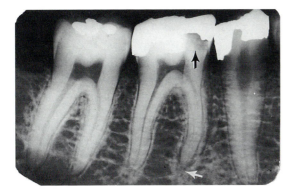

Figure 18.4. Acute Apical Abscess. Note thickening of periodontal ligament space of mesial root of lower first molar. Tooth has large, recurrent (secondary) carious lesion under mesial portion of restoration of this tooth. The tooth is mobile, nonvital, and has percussion pain, with swelling and tenderness to palpation. On removal of restoration and entry into the pulp, a purulent exudate (pus) drained from the access opening; the pain subsided almost immediately.

flammation stage. The pulp is nonvital and associated with painful percussion tests. Palpation of the facial surface of the soft tissue of the offending tooth root reveals swelling and pain. In the later stages as the abscess develops, the pain becomes more intense and continuous; the tooth becomes loosened and protrudes in the socket. The initial treatment of AAA is the establishment of drainage that will relieve acute symptoms at once. Radiographically, the periapical tissue of AAA may appear normal, because fulminating infections may not have had sufficient time (10 days or more) to erode enough cortical bone to cause a radiolucency. However, only a slight widening of the periodontal ligament is usually present (Fig. 18.4).

CHRONIC APICAL (PERIAPICAL) PERIODONTITIS

Chronic apical periodontitis can be subdivided into the following four subtypes: apical granuloma, apical cyst, chronic apical abscess, and condensing osteitis (Fig. 18.5).

APICAL GRANULOMA (PERIAPICAL GRANULOMA, DENTAL GRANULOMA)

An apical granuloma is an advanced form of chronic apical periodontitis characterized by a growth of granulomatous tissue (chronic inflammatory tissue) continuous with the periapical ligament, resulting from death of the pulp, with diffusion of mild infection or irritation of the periapical tissue, stimulating a productive cellular reaction. Basically, the apical granuloma may be looked on

as a successful attempt by the periapical tissue to neutralize and confine the irritating toxic products that are escaping from the root canal. The term granuloma is a misnomer because the tissue referred to is composed principally of chronic inflammatory tissue (granulomatous tissue); it is not a tumor, as is intimated. The term apical or dental granuloma is in common usage and, until a more appropriate term is found, we will use it in our classification.

Apical granulomas are the most common periapical radiolucency found in dental practice. They are asymptomatic, except in rare cases they break down and undergo suppuration (pus formation). The teeth will not respond to thermal or electrical pulp tests. When an apical granuloma is present, root canal therapy is usually the treatment of choice if the tooth is to be retained. Radiographically, the apical granuloma appears as a radiolucent, circular to ovoid area that encloses the root end and extends periapically from it. Trabeculations of the alveolar bone may be seen superimposed over the lesion, because the lesion has a grayish appearance and is not dark (Fig. 18.6). In a long-standing lesion, the margin may become clearly defined. Because the apical granuloma and apical cyst may have identical radiographic appearances, the apical cyst sometimes may be differentiated from the granuloma by virtue of its size. The apical granuloma is usually smaller than 1 cm in diameter, whereas the apical cyst may become as large as 10 cm and may, in rare instances, fill an entire jaw. In clinical practice, it usually is not necessary to differentiate between an apical granuloma and an apical cyst radiographically, because both respond well to root canal therapy without surgical intervention.

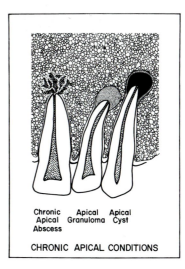

Figure 18.5. Chronic Apical Lesions. Radiographic appearance of three chronic apical lesions. (The fourth chronic periapical lesion, condensing osteitis, is not shown).

415

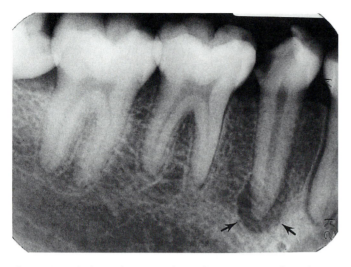

Figure 18.6. Apical Granuloma. Radiographic appearance of apical granuloma of nonvital mandibular second premolar. The lesion is somewhat rounded and well circumscribed, and bony trabeculations are superimposed over the lesion giving it a gray appearance.

APICAL CYST (RADICULAR CYST, ROOT END CYST, PERIAPICAL CYST, ALVEOLAR CYST)

The apical cyst is a true cyst in that it is an abnormal pathologic space within bone lined by stratified squamous epithelium and filled with a fluid or semifluid. Apical cysts are the most common cysts of the jaws. They are painless unless infected. They do not respond to pulp tests.

Practically all apical cysts originate from preexisting apical granulomas, and their pathogenesis depends on an inflammatory response. Histologically, the apical cyst can be described as a cyst within a granuloma (granulomatous tissue). Cysts expand slowly, the fluid that is formed within cysts raises the interstitial (interspaces of tissue) pressure abutting the bone margins, and resorption results. Eventually, the lesion may reach a large size. An apical cyst is usually treated by removal of necrotic pulpal irritants and complete obturation of the root canal system. The healing pattern is similar to the apical granuloma, although it may be more prolonged if the apical cyst is large. The radiologic appearance of the apical cyst is a more circumscribed area of radiolucency than apical granuloma, and it is usually bounded by a thin unbroken line of sclerotic bone. The radiolucent area is generally round in outline except where it approximates adjacent teeth, in which case it may be flattened in outline (oval pattern). Because the apical cyst is a cavity in bone that contains fluid, it appears as a dark radiolucent area with little signs of bone trabeculation (Fig. 18.7). They are usually larger than apical granulomas. If the radiolucency is more than 1 cm in diameter, it is more likely to be an apical cyst.

CHRONIC APICAL ABSCESS (SUPPURATIVE PERIAPICAL PERIODONTITIS, CHRONIC PERIAPICAL ABSCESS, CHRONIC DENTOALVEOLAR ABSCESS, SUBACUTE PERIAPICAL ABSCESS)

The chronic apical abscess is a long-standing, low-grade inflammatory reaction to irritating products from a necrotic pulp. It is characterized by the formation of

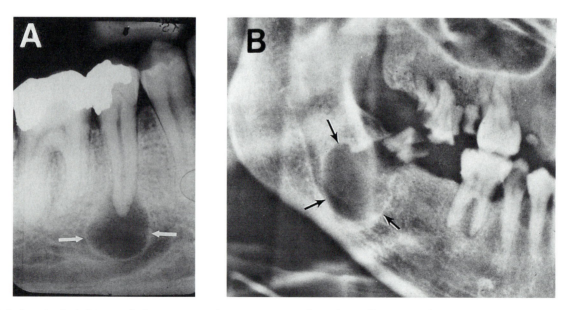

Figure 18.7. Apical cyst (Periapical Cyst, Radicular Cyst). **(A)** Classic appearance of apical cyst of lower second premolar. **(B)** Large apical cyst of retained roots of mandibular third molar (*arrows*).

an abscess (pus) at the periapical region of a tooth. On examination, the tooth may be slightly loose or tender to percussion. On palpation, the periapical soft tissue may be slightly swollen and tender. Often a gum boil (parulis) is found. The tooth shows no reaction to electric pulp testing. The microscopic picture varies but depending on the stage of infection, it basically consists of an abscess in the center of granulomatous tissue. There are two types of chronic apical abscess: one with a fistula (abnormal passage) and one without a fistula. The chronic apical abscess heals spontaneously after adequate root canal treatment.

The **chronic apical abscess with a fistula** is the most common of the two chronic apical abscesses. It is characterized by active pus formation draining through a fistulous opening (sinus tract stoma) at the surface of the oral mucosa or the skin of the face (Fig. 18.8). A small proliferation of granulomatous tissue often forms on the mucosal surface and is referred to as a gum boil or parulis,

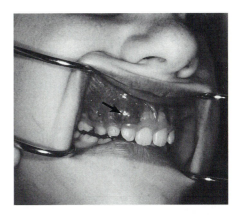

Figure 18.9. Parulis or Gum Boil. This is the classic sign of a chronic apical abscess. This is a young patient who had previously experienced all the acute symptoms of an acute apical abscess of upper lateral incisor. After free drainage of pus from the gum boil, the acute symptoms subsided.

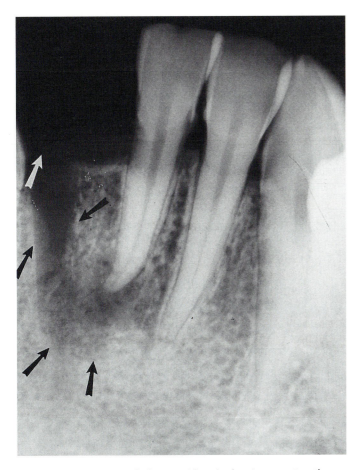

Figure 18.8. Chronic Apical Abscess With a Fistula (Sinus Tract). Chronic apical abscess originating from acute apical abscess of lower lateral incisor. Note radiolucent fistulous tract (*black arrows*) through alveolar bone to opening at surface of oral mucosa (*white arrow*).

which is also frequently observed in conjunction with infection of primary teeth (Fig. 18.9). As soon as drainage is established through the mucoperiosteal tissue in an AAA, either by incision or by a fistulous tract, symptoms subside and a chronic apical abscess is formed with a fistulous tract.

The **chronic apical abscess without a fistula** seldom develops directly from an AAA. It probably occurs as a natural developmental sequence of the death of the pulp with extension of the infective process periapically, in which the virulence and number of the bacterial organisms are low and the host resistance is high. Although mild, painful symptoms may occur, it is usually symptom free. When the production of pus commences, it begins a slow route that yields the least resistance through bone. When no fistula is present, the toxic products are sometimes absorbed through the blood and lymph channels, a condition sometimes referred to as a "blind abscess." Radiographically, the chronic apical abscess without a fistula will demonstrate diffuse, irregular borders (Fig. 18.10). The radiolucent area fades indistinctly into normal bone and is usually represented by an area of lesser density than the granuloma or cyst.

APICAL CONDENSING OSTEITIS (FOCAL SCLEROSING OSTEOMYELITIS)

ACO (focal sclerosing osteomyelitis) is a variant of chronic apical periodontitis and is a reaction of bone to a mild bacterial infection of periapical bone in persons who have a high degree of tissue resistance and tissue reactivity. Periapical bone reacts to the infection by a diffuse increase in trabecular bone rather than destruction. Therefore, the infection acts as a stimulus rather than an

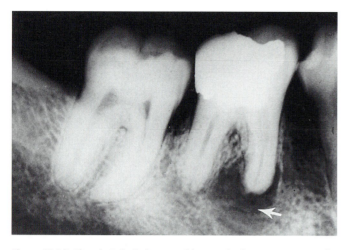

Figure 18.10. Chronic Apical Abscess Without a Fistulous Tract. Note the diffuse area of radiolucency of the mesial root of the lower first molar (*arrow*). The apical granuloma and the apical cyst have more definite circumscribed area of radiolucency than the chronic apical abscess.

irritant. ACO is usually found in patients younger than 20 years of age around the apices of mandibular first molar teeth with large carious lesions and chronically inflamed pulps; however, ACO may occur around the apex of any tooth. Depending on the cause (pulpitis or pulpal necrosis), ACO—although usually asymptomatic—may be associated with pain and discomfort. There are usually no signs or symptoms of disease other than mild pain associated with an infected pulp. The pulp tissue of these teeth with ACO usually does not respond to electrical or thermal stimuli. In addition, these teeth generally will not be sensitive to palpation or percussion. A return to the normal trabecular pattern may occur after

root canal therapy, although the sclerotic bone may remain as bone scar. Radiographically, ACO appears as a pathognomonic, well-circumscribed radiopaque mass of sclerotic (hard, compact) bone surrounding and extending below the apex of one or both roots (Fig. 18.11). There is usually a radiolucency immediately adjacent to the periapical end of the involved tooth.

OTHER APICAL (PERIAPICAL) CONDITIONS

APICAL CEMENTOMA (PERIAPICAL CEMENTOMA, PERIAPICAL CEMENTAL DYSPLASIA)

The apical cementoma (periapical cemental dysplasia) is a benign, slowly growing, connective tissue proliferation thought to originate from cellular elements in periodontal ligament. Developing lesions destroy the lamina dura and spread periapically, replacing the surrounding normal trabecular bone with a fibrous tissue mass (radiolucent) within which varying amounts of radiopaque material (cementum) may be observed, especially as the lesion matures. It has limited growth potential with a long duration. It is most often seen in middle-aged African-American and Asian females. The mandibular teeth are most frequently involved, and the teeth are **vital**. (No treatment is indicated.) In the early stages of the apical cementoma, the radiologic appearance varies from a thickened periapical periodontal membrane space associated with destruction of the lamina dura to a well-defined radiolucent lesion similar to a chronic inflammatory periapical lesion (Fig. 18.12). However, in the case of the periapical cementoma,

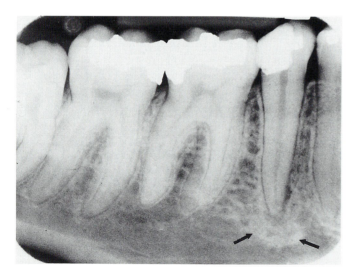

Figure 18.11. Apical Condensing Osteitis. Condensing osteitis of lower second premolar with large restoration (*arrows*).

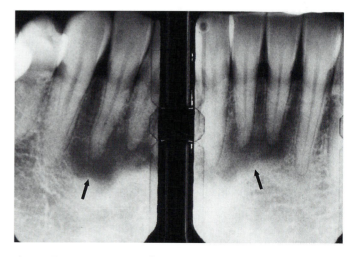

Figure 18.12. Immature Apical Cementoma (Periapical Cemental Dysplasia). Immature apical cementomas are radiolucent lesions. The mandibular incisor teeth are vital. The immature apical cementomas are "filling in" with radiopaque material (*arrows*).

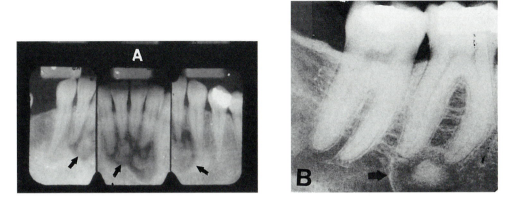

Figure 18.13. Mature Apical Cementoma (Periapical Cemental Dysplasia). **(A)** Mature cementoblastic stage of apical cementoma of vital mandibular incisors (*arrows*). **(B)** Target lesion (opacity with lucent halo) of apical cementoma (*arrow*).

the pulps of the teeth are **vital**. In later stages, increasing amounts of radiopaque material are laid down in the lesion (Fig. 18.13).

HYPERCEMENTOSIS

Cementum is formed on permanent teeth throughout life. Hypercementosis is the excessive formation of secondary cementum on the root surfaces. It is the abnormal increase in the thickness of cementum that may affect single teeth or the entire dentition. It produces no clinical signs or symptoms. The increased formation of cementum occurs mainly as a generalized type of hypercementosis producing a radiographic appearance of a symmetric enlargement of the entire root (Fig. 18.14). There are two

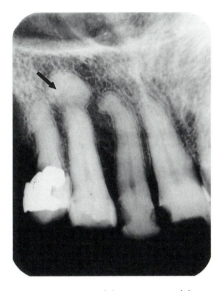

Figure 18.15. Hypercementosis (Nodular Type). Nodular type of hypercementosis on root tips of canine and lateral. (Also note attrition and silicate restorations.)

generalized types of hypercementosis. In some instances of hypercementosis, the cementum formation is focal, appearing on the radiograph as a nodular or bulbous enlargement near or at the root apex (Fig. 18.15).

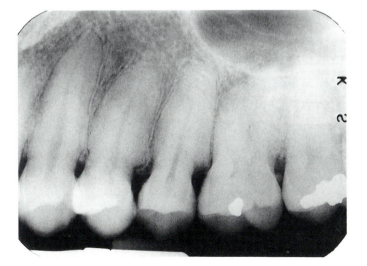

Figure 18.14. Hypercementosis. Increased formation of hypercementosis forming a generalized type producing symmetrical enlargement of entire roots of premolars.

REVIEW QUESTIONS

1. Which of the following is most common?

   A. Chronic periapical abscess.
   B. Periapical cyst.
   C. Dental granuloma.

D. Condensing osteitis.
E. Residual cyst.

2. Which of the following usually is (are) associated with nonvital pulps of teeth?

   A. Hypercementosis.
   B. Cementoma (periapical cemental dysplasia).
   C. Periapical cyst.
   D. Periapical osteosclerosis.
   E. All of the above.

3. Which of the following would best differentiate condensing osteitis from a periapical cementoma (periapical cemental dysplasia)?

   A. Pulp of tooth is nonvital in condensing osteitis, and pulp of tooth is vital when associated with periapical cementoma.
   B. Condensing osteitis affects mandibular incisors 80% of the time.
   C. Condensing osteitis is seen mostly in women in the postmenopausal age group.
   D. Periapical cementomas (periapical cemental dysplasia) are attached to root, whereas condensing osteitis is not.
   E. Periapical cementomas (periapical cemental dysplasia) are seen mostly in teen-agers and are usually associated with a carious mandibular first molar.

4. Which of the following would most likely cause the most pain and many times would **not** be seen on the radiograph?

   A. Periapical granuloma.
   B. Periapical cementoma.
   C. Chronic apical abscess.
   D. Acute apical abscess.
   E. Periapical cyst.

5. Which of the following can mimic a periapical radiolucent lesion on the dental radiograph?

   1. Periapical foramen of tooth not closed in an immature tooth.
   2. Mental foramen.
   3. Nasopalatine foramen.
   4. Greater palatine foramen.
   A. 1, 2, 3, and 4.
   B. 1, 2, and 4.
   C. 1, 2, and 3.
   D. 3 and 4.
   E. 1 and 2.

CASE-BASED QUESTIONS

CASE 18.1

This patient has a toothache. All the teeth have onlays or crowns and are difficult to pulp test.

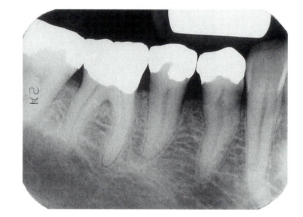

1. Which tooth do you think is the culprit?

   A. First premolar.
   B. Second premolar.
   C. First molar.
   D. Some other tooth.

CASE 18.2

This is a 28-year-old beach volleyball player. The left central incisor is nonvital; the cause was previous trauma.

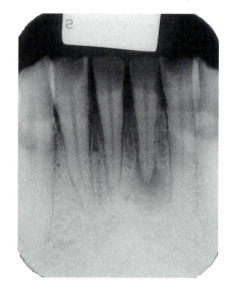

1. The resorption at the apex indicates the lesion is most likely an:

   A. Apical granuloma.
   B. Apical cyst.

C. Apical abscess.

D. Apical cementoma.

CASE 18.3

This 13-year-old boy fell off his skateboard some time ago. The tooth is nonvital.

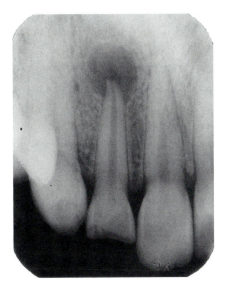

1. The thin sclerotic line around the periapical radiolucency indicates the lesion is most likely an:

    A. Apical granuloma.
    B. Apical cyst.
    C. Apical abscess.
    D. Apical cementoma.

CASE 18.4

This patient is a 6-year-old boy with a gum boil adjacent to the left second primary molar.

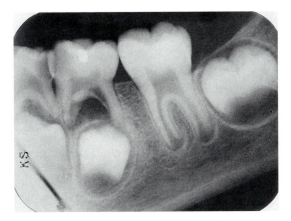

1. The furcal radiolucency is:

    A. Of periodontal origin.
    B. Of pulpal origin.
    C. Resorption due to the erupting second premolar.
    D. Normal for this age.

2. The erupting second premolar:

    A. Will probably be normal.
    B. May develop preeruption caries.
    C. May develop Turner's hypoplasia.
    D. May become cystic.
    E. C and D.

CASE 18.5

This 12-year-old girl has a large carious lesion in the first premolar.

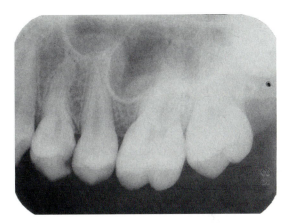

1. A sign of pulpal involvement is:

    A. Caries.
    B. Strange-looking apex.
    C. Localized antral mucositis.
    D. Not seen on this radiograph.

CASE 18.6

This 21-year-old college student has a toothache. There is caries in all three of these teeth.

Questions

1. Which tooth do you think is the culprit?

    A. Second premolar.
    B. First molar.
    C. Second molar.
    D. All of the above.

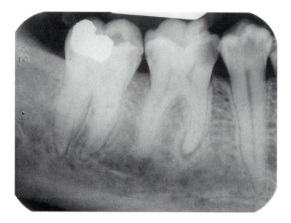

2. What periapical changes suggesting irreversible pulpitis are present?

    A. Loss of the lamina dura.
    B. Thickened apical periodontal ligament space.
    C. Resorption of apical bone.
    D. Condensing osteitis.
    E. All of the above.

CASE 18.7

This 11-year-old boy has a tooth that is sensitive to hot, cold, and sweets. You note the deep occlusal caries and periapical radiolucencies in the first molar.

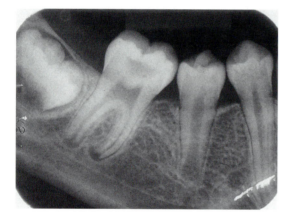

1. Your conclusion is:

    A. The tooth is vital and the apices are not yet closed.
    B. The tooth is nonvital with apical involvement.
    C. Neither of the above.
    D. It is too early to decide; place a sedative dressing.

BIBLIOGRAPHY

Bhaskar SN. Periapical lesion-types, incidence, and clinical features. Oral Surg 1966;21:657–665.

Block RM, Bushell A, Rodrigues H, et al. A histopathologic, bacteriologic and radiographic study of periapical endodontic surgical specimens. Oral Surg 1976;42:656–678.

Grossman LI. Endodontic practice. 8th ed. Philadelphia: Lea & Febiger, 1974:68, 87–93.

Hedin M, Polhagen L. Follow-up study of periradicular bone condensation. J Dent Res 1971;79:436–441.

Ingle JI. Endodontics. Philadelphia: Lea & Febiger, 1965.

Lalonde ER. A new estimate for the management of periapical granulomas and cysts: an evaluation of histopathological and radiologic findings. J Am Dent Assoc 1970;80:1056–1063.

Ludlow MO. Endodontic first aid for the patient with odontalgia. Dental Surg 1959;42:25, 54–60.

McKinney RV. Clarification of the terms granulomatous and granulation tissue. J Oral Pathol 1981;10:307–310. Letter to the Editor.

Natkin E, Oswald RJ, Carnes LI. The relationship of lesion size to diagnosis, incidence, and treatment of periapical cysts and granulomas. Oral Surg 1984;57:82.

Priebe R, Lazansky S, Wuehrmann A. Histology of periapical lesions. Oral Surg 1954;7:979–983.

Ross PN, Birch BS. A clinical histopathologic study of conservative endodontic failures. J Dent Res 1976;Special issue B. Abstract no. 271.

Shafer W, Hine M, Levy B. Textbook of oral pathology. Philadelphia: WB Saunders, 1974:433–462.

Shah N. Nonsurgical management of periapical lesions. Oral Surg 1988;66:365–371.

Slowey RR. Radiographic aids in the detection of extra root canals. Oral Surg 1974;37:762–772.

Smulson MH, Hagen JC. Pulpoperiapical pathology and immunologic considerations. In: Weine F, ed. Endodontic therapy. 4th ed. St. Louis: CV Mosby, 1989:173–174.

Stockdale CR, Chandler NP. The nature of the periapical lesion: a review of 1108 cases. J Dent 1988;16:123–129.

Strindberg LZ. Periapical lesions. Acta Odont Scand 1956;14:100–107.

Walton RE. Endodontic radiographic technics. Dent Radiogr Photogr 1973;46:51–59.

Weine FS. Endodontic therapy. 4th ed. St. Louis: CV Mosby, 1989:171, 449–451.

Glossary

A

Abrasion: Abnormal wearing away of tooth substance by a mechanical process.

Accelerators: This chemical serves to swell the film emulsion and provides an alkaline medium during processing.

Activator: This gives the solution the proper pH and neutralizes any remaining developer on the film. It also acts to aid the other processing chemicals in their activity.

Acute: Having a rapid onset, short severe course, and pronounced symptoms; opposite of chronic.

Acute effects: Effects that are usually the result of high doses of radiation (usually over the whole body). The symptoms of these acute effects may include nausea, vomiting, hemorrhage, diarrhea, fever, loss of hair, and death.

Ala: The wing of the nose. In dental radiography, the depression at which the nostril connects with the cheek.

Ala-tragus line: An imaginary line that intersects the ala of the nose and the tragus of the ear; used in positioning a patient for a panoramic film (ala is the tissue that surrounds the nostril; tragus is a cartilaginous projection anterior to the external opening of the ear).

ALARA concept: This principle emphasizes that the dose to the patient should be kept as low as reasonably achievable under a given set of circumstances.

Alpha particle (symbol α): The nucleus of a helium atom ejected from a radioactive nucleus when it disintegrates.

Alternating current: A flow of electrons in one direction followed by a flow of electrons in the opposite direction.

Alveolar bone: That portion of the maxillary or mandibular bone that surrounds and supports the roots of the dentition.

Alveolar crest: The most coronal portion of alveolar bone found between the teeth; it is composed of dense cortical bone and appears radiopaque.

Ampere (A): The unit of intensity of an electric current produced by 1 volt (V) acting through a resistance of 1 ohm (Ω).

Anode: The positive terminal of an x-ray tube; a tungsten block embedded in a copper stem and set at an angle to the cathode. The anode emits x-rays from the point of impact of the electron stream from the cathode.

Anomaly: A significant deviation from the normal or a departure from the regular order of things.

Anterior nasal spine (ANS): This structure appears as a radiopaque area at the base of the nasal septum. It represents a bony protuberance to which the nasal cartilage is attached.

Atom: The smallest particle of an element that has the characteristic properties of that element.

Atomic number (Z): The number of protons in the nucleus of an atom.

Attenuation: In radiography, the process by which a beam of radiation is reduced in energy when passing through matter.

Attrition: Physiologic wearing away of teeth as a result of tooth-to-tooth contact as in mastication, clenching, and bruxism.

B

Background radiation: Radiation that occurs naturally in the environment.

Backscatter: Radiation that is scattered backward into the path of the original beam.

Beta particle (symbol β-): Electrons, positive or negative, emitted by the nucleus of a radioactive atom when it disintegrates.

Benign: Harmless or nonmalignant.

Binding energy: The energy needed to eject an electron from the atom.

Bremsstrahlung radiation (white radiation): A spectral distribution of x-rays ranging from very–low-energy photons to those produced by the peak kilovoltage applied across an x-ray tube. Bremsstrahlung or braking radiation, refers to the sudden deceleration of electrons (cathode rays) as they interact with highly positively charged (high atomic number) nuclei such as tungsten.

C

Calculus: In dentistry, a deposition of mineral salts to form a concretion or ring around the root of a tooth or to cover parts of the crown.

Cancellous (spongy) bone: This bone surrounds the lamina dura and tooth socket. It is composed of thin strands of bone called trabeculae that cross one another in an irregular manner. Separating the trabeculae are spaces containing bone marrow.

Canthus: The angle at either end of the slit that separates the eyelids. In radiography, the inner canthus is the part of the slit nearest to the nose; the outer canthus is the part farthest from the nose.

Cassette: A light-tight case, usually made of thin, low–x-ray absorption plastic for holding x-ray film. One or two intensifying screens for the conversion of x-rays to visible light photons are mounted inside the cassette in close contact with the film.

Cathode: The negatively charged component of an x-ray tube that repels electrons toward the anode.

Cathode rays: A stream of electrons passing from the hot filament of the cathode to the anode in an x-ray tube.

Central ray: The theoretical center of the x-ray beam. This term is used to designate the direction of the x-rays in a given projection; may be considered to extend from the focal spot of the x-ray film.

Cervical: Pertaining to the neck or cervical vertebrae. Pertaining to the cementoenamel junction area of a tooth.

Cervical burnout: A radiolucent artifact seen on a dental radiograph resulting from the differences in densities of adjacent tissues.

Characteristic curve: A type of input-output response curve. In radiography, this curve expresses the change in optical density (output) with the change in exposure of x-ray film; also called H & D curve or sensitometric curve.

Characteristic radiation: A form of radiation originating from an atom following removal of an electron or excitation of the atom. The wavelength of the emitted radiation is specific for the element concerned and the particular energy levels that are involved.

Chronic effects (because of radiation exposure): These effects, which are usually shown as a decrease in the tissue to resist trauma and infection, are usually produced over a long period of time.

Clearing agent: The agent in the fixer solution that dissolves the unexposed, undeveloped silver halide crystals, leaving the black metallic silver in the exposed and developed areas of the film more readily discernible; also called hypo.

Collimator: A common term for a variable-aperture, beam-limiting device for restricting the field of x-ray photons in a beam to a desired shape and size.

Compton scatter radiation (scatter radiation): The incident radiation has sufficient energy to dislodge a bound electron but attacks a loosely bound electron. The remaining radiation energy proceeds in a different direction as scatter radiation.

Contrast: The difference in image density appearing on a radiograph, representing various degrees of beam attenuation.

Film contrast: A characteristic inherent in the type of film used.

Long-scale contrast: An increased range of grays between the blacks and whites on a radiograph. Higher kilovoltages increase this range.

Short-scale contrast: A reduced range of grays between the blacks and whites on a radiograph. Lower kilovoltages decrease this range.

Subject contrast: The relative differences in density and thickness of the components of the radiographed subject, as evidenced by the varied radiographic densities caused by the differences in absorbing power of the different kinds of material traversed by an x-ray beam.

Contrast, radiographic: The difference in optical density (film blackening) between areas of interest in a radiograph. The combination of subject contrast and film contrast determines radiographic contrast.

Corpuscular radiation: Minute subatomic particles such as protons, electrons, and neutrons; also alpha and beta particles. These particles occupy space, have mass and weight, and with the exception of neutrons have an electrical charge.

Cortical bone: Compact bone that forms the outer and inner plates of the alveolar process.

Crestal bone: That portion of the alveolar bone that extends from tooth to tooth. It appears radiopaque.

Current: The flow of charged particles, for example, electrons.

D

Definition: In radiography, the sharpness and clarity of the outline of the structures on the image shown on the film. Poor definition is generally caused by movement of the patient, film, or the tubehead during exposure.

Densitometer: A device consisting of a light source, an aperture, and a light sensor used to measure optical density.

Density: The degree of darkening of exposed and processed photographic or x-ray film.

Density, optical: The degree of blackening of film after exposure and processing.

Density, physical: The mass of a substance per unit volume. For example, g/cm^3.

Detail: The point-by-point delineation of the minute structures visible in the shadow images on the radiograph. Detail may be good or poor.

Developer: A chemical solution that converts the latent image on film to a visible image.

Developer agent: Elon and hydroquinone; substances that reduce the halides in the film emulsion to metallic silver. Elon brings out the details, and hydroquinone brings out the contrast in the film.

Direct current: Electric current that flows continuously in one direction. Unidirectional current is produced in batteries but cannot be used in x-ray machines unless they are modified.

Distal: Remote; farther from any point of reference; e.g., midline.

Disto-oblique radiograph: An image useful for viewing the most posterior areas of the mouth, such as impacted third molars.

Distortion: An inaccuracy in the size or shape of an object as it is displayed in the radiograph. Distortion is brought about by misalignment of the cone relative to the object or by excessive film-object distance.

Dose (dosage of radiation): The amount of energy absorbed per unit mass of tissue at a site of interest.

Absorbed dose: The amount of energy imparted by ionizing radiation to a unit mass of irradiated material at a place of interest. The unit of absorbed dose in the traditional system is the rad (100 erg/g). The currently accepted unit of absorbed dose is the gray (Gy) (1 Gy = 1 J/kg).

Cumulative dose: The total dose resulting from repeated exposures to radiation of the same region or of the whole body.

Doubling dose: The amount of ionizing radiation absorbed by the gonads of the average person in a population over several generations that will result in a doubling of the current rate of spontaneous mutations.

Erythema dose: Antiquated approach to radiation measurement based on the amount of radiation to cause erythema (redness) of the skin.

Exit dose: Dose of radiation at the surface of body opposite to that on which the beam is incident.

Threshold dose: The minimum dose that will produce a detectable degree of any given effect.

Dose equivalent: The product of absorbed dose and modifying factors, namely the quality factor, distribution factor, and any other necessary factors. The traditional unit of dose equivalence is the rem (rads × qualifying factors). The International System (SI) (mks) unit of dose equivalence is the sievert (grays × qualifying factors).

Dosimeter (radiation meter): An instrument used to detect and measure an accumulated dosage of radiation.

E

Effective dose equivalent: The purpose of the effective dose equivalent is to relate exposure to risk. In an attempt to make some comparison in the risk assessment for all types of exposures, the concept of effective dose equivalent was developed. The unit of effective dose equivalent is the sievert.

Electromagnetic radiation: Forms of energy propelled by wave motion as photons of energy. This is a combination of electric and magnetic energy.

Electromagnetic spectrum: The range of all electromagnetic radiations according to their energy.

Electron: A minute, negatively charged particle that revolves around the positively charged nucleus in assigned orbits or shells.

Electron volt (eV): The kinetic energy gained by an electron falling through a potential difference of 1 volt.

Element: A substance that is composed exclusively of atoms having the same atomic number, which cannot be separated into simpler substances by ordinary chemical means.

Emulsion, film: A mixture of gelatin and silver halide crystals (in suspension) in which latent image formation takes place.

Energy: The ability to do work.

Excited state: The addition of energy to a system, thereby transforming it from its ground state to an excited state.

Exposure: A measure of the amount of ionization produced in air by an x-ray beam; measured in milliroentgens (mR) or Roentgens (R).

External oblique ridge: A ridge originating from the anterior border of the ramus of the mandible extending to the lateral body of the mandible in the molar region.

F

Filament: A coiled tungsten wire that, when heated to incandescence, emits electrons.

Film speed: The sensitivity of film emulsion to x-ray or light exposure. The amount of exposure the light or x-rays require to produce a given image density.

Filter: Material (usually aluminum) placed in the path of the useful beam to preferentially absorb the less-energetic (less-penetrating) x-rays.

Filtration, added: A material or device inserted between the x-ray tube and the patient to preferentially absorb lower-energy photons from an x-ray beam.

Filtration, total: The equivalent amount of filtering material (usually stated in millimeters of aluminum [mm Al]) between the focal spot and the object being radiographed; also the sum of the added and inherent filtration that is usually from glass of x-ray tube (0.5 mm Al equivalent).

Fixer: A chemical solution that both removes the unexposed and undeveloped silver halide crystals from the coated film emulsion and hardens the gelatin.

Fluorescence: The property of a phosphor to emit light in the visible region of the electromagnetic spectrum as a result of absorbing higher-energy radiation, such as x-rays.

Focal spot: That part of the target anode of an x-ray tube that is bombarded by the focused electron stream when the tube is energized.

Focal trough: In panoramic radiography, a three-dimensional curved zone or image layer in which structures are reasonably well defined; a patient must be positioned so that the dental arches are located within the focal trough area.

Focusing cup: Along with the filament, the focusing cup determines the size and shape of the target (focal) spot. The cup is constructed of molybdenum.

Fog (fogging): A darkening of the whole or part of a radiograph by sources other than the radiation of the primary beam to which the film was exposed.

Foramen: A naturally formed hole or passage through a bone or tooth. Often the opening for a canal through which blood vessels and nerves pass. Appears radiolucent on radiograph.

Fossa: A broad, shallow, scooped-out or depressed area of bone; appears radiolucent.

Frankfort plane: A term used in cephalometric radiography. The horizontal plane between the porion and the orbitale.

Frequency: The number of crests of a wavelength passing a given point per second. This provides an indication of the energy of the radiation. The higher the frequency, the shorter the wavelength. The shortest wavelengths have the most energy and penetrating ability.

G

Gamma radiation: Short wavelength electromagnetic radiation of nuclear origin.

Generator: A machine that converts alternating current electrical power into a waveform suitable for the production of x-rays.

Genetic effect: Changes produced in the genes and chromosomes of all nucleated body cells. In customary usage, the term relates to the effect produced in the reproductive cells.

Genial tubercles: Tiny bumps of bone in the anterior region of the mandible that serve as attachment sites for the genioglossus and geniohyoid muscles; appear radiopaque.

Gray (Gy): A unit of absorbed dose or energy deposited in tissue; 1 Gy = 100 rad.

H

H & D curve: A characteristic curve of a photographic emulsion obtained by plotting film density against the logarithm of the exposure; named after the British scientists and founders, Hurter and Driffield.

Half-value layer (HVL): The thickness of a given material required to reduce the ionizing effect of the primary beam of radiation to one-half its original (unattenuated) value.

Hamulus: This bony projection appears radiopaque and extends downward from the medial pterygoid plate. It is located behind the maxillary tuberosity region.

Hardener: Hardeners help to toughen and shrink the gelatin in the film emulsion. This also helps to reduce the drying time needed at the completion of the processing.

Hertz (Hz): Unit of measurement of frequency of electromagnetic radiation; 1 Hz = 1 cycle/sec.

Heterogeneous radiation: Radiation consisting of various wavelengths and energies.

Homogeneous radiation: Radiation that consists of only one wavelength and energy.

Horizontal angulation: The position of the cone/position-indicating device, with movement occurring in a right-to-left direction (horizontal).

Hydroquinone: This is responsible for blackening the exposed silver halide crystal and for bringing out the contrast.

I

Impulse: In dental radiography, a measure of exposure time. Many of the newer x-ray machines are calibrated to make the exposure in impulses instead of fractions of a second. There are 60 impulses per second.

Incisive foramen: This structure is an opening through which the nasopalatine nerves and artery pass. This area appears as a radiolucent, oval-shaped structure between the central incisors.

Intensifying screen: A device used to convert x-ray energy to light energy. It consists of a card or plastic sheet coated with fluorescent material, positioned singly or in pairs in a cassette to contact the film. When the cassette is exposed to x-radiation, the light emitted from the fluorescent screen exposes the film and produces the latent image.

Interproximal: The mesial and distal surfaces of the tooth crown where the adjacent tooth touches.

Inverse Square Law: The relationship between distance and radiation intensity in which the exposure varies inversely as the square of the distance from the source.

Ion: An atomic particle, atom, or chemical radical bearing an electrical charge, either negative or positive.

Ionization: The process or the result of a process by which a neutral atom or molecule acquires either a positive or a negative charge.

Ionizing chamber: A cylinder or enclosure in a monitoring device that contains electrodes. An electric field is maintained between them for the purpose of collecting the charge when the gas or air in the chamber is ionized during exposure to radiation.

Ion pair: A pair of ions, one positive and one negative, that results when an electron is removed from an atom in the ionization process.

J

Joule (J): Unit of work and energy equal to 1 Newton (N) expended along a distance of 1 meter (m).

K

Kilo: A prefix used with a unit of measure indicating that the unit should be multiplied by 1000. For example, 1 kilovolt (kV) is equivalent to 1000 volts (V).

Kiloelectron volts (keV): One thousand electron volts.

Kilovoltage, peak (kVp): The maximum potential difference between anode and cathode in an x-ray tube.

Kinetic energy: The energy possessed by a mass because of its motion.

L

Latitude, exposure: A measure of the tolerance allowed in the choice of exposure values required to produce the desired density range.

Latitude, film: The capability of a film emulsion to record a wide range of exposures, resulting in the film having long-scale contrast.

Latent image: The invisible change produced in an x-ray or photographic film emulsion by the action of x-radiation or light, from which a visible image is produced on the film by chemical processing.

Latent period: The period between the time of exposure of tissue to an injurious agent (e.g., radiation) and the clinical manifestation of a particular response.

Lateral fossa: A smooth, depressed area of the maxilla located between the canine and lateral incisor; appears radiolucent.

Linear energy transfer (LET): The linear rate of loss of energy by an ionizing particle traversing a medium.

Lingual foramen: A very small opening through which a branch of the incisive artery emerges. It is located in the center of the genial tubercles on the lingual side of the mandible.

M

Mach band effect: A simulated, false appearance of caries due to the optical illusion presented from a light and dark object (e.g., enamel and dentin) placed next to one another.

Magnification, radiographic: The equal enlargement of a radiographic image recorded on film emulsion, minimized by reducing the object-to-film distance and increasing the focus-film distance.

Mass number (symbol Å): The number of nucleons (protons and neutrons) in the nucleus of an atom.

Maxillary sinus: Paired air-filled cavities or compartments of bone located within the maxilla; above the premolars and molars. Appears radiolucent.

Maxillary tuberosity: This bony structure appears as a bulge distal to the maxillary molars and at the end of the maxillary alveolar ridges.

Mental foramen: This structure provides a means for the blood vessels and nerves to supply the lower lip. It appears as a radiolucent, round, or oval-shaped area located near the apices of the mandibular premolars.

Mental ridge: The mental ridge is a bony prominence on the external portion of the mandible, which extends in a sloping fashion from the premolar area to the central incisors. It appears as a radiopaque, curved ridge below the mandibular anterior teeth.

Mesial: The interproximal surface of the tooth toward the center of the dental arch.

MeV: Million electron volts.

Midsagittal plane (midsagittal line): An imaginary vertical line or plane passing through the center of the body that divides it into a right and left half.

Milli: A prefix used with a unit of measure indicating that the unit should be multiplied by one one-thousandth. For example, 1 millisecond (ms) equals one one-thousandth of a second.

Milliamperage (mA): A measure of the number of electrons flowing per second; also called milliamperes.

Milliampere-seconds (mAs): The product of the factors milliamperes and time, used to calculate changes in exposure; mAs = mA X time (sec).

Molecule: The smallest quantity of matter that can exist by itself and retain its chemical properties. It is composed of one or more atoms.

Mutation: A departure from the parent type, as when an organism differs from its parents in one or more heritable characteristics, as a result of genetic change.

N

Nanometer (nm): Approximately one-billionth of an inch or one millionth of a millimeter.

Negatron: Term used for an electron to emphasize its negative charge in contradistinction to the positive charge carried by the otherwise similar positron.

Neoplasm: A tumor or any new or abnormal growth in which cell multiplication is uncontrolled.

Neutrons: An atomic particle with no charge that is similar in mass to the proton; neutrons are constituents of all atomic nuclei except that of hydrogen.

Newton: Unit of force that when applied to a mass of 1 kilogram will accelerate 1 meter/second/second.

Nonstochastic effects: These have threshold doses. It is believed that below these threshold doses, the effects do not occur. In addition, the severity of the effect is increased as the dose is increased. An example of this is erythema of the skin.

Nutrient canals: These canals provide a means for the blood vessels and nerves to reach the teeth. Nutrient canals can be seen as radiolucent lines extending downward from the mandibular anterior teeth.

O

Occlusal radiographs: A radiograph made with a film designed for placement between the occlusal surfaces of the teeth, with the x-ray beam directed vertically superiorly or inferiorly.

P

Palate: The roof of the mouth.

Panoramic film: A radiograph that shows a large area of the mandible and maxilla on a single film.

Parulis: A raised swollen area indicating an abscess of the gum. Often called a gum boil. A fistula (narrow canal) often connects the parulis with the core of the abscess at the apex of the root in the alveolus (tooth socket).

Penumbra: A penumbra, produced by light, is the secondary shadow that is the periphery of the primary shadow. In radiography, the penumbra is the blurred or ill-defined margin of an image detail; also called geometric unsharpness.

Periapical projection: A radiograph made by intraoral placement of film for recording shadow images of the outline and the position and mesiodistal extent of the teeth and surrounding tissue. It is the best means available for revealing the apices of the teeth and their contiguous tissues.

Periodontal disease: A group of diseases that affects the tissues surrounding the teeth.

Periodontal ligament space: A radiolucent space that exists between the root of the tooth and bone.

Periodontitis: Inflammation of the tissues that support the teeth; results in the destruction of the periodontium.

Photoelectric effect: The ejection of bound electrons by an incident x-ray photon such that the whole energy of the x-ray photon is absorbed and characteristic x-radiation is produced.

Photon: A quantum (bundle of energy) of electromagnetic radiation.

Proton: An elementary nuclear particle with a protective electric charge.

Polychromatic: Having many colors. This term is used in dental radiography to describe the x-ray beam that is composed of many wavelengths of different intensity.

Positron (symbol β+): A particle equal in mass to the electron but having an equal but opposite (positive) charge.

Preservatives: Chemicals that inhibit oxidation of the reducing agents (developing agents) by air. Sodium sulfite is the chemical usually used.

Proton: An elementary particle in the atomic nucleus that has a positive charge equal to that of the electron but with much greater mass.

Q

Quality factor (QF): A term that expresses the differences in biologic effectiveness of various types of radiation compared with ordinary x-rays.

Quantum: A packet or bundle of electromagnetic energy.

Quantum theory: The theory that electromagnetic energy is transferred in discrete quanta or photons.

R

Radiation absorbed dose (rad): A unit of measurement for the absorbed dose of any type of ionizing radiation in any medium; 1 rad is the energy absorption of 100 erg/g.

Radiolucent: A black or dark area seen on a radiograph; structures that appear radiolucent lack density and permit the passage of the x-ray beam.

Radiopaque: A white or light area on a radiograph; structures that appear radiopaque are dense and resist the passage of the x-ray beam.

Rarefaction: The state of being or becoming less dense, usually as a result of some disease process, indicated by radiolucent areas in the bone structures shown on radiographs.

Rectification: Conversion of alternating current to direct current.

Reducing agents: Chemicals that "reduce" (or change) the exposed silver halide crystal to black metallic silver.

Rem (Roentgen equivalent man): a unit of dose of any radiation to body tissue in terms of its estimated biologic effects relative to an exposure of 1 Roentgen of x- or gamma-radiation.

Replenisher: A superconcentrated solution of developer or fixer that is added daily or as indicated to the developer or fixer in the processing tank to compensate for loss of volume and loss of strength from oxidation.

Resolution: A term that relates to the ability of a film to record a true image. This is often seen as the ability of the radiographic image to discern the boundaries between two objects that are close together.

Restrainers (antifogging agents): The restrainers act to block the action of the reducing agent on unexposed crystals. Without this chemical, the processed radiographic film would be totally black.

Roentgen (R): A unit of radiation exposure measured in air that was named after Wilhelm Conrad Roentgen, who discovered x-rays in 1895.

Rule of isometry: A geometric theorem which states that two triangles with two equal angles and a common side are equal triangles.

S

Sagittal plane: An imaginary vertical line or plane that bisects the body into a right and left portion. If the plane is exactly at the midline, it is referred to as the **midsagittal plane**.

Scatter radiation: Radiation that has been deflected from its path by impact during its passage through matter. This form of secondary radiation is emitted or deflected in all directions by the tissues of the patient's head during exposure to x-radiation.

Secondary radiation: This is a form of radiation that is created at the instant the primary x-ray beam interacts with matter and gives off some of its energy, forming new and less-powerful wavelengths.

Self-rectification: Suppression of half the sine wave of the alternating current across an x-ray tube. This results from the absence of electrons at the anode side when the polarity is reversed.

Sensitometer: A device that exposes film to a controlled set of light exposures. It is used to evaluate a film's response to exposure.

Sievert (Sv): The SI unit associated with a rem; 1 rem = 100 Sv. It is a dose equivalent unit defined as the absorbed dose Gray (Gy), times the quality factor (QF). For dental x-rays, 1 Sv = 1 Gy.

Silver halide: A salt compound used in photographic emulsions because of its sensitivity to light and other forms of radiation. Halides are compounds of metals with halogen elements of bromine, chlorine, and iodine.

Solvent: A liquid that dissolves another solution. Water is the solvent used as the vehicle for mixing chemicals in the developer and the fixer.

Somatic cells: All body cells except the reproductive cells.

Somatic effects: In radiography, the effect of radiation on all body cells except the reproductive cells, especially the effect on the blood, the soft muscular tissues, and the bone.

Source: In radiography, the place where the x-ray photons originate. This is the focal spot on the target of the anode inside the x-ray tube.

Speed: A measure of the exposure needed to produce a given density on film.

Step-wedge: A device with graduated thicknesses (usually of aluminum) that is used to demonstrate or test various degrees of x-ray penetration.

Stochastic effects: Those effects in which the risk of getting the effects is dependent on the dose of radiation received. There is no known threshold below which the effects do not occur. An example of stochastic effect is cancer.

T

Target (x-ray tube): The part of the anode in an x-ray tube toward which electrons from the cathode are focused and attracted and where they interact to produce x-radiation.

Target theory: A theory that explains some biologic effects of radiation on the basis of ionization in a very small, sensitive region within the cell.

Thermionic emission: The escape of electrons from the heated filament in the cathode of an x-ray tube.

Threshold dose: The minimum exposure that will produce a detectable degree of any given effect.

Tomography: A special radiographic technique used to show in detail images of structures located within a predetermined plane of tissue while eliminating or blurring those structures in the planes not selected.

Topographic occlusal: A radiograph that demonstrates the anterior area of the maxillary arch.

Trabecular bone (cancellous bone): The softer spongy bone that makes up the bulk of the inside portion of most bones.

Tragus: The small cartilaginous prominence of tissues located near the center and in front of the acoustic meatus (outer ear opening).

Transformer: One of several types of electrical devices capable of increasing or decreasing the voltage of an alternating current by mutual induction between primary and secondary coils or windings on cores of metal.

U

Umbra: A complete shadow produced by light, with sharply demarcated margins. In radiography, a sharply delineated image detail.

V

Valence electrons: Number of electrons in the outer shell of the atom that determines the combining power of one atom of an element (or a radical).

W

Wave propagation: Energy manifested by movements in an advancing series of alternating elevations and depressions traveling through space or a medium.

Wavelength: The distance between the peaks of waves in any waveform. The distance between the crest of one wave to the crest of the next wave determines the energy and penetrating power of the radiation, such as light or x-rays.

X

X-ray (Roentgen rays): A type of electromagnetic radiation characterized by wavelengths of 100 Angstroms ($\mathring{A}$) or less.

X-ray tube: An electronic tube in which x-rays are generated.

Y

Yoke: The curved portion of the x-ray machine that can revolve 360° horizontally where it is connected to the extension arm. The tubehead is suspended within the yoke and can be rotated vertically within it.

Z

Zygomatic (malar) bone: Cheek bone (sometimes called the zygoma) that appears as a U-shaped radiopacity above the maxillary molar teeth.

Z number: Symbolic number referring to the number of protons in an atomic nucleus.

Sample National Board/ State Board/Certification Examination Multiple Choice and Case-Based Questions

MULTIPLE CHOICE QUESTIONS

1. Which of the following is not a characteristic of an x-ray photon?

   A. It travels with a wave-like motion.
   B. It travels at 186,000 miles/second in a vacuum.
   C. It causes ionization in matter.
   D. It has a mass equal to its density.

2. If a machine could produce 10,000 x-ray photons in 1 second, but you wanted it to produce more than that in 1 second, what would you change to produce more than 10,000 x-ray photons in 1 second?

   A. The milliamperage.
   B. The exposure time.
   C. The kilovoltage.
   D. The thickness of filtration.

3. A car at high speed brakes or loses some of its speed (energy) turning a sharp corner. Similarly, a high-speed electron is said to loose energy. Yet, we know that in reality the energy is not really lost, but transferred to another form called an x-ray photon. This phenomenon is called:

   A. Characteristic radiation.
   B. Radioactive decay.
   C. Particulate gamma radiation.
   D. Bremsstrahlung radiation.

4. The beam of radiation emitted from the constant potential x-ray tubehead consists of:

   A. X-ray photons of many different energies and wavelengths.
   B. X-ray photons of uniform energies and wavelengths.
   C. X-ray photons of the same energy but different wavelengths.
   D. Cathode rays of varying intensities.
   E. A larger percentage of characteristic radiation than any other type of radiation.

5. Which of the following series shows the correct progression of energy transformation in the production of x-ray photons?

   A. Kinetic energy, electrical energy, and radiation.
   B. Kinetic energy, radiation, and electrical energy.
   C. Electrical energy, kinetic energy, and radiation.
   D. Electrical energy, radiation, and kinetic energy.

6. X-radiation:

   1. Is absorbed by the tissues.
   2. Scatters.
   3. Passes through the patient.
   4. Imparts some or all of its energy to any material through which it passes.
   A. 1 and 2.
   B. 2 and 3.
   C. 2 and 4.
   D. 1, 3, and 4.
   E. All of the above.

7. A dentist has been using film speed E at 65 kVp, 10 mA, and 0.5-second exposure for a maxillary molar region. His or her assistant decides to use 15 mA. What will the new exposure time be?

   A. 0.25-second.
   B. 0.33-second.
   C. 0.7-second.
   D. 1.0-second.

8. The number of electrons in a dental x-ray tube is determined by the:

   A. Kilovoltage used.
   B. Distance between the filament and the target.
   C. Step-up transformer.
   D. Size of the focusing cup.
   E. Low-voltage circuit.

9. X-rays are known as ionizing radiation. Ionization is:

   A. The separation of the nucleus into positive and negative ions.
   B. Produced by photoelectric absorption only.
   C. Produced by the Compton effect and Bremsstrahlung only.
   D. Produced by photoelectric absorption and Compton scatter.

10. Which of the following statements describes Compton scatter?

   A. The photon uses some of its energy to remove an electron from its orbit and then transfers the remaining energy to the electron in the form of kinetic energy, which is capable of ionizing molecules.
   B. The photon give up some of its energy in ejecting an orbiting electron and is then deflected with a longer wavelength.
   C. A high-energy photon passes close to a nucleus, releasing an electron and a positron. Some of the energy is used to give kinetic energy to the two particles.
   D. None of the above.

11. Radiopaque tissues:

   A. Absorb little of the x-rays.
   B. Absorb x-rays more fully.
   C. Are hollow regions.

   D. Are cysts, granulomas, or abscesses.
   E. None of the above.

12. Which property of x-radiation must be utilized to control magnification of the radiographic image?

   A. X-rays travel in divergent paths from their source.
   B. X-rays penetrate opaque objects.
   C. X-rays cannot be focused.
   D. X-rays cause secondary radiation when they strike the patient's face.

13. Which of the following would you do to increase film density?

   1. Increase the mA.
   2. Increase the kVp.
   3. Increase the time.
   4. Decrease the distance.
   5. Increase the distance.
   A. 1, 2, and 4.
   B. 1, 2, and 5.
   C. 1, 3, and 4.
   D. 1, 3, and 5.
   E. 1, 2, 3, and 4.

14. Increasing the kVp results in:

   A. Low contrast (long-scale contrast).
   B. High contrast (short-scale contrast).
   C. Lighter film density (medium-scale contrast).
   D. None of the above.

15. Disease is transmitted in oral and maxillofacial procedures by which of the following?

   A. Direct contact with saliva.
   B. Contamination from an infected intraoral film packet.
   C. Contamination from infected processing solutions.
   D. A and B only.
   E. A, B, and C.

16. According to OSHA, the hands **must** be washed.

   A. Before donning gloves.
   B. After removing gloves.
   C. When gloves are perforated.
   D. A and C.
   E. B and C.

17. One way to avoid placing a barrier on the exposure switch is to:

    A. Spray it with an EPA-registered solution.
    B. Have the patient hold the switch.
    C. Install a remote, "switchless" control.
    D. Use a foot switch.

18. During mouth-rinsing before taking the radiographs, there is destruction of microorganisms on living tissues as long as there is contact between the tissues and the antimicrobial agent; this denotes:

    A. Sanitization.
    B. Antisepsis.
    C. Sterilization.
    D. Disinfection.
    E. Pasteurization.

19. Which statement is most correct?

    A. The long cone can be used with either the paralleling or the bisecting-angle technique.
    B. The long cone is used with the paralleling technique only.
    C. The short cone is used satisfactorily with either the paralleling or the bisecting-angle technique.
    D. Film-holders are not necessary with the paralleling technique.

20. As used in intraoral radiography, the bisecting-angle technique is one in which the central ray x-ray beam is directed:

    A. Perpendicular to the long axis of the object.
    B. Parallel to the long axis of the object.
    C. Perpendicular to the "bisecting line."
    D. Perpendicular to the long axis of the film packet.

21. The premolar bitewing radiograph should be placed to include which of the following anatomical structures?

    A. All of the crown of the maxillary first premolar crown.
    B. All of the mandibular canine crown.
    C. The distal half of the maxillary canine crown.
    D. The mesial half of the maxillary first molar crown.

22. X-ray intensity (I), like light, is related to its distance (D) from the source. This is expressed as the inverse square law and is formulated as:

$$\frac{I_1}{I_2} = \frac{(D_2)^2}{(D_1)^2}$$

If the distance from the source to the object is tripled, the intensity of the x-ray beam at the new distance (D_2) would be:

    A. One ninth the original distance (D_1).
    B. One sixth the original distance.
    C. One third the original distance.
    D. One half the original distance.

23. The radiation output of a machine at a 16-inch source-film distance is 250 mR per second. Under identical exposure conditions, if the source-film distance is changed to 8 inches, what will be the new output per second?

    A. 500 mR.
    B. 125 mR.
    C. 1000 mR.
    D. 2000 mR.

24. The embossed, raised dot on the intraoral periapical film is important because it:

    A. Identifies the side of the film toward the tongue.
    B. Identifies the facial and lingual surfaces of teeth.
    C. Identifies the apices of roots of teeth.
    D. Identifies the left and right sides of patient.
    E. Identifies the side of film to place into the processor first.

25. Which of the following is important concerning the safelight in the darkroom?

    A. Wattage of bulb.
    B. Distance of safelight from working area.
    C. Color of filter.
    D. Length of time film is exposed to safelight.
    E. All of the above.

26. The most efficient source of light in a film duplicator is which of the following?

    A. 15-watt bulb.
    B. Fluorescent light.
    C. Flood lamp.
    D. Ultraviolet fluorescent light.

27. The latent image consists of the accumulation of:

    A. Electrons in exposed silver bromide crystals.
    B. Atomic silver at the sensitization specks.
    C. Atomic silver in gelatin molecules.
    D. Electrons in photoconductance bands.

28. Which of the following factors contribute to fog with a resultant degradation of film quality?

    1. Unsafe safelight.
    2. Unsafe storage following exposure.
    3. Overdevelopment.
    4. High temperature development with no change in processing time.
    5. Outdated emulsion.
    6. White light leaks in the darkroom.
    A. 1, 2, 3, and 4.
    B. 1, 3, 5, and 6.
    C. 1, 2, 3, 5, and 6.
    D. 1, 3, 4, 5, and 6.
    E. All of the above.

29. In your office, the radiographs turn brown with age almost all of the time. What corrective action will you take?

    A. Develop the films adequately.
    B. Change the solutions more regularly.
    C. Wash the films properly after fixing.
    D. Fix the films adequately.
    E. None of the above.

30. You turn on the water in the manual tanks at the beginning of the day, stir the solution, check the temperature, and set a developing time to go with the temperature. You take a set of films at about 9:00 a.m. that appear fine. About 2:00 p.m., you process another set of films, which are so dark you can hardly read them. What most likely happened with the second set of films?

    A. Your exposure time was too long.
    B. Your darkroom has a light leak.
    C. Your water temperature is too hot.
    D. Your chemicals are contaminated.

31. The use of outdated films may result in images that are:

    A. Gray.
    B. Low in contrast.
    C. Brownish.

    D. A and B.
    E. A, B, and C.

32. When a piece of rare earth screen is used to ensure that the beam is restricted to the diameter of the BID tip, you are checking the:

    A. Filter.
    B. Benson line focus.
    C. Focal spot integrity.
    D. Collimator.

33. Resolution in line pairs per millimeter is the basis for a test device that checks the:

    A. Focal spot integrity.
    B. Alignment of the collimator.
    C. Ideal BID length.
    D. Benson line focus alignment.

34. The sensitometer is a device to check processing in a Class III facility. It is used to detect:

    A. Fog.
    B. Density changes.
    C. Contrast changes.
    D. All of the above.

35. The half-value layer (HVL) can be defined as:

    A. The amount of tissue that reduces beam intensity by half.
    B. The added aluminum filtration in the unit.
    C. The thickness of a material that cuts the exposure time by half.
    D. The thickness of a standardized material that absorbs half the output.

36. A patient has a supernumerary mandibular premolar that has erupted lingual to the normal premolars and is not seen in the panoramic image. The reason for this is:

    A. Mechanical malfunction.
    B. Processing error.
    C. Premolar not in layer.
    D. Supernumerary obscured by the normal premolars.

37. In panoramic radiology, spreading out of the turbinate is:

A. Undesirable and caused by positioning errors.
B. Desirable and part of the normal panoramic projection.
C. Inevitable, especially in allergic patients.
D. Not seen in panoramic radiology.

38. In panoramic radiology, double images are real images of objects falling within the diamond-shaped area and:

A. In front of it.
B. In back of it.
C. In front and back of it.
D. In the midline region.

39. Which of the following statements is/are true, with regard to the panoramic image?

1. Air obscures hard tissue.
2. Soft tissue obscures air.
3. Hard tissue obscures soft tissue.
4. Ghost images obscure everything.
A. A and B.
B. B and C.
C. D only.
D. All of the above.

40. When one condyle is higher and bigger than the other in the panoramic image, the patient is:

A. Twisted.
B. Tilted.
C. Positioned with the chin too low.
D. Slumped.

41. In the panoramic image, widening of the anterior teeth along with ghosting of the contralateral rami occurs when the patient is positioned:

A. Too far forward.
B. Too far back.
C. With the chin raised too high.
D. With the chin depressed too low.

42. In panoramic radiology, streaking out and ghosting of the hyoid bone occurs when the patient is positioned:

A. Too far forward.
B. Too far back.
C. With the chin raised too high.
D. With the chin depressed too low.

43. In the panoramic image, when the "smile" line of the teeth is exaggerated and the condyles go off the top of the film, the patient is:

A. Twisted.
B. Tilted.
C. Positioned with the chin too low.
D. Positioned with the chin too high.

44. Extraoral films are:

1. Used when large areas of the skull need to be radiographed.
2. Loaded in cassettes.
3. Often used when fractures of the skull are suspected.
4. Used in conjunction with intensifying screens.
A. 2 and 4.
B. 3 and 4.
C. 1, 2, and 3.
D. 2, 3, and 4.
E. 1, 2, 3, and 4.

45. A radiographic technique for evaluation of the maxillary sinuses is the:

A. Submentovertex view.
B. Caldwell view.
C. Transorbital view.
D. Waters view.

46. Which of the following best describes a slow-speed intensifying screen compared with a fast-speed intensifying screen? The slow-speed screen has:

A. Thick phosphor layers and produces an unsharp image.
B. Thick phosphor layers and produces a sharp image.
C. Thin phosphor layers and produces an unsharp image.
D. Thin phosphor layers and produces a sharp image.

47. Intensifying screens:

1. Aid in reducing radiation exposure times.
2. Contain phosphor crystals.
3. Contain silver bromide crystals.
4. Consist of x-ray–penetrable base material.
A. 2 and 3.
B. 3 and 4.
C. 1, 2, and 3.

D. 1, 2, and 4.
E. All of the above.

48. Following an exposure to radiation, the residual biologic damage that remains is what type of effect?

A. Direct.
B. Indirect.
C. Tolerance.
D. Cumulative.
E. Fractionation.

49. It is well documented that x-rays react at the cellular level and can cause biologic damage. When a photon interacts with one molecule of water, it results in:

A. Excitation.
B. Electrolyte formation.
C. Attenuation.
D. Free radical formation.

50. The latent period related to radiation biology is that period between:

A. Exposure of the film and development of the images.
B. Exposure to x-radiation and the appearance of clinical symptoms.
C. The states of cell rest and cell mitosis.
D. Subsequent doses of x-radiation.

51. The annual whole-body effective radiation dose emitted for the general population (infrequent exposure) is:

A. 5 mSv.
B. 10 mSv.
C. 1 mSv.
D. Not specified.

52. The majority of biologic damage produced by ionizing radiation is generally believed to result from:

A. Direct interactions of ionizing radiation with DNA.
B. Multi-hit direct inactivation of ribosomes.
C. Damage inflicted by free radicals.
D. Leakage of ATP from irradiated cells.

53. Mutations from radiation exposure may occur:

A. Only in reproductive organs as genetic abnormalities.
B. In both somatic and reproductive tissue.

C. Only in the critical organs.
D. Only in the cytoplasm.

54. Collars are attached to leaded aprons or separate collars are used in conjunction with leaded aprons in dental radiography to protect what specific area of the body?

A. Spinal cord.
B. Thyroid gland.
C. Neck region.
D. Gonads.

55. Which one of the following factors will reduce the patient's somatic exposure by the greatest amount?

A. Leaded apron.
B. Short, pointed, plastic cone.
C. Short, lead-lined, open-ended cylinder.
D. Long, lead-lined, open-ended cylinder.
E. Long, lead-lined, rectangular beam indicating device.

56. Which of the following is least effective in reducing patient radiation dose?

A. Fast films.
B. Higher kilovoltage.
C. Proper collimation.
D. Increased filtration.

57. The hazards to the operator in radiographic work are:

1. Exposure to the radiation coming directly from the x-ray cones.
2. Exposure to tubehead leakage.
3. Exposure to secondary radiation emitted from the patient during an exposure.
4. Radiation coming from an adjacent room.
A. 1, 2, and 3.
B. 1, 3, and 4.
C. 2, 3, and 4.
D. All of the above.

58. The benefits of x-ray beam collimation include:

1. Increasing the mean energy of the beam.
2. Restriction of the beam size.
3. Decreased patient dose.
4. Increased quality of the resultant image.
A. 1 and 2.
B. 3 and 4.

C. 1, 2, and 3.
D. 2, 3, and 4.

59. If you receive more than 1 mSv in a week as a radiation worker, you should:

   A. Evaluate the radiation protection measures used in your dental office.
   B. Do not work with radiation until you dissipate the 1 mSv.
   C. Go on a vacation.
   D. Find another job.

60. Which of the following normal anatomical structures is radiolucent and usually found on a periapical radiograph of the maxillary central region?

   A. Anterior nasal spine.
   B. Incisive foramen.
   C. Lingual foramen.
   D. Nasal fossa.

61. The coronoid process of the mandible is frequently visible on a periapical radiograph of the:

   A. Maxillary second premolar region.
   B. Maxillary second molar region.
   C. Mandibular second molar region.
   D. Maxillary central incisor region.

62. Which of the following statements are **true** concerning the use of the dental radiograph in periodontal disease diagnosis?

   1. Does reveal soft-to-hard tissue relationships.
   2. Does not record morphology of bone deformities.
   3. Does not reveal facial or lingual aspects of the tooth.
   4. Does detect overhanging restorations.
   5. Does not detect crown-root ratio.
   A. 1 and 2.
   B. 2 and 4.
   C. 1, 3, and 5.
   D. 2, 3, and 5.
   E. 2, 3, and 4.

63. Which of the following anomalies are called ghost teeth because of defective calcified tooth structures?

   A. Regional odontodysplasia.
   B. Dental dysplasia.
   C. Shell teeth.
   D. Amelogenesis imperfecta.
   E. Dentinogenesis imperfecta.

64. Which of the statements are true?

   1. Germination is associated with the correct number of teeth in the dental arch.
   2. Fusion leads to a reduced number of teeth in the dental arch.
   3. Concrescence denotes dentinal union of two fully formed teeth.
   4. Teeth with taurodontism usually have obliterated pulps.
   5. Dens invaginatus is usually found in premolars.
   A. 1 and 2.
   B. 1 and 3.
   C. 2 and 3.
   D. 3, 4, and 5.
   E. 2, 3, and 5.

65. Which of the following conditions have pulpal enlargement?

   A. Regional odontodysplasia.
   B. Taurodontism.
   C. Shell teeth.
   D. Hypophosphatemia.
   E. All of the above.

66. Which of the following usually are associated with nonvital pulps of teeth?

   A. Hypercementosis.
   B. Apical cementoma (apical cemental dysplasia).
   C. Apical cyst.
   D. Apical osteosclerosis.
   E. All of the above.

67. Which of the following explains why the size of the interproximal carious lesion, as seen radiographically, is usually smaller than seen microscopically or after clinical excavation of the caries?

   1. Radiographic evidence will not be observed until there is sufficient decalcification of the tooth.
   2. The ratio of sound tooth structure to the carious lesion varies in different areas of the tooth.
   3. The difference in root configuration and shape of cementoenamel contour.
   4. The differences in density (mass/volume) of enamel and dentin.
   A. 1 and 2.
   B. 2 and 4.

C. 1, 2, and 4.
D. 2, 3, and 4.
E. 2 only.

68. What causes cervical burnout?

A. A "burning out" of the peripheral surface of the tooth by increased kilovoltages.
B. Differences in the ratio of sound tooth structure to the carious lesion.
C. Depends on shape of interproximal enamel surfaces of teeth.
D. Density differences at cementoenamel junction.
E. None of the above.

69. Which of the following apical lesions have the potential for the most destruction to the alveolar bone?

A. Chronic apical abscess.
B. Apical cementoma.
C. Apical cyst.
D. Apical granuloma.
E. Condensing osteitis.

70. Which of the following statements are true concerning periapical disease?

1. It is possible to differentiate the chronic abscess, apical granuloma, or apical cyst by use of the radiograph.
2. The apical granuloma is a tumor of granulomatous tissue.
3. The apical cyst is the most common cyst of the jaws.
4. Chronic periapical lesions are usually involved with nonvital teeth and are asymptomatic.
5. The apical cementoma (periapical cemental dysplasia) is most often seen in males younger than 25 years of age.
   A. 1, 2, 3, and 5.
   B. 1, 3, and 4.
   C. 3 and 4.
   D. 2 and 4.
   E. 2 and 5.

71. The radiolucency occurring in the bone from an infected primary molar, as studied radiographically, most frequently appears:

A. Around the apices.
B. Between two teeth.
C. In the bifurcation.
D. Around the developing permanent tooth.

E. As a uniform widening of the periodontal ligament space.

CASE-BASED QUESTIONS

Case No. 1
This patient complained of intermittent pain and swelling in the right submandibular gland, especially at meal times. A sialolith (stone) was found in the right Wharton's duct.

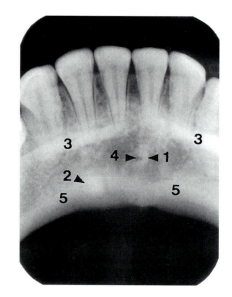

Questions:

1. To obtain this image:

A. The film was not placed parallel to the teeth.
B. The patient bit down more firmly on the bite-block.
C. The film was tilted on a downward angle, and the central ray was perpendicular to the teeth.
D. The negative vertical angulations of the cone (BID) was increased too much.
E. A and D

2. Matching the columns, identify the following:

Column A	Column B
1. _____	A. Lingual foramen.
2. _____	B. Mental ridge.
3. _____	C. Sialolith.
4. _____	D. Genial tubercles.
5. _____	E. Inferior cortex.

Case No. 2

This 22-year-old, male college student developed a spontaneous, persistent toothache while watching a football game. A molar radiograph was taken by a dental hygienist at his dentist's office.

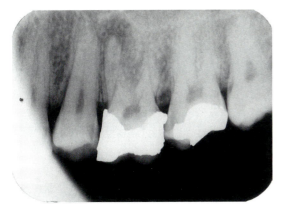

Questions

1. The errors that occurred while taking this molar radiograph consisted of:

   A. Cone-cut.
   B. Improper film placement.
   C. Insufficient vertical angulation.
   D. A and B.
   E. A, B, and C.

2. Despite the errors, the problematic tooth was likely the:

   A. Second premolar because it is carious.
   B. The first molar because the overhangs cause periodontal problems.
   C. The first molar because of periapical pathology.
   D. The second molar because it is carious.

Case No. 3

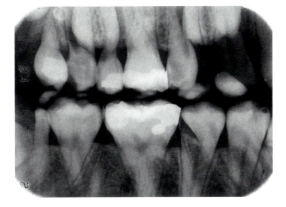

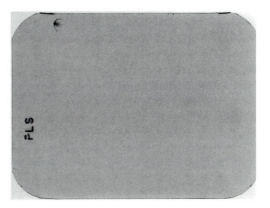

Question

1. The hygienist was asked to take a set of two bitewings on the patient's right side. These two images were the result of:

   A. Two films overlapped in the processor, and the blank film was exposed to light.
   B. One film was double exposed, and the other was exposed to light.
   C. One film was double exposed, and the other was not exposed.
   D. Two films overlapped in the processor, and the emulsion from the blank film stuck on top of the other.

Case No. 4

One concept of panoramic radiology is that whenever a structure is positioned **behind** the rotation center, it produces a real image on one side of the film and a ghost image on the other side of the film. Ghost image formation by anatomical structures is often associated with errors in patient positioning in the machine.

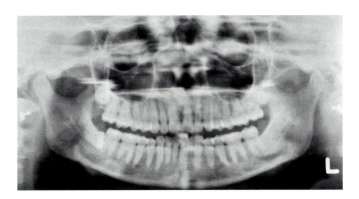

Question

1. Objects such as earrings and necklaces or napkin chains can produce ghost images, and this is why they should be removed before exposure. Note the ghost images produced by the two earrings left on this patient. With respect to the features of ghost images, indicate which statements are true or false.

   A. The ghost image is on the same side as the real image.
   B. The ghost image is usually smaller than the real image.
   C. In the ghost image only, horizontal elements are more prominent than vertical elements.
   D. The ghost image is usually sharper than the real image.
   E. The ghost image is usually above the real image.

Case No. 5

This is a good panoramic image. There are some key anatomical structures we need to learn to identify.

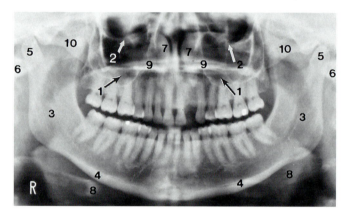

Question

1. Identify the anatomical structures by matching the numbered structures in Column A with Column B.

Column A	Column B
1. _____	A. Maxillary sinus
2. _____	B. Ramus
3. _____	C. Condyles
4. _____	D. Inferior cortex mandible
5. _____	E. Turbinates
6. _____	F. Spine
7. _____	G. Hard palate images
8. _____	H. Floor of orbit/roof of sinus
9. _____	I. Hyoid bone
10. _____	J. Zygomatic arch

Case No. 6

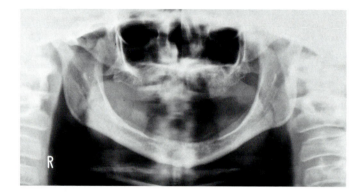

Question

1. The positioning error in this case is:

   A. Movement.
   B. Too far back.
   C. Chin too high.
   D. Twisted.
   E. A and D.

Case No. 7

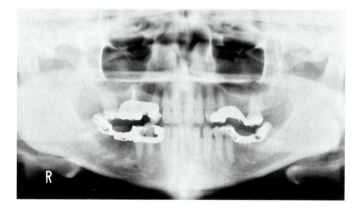

Question

1. The error(s) in this case is (are):

   A. Partials left in.
   B. Partials left in, too far back.
   C. Partials left in, too far back, chin too high.
   D. Partials left in, too far back, chin too high, slumped.

Case No. 8

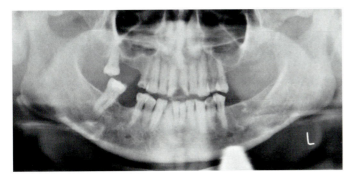

Question

1. The error(s) in this case is (are):

   A. Real image of neck jewelry.
   B. Apron artifact.
   C. Cassette leak.
   D. Fixer artifact.
   E. Chin alignment rod.

Case No. 9

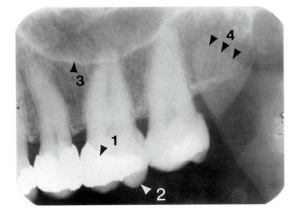

Question

1. Identify the anatomical structures and materials by matching the columns.

Column A	Column B
1. _____	A. Coronoid process.
2. _____	B. Floor of sinus.
3. _____	C. Buccal cusp.
4. _____	D. Lingual cusp.
	E. Zygomatic bone.
	F. Maxillary tuberosity.
	G. Amalgam restoration.
	H. Composite restoration.

Case No. 10

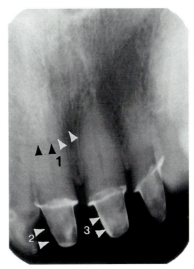

Question

1. Identify the materials/structures by matching the columns.

Column A	Column B
1. _____	A. Porcelain crown.
2. _____	B. Acrylic crown.
3. _____	C. Soft tissue of nose.
	D. Alveolar bone level.
	E. Cement.

Case No. 11

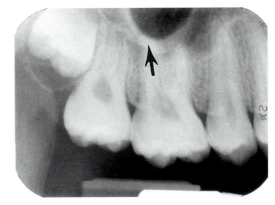

Question

1. What is the radiopaque U-shaped structure identified by the arrow? The teeth are vital.

   A. Floor of the maxillary sinus.
   B. Sclerotic border of apical cyst.

C. Zygomatic process of temporal bone.
D. Inferior border of zygomatic bone.
E. Septum in maxillary sinus.

Case No. 12

This patient is a 38-year-old woman. She has a collagen disease with a positive rheumatoid factor.

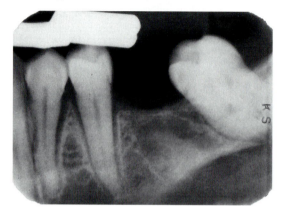

Question

1. Although she is asymptomatic, the periodontal membrane spaces are significantly widened because:

   A. Her teeth are mobile.
   B. She has scleroderma.
   C. She has periodontitis.
   D. She has had orthodontics treatment.
   E. The widening is at the outer range of normalcy.

Case No. 13

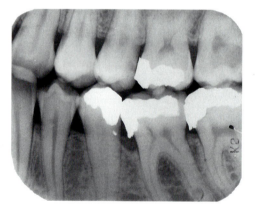

Question

1. This radiograph reveals definite radiographic evidence of periodontal disease between which of the following teeth?

1. Maxillary first and second premolar.
2. Maxillary second premolar and first molar.
3. Mandibular first and second premolar.
4. Mandibular second premolar and first molar.
5. Mandibular first and second molar.
A. 1, 2, and 4.
B. 2 and 3.
C. None of the areas identified above.
D. 4 only.
E. All of the areas identified above.

Case No. 14

A 60-year-old, female, retired school teacher visits your clinic for a routine check-up; her dentist of 30 years has died. In completing the periodontal examination, a radiograph was taken of the maxillary premolar region.

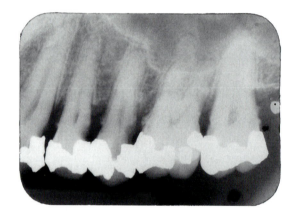

Questions

1. Radiographically, what is the most appropriate classification of this person's periodontal condition?

   A. Moderate generalized horizontal bone loss.
   B. Advanced generalized horizontal bone loss.
   C. Moderate localized horizontal bone loss.
   D. Advanced generalized vertical bone loss.
   E. Moderate localized vertical bone loss.

2. What is (are) the contributory factors to this person's periodontal condition, as seen radiographically.

   1. Deficient contact between canine and first premolar.
   2. Recurrent root caries, a sign of poor flossing.
   3. Multiple areas of interproximal calculus.
   4. Overhanging restorations.
   5. Occlusal trauma.
   A. 2, 3, and 4.
   B. 1, 4, and 5.

C. 2, 3, and 5.
D. 1, 2, 3, and 4.
E. 1 and 5 only.

Case No. 15

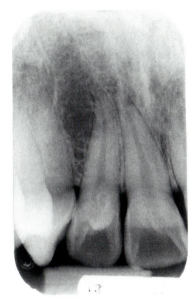

Question

1. What are the developmental abnormalities of the teeth that are seen in this radiograph?

    1. Shovel-shaped incisors.
    2. Dens invaginatus.
    3. Dental dysplasia.
    4. Talon cusp.
    5. Abnormally enlarged pulp.
    A. 3, 4, and 5.
    B. 1, 2, and 4.
    C. 2, 3, and 5.
    D. 1, 2, 3, and 5.
    E. 2, 3, and 4.

Case No. 16

Question

1. Which of the following anomalies are represented by this radiograph?

    A. Concrescence.
    B. Supernumerary tooth.
    C. Fusion.
    D. Gemination.
    E. Supernumerary cusps.

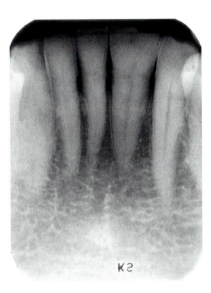

Case No. 17

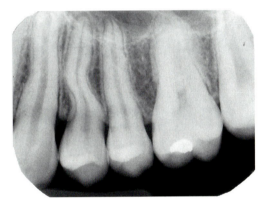

Questions

1. What is the significance of the anomaly of the upper premolar in this radiograph?

    1. Difficulty in endodontic procedure.
    2. Difficulty in crown preparation.
    3. Difficulty in extraction.
    4. Tooth is more subject to periodontal disease.
    5. Tooth is more subject to caries.
    A. 1, 2, and 3.
    B. 4 and 5.
    C. 1, 2, 3, 4, and 5.
    D. 1 and 3.
    E. 2, 4, and 5.

2. The anomaly is known as:

    A. Diastema.
    B. Concrescence.

C. Dilaceration.

D. Transposition.

Case No. 18

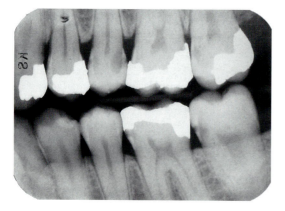

Question

1. Which of the following teeth have definite radiographic evidence of dentinal caries?

1. Upper second premolar.
2. Upper second molar.
3. Lower second premolar.
4. Lower first molar.
5. Lower second molar.
A. 2, 3, and 5.
B. 1, 2, 4, and 5.
C. 3, 4, and 5.
D. 1, 2, and 3.
E. 1, 2, 3, and 4.

Case No. 19

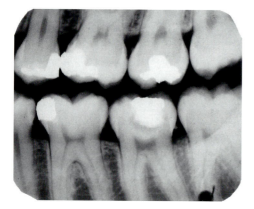

Question

1. This 35-year-old man has a dull toothache on the left side of his jaws. He cannot localize the pain. Which one of the following teeth, from the radiograph alone, is most likely the cause of the toothache?

A. Upper left second premolar.
B. Upper left first molar.
C. Upper left second molar.
D. Lower left second molar.
E. Lower left first molar.

Case No. 20

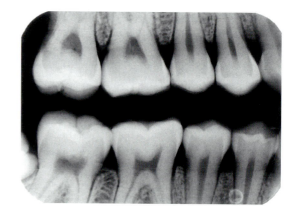

Question

1. There is radiographic evidence of how many carious lesions on this radiograph?

A. One.
B. Two.
C. Three.
D. Four.
E. None.

Case No. 21

This patient is a 35-year-old, African-American woman. Although she once fell on her jaw during a track meet at an early age, the teeth are vital.

Questions

1. The condition affecting the incisors is:

A. Traumatic cysts.
B. Apical granulomas.

Question

1. This patient is a teen-ager with a large carious lesion in the mandibular first molar. The tooth is nonvital. Most likely, what is the lesion at the apical end of the mesial root?

   A. Condensing osteitis.
   B. Idiopathic osteosclerosis.
   C. Apical cementoma.
   D. Osteoma.
   E. Benign cementoblastoma.

Case No. 23

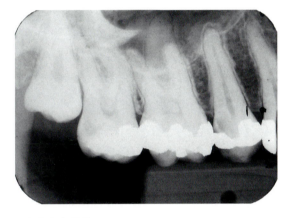

C. Apical cementomas.
D. Chemical stains (developer).

2. What is the black spot identified by the arrow?

   A. Developer artifact.
   B. Fixer artifact.
   C. Water mark.
   D. Film clip mark.
   E. None of the above.

Case No. 22

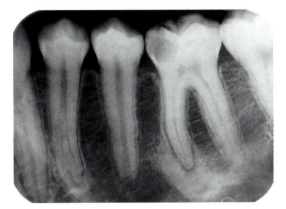

Question

1. A 17-year-old girl has a toothache in this quadrant. Based on what you can see in this radiograph alone, which one of the teeth is most likely to be the cause of the toothache?

   A. Second premolar.
   B. First molar.
   C. Second molar.
   D. Third molar.
   E. All of them.

Appendix 1

ANSWERS TO REVIEW AND CASE-BASED QUESTIONS AT THE ENDS OF THE CHAPTERS

CHAPTER 1:
Answers to
Review Questions

1. C
2. C
3. E
4. B
5. C
6. B
7. A
8. A
9. B
10. C
11. B
12. B
13. A
14. B
15. A
16. E

CHAPTER 2:
Answers to
Review Questions

1. D
2. B
3. C
4. C
5. C
6. C
7. C
8. A
9. B
10. C
11. E
12. C
13. B
14. E
15. E

CHAPTER 3:
Answers to
Review Questions

1. A
2. A
3. B
4. A
5. C
6. C
7. D
8. D
9. C
10. D
11. B
12. A
13. B

CHAPTER 4:
Answers to
Review Questions

1. D
2. E
3. C
4. E
5. A
6. B
7. C
8. E
9. E

CHAPTER 5:
Answers to
Review Questions

1. B
2. D
3. C
4. B
5. B
6. B
7. B
8. B

9. C
10. B

CHAPTER 5:
Answers to
Case-Based
Questions

Case 5.1
1. D
2. D
3. Arrow 1—B
   Arrow 2—C
   Arrow 3—A
   Arrow 4—D

Case 5.2
1. B
2. Arrow 1—B
   Arrow 2—D
   Arrow 3—A
   Arrow 4—C
   Arrow 5—E

CHAPTER 6:
Answers to
Review Questions

1. B
2. A
3. C
4. B
5. B
6. B
7. D
8. D
9. A
10. B
11. E
12. D
13. B
14. C

CHAPTER 7:
Answers to
Review Questions

1. E
2. B
3. B
4. D

CHAPTER 7:
Answers to
Case-Based
Questions

Case 7.1
B

Case 7.2
B

Case 7.3
D

Case 7.4
D

Case 7.5
C

Case 7.6
C

Case 7.7
C

CHAPTER 8:
Answers to
Review Questions

1. B
2. E
3. D
4. D

5. C
6. B
7. E
8. D
9. B
10. A
11. A

CHAPTER 9:
Answers to
Review Questions

1. C
2. A
3. D
4. A
5. C
6. B
7. B
8. C
9. B

CHAPTER 9:
Answers to
Case-Based
Questions

Case 9.1
1. B
2. C

Case 9.2
1. True
2. True
3. False
4. True
5. False
6. True
7. True
8. False
9. True
10. True

Case 9.3
1. True
2. True
3. True
4. False
5. True
6. False
7. False

8. True
9. True
10. False

Matching
Arrows 1—C
Arrow 2—H
Arrows 3—D
Arrows 4—A
Arrow 5—F
Arrows 6—B
Arrows 7—G
Arrows 8—E
Arrows 9—I

Case 9.4
1. B

Case 9.5

Matching
1. F
2. L
3. B
4. I
5. D
6. H
7. J
8. A
9. K
10. G
11. E
12. C

CHAPTER 10:
Answers to
Review Questions

1. D
2. E
3. D
4. C
5. D
6. B
7. C

CHAPTER 10:
Answers to
Case-Based
Questions

Case 10.1
1. A
2. A

Case 10.2
1. C

Case 10.3
1. D

Case 10.4
1. D

Case 10.5
1. E

Case 10.6
1. C

CHAPTER 11:
Answers to
Review Questions

1. C
2. D
3. B
4. D
5. C
6. D
7. B
8. D
9. C
10. B
11. A

CHAPTER 12:
Answers to
Review Questions

1. A
2. D
3. B
4. D
5. B
6. B

7. A
8. D
9. A
10. B
11. C
12. A

CHAPTER 13:
Answers to
Review Questions

1. D
2. B
3. D
4. C
5. C
6. B
7. D
8. D
9. D
10. D
11. D
12. B
13. C
14. B
15. C

CHAPTER 14:
Answers to
Review Questions

1. A
2. B
3. A
4. D

5. Matching
1. B
2. D
3. A
4. C
5. F
6. G
7. H
8. E
6. D

CHAPTER 14:
Answers to
Case-Based
Questions

Case 14.1

Column A	Column B
Arrow 1	D
Arrow 2	C
Arrow 3	E
Arrow 4	B
Arrow 5	A

Case 14.2
1. B

Case 14.3
1. D

Case 14.4
1. A

Case 14.5
1. C

Case 14.6
1. D

Case 14.7
1. C

Case 14.8
1. C

CHAPTER 15:
Answers to
Review Questions

1. B
2. B
3. E

CHAPTER 15:
Answers to
Case-Based
Questions

Case 15.1
1. E

Case 15.2
1. D

Case 15.3
1. A

Case 15.4
1. E

Case 15.5
1. A

Case 15.6
1. E

CHAPTER 16:
Answers to
Review Questions

1. C
2. D
3. D
4. C
5. A
6. C
7. B
8. C
9. B

CHAPTER 16:
Answers to
Case-Based
Questions

Case 16.1
1. E
2. C

Case 16.2
1. B

Case 16.3
1. A
2. A

Case 16.4
1. D

Case 16.5
1. B
2. D

Case 16.6
1. C

CHAPTER 17:
Answers to
Review Questions

1. A
2. B
3. E
4. D
5. B

CHAPTER 17:
Answers to
Case-Based
Questions

Case 17.1
1. E
2. D
3. C

Case 17.2
1. C

Case 17.3
1. D

Case 17.4
1. C

Case 17.5
1. C
2. E

Case 17.6
1. A

Case 17.7
1. D

Case 17.8
1. D
2. D

CHAPTER 18:
Answers to
Review Questions

1. C
2. C
3. A
4. D
5. A

CHAPTER 18:
Answers to
Case-Based
Questions

Case 18.1
1. C

Case 18.2
1. A

Case 18.3
1. B

Case 18.4
1. B
2. C

Case 18.5
1. C

Case 18.6
1. B
2. E

Case 18.7
1. A

Appendix 2

ANSWERS TO SAMPLE NATIONAL BOARD/STATE BOARD/CERTIFICATION EXAMINATION MULTIPLE CHOICE AND CASE-BASED QUESTIONS

Answers to Sample National Board/State Board/Certification Examination: Multiple Choice Questions

		14.	A	34.	D	54.	B
		15.	E	35.	D	55.	E
		16.	E	36.	C	56.	B
		17.	D	37.	A	57.	D
		18.	B	38.	D	58.	D
		19.	A	39.	D	59.	A
		20.	C	40.	B	60.	B
1.	D	21.	C	41.	B	61.	B
2.	A	22.	A	42.	D	62.	E
3.	D	23.	C	43.	C	63.	A
4.	B	24.	D	44.	E	64.	A
5.	C	25.	E	45.	D	65.	E
6.	E	26.	D	46.	D	66.	C
7.	B	27.	B	47.	D	67.	A
8.	E	28.	E	48.	D	68.	D
9.	D	29.	C	49.	D	69.	C
10.	B	30.	A	50.	B	70.	C
11.	B	31.	D	51.	A	71.	C
12.	A	32.	D	52.	C		
13.	E	33.	A	53.	A		

Answers to Sample National Board/State Board/Certification Examination: Case-Based Questions

Case No. 1
1. E
2. Matching
   1. D
   2. C
   3. B
   4. A
   5. E

Case No. 2
1. D
2. C

Case No. 3
1. C

Case No. 4
A. False.
B. False.
C. True.
D. False.
E. True.

Case No. 5
1. A
2. H
3. B
4. D
5. C
6. F
7. E

8. I
9. G
10. J

Case No. 6
1. E

Case No. 7
1. D

Case No. 8
1. B

Case No. 9
1. G
2. C
3. B
4. A

Case No. 10
1. C
2. B
3. E

Case No. 11
1. D

Case No. 12
1. B

Case No. 13
1. D

Case No. 14
1. B
2. D

Case No. 15
1. B

Case No. 16
1. C

Case No. 17
1. D
2. C

Case No. 18
1. B

Case No. 19
1. D

Case No. 20
1. E

Case No. 21
1. C
2. A

Case No. 22
1. A

Case No. 23
1. A

Index